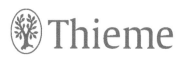

Neck Dissection

Brendan C. Stack, Jr., MD, FACS, FACE
Professor
Department of Otolaryngology – Head and Neck Surgery
University of Arkansas for Medical Sciences
Little Rock, Arkansas

Mauricio A. Moreno, MD
Associate Professor
Director, Head & Neck Division
Department of Otolaryngology – Head and Neck Surgery
Vice Chair, Adult Services
University of Arkansas for Medical Sciences
Little Rock, Arkansas

242 illustrations

Thieme
New York • Stuttgart • Delhi • Rio de Janeiro

Executive Editor: Timothy Y. Hiscock
Managing Editor: Nikole Y. Connors
Director, Editorial Services: Mary Jo Casey
Production Editor: Naamah Schwartz
International Production Director: Andreas Schabert
Editorial Director: Sue Hodgson
International Marketing Director: Fiona Henderson
International Sales Director: Louisa Turrell
Director of Institutional Sales: Adam Bernacki
Senior Vice President and Chief Operating Officer: Sarah Vanderbilt
President: Brian D. Scanlan

Library of Congress Cataloging-in-Publication Data

Names: Stack, Brendan C., Jr., 1963- editor. | Moreno, Mauricio A., editor.
Title: Neck dissection / [edited by] Brendan C. Stack, Jr., MD, CACS, FACE, Professor, Department of Otolaryngology – Head and Neck Surgery, University of Arkansas for Medical Sciences, Little Rock, Arkansas, Mauricio A. Moreno, MD, Associate Professor, Director Head & Neck Division, Department of Otolaryngology – Head and Neck Surgery, Little Rock, Arkansas.
Description: First edition. | New York, NY : Thieme Medical Publishers, Inc., [2019] | Includes bibliographic references. |
Identifiers: LCCN 2018041348 (print) | LCCN 2018050310 (ebook) | ISBN 9781626238350 (e-book) | ISBN 9781626238343 (print) | ISBN 9781626238350 (eISBN)
Subjects: LCSH: Neck–Cancer–Surgery–Handbooks, manuals, etc.
Classification: LCC RC280.N35 (ebook) | LCC RC280.N35 N43 2019 (print) | DDC 616.99/493–dc23
LC record available at https://lccn.loc.gov/2018041348

We dedicate this book to the tens of thousands of patients we as editors and authors have treated over our careers, especially to those we performed neck dissections upon. We always did our best in the care we provided, and you allowed us to learn from our experiences caring for you and use that knowledge to help others in need.

Contents

Foreword I

Neck dissection may be required for malignant diseases of the skin, aerodigestive tract, thyroid, and salivary glands. Diseases involving the cervical lymphatics of the head and neck may be treated surgically, but may need interdisciplinary knowledge and cooperation in cases of extensive burden of disease or in the setting of a recurrence. This book is a well-constructed, comprehensive, and current summary of anatomic, medical and surgical aspects of cervical lymphatic diseases of all origins. Because many types of malignancy may metastasize to the cervical lymphatics, each respective disease is addressed with its particular anatomic and pathophysiologic nuances. These include squamous cell carcinoma, thyroid cancers, salivary gland malignancies, and skin cancers (melanoma).

The editors of this text have engaged many of the world leaders in head and neck surgery to create in-depth, evidence-based summaries of the principles of surgery for cervical lymphadenopathy. During the past decade, several advances in the understanding of and treatment for many of the primary malignancies of the head and neck have come to fruition. This text therefore comes at an appropriate time. It will serve as an excellent reference guide for a wide range of medical and surgical experts involved in the interdisciplinary diagnosis and treatment. Although the fund of information is primarily related to clinical management, the chapters are succinct and concise, making them highly valuable not only for clinicians but also for those involved in preclinical, molecular and laboratory, as well as in postsurgical evaluation of lymphadenopathy patients. Overall, this book is an outstanding resource for an evidence-based, yet personalized, management of cervical lymphadenopathy and should have an active place in the current library of all physicians dealing with head and neck patients.

Prof. Dr. med. Dr. h.c. mult. Henning Dralle, FRCS, FACS, FEBS
University Hospital Essen
Head of the Section of Endocrine Surgery
Department of General, Visceral and Transplantation Surgery
Essen, Germany

Foreword II

Successful treatment of cancers arising in the head and neck region most often requires consideration of potential or actual metastases to lymph nodes in the neck. The finding of metastatic lymph nodes and extension of metastatic cancer beyond the lymph node capsule known as extracapsular spread (ECS) or extra-nodal extension (ENE) are the most reliable predictors of decreased survival in patients with cancers of the upper aerodigestive tract, skin of the head and neck region, and salivary and thyroid glands. Therefore, the assessment and elective evaluation or therapeutic treatment of the neck by neck dissection remains a critical component of head and neck cancer management that has not been addressed as comprehensively heretofore as it is in the text book titled *Neck Dissection*. This book has been edited by Drs. Mauricio Moreno and Brendan Stack, Associate Professor and Professor of Otolaryngology-Head and Neck Surgery, respectively, at the University of Arkansas Medical School (UAMS).

I got to know Dr. Stack well through the American Head and Neck Society (AHNS) when I was Vice President of that organization and he was working with colleagues to develop an Endocrine Surgery Section of the AHNS. I was very impressed by his passion for the comprehensive management of thyroid cancers, inclusive of management of the neck in well-differentiated and aggressive thyroid cancers. Dr. Moreno was a clinical fellow for several years in the Department of Head and Neck Surgery at the University of Texas MD Anderson Cancer Center, which I now chair, through which I acquired firsthand evidence of his intense commitment to patient care, education, and technical precision in the operating room. I have proudly watched him from a distance mature from Assistant Professor to Associate Professor and Vice Chair of Adult Services at UAMS. These two colleagues have taken a very scholarly and comprehensive approach in putting together a much-needed text on neck dissection for trainees, faculty, practitioners, and allied health professionals caring for patients with head and neck cancer.

The title "*Neck Dissection*" suggests that this book might be a description of a series of surgical procedures of the same name or a surgical atlas outlining the steps of several operations considered under the general rubric of neck dissection, and it is; but it is also much, much more than that. This book contains chapters written by a collection of well-established and emerging international experts from around the world that cover a range of relevant subjects. These include the biology of cervical metastases of head and neck cancers, the non-operative evaluation and staging of lymph nodes of the neck by a variety of methods, and the treatment of the neck using multiple modalities inclusive of surgery, radiotherapy, and systemic therapy. In addition, it provides the unique consideration of nodal spread from cancers of the head and neck region that arise from a variety of tissue types including mucosal and cutaneous epithelia, thyroid and salivary glands, and neural crest derived melanocytes. A major highlight is the step by step description with accompanying surgical photos that outline the basic steps of each of the major neck dissections used today by head and neck surgeons around the globe. More contemporary topics including i) sentinel lymph node biopsy, ii) surgical quality measures, and iii) functional outcomes and rehabilitation are also covered by experts in these areas.

In summary, Drs. Stack and Moreno have added significant value to our field with their new text titled *Neck Dissection*, which will be particularly useful for head and neck surgical oncologists and trainees in the field, but will also benefit other head and neck oncologists and supportive care providers.

Jeffrey N. Myers, MD, PhD, FACS
Chair, Department of Head and Neck Surgery
Alando J. Ballantyne Distinguished Chair of Head and Neck Surgery
University of Texas MD Anderson Cancer Center
Houston, Texas, USA

Preface

The dissection of critical structures of the neck is an integral part of all aspects of head and neck surgery, for both benign and malignant diagnoses of the head, skull base, neck, and cervicothoracic junction. An appreciation for neck anatomy is the foundation for success in executing surgery of the head and neck well. This anatomic understanding, married to fastidious surgical technique and extensive operative experience, can result in excellent outcomes when managing a broad spectrum of head and neck conditions. Moreover, a broad experience with the breadth of head and neck diseases is essential for comprehensive head and neck surgical care.

It is the aspiration of the editors and authors of this book to present a complete treatment of the topic of neck dissection in its many applications. This book starts from the fundamentals and expands to all possible applications for deploying neck dissections and the procedure's evolution to the current state of the art.

Brendan C. Stack, Jr., MD, FACS, FACE
Mauricio A. Moreno, MD

Acknowledgments

I wish to publicly thank the support of my wife Cynthia and family of 4 daughters and 3 sons, my clinic support staff and colleagues at the University of Arkansas for Medical Sciences, and my excellent group of fifteen Otolaryngology-Head and Neck Surgery residents. All have been supportive of my pursuits of new knowledge and excellence in clinical care over my career. I extend my deepest gratitude and heartfelt humility for their support.

Brendan C. Stack, Jr.

I would like to thank my wife Patricia, and my two beautiful daughters, Sofia and Emma, for their relentless support, and for being a constant source of inspiration in every aspect of my life; and my parents, Alejo and Teresa, for fostering my desire to learn, and for engraving in me the work ethic needed to succeed.

Mauricio A. Moreno

Contributors

Misha Amoils, MD
Adjunct Clinical Assistant Professor
Santa Clara Valley Medical Center
Department of Otolaryngology – Head and Neck Surgery
Stanford University
Stanford, California

Konstantinos Arnaoutakis, MD
Associate Professor
Department of Medicine
Division of Oncology
Winthrop P Rockefeller Cancer Research Institute
University of Arkansas for Medical Sciences
Little Rock, Arkansas

Twyla B. Bartel, DO, MBA
Radiologist
Global Advances Imaging, PLLC
Little Rock, Arkansas

Donald Bodenner, MD, PhD
Professor
Department of Geriatrics
Director
Thyroid Unit
Chief
Endocrine Oncology
University of Arkansas for Medical Sciences
Little Rock, Arkansas

Estelle Eun Hae Chang, MDCM, MPH
Professor
Department of Otolaryngology – Head and Neck Surgery
University of Nebraska Medical Center
Omaha, Nebraska

Chien Chen, MD, PhD
Associate Professor
Department of Pathology
University of Arkansas for Medical Sciences
Little Rock, Arkansas

Douglas B. Chepeha, MD, MScPH, FACS, FRCS (C)
Professor
Department of Otolaryngology
University of Toronto
Toronto, Ontario, Canada

Francisco Civantos, MD, FACS
Professor
Department of Otolaryngology
University of Miami
Miami, Florida

Anil K.D. Cruz, MS, DNB, FRCS(Hon)
Professor and Surgeon
Chief, Head and Neck Services
Tata Memorial Hospital
Parel, Mumbai, India

Harsh Dhar, MS, M Ch (Head Neck Surgery)
Specialist Senior Resident
Department of Head and Neck Surgery
Tata Memorial Hospital
Parel, Mumbai, India

Vasu Divi, MD
Assistant Professor
Department of Otolaryngology – Head and Neck Surgery
Stanford University
Stanford, California

Quinn A. Dunlap, MD
Resident
Department of Otolaryngology – Head and Neck Surgery
University of Arkansas for Medical Sciences
Little Rock, Arkansas

Jamie Ferguson, MNSc, APRN, AGPCNP-C
Nurse Practitioner
Department of Head and Neck Oncology
University of Arkansas for Medical Sciences
Little Rock, Arkansas

Marcelo F. Figari, MD, FACS
Section of Head and Neck Surgery
Department of Surgery
Hospital Italiano
Ciudad Autónoma de Buenos Aires
Buenos Aires, Argentina

Ryan T. Fitzgerald, MD
Radiology Consultants
Adjunct Associate Professor
Department of Radiology, Neuroradiology Division
University of Arkansas for Medical Sciences
Little Rock, Arkansas

Chad E. Galer, MD, FACS
Chief
Department of Otolaryngology – Head and Neck Surgery
Richard L Roudebush VA Medical Center
Assistant Professor
Department of Otolaryngology – Head and Neck Surgery
Indiana University
Indianapolis, Indiana

Rachel Giese, MD
Fellow
Department of Head and Neck Surgery
Memorial Sloan Kettering Cancer Center
New York, New York

M. Kürşat Gökcan, MD
Associate Professor
Department of Otorhinolaryngology, Head and Neck Surgery
Ankara University
Ankara, Turkey

William Harris, MD
Resident
Department of Otolaryngology
Tulane University
New Orleans, Louisiana

David J. Hernandez, MD
Assistant Professor
Department of Otolaryngology – Head and Neck Surgery
Baylor College of Medicine
Houston, Texas

Andrew J. Johnsrud, MD
Department of Medicine
Division of Oncology
Winthrop P Rockefeller Cancer Research Institute
University of Arkansas for Medical Sciences
Little Rock, Arkansas

Dipti Kamani, MD
Director of Research
Division of Thyroid and Parathyroid Surgery
Department of Otolaryngology
Massachusetts Eye and Ear Infirmary
Boston, Massachusetts

Yoon Woo Koh, MD
Professor
Department of Otorhinolaryngology
Yonsei Head and Neck Cancer Center
Yonsei University College of Medicine
Seoul, Korea

Michael Kubala, MD
Resident
Department of Otolaryngology – Head and Neck Surgery
University of Arkansas for Medical Sciences
Little Rock, Arkansas

Bradley R. Lawson, MD
Physician
Licking Memorial Health Systems
Newark, Ohio

Kang Dae Lee, MD
Professor
Department of Otolaryngology – Head and Neck Surgery
Kosin University College of Medicine
Busan, South Korea

Eric J. Lentsch, MD, FACS
Professor
Department of Otolaryngology – Head and Neck Surgery
Medical University of South Carolina
Charleston, South Carolina

Mingyann Lim, MD
Consultant
Department of Otolaryngology
Tan Tock Seng Hospital
Singapore, China

Shivangi Lohia, MD
Resident
Department of Otolaryngology – Head and Neck Surgery
Medical University of South Carolina
Charleston, South Carolina

Manish Mair, MS, M Ch (Head Neck Surgery)
Specialist Senior Resident
Department of Head and Neck Surgery
Tata Memorial Hospital
Parel, Mumbai, India

Jesus E. Medina, MD, FACS
Professor
Department of Otorhinolaryngology
Stephenson Cancer Center
University of Oklahoma
Oklahoma City, Oklahoma

William M. Mendenhall, MD
Professor
Department of Radiation Oncology
University of Florida College of Medicine
Gainesville, Florida

Catherine E. Mercado, MD
Resident
Department of Radiation Oncology
University of Florida College of Medicine
Gainesville, Florida

Brian Moore, MD
Chairman
Department of Otorhinolaryngology and Communication Sciences
Ochsner Medical Center
New Orleans, Louisiana

Mauricio A. Moreno, MD
Associate Professor
Director, Head & Neck Division
Department of Otolaryngology – Head and Neck
  Surgery
Vice Chair, Adult Services
University of Arkansas for Medical Sciences
Little Rock, Arkansas

Brian Nussenbaum, MD
Professor
Department of Otolaryngology – Head and Neck
  Surgery
Washington University
Saint Louis, Missouri

Angela M. Osmolak, MD
Head and Neck Surgical Oncologist
Nebraska Methodist Health System
Omaha, Nebraska

Patrik Pipkorn, MD
Professor
Department of Head and Neck Surgery
Department of Otolaryngology – Head and Neck
  Surgery
Washington University
Saint Louis, Missouri

Kristen Pytynia, MD, MPH
Professor
Department of Head and Neck Surgery
University of Texas MD Anderson Cancer Center
Houston, Texas

Gregory W. Randolph, MD, FACS, FACE
Professor
Department of Otolaryngology
Claire and John Bertucci Endowed Chair in Thyroid
  Surgical Oncology
Harvard Medical School
Division Chief
General and Thyroid/Parathyroid Endocrine Surgical
  Divisions
Massachusetts Eye and Ear
President
American Academy of Otolaryngology—Head and
  Neck Surgery
Boston, Massachusetts

Brendan C. Stack, Jr., MD, FACS, FACE
Professor
Department of Otolaryngology – Head and
  Neck Surgery
University of Arkansas for Medical Sciences
Little Rock, Arkansas

Jumin Sunde, MD
Clinical Lecturer
Department of Otolaryngology
University of Michigan
Ann Arbor, Michigan

Samuel J. Trosman, MD
Assistant Professor
Department of Otolaryngology/Head and Neck Surgery
Icahn School of Medicine at Mount Sinai
New York, New York

Vincent Vander Poorten, MD PhD MSc
Full Professor and Clinical Head
Department of Otorhinolaryngology, Head and Neck
  Surgery
University Hospitals
Leuven, Belgium
Section Head of Head and Neck Oncology
Department of Oncology
KU Leuven, Belgium
Otorhinolaryngology, Head and Neck Surgery
Department of Oncology, section Head and Neck Oncology
University Hospitals Leuven
Leuven, Belgium

Kathryn M. Vorwald, DDS, MD
Surgeon
Department of Head and Neck – Endocrine Oncology
H. Lee Moffitt Cancer Center and Research Institute
Tampa, Florida

Peter S. Vosler, MD, PhD
Fellow
Department of Otolaryngology – Head and Neck Surgery
University of Toronto
Toronto, Ontario, Canada

Emre A. Vural, MD, FACS
Professor
Department of Otolaryngology – Head and Neck Surgery
University of Arkansas for Medical Sciences
Little Rock, Arkansas

J. Trad Wadsworth, MD, MBA
Department of Head and Neck – Endocrine Oncology
H. Lee Moffitt Cancer Center & Research Institute
Tampa, Florida

Richard Wong, MD, FACS
Chief
Head and Neck Services
Memorial Sloan Kettering Cancer Center
New York, New York

Tracy L. Yarbrough, MD, PhD
Associate Professor
Department of Physiology
California Northstate University College of Medicine
Elk Grove, California

Mark Zafereo, MD
Associate Professor
Department of Head and Neck Surgery
MD Anderson Cancer Center
Houston, Texas

Joseph Zenga, MD
Department of Otolaryngology – Head and Neck Surgery
Washington University
Saint Louis, Missouri

1 Clinical Assessment of Neck Lymphadenopathies

M. Kürşat Gökcan and Emre A. Vural

Abstract

Cervical lymphadenopathy is a common cause of clinic visits, which necessitates rapid and efficient diagnosis. The key requirement for this practice is the combination of the recognition of various risk factors in patients' history with the understanding of neck anatomy and appropriate usage of diagnostic tools such as imaging and biopsies. This chapter aims to provide necessary information for clinicians in obtaining a thorough history and head and neck examination, as well as employing the correct imaging algorithm and the differential diagnosis in patients with cervical lymphadenopathy.

Keywords: neck mass, lymphadenopathy, differential diagnosis, diagnostic imaging, pediatric lymphadenopathy, congenital lesions, neoplasms of the neck, carcinoma of unknown primary

1.1 Introduction

Neck is the bridge between the head and the trunk. Besides conveying spinal cord in a chamber made of vertebrae and muscles, neck contains important vasculature, nerves, fat and lymphatics, and elements of upper aerodigestive tract, as well as salivary, thyroid, and parathyroid glands. Seeing a lump or a swelling in the neck is a very common clinical finding in all age groups, which can be related to the structures in the neck or can be part of an infectious, inflammatory, or a neoplastic process. Therefore, diagnostic workup may pose a major challenge in the daily practice of any physician.

The scope of this chapter is to provide a systematical approach for the evaluation of neck masses, specifically cervical lymphadenopathies, which entails obtaining a thorough history from the patient, performing a complete physical examination including endoscopy, utilizing relevant imaging modalities, and performing biopsies in the form of needle aspiration or excision as necessary. Many characteristics of the patient and the findings in the history are invaluable in presumptive diagnosis, and may help direct the subsequent physical examination and in selecting the appropriate laboratory and imaging studies. Detailed head and neck physical examination is the crucial step for proper diagnosis and management. Imaging should be directed for better delineation of pathology and/or involved nodal groups.

1.2 History and Physical Examination

A mass in the neck is a very common finding in patients of all age groups. Despite significant progress in clinical diagnostic and imaging modalities, history and physical examination of a patient with neck mass still remains the mainstay of diagnosis. A rapidly growing, tender mass in a child usually consists of reactive lymph nodes that are caused by inflammation after infections. On the other hand, a slow-growing, firm mass in a heavy drinker and smoker elderly male could be metastatic lymph node from a primary malignancy in the upper aerodigestive tract. More than 90% of all neck masses were estimated to be benign in pediatric age group, while—excluding thyroid masses —80% of adult neck masses are neoplastic and 80% of those are malignant.[1] Therefore, every piece of information gathered from history of the patient and the present illness is not only important for obtaining a proper diagnosis, but may also save time by preventing unnecessary tests.

History taking should be concentrated on the history of the present illness, onset and duration of the neck mass, and any associated symptoms such as pain, fever, anorexia, weight loss, night sweats, fatigue, otalgia, throat pain, dysphonia, dysphagia, odynophagia, hoarseness, and/or dyspnea. Past medical, surgical, social, and family histories are important parts of patient's evaluation. Patient's tobacco and/or alcohol consumption, its duration and intensity, and occupational exposures to environmental toxins, recent travels especially to exotic regions, exposure to animals and sexually transmitted diseases such as human papillomavirus (HPV), and any history of radiation to the head and neck should also be noted.

After obtaining a detailed history, a careful head and neck physical examination should be carried out for evaluation of craniofacial skin, eyes, oral cavity, oropharynx, larynx, hypopharynx, ears, nasal cavity, and nasopharynx. Palpation of neck nodal basins, salivary glands, and thyroid, and bimanual palpation of tongue, tonsil, and floor of mouth should be part of the physical examination. A key adjunct to visual inspection is the fiberoptic endoscopy, which not only allows a thorough examination of the upper aerodigestive tract with illumination and magnification, but also provides a dynamic evaluation of swallowing and airway.

Features of a palpable mass include mobility, tenderness, location in the neck, firmness, fluctuance, overlying erythema, pulsation, and palpable bruits.[1] Several features may help in differentiating a benign reactive lymphadenopathy from a lymph node harboring malignancy. Cervical lymphadenopathy associated with viral infections is often soft, small, bilateral, mobile, nontender, and without overlying skin changes, although this general rule may not be true with some of the more subacute and chronic viral infections, such as Epstein–Barr virus (EBV) and cytomegalovirus.[2,3] Cervical lymphadenopathy associated with bacterial infections is usually of acute onset and unilateral. Bacterial lymphadenitis develops more commonly in submandibular (50–60%) or upper cervical (25–30%) regions compared with other cervical lymph node subsites.[3] Up to 25% of patients with acute bacterial lymphadenitis will demonstrate fluctuance on physical examination, and this is especially true with *Staphylococcus aureus* lymphadenitis.[3] Concerning findings that may suggest malignancy include nodes that are rapidly enlarging, firm, nontender, and fixed-to-the-skin or underlying structures. Also, generalized lymphadenopathy, supraclavicular nodes regardless of size, lower cervical nodes, lymph nodes greater than 2 to 3 cm, and accompanying hepatosplenomegaly are associated with increased risk of malignancy.[4]

One should always keep in mind that a neck mass is maybe part of a systemic illness, especially in the absence of an obvious etiology within the head and neck.[1]

1.3 Relevant Anatomy and Nodal Classification

Although detailed surgical anatomy and patterns of nodal spread are given elsewhere in this book, it is crucial to review anatomy of the neck for proper documentation of the findings and differential diagnosis. Localization of cervical lymphadenopathy is closely associated with the origin of the pathology, and allows for a focused clinical examination with efficient use of diagnostic tools. It is also very important to organize physical examination findings in an order and understanding of the neck's triangles and nodal levels. Therefore, relevant anatomy and nodal classification will be touched upon for these purposes.

1.3.1 Triangles of the Neck

Most physicians find it helpful to define the neck in terms of triangles when communicating the location of physical findings.[5] Each side of the neck is bordered by the inferior edge of the mandible superiorly, trapezius muscle posteriorly, clavicle inferiorly, and midline medially. The sternocleidomastoid muscle (SCM) divides the neck into a posterior and an anterior triangle. The posterior triangle is then subdivided by the inferior belly of omohyoid muscle into the supraclavicular triangle inferiorly and the occipital triangle superiorly. The anterior triangle is further divided into four smaller triangles, which are submandibular, submental, muscular, and carotid triangles. The submandibular triangle is formed by the two bellies of digastric muscle and the inferior border of the mandible. The submental triangle lies between the anterior bellies of digastric muscles and the hyoid bone. The muscular triangle is bordered by the SCM, superior belly of the omohyoid muscle, and the midline. The carotid triangle is the area between the anterior border of SCM, superior belly of the omohyoid, and posterior belly of the digastric muscles.

1.3.2 Lymph Node Regions

Lymph nodes tend to be organized into groups or chains that drain discrete anatomic regions.[6] Several classifications have been proposed to organize cervical lymph nodes into nodal regions that enable reliable localization of pathologic lymph nodes, effective communication among clinicians, and accurate cancer staging. The most widely used schemes historically have been those, such as that of Rouviere, describing nodal groups

based on proximity to adjacent structures.[7] This system was based on palpation and inspection of lymph nodes. With the development of cross-sectional imaging systems, a "level"-based classification was proposed[8] and adopted by the American Joint Committee on Cancer for both radiologists and clinicians involved in the care of head and neck cancer patients in order to reliably communicate the location of pathologic lymph nodes and for cancer staging.[6] Nodal basins of the neck will be discussed in detail in another chapter of this book.

1.4 Diagnostic Testing

After acquiring a detailed history and necessary evidence from physical examination, it may be necessary to run additional diagnostic testing and/or imaging for accurate diagnosis. It is usually unnecessary and inefficient to run all imaging and diagnostic tests in every patient; the practitioner should have the knowledge on the indications, advantages, and pitfalls of each modality.

1.5 Laboratory Testing

Laboratory testing can usually be an adjunct to other findings in the differential diagnosis. Complete blood cell count can be useful to identify markers of infection, as elevated white blood cell count with neutrophil predominance. Elevated erythrocyte sedimentation rate and C-reactive protein (CRP) levels not only are useful in supporting the clinical suspicion of an infectious or an inflammatory mass, but also are used to monitor the response to treatment. Serologic testing can be necessary in the diagnosis or differential diagnosis of certain infectious diseases, such as tuberculosis, infectious mononucleosis, and brucellosis.

1.5.1 Imaging

Evaluation of a neck mass usually involves an imaging modality that confirms the presumed diagnosis or provides a differential diagnosis. The preferred imaging modality in the workup of a neck mass may differ mainly based on physical examination findings and associated conditions that may exclude utilization of certain modalities such as kidney failure that may exclude administration of iodine contrast in computed tomography (CT) or an implanted pacemaker that eliminates the option of performing a magnetic resonance imaging (MRI). Details of anatomic imaging and imaging criteria for characterization of metastatic lymph nodes are given elsewhere in this book. However, brief description of advantages and disadvantages of frequently used imaging modalities in differential diagnosis of neck masses are provided in this chapter (▶ Table 1.1).

Table 1.1 Brief description of frequently used imaging modalities in differential diagnosis of cervical masses

Modality	Basic indication	Advantages	Disadvantages
Ultrasound	First-line imaging in the evaluation of thyroid nodules and pediatric neck masses. Useful in salivary gland imaging	Inexpensive and quick. No ionizing radiation. Can be utilized without sedation. Can readily distinguish between a solid and a fluid-filled mass. Can be used in conjunction with fine-needle aspiration biopsy	Operator dependent. Limited use in imaging of deep structures and parapharyngeal space due to acoustic shadowing. Cannot provide anatomic details as a cross-sectional imaging modality
Computed tomography	Most frequently utilized imaging in adult neck masses. Iodinated contrast enhancement is usually necessary for better delineation of anatomic characteristics of bone, airway, soft tissues, and vasculature of the neck	Provides three-dimensional relationships of lymph nodes with other structures. Best for discretion of bone invasion or evaluation of bony lesions	May pose significant risk of radiation exposure, especially in pediatric population or in repeated utilization. Iodine contrast may cause allergic reaction or nephrotoxicity
Magnetic resonance imaging	Important part of treatment planning in salivary gland and oral cavity neoplasms	Provides best soft-tissue delineation. Good for depicting soft-tissue invasion and vascular invasion. Only imaging modality to show perineural invasion. No ionizing radiation	Expensive and time-consuming. May require sedation or anesthesia in pediatric population. May not be tolerated by claustrophobics
Positron emission tomography	Useful for staging and follow-up of malignant diseases. Can be used in the search of unknown primary in neck metastases	Provides whole-body scanning	Narrow indication. Cost
Angiography	Evaluation and preoperative assessment of vascular lesions or malignant lesions invading vascular structures	Digital subtraction angiography may be used for embolization of feeding vessels in paragangliomas	Narrow indication

Ultrasound (US) is typically the initial imaging performed for evaluation of a palpable neck mass as it utilizes no radiation, requires no sedation or intravenous contrast, is easily accessible, and is relatively low in cost. Advances in technology allowed clinicians to access more compact US devices with higher resolution at lower cost and helped popularizing clinician performed US examinations at office. US can provide information about the size and location of the lesion as well as its cystic or solid nature. Doppler feature can be utilized to identify vascularity of the mass.[9] Certain findings in the US examination may provide clues in differentiating a normal or reactive lymph node from a malignant one, and also guide the examiner in performing needle biopsies for cytological evaluation. Normal lymph nodes are typically ovoid to kidney shaped in shape and are slightly hypoechoic when compared to the surrounding soft tissues with a hyperechoic region that represents the fatty hilum of the lymph node. On color Doppler examination, there is flow in normal lymph nodes, which is relatively increased near the hilum.[9] Reactive lymph nodes are typically less than 1 to 1.5 cm in greatest diameter, and usually keep the fusiform shape with a short-to-long axis ratio of less than 0.5. Malignant lymph nodes are usually rounded in shape and increased in size, and have lost their characteristic architecture with lack of an echogenic fatty hilum, and distortion or displacement of normal vascularization.[10]

Despite being an excellent screening tool, US examination has several limitations and flaws in evaluation of neck masses. Penetration of high-frequency linear probe may be reduced at deep neck structures, especially at short and/or thick necks. Also, acoustic shadowing hinders evaluation of retrosternal, retropharyngeal lymph nodes, and parapharyngeal lesions. Proper US evaluation is also highly dependent on the skills and the proficiency of the examiner, especially in the pediatric age group.

For the adult population, the diagnostic algorithm usually continues with a cross-sectional imaging modality such as CT and/or MRI. CT continues to be the most frequently utilized modality. Discrimination of fine anatomic characteristics of bone and of the soft tissues of the neck is particularly facilitated by the use of iodinated contrast studies (▶ Fig. 1.1). On the one hand, CT scans may provide excellent details about the head and neck mucosal sites, locate masses within or outside of glands or nodal chains, and give relation of the mass to lymph nodes, major blood vessels, airway, and bony structures such as the mandible and vertebral column.[1] On the other hand, CT scans may expose the individual to radiation, which can be an important issue in pediatric cases or with repeated scans. Also, iodine contrast may cause allergic/anaphylactic reaction in susceptible individuals and may cause nephrotoxicity, particularly if utilized in a dehydrated patient.

MRI provides better soft-tissue delineation, with better appreciation of vascular and/or perineural invasion. MRI carries no risk of radiation; it can be safely used in pregnant or pediatric patients. On the other hand, MRI is less readily available and more expensive than the aforementioned studies.

CT and MRI are not substitutes for each other, but are complementary to each other in the evaluation of malignant neck masses. Physician chooses one or both, depending on the suspected pathology. CT and MRI are usually ordered together in the evaluation of masses involving oral cavity, skull base, pharynx, and parapharyngeal space.

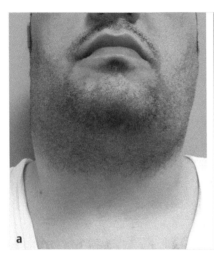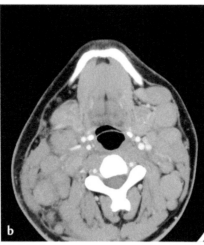

Fig. 1.1 Discretization of cervical lymphadenopathies can be difficult in short and thick necks (**a**). Computed tomography with iodine contrast provides detailed information of lymph nodes regarding their size, location, and relationship to other structures (**b**).

Positron emission tomography (PET) is another important imaging modality in evaluation of cervical lymphadenopathy, especially in the presence of a primary tumor in the head and neck. PET provides important information in head and neck oncology, especially in initial staging and in evaluation of the treatment response.

1.5.2 Fine-Needle Aspiration Biopsy and Cytological Analysis

Fine-needle aspiration biopsy (FNAB) has become an essential tool in the diagnosis of neck masses. Imaging can be highly suggestive in the diagnosis of certain neck masses with vascular, infectious, or congenital origin (i.e., thyroglossal duct cyst [TDC] or branchial cleft cyst), but cytopathological evaluation is usually necessary for most neck masses in adult patients. The procedure is quick and safe. Generally, a 22- to 25-gauge needle with 10-mL syringe is inserted into the mass, and multiple passes through the lesion are made with or without the suction of the syringe plunger. The aspirate is transferred on a microscope slide and dried on air, or inserted to a liquid medium and transferred to the laboratory depending on the practice of the institution. This can also allow staining of the tissue block obtained during the aspiration process. FNAB cytology is highly sensitive and specific in differentiating cystic masses from solid, benign masses from malignant, and epithelial metastases from lymphoid infiltration. Analysis of tissue architecture with immunohistochemistry and/ or flow cytometry is usually required for the diagnosis of lymphoma and other pathologies of lymphoid origin. Therefore, core needle biopsy or open biopsy may be warranted for further identification of such lesions. Occasionally, CT- or MRI-guided FNAB may be necessary where US guidance is not adequate for targeting masses in locations with difficult access such as retropharyngeal space or the pterygopalatine fossa.

1.6 Differential Diagnosis of Neck Masses

The differential diagnosis of the neck masses can be listed under three main categories:
- Infectious and inflammatory lesions.
- Congenital lesions.
- Neoplasms of the neck.

1.6.1 Infectious and Inflammatory Lesions

Infectious and inflammatory lesions are the most frequently encountered neck masses in both adults and children. The neck has an extensive capillary lymphatic network that drains skin, upper aerodigestive tract, salivary glands, and thyroid gland. Approximately 40% of all the lymph nodes in the body are located in the head and neck.[6] Thus, it is quite common to encounter enlarged submandibular masses as reactive lymphadenopathy in the neck, after a viral or bacterial upper respiratory tract infection or a dental infection. Often, these reactive nodes will manifest as palpable, mobile, and tender masses, and the patient may report fever, upper respiratory infection symptoms, tooth pain, or dysphagia.[1] Occasionally, these lymph nodes will become necrotic in the course of a bacterial infection, and an abscess forms. US is usually the preferred imaging modality in such case, which will readily show the necrotic area in the lymph node, and enable aspiration of fluid for culture and cytology. CT scan with iodine contrast is best for delineating diffuse lymphadenopathy or an abscess formation in parapharyngeal, retropharyngeal, or masticatory spaces.

Granulomatous diseases include a wide variety of pathologies, which may occasionally present as a neck mass. These include infectious or autoimmune diseases such as sarcoidosis, tuberculosis, atypical mycobacterial infections, cat-scratch disease, or Kawasaki's disease. US-guided FNAB cytology may reveal important features of the disease or exclude a malignant process. Excisional or incisional biopsies are a last resort because of the concern for creation of a chronically draining wound.[1]

Infection or inflammation of the salivary or thyroid glands is not uncommon. Obstruction of Wharton's or Stensen's ducts by sialolithiasis or mucus plugs causes tender and swollen glands with warmth and hyperemia. The symptoms are usually unilateral and confined to one gland, and are usually exacerbated with ingestion of food or drinks. Infection may ensue behind the obstruction, and thus, examiner can see purulent discharge from the orifice of the salivary duct upon massage to the respective salivary gland. US shows signs of inflamed parenchyma and often dilated duct with calculi in it. CT scan may better show the place of calculi deposits, and often ordered if surgical treatment is anticipated.

Inflammatory diseases of thyroid gland can be encountered in the differential diagnosis of anterior neck masses. Three broad categories of thyroiditis are defined: (1) acute suppurative thyroiditis, which is due to bacterial infection; (2) subacute thyroiditis, which results from a viral infection of the gland; and (3) chronic thyroiditis, which is usually autoimmune in nature. Acute thyroiditis is characterized with painful palpable thyroid gland with signs of infection. The pain worsens with extension of the neck. Subacute thyroiditis can also cause a tender and palpable thyroid gland, with systemic symptoms as fatigue, malaise, and low-grade fever. Chronic autoimmune thyroiditis has a slower course and results in a diffuse, nontender goiter. Diagnosis is usually done on clinical and laboratory findings. US is the preferred imaging modality for diagnosis and follow-up.

1.6.2 Congenital Lesions

Congenital lesions are an important cause of neck masses in childhood or early adulthood period. Detailed description of embryological development of the neck is beyond the scope of this chapter, but understanding certain features of congenital lesions is usually required for differential diagnosis and treatment.

Thyroglossal Duct Cyst

TDC is the most common congenital neck mass in children, which presents as a midline cystic mass. It represents 70% of all congenital neck masses.[1] TDCs are formed due to a congenital defect in the closure of embryonic descent route of the thyroid gland. This route originates from foramen cecum, in the base of tongue, and courses in the anterior neck, close to the midline, usually deep to the hyoid bone and the strap muscles, to the isthmus of the thyroid gland. Remnants of the thyroglossal duct are actually found in approximately 7% of the population, but only a small number of these ever become symptomatic.[11] TDCs usually become evident in childhood as a midline cystic neck mass that elevates in the neck with tongue protrusion or swallowing. Occasionally, cyst fluid gets infected, and presents as a painful and inflamed midline mass.

Evaluation of thyroid function and US imaging is necessary to rule out lingual ectopic thyroid tissue. Acute infection of TDC is treated with aspiration of cyst contents and antibiotics. Complete removal of descent route by the Sistrunk procedure is recommended for definitive treatment.

Branchial Cleft Anomalies

Branchial cleft anomalies are also common both in pediatric and in young adult populations. One-third of all congenital neck masses are the result of incompletely obliterated embryonic branchial tissue, which may be in the form of a cyst, sinus, or a fistula.[1,11] Evaluation of their location and course requires understanding the branchial cleft embryonic development. First-arch anomalies represent about 1% of all branchial arch anomalies and are classified as type 1 or type 2. Type 1 anomalies are duplications of the external auditory canal, and they can have attachments to the skin of the external auditory canal. Type 2 anomalies are found within the parotid gland deep to the facial nerve. Their relation with the facial nerve makes the management difficult.[1]

Anomalies of the second arch are by far the most common (representing 95% of all branchial cleft anomalies) and typically manifest as a submandibular cystic mass, anterior to the SCM (▶ Fig. 1.2). The course runs always lateral to the internal carotid artery. If it is in the form of sinus or fistula, it enters the pharynx at the tonsillar fossa. It may get infected during the course of an upper respiratory tract infection. Differential diagnosis may be required from cystic metastatic lymph nodes, especially in the young adults.

Third- and fourth-arch anomalies are extremely rare. Third-arch anomalies run deep to the internal carotid artery and open into the piriform sinus through the thyrohyoid membrane. They are superior to the superior laryngeal nerve. Fourth-arch anomalies are side dependent: on the right, they lie deep to the subclavian artery, whereas on the left they course under the aortic arch. Ultimately, they can enter the piriform sinus, inferior to the superior laryngeal nerve, and can be intimately associated with the thyroid gland.[1]

Evaluation of branchial cleft anomalies usually requires CT scan and US. US shows the cyst structure and enables aspiration and drainage, if required. CT scan with contrast shows the anatomic relations in the neck including the carotid artery.

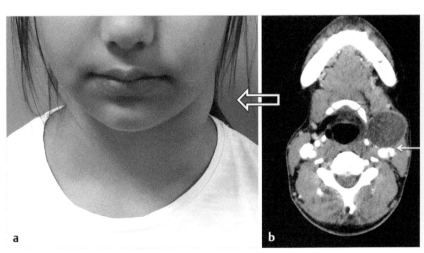

Fig. 1.2 (a) Second branchial arch cyst represents as a mass in lateral neck compartment (*thick arrow*). **(b)** Contrast-enhanced computed tomography shows the location of the cyst and its relation to internal carotid artery. *Arrow* indicates the cyst structure displacing the carotid sheath and its components, posteriorly.

a

b

Teratoma and Dermoid Cysts

Teratomas are developed from embryonic remnants of all three germ layers. Head and neck teratomas comprise approximately 2% of all teratomas.[12] They start to form in utero, during the second trimester, and present at birth as firm, midline neck masses. Occasionally, they can be diagnosed prenatally as cystic soft-tissue masses containing calcifications on imaging. The presence of calcifications within a neck mass is strongly suggestive of a teratoma. In neonates, a teratoma can present as a rapidly expanding neck mass that may compromise airway or deglutition. Surgical excision is the treatment of choice.

Dermoid cysts are the result of trapped rests of epithelial elements along natural lines of embryonic fusion, and are usually found in the midline or just lateral of midline. These cysts contain both ectodermal and endodermal elements. They are lined by epithelium but contain endodermal elements as hair follicles and sebaceous glands, which grow slowly due to accumulation of the sebaceous content. Infection of the cyst content is rare. They are usually diagnosed prior to 3 years of age.[12]

Hemangiomas and Lymphangiomas

Hemangiomas are bluish-purple colored, soft, compressible lesions, commonly presented within the first few months of life. These lesions are caused by the proliferation of vascular endothelial cells, and commonly encountered in the head and neck. Clinically, they show three phases of growth: a rapid, proliferative phase is followed by a stable phase, and then involution. Complete involution can be seen in half of patients before the age of 5, and nearly all tumors regress by ages 10 to 12.[11]

Vascular malformations are classified according to dominant type of vascular flow. Arteriovenous fistula and arteriovenous malformation are high-flow lesions with aberrant arterial and venous connections that lack parenchyma. Besides causing a mass with poor cosmetic appearance, they may result in ischemic ulcers or even congestive heart failure.[11] Doppler US and MRI angiography are excellent modalities for visualization of these lesions. Low-flow vascular malformations encompass venous malformations and lymphatic malformations. Venous malformations are made from dysplastic venous channels that present as blue or purple masses that feel spongy to palpation. Often, they will enlarge with Valsalva's maneuvers, and they are easily differentiated from lymphatic malformations with MRI angiography.

Lymphangiomas are also soft, compressible masses of benign hamartomatous lymphatic vessels and channels. They are commonly seen at birth or before age 2 years, and located most commonly in the posterior triangle of the neck.[11] They can often enlarge within the course of upper respiratory infections, but do not increase in size with Valsalva's maneuvers. Bleeding can be seen into the cystic spaces, which may result in dense phleboliths. Diagnosis is usually done with history and clinical examination findings. Evaluation is usually done by MRI and US.

1.6.3 Neoplasms of the Neck

Paragangliomas

Paraganglia are collections of cells of neuroectodermal origin that secrete catecholamines. They have an important functional role during embryogenesis, when they serve as the major source of catecholamines. After birth, most paraganglia nests disappear, with the exception of the adrenal medulla and the sites around the autonomic nervous system. In the adult, the function of the paraganglia is to help the autonomic nervous system respond to stressors such as hypercapnia, hypoxia, or decreased pH.[11]

Paragangliomas are highly vascular, slow-growing, mostly benign lesions originating from the nests of paraganglia, with less than 10% thought to be malignant. In the head and neck, they occur in three main locations and their presentations differ accordingly: carotid body, jugulotympanic region, and vagus nerve paragangliomas. Carotid body tumors are located in bifurcation of the carotid, and typically present as a painless, slowly enlarging neck mass (▶ Fig. 1.3). The classic diagnostic features are a nontender mass at the carotid triangle that is mobile horizontally, but fixed vertically, which has an associated

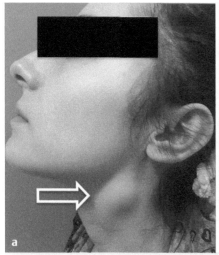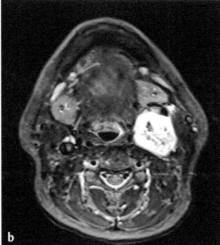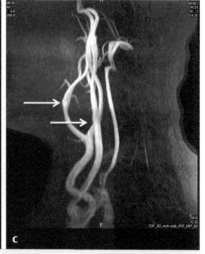

Fig. 1.3 (a) Carotid body tumor is a slow-growing, pulsatile mass in the lateral neck, located within the carotid triangle (*thick arrow*). (b) Magnetic resonance imaging with angiography shows typical location at the carotid bifurcation. (c) *Arrows* indicate the characteristic displacement of carotid arteries due to tumor structure (Lyre's sign).

bruit or vascular thrill. As these lesions enlarge, they may also cause cranial nerve or sympathetic chain neuropathies. Vagal paragangliomas will have a similar presentation but may have an increased incidence of hoarseness, pharyngeal fullness, or dysphagia at presentation. Proper evaluation and differential diagnosis is done with angiography, CT angiography, and MRI angiography. These lesions should be diagnosed by physical examination and imaging, and FNAB should be avoided.[11]

Neurogenic Neoplasms

Neurogenic neoplasms of the neck can be schwannomas, neurofibromas, malignant peripheral nerve sheath tumors, or tumors of neuroblastic origin such as neuroblastoma or ganglioneuroblastoma. Schwannomas are the benign tumors of Schwann cell origin, and are the most common solitary neurogenic tumors of the neck. These lesions occur in patients who are 20 to 50 years old, and 25 to 45% of extracranial schwannomas occur in the neck.[11] Schwannomas can originate from the cranial nerves, sympathetic chain, or spinal nerve roots, and therefore can commonly be encountered as a parapharyngeal masses. Clinical course can be asymptomatic, until compressive symptoms occur. Radiological differential diagnosis from other parapharyngeal masses can be best done with MRI, since cervical schwannomas—like paragangliomas of the neck—typically develop in the poststyloid parapharyngeal space, displacing carotid sheath contents anteriorly.

Neuromas typically result from traumatized nerve endings of sensory nerves. They are commonly encountered after neck dissection or parotidectomy, from the scarified nerve endings of greater auricular nerve or cervical plexus. Patients usually present with a painful neck mass, radiating to shoulder or temporal area.

Lipoma

Lipomas represent the most common subcutaneous soft-tissue tumor of adults.[11] They are slow-growing, benign tumors composed of adipocytes, which commonly occur in the posterior triangle but can occur throughout the neck and face. Lipomas are most often asymptomatic. When they arise from subcutaneous fat, palpation yields a sliding, lobulated mass with normal skin on it, which helps differentiate it from a sebaceous cyst or abscess. Deep lipomas have a firm to rubbery consistency on palpation. Differentiation of deep lipomas from low-grade liposarcomas is difficult; therefore, serial imaging with MRI or CT or complete surgical excision of enlarged lipomas is recommended.

Neoplasms of Salivary Glands

Salivary gland tumors represent a small percentage (about 1%) of all head and neck masses, but are the source of diverse group of pathologies, and, thus, are important to review. Besides major salivary glands (parotid, submandibular, and sublingual), there are numerous minor salivary glands found throughout the upper aerodigestive tract. However, the majority of salivary gland neoplasms occur in parotid gland, and among those, the majority are benign neoplasms. In adults, 80% of parotid lesions are benign; the majority of these are pleomorphic adenomas.

Only 15 to 20% of salivary gland tumors arise in submandibular and sublingual glands, but up to 50 to 75% of those are malignant. Although it is also uncommon to diagnose a salivary gland tumor in pediatric age group, a greater percentage of those are malignant. Hemangiomas represent the most common benign lesions of the parotid glands in children. Mucoepidermoid carcinomas are the most common salivary gland malignancies in all groups.[1,11] Parotid or minor salivary gland tumors may also present as parapharyngeal space masses and are typically located at the prestyloid compartment displacing the carotid artery posteriorly.

US imaging and US-guided FNAB cytology are the preferred diagnostic utilities in salivary gland tumors. CT or MRI may be useful in surgical planning and showing invasion into surrounding structures and/or lymph node metastasis, in the treatment of malignant salivary gland tumors.

Thyroid Neoplasms

Neoplasms of the thyroid gland are an important cause of neck mass among all age groups. The thyroid gland may host pathologies differing from a benign goiter to a thyroid carcinoma. Thyroid carcinoma is also an important cause of metastatic lymphadenopathy in the neck. US-guided FNAB is the gold standard diagnostic modality in the evaluation of a thyroid nodule.

Malignancy Harboring Lymph Nodes in the Neck

Malignancy harboring lymph nodes in the neck can represent as primary lymph node malignancies such as various types of lymphoma, regional metastatic disease from a primary source in the head and neck, or distant metastatic disease from a primary outside of the head and neck region.

Lymphoma

Both types of lymphoma (Hodgkin's and non-Hodgkin's) present commonly as a neck mass; therefore, the otolaryngologist is often the first physician to evaluate a patient with lymphoma. Lymphoma represents the most common type of head and neck malignancy in the pediatric population and is the second most common type in adults.[11] Being a highly curable malignancy—if treated properly—differentiation of a benign, reactive lymphadenopathy from a lymphoma is an important task, especially in the pediatric age group.

Eighty percent of patients with Hodgkin's disease (HD) have cervical nodal disease, whereas only about 33% of those with non-Hodgkin lymphoma (NHL) have involved cervical lymph nodes. NHL, however, is approximately five times more common than HD in the head and neck.[11] The majority of lymph nodes associated with lymphoma presents as a nontender mass of greater than 2 weeks' duration, usually at supraclavicular area or posterior neck triangle. HD is primarily a disease confined to lymph nodes, but NHL may present at extra nodal sites as Waldeyer's ring, salivary glands, or thyroid, in 25 to 40% of patients at initial diagnosis.[13]

Diagnosis of lymphoma involves combination of history, physical examination, imaging, and biopsy. Lymphoma usually shows systemic involvement with multiple lymph nodes in other areas (axilla, mediastinum, abdomen, or groin) and/or hepatosplenomegaly. Thus, systemic involvement should be questioned and examined. Systemic symptoms (also known as B symptoms) include fever greater than 38 °C, night sweats, and unintentional weight loss; these may also exist during presentation of the patient. Indirect mirror or flexible endoscopic examination should be employed to rule out Waldeyer's ring involvement in NHL. A complete blood count with differential and peripheral smear is usually warranted. Bone marrow aspiration biopsy is usually performed by oncologists. Serum lactate dehydrogenase level may be found elevated in both types of lymphomas, and is an important prognostic factor for indicating treatment response.[14]

US is usually the preferred first-line imaging modality in evaluation of lymph nodes in pediatric age group. US shows rounded lymph nodes in HD and enlarged lymph node masses, often conglomerated lymph nodes with ill-defined borders in NHL. Contrast-enhanced CT is the gold standard in evaluation of lymphoma. US-guided FNAB or core needle biopsy may be ordered before an open biopsy, which may direct clinicians to a neoplasm of lymphoid lineage. However, an incisional or excisional open biopsy is often required for definitive histopathological diagnosis and classification. Whole-body scan with 18-fluorodeoxyglucose (18-FDG) PET-CT or cranial–neck–thorax–abdomen–pelvic CT with contrast is ordered for staging of the disease.

Regional and Distant Metastasis of the Neck, Carcinoma of Unknown Primary

Regional metastasis to the neck is a common finding in squamous cell carcinoma (SCC) of the upper aerodigestive tract in smokers and elderly males. However, its incidence is increasing in the younger, nonsmoker population, mostly due to HPV infection. Additionally, malignant thyroid and salivary gland adenocarcinomas are also commonly encountered with metastatic lymph nodes in the neck. Distant metastasis as a neck mass is a relatively rare condition, although hundreds of neoplasms have been described that can metastasize to the neck. The most common distant sites include the lung, esophagus, kidney, ovary, cervix, and prostate.[15] Each condition is managed

in accordance with the oncologic principles for treating the given malignancy. However, metastasis in the lymphatic structures of the neck without a given primary site is a challenge for the clinician in the management.

Principles of management of metastatic lymph nodes with unknown primary involves the same steps with any other mass in the neck; biopsy follows history, physical examination, and imaging. This examination should consist of careful inspection and palpation of all mucosal subsites of the oral cavity and oropharynx, as well as fiberoptic flexible and/or rigid endoscopy. During endoscopy, particular attention should be paid to the common sites of occult primary origin such as nasopharynx, palatine tonsils, tongue base, supraglottic larynx, hypopharynx, and the floor of the mouth (▶ Fig. 1.4).

Contrast-enhanced CT from cranium to abdomen and US of the neck are the first-line imaging modalities both for defining the characteristics of metastatic mass and for revealing the site of primary. Gadolinium-enhanced MRI may be preferred for better definition of soft tissues. 18-FDG PET-CT is popularized in determining the site of origin and directing biopsies.

Diagnosis of a metastatic carcinoma in the neck is typically performed by cytopathological evaluation of an FNAB specimen obtained with or without US or CT guidance. Occasionally, the diagnosis is obtained by performing an incisional or excisional biopsy. Cytopathological or histopathological findings in the metastatic node may assist in determining the primary site. A diagnosis of adenocarcinoma usually reveals its primary in lung, bronchi, stomach, prostate, or intestines. Metastasis from a thyroid carcinoma is usually a straightforward diagnosis with typical US, cytological, and immunohistochemistry findings. SCC is the most common type of histology among the metastasis with unknown primary. Upper aerodigestive tract sites should be examined thoroughly, with special emphasis on the common sites of occult origin, especially with fiberoptic endoscopy. Molecular and/or genetic demonstration of HPV or EBV genomes in metastatic lymph node aspirates provide important clues in the subsite of origin of the primary.

The location of the metastatic lymph node also offers important diagnostic information on the location of the primary site. Regional metastases from primary lesions of the oral cavity are

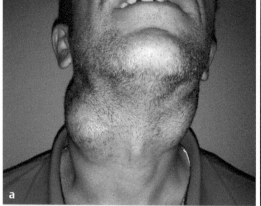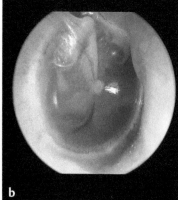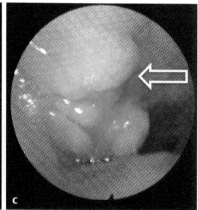

Fig. 1.4 Detailed head and neck examination in the evaluation of bilaterally enlarged cervical lymph nodes (a) may provide vital information regarding the source of the problem. An otoscopic examination revealing otitis media with effusion (b) may lead the clinician directly to perform a directed fiberoptic examination of the nasopharynx revealing a lesion (*thick arrow*) (c).

typically found in levels I, II, and III, while primary malignancies of oropharynx, hypopharynx, and larynx are found at levels II, III, and IV. Nasopharyngeal cancer typically metastasizes to level V.[15] When the mass presents in the supraclavicular region, esophageal and pulmonary primary sites should be considered in addition to abdominal and pelvic locations.[15]

If no primary site can be revealed with physical examination and imaging, a diagnostic panendoscopy and biopsy is required under general anesthesia. The physician examines the whole upper aerodigestive tract, under the illumination and magnification of endoscope and/or operating microscope, and palpates carefully the floor of mouth and oropharyngeal subsites including the tongue base, palatine tonsils, and glossotonsillar sulcus. Any mucosal or submucosal lesions should be biopsied, as well as blind biopsies from common occult primary sites such as Rosenmüller fossae of nasopharynx, ipsilateral palatine tonsil, tongue base, piriform sinus, and postcricoid region. The ipsilateral tonsil has been reported to harbor the occult primary in 20 to 40% of cases. The next most common subsite is the tongue base. PET-CT maybe helpful in the diagnosis of an occult primary malignancy in the head and neck; however, the clinician should keep in mind that this modality should be employed before performing any biopsies, since biopsy-related inflammatory response may cause false-positives.

1.7 Conclusion

Neck masses are common in the general population and represent a wide array of pathologies including enlarged lymph nodes. Both benign and malignant lesions can present as a mass in the neck, which makes a careful approach to these lesions important. The likelihood of malignancy increases in an elderly, male patient who consumes alcohol and tobacco products. On the other hand, inflammatory neck masses are the most common neck masses in pediatric and young adult age groups. A thorough head and neck examination (with flexible endoscopy, where indicated) is the crucial step for diagnosis. Neck imaging in the form of US, CT, MRI, or PET-CT is usually employed as additional diagnostic tools depending on

differential diagnoses. FNAB is the key step toward tissue diagnosis. There is a wide variety of neck masses that may mimic an enlarged lymph node, and every clinician should be knowledgeable in the process of differential diagnosis for a mass in the neck.

References

[1] Nugent A, El-Deiry M. Differential diagnosis of neck masses. In: Flint PW, Haughey BH, Lund V, et al, eds. Cummings Otolaryngology: Head and Neck Surgery. Philadelphia, PA: Elsevier Health Sciences; 2014:1767–1772

[2] Rajasekaran K, Krakovitz P. Enlarged neck lymph nodes in children. Pediatr Clin North Am. 2013; 60(4):923–936

[3] Kelly CS, Kelly RE, Jr. Lymphadenopathy in children. Pediatr Clin North Am. 1998; 45(4):875–888

[4] Rosenberg TL, Nolder AR. Pediatric cervical lymphadenopathy. Otolaryngol Clin North Am. 2014; 47(5):721–731

[5] Couch ME. History, physical examination, and the preoperative evaluation. In: Flint PW, Haughey BH, Lund V, et al, eds. Cummings Otolaryngology: Head and Neck Surgery, 3 Vol. Philadelphia, PA: Elsevier Health Sciences; 2010:93–107

[6] Forghani R, Yu E, Levental M, Som PM, Curtin HD. Imaging evaluation of lymphadenopathy and patterns of lymph node spread in head and neck cancer. Expert Rev Anticancer Ther. 2015; 15(2):207–224

[7] Edge S, Byrd DR, Compton CC, Fritz AG, Greene F, Trotti A, eds. AJCC Cancer Staging Handbook: From the AJCC Cancer Staging Manual. New York, NY: Springer; 2010

[8] Som PM, Curtin HD, Mancuso AA. An imaging-based classification for the cervical nodes designed as an adjunct to recent clinically based nodal classifications. Arch Otolaryngol Head Neck Surg. 1999; 125(4):388–396

[9] Stern JS, Ginat DT, Nicholas JL, Ryan ME. Imaging of pediatric head and neck masses. Otolaryngol Clin North Am. 2015; 48(1):225–246

[10] Sofferman RA. Interpretation of ultrasound. Otolaryngol Clin North Am. 2010; 43(6):1171–1202, v–vi

[11] Chen A, Otto KJ. Differential Diagnosis of Neck Masses. In: Flint PW, Haughey BH, Lund V, et al, eds. Cummings Otolaryngology: Head and Neck Surgery. 3 Vol. Philadelphia, PA: Elsevier Health Sciences; 2010:1636–1655

[12] Kamat AR, Schantz SP. Evaluation and management of the solitary neck mass. In: Sclafani AP, ed. Total Otolaryngology-Head and Neck Surgery. New York, NY: Thieme; 2015:306–311

[13] Alexander DD, Mink PJ, Adami HO, et al. The non-Hodgkin lymphomas: a review of the epidemiologic literature. Int J Cancer. 2007; 120 Suppl 12:1–39

[14] Chai RL, Tassler AB, Kim S. Lymphomas of the head and neck. In: Johnson J, Rosen CA, eds. Bailey's Head and Neck Surgery: Otolaryngology. Philadelphia, PA: Lippincott Williams & Wilkins; 2014:2032–2043

[15] Day TA, Bewley AF, Joe JK. Neoplasms of the neck. In: Flint PW, Haughey BH, Lund V, et al, eds. Cummings Otolaryngology-Head and Neck Surgery. Philadelphia, PA: Elsevier Health Sciences; 2014:1787–1804

2 History/Classification of Nodal Levels and Neck Dissections

Angela M. Osmolak and Jesus E. Medina

Abstract

The management of the cervical lymph nodes in patients with squamous cell carcinoma of the upper aero-digestive tract has evolved, since the beginning of the 20th century, along with the evolution of the neck dissection. In addition to a historical review of this evolution, this chapter presents a detailed review of two of the key elements that have driven the evolution of the radical neck dissection into several neck dissections, each of which has different indications. These elements are (1) a progressive understanding of the anatomy of the lymphatic drainage of the head and neck region and (2) clinical and histopathological observations of the patterns of lymph node metastases of cancers in the different areas of the upper aero-digestive tract and of the skin of the head and neck. The chapter concludes with a description of the different neck dissections, the nomenclature used to designate them, and the different classification systems that have been proposed to date.

Keywords: neck dissection, neck

2.1 History and Evolution of the Neck Dissection

The spread of cancer of the mouth to the "lymph glands" was mentioned in the literature as early as the mid-1800s only to point out that once this had occurred, removal of the disease and cure were not possible. A thorough historical review of surgical procedures to remove "cancer in the neck" nodes, prior to 1951, can be found in Hayes Martin's landmark paper on "Neck dissection."[1] In this review, Martin mentions an attempt to remove "cancer of the neck with an incision from the masseter to the clavicle," reported by Warren in 1847. He adds the comment that this operation was improvised rather than a planned procedure based on anatomical considerations. He also mentions an operation, described by Kocher in 1880, in which a tongue cancer was removed incidentally through the submaxillary triangle first, "clearing out the lymphatic glands and the sublingual and submaxillary salivary glands." Subsequently, Kocher proposed the notion that cervical lymph nodes involved with cancer should be removed more widely, and he introduced the Y-shaped "Kocher incision." In the literature of the latter part of the 19th century and very early in the 20th century, there were several mentions of operations to remove cancer in the cervical lymph nodes, which were in essence nonsystematic, variably extensive "extirpations" of cervical lymph nodes.

It appears that an operation first labeled as a "radical neck dissection" (RND) was performed in 1888 by a Polish surgeon by the name of Fr. Jawdinsky. In that regard, Edward Towpik, MD, PhD, wrote in the Gazeta Lekarska in 1888[2] (▶ Fig. 2.1):

Although not the first to perform the operation, Jawdynski was, to my knowledge, the first to describe the technique and

extent of radical en-bloc neck dissection. Published in a Polish medical journal, his contribution remained virtually unknown abroad. Jawdynski himself was apparently not aware of the true importance of his operation; he never mentioned its potential application in removing lymph node metastases.

The first description of a systematic blocklike removal of the lymphatics of the neck for lymph node metastases was published by Crile in 1906.[3] He actually attempted a complete removal of the cervical lymphatics, the sternocleidomastoid muscle (SCM), the internal jugular vein (IJV), and all of the areolar and lymphatic tissue of the various triangles of the neck. Interestingly, however, the drawings that illustrate Crile's publication depict the spinal accessory nerve (SAN) and the ansa hypoglossi being preserved (▶ Fig. 2.2).

Removal of the SAN during cervical lymphadenectomy was actually advocated by Blair and Brown in 1933[4] as a means to decrease operating time and, more importantly, to assure a complete removal of the cervical lymph nodes. In subsequent years, other clinicians concurred with the desirability of removing

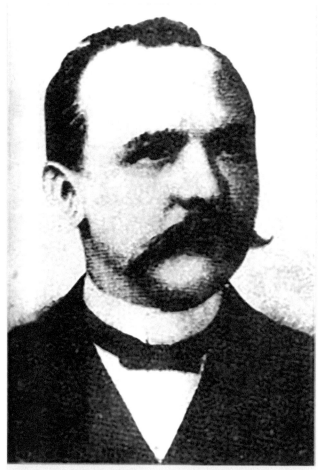

Fig. 2.1 Polish surgeon Fr. Jawdinsky.

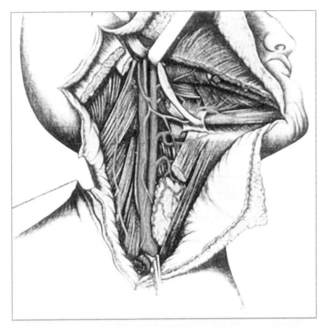

Fig. 2.2 Crile's neck dissection. (Reproduced with permission of Crile.[3])

the SAN.[5] However, this concept was championed and popularized in the 1950s by Martin,[6] who stated: "Any technique that is designed to preserve the spinal accessory nerve should be condemned unequivocally." As Chief of the Head and Neck Surgery Service at Memorial Sloan Kettering, he was very influential at the time. His book *Surgery of Head and Neck Tumors* published in 1957 was a benchmark in head and neck surgery for at least a couple of decades since.[6] As a result, the RND was considered for many years the only acceptable operation for the treatment of the neck in patients with cancer.

At the same time, however, the observation that resection of the SAN results in significant postoperative shoulder dysfunction prompted clinicians like Ward and Roben[7] to modify the operation by preserving the SAN, whenever possible, in order to prevent postoperative shoulder drop.

In 1963, Suarez published a landmark paper entitled "El Problema de las Metastases Ganglionares y Alejadas" (The Problem of the Lymphatic and Distant Metastases).[8] In it, he presented the results of a study of the lymphatics of the larynx and hypopharynx in 1,318 cases with neoplasms of these sites in whom he performed 532 therapeutic neck dissections and 271 "prophylactic" neck dissections. His observations resulted in what is, arguably, the most detailed description of the lymphatics within the larynx and hypopharynx. He noted that the lymphatic vessels are not within the fascia that envelops muscles like the SCM, do not traverse the muscles per se (instead they are located and run within the connective tissue), and they are not a part of the adventitia of neighboring veins, but are located outside of it. Suarez then described an operation that "eliminates all the areolar tissue, fascia and lymph nodes and leaves the muscles, great vessels and noble parts without mutilation." He called it "functional dissection." Although Suarez did not report specific outcomes, he indicated in this paper that he obtained good results with the technique he described. Nevertheless, the functional neck dissection was adopted and popularized in America and particularly in Europe, and the oncologic and functional results reported by several clinicians

were excellent in the treatment of both the N0 and the N + neck. The feasibility and effectiveness of the functional neck dissection were validated by other clinicians, and this operation became the mainstay of the surgical treatment of the neck in patients with larynx cancer in Europe, South America, and, to a lesser extent, the United States.

Undoubtedly, the observations of Suarez were truly seminal and influenced open-minded clinicians at the MD Anderson Cancer Institute like Alando Ballantyne, Richard Jesse, Robert Byers, and Robert Lindberg who, in addition, noted that metastases were more likely to occur to certain lymph nodes in the neck, depending on the location of the primary tumor. These surgeons began to remove only those lymph node groups that were at highest risk of containing metastases.[9]

These operations were eventually called "selective neck dissections" (SNDs).[10] The rationale for these neck dissections has been validated by anatomic,[11] pathologic,[12,13] and clinical investigations,[14,15,16,17] demonstrating that cervical lymph node metastases do, indeed, occur in predictable patterns in patients with squamous cell carcinomas of the head and neck. Tumors of the oral cavity metastasize most frequently to the neck nodes in levels I, II, and III, whereas carcinomas of the oropharynx, hypopharynx, and larynx involve mainly the nodes in levels II, III, and IV. These observations coupled with the results of several retrospective and prospective clinical studies showing that, when an SND is utilized for the elective treatment of the regional lymphatics, regional control and survival rates are similar to those obtained with more extensive neck dissections[16,18, 19,20,21,22,23,24] were responsible for the current near universal acceptance of SND for the management of the N0 neck.

Recent studies have shown that the predictability of lymphatic spread applies to both occult (N0 neck) and clinically evident (N + neck) lymph node metastases.[13,18,25] As a result, SNDs are now being used in the treatment of selected N + patients. SNDs are associated with less postoperative dysfunction of the trapezius muscle, which, when it occurs, is usually temporary and reversible.[26,27,28,29,30,31] Furthermore, in the last couple of decades the role of neck dissection has evolved toward that of a staging procedure; the findings on the histopathological examination of the neck dissection specimen are now used for decision-making regarding the need for adjuvant postoperative radiation therapy[32,33] and in some instances chemotherapy.[34,35]

2.2 Classification of Nodal Levels

The lymph nodes of the head and neck region have been designated in various ways over the years. The first fundamental nomenclature of the neck is derived from the work of Henri Rouvière. His 1932 publication, *Anatomie des Lymphatiques de l'Homme*, eloquently and anatomically details the 10 principal lymph node groups of the head and neck. The six groups that lie within the neck are as follows[36,37]:

• Occipital nodes: These are nodes located at the junction of the nape of the neck and the cranial vault. They are divided into three groups: suprafascial/superficial, subfascial, and submuscular/subsplenius. The suprafascial/superficial nodes are intimately related to the third part of the occipital artery and the great occipital nerve. They are located on the posterosuperior angle of the SCM and on the fibrotendinous tissue covering the occipital bone between the insertions of the SCM and trapezius muscles. The subfascial node is located on the splenius muscle beneath the superficial layer of the deep cervical fascia, near the superior curved line of the occipital bone. The submuscular/subsplenius nodes are located beneath the splenius capitis along its superior insertion, above the obliquus capitis superior muscle and medial to the longissimus capitis muscle.

- Submaxillary nodes: These nodes are located around the submaxillary gland. They are divided into five groups: preglandular, prevascular, retrovascular, retroglandular, and intracapsular. The preglandular nodes are intimately related to the submental vessels and are located in the triangular space in front of the gland, bordered by the mandible, the lateral border of the anterior belly of the digastric, and the anterior extremity of the submaxillary gland. The prevascular nodes are located on the submaxillary artery in front of the anterior facial vein. The retrovascular nodes are located behind the anterior facial vein and sometimes along the posterior border of the submaxillary gland. The retroglandular nodes are located behind the submaxillary gland and the retrovascular nodes, medial and slightly below the angle of the mandible. The intracapsular nodes lie within the capsule of the submaxillary gland.
- Submental nodes: These are nodes that are located directly on the mylohyoid, in the region bordered by the mandible, the hyoid, and the anterior bellies of the digastric muscles. They are divided into three groups: anterior, middle, and posterior.
- Retropharyngeal nodes: These nodes are divided into lateral and median groups. The lateral nodes are located bilaterally in the lateropharyngeal space between the posterior wall of the pharynx and the prevertebral fascia. Anteriorly, these nodes project across the superior aspect of the oropharynx onto the soft palate and palatine tonsils. Laterally, they course along the internal carotid artery near its entrance into the carotid canal and along the superior pole of the superior cervical ganglion of the sympathetics. The median nodes are located at the midline, directly on the posterior surface of the pharynx from the base of the skull to the level of the plane drawn through the extremities of the greater cornua of the hyoid bone.
- Anterior cervical nodes: These nodes are located below the hyoid bone and between the two carotid sheaths. They are divided into two groups: the anterior jugular chain and the juxtavisceral chain. The anterior jugular chain nodes are located along the anterior jugular vein in the space bordered by the superficial layer of the deep cervical fascia and the SCM and the pretracheal layer of the deep cervical fascia and the infrahyoid muscles. The juxtavisceral chain nodes are located in front of the larynx and the thyroid gland and in front of and along the lateral surfaces of the trachea along the recurrent laryngeal nerves (RLN). This chain is further divided into four subgroups: prelaryngeal, prethyroid, pretracheal, and latero(para)tracheal. The prelaryngeal nodes include the interthyroid aggregation in front of the thyrohyoid membrane, the thyroid aggregation in front of the middle part of the thyroid cartilage, and the intercricothyroid aggregation in front of the cricothyroid membrane. The prethyroid nodes are located in front of the thyroid gland isthmus. The pretracheal nodes are located in front of the trachea between the inferior aspect of the thyroid gland and the innominate vein. The laterotracheal nodes are located bilaterally along the RLNs.

- Lateral cervical nodes: These nodes are divided into superficial and deep groups. The superficial nodes lie along the external jugular vein (EJV) on the outer surface of the SCM. The deep nodes include the internal jugular chain, the spinal accessory chain, and the transverse cervical chain. The internal jugular chain is divided into lateral and anterior. The lateral nodes extend along the lateral border of the IJV from the posterior belly of the digastric to the junction of the IJV and the omohyoid muscle. The anterior nodes are divided into three groups: superior, middle, and inferior. The superior group lies between the inferior border of the posterior belly of the digastric and the thyrolinguofacial venous trunk. The middle group lies between the thyrolinguofacial venous trunk and the omohyoid muscle. The inferior group lies between the omohyoid muscle and the termination of the IJV. The spinal accessory chain extends along the SAN from the superior portion of the SCM to the deep aspect of the trapezius. The transverse cervical chain accompanies the transverse cervical artery and veins and extends from the inferior extremity of the spinal accessory chain to the jugulosubclavian junction.

Hayes Martin and George Pack also divided the lymph nodes of the head and neck into anatomic systems. In his 1951 paper, "Neck Dissection," Martin divides the cervical lymphatics into three chains and three nodal groups. His descriptions of the submental nodal group, submaxillary nodal group, deep cervical/ internal jugular chain, spinal accessory chain, and transverse cervical chain reflect those of Rouvière. He is the first, however, to separately describe the subdigastric nodal group, which includes nodes located just below the posterior belly of the digastric muscle. Additionally, he delineates three nodal groups associated with the IJV[1] (▶ Fig. 2.3). Then in 1962, Pack and Ariel divided the lymph nodes of the head and neck into circular and vertical chains. The majority of these regions again reflect those described by Rouvière. The circular chain comprises nine regions, five of which are in the neck (▶ Fig. 2.4, ▶ Fig. 2.5; Pack II). These regions include the occipital, superficial cervical, submental, submaxillary, and anterior cervical. The vertical chain includes the retropharyngeal, supraclavicular/ transcervical, accessory chain, inferior deep cervical, tonsillar/jugulodigastric, and supraomohyoid nodes.[38]

A topographical division of the head and neck lymph nodes is first seen in the early 1970s. In his 1972 paper, "Distribution of Cervical Lymph Node Metastases from Squamous Cell Carcinoma of the Upper Respiratory and Digestive Tracts," Lindberg divides each side of the neck into nine nodal regions based on pathophysiological mechanisms (▶ Fig. 2.6). These nine regions include submental, submaxillary triangle, subdigastric, midjugular, low jugular, upper posterior cervical, midposterior cervical, low posterior cervical, and supraclavicular nodes.[14]

Around the same time, the first papers referencing cervical metastases by five anatomical levels utilizing Roman numerals (I–V) were published. The system that was started by the Head and Neck Service at Memorial Sloan Kettering Cancer Center (MSKCC), some time after the publication of Martin's paper, "Neck Dissection," in 1951, defines the following levels:

- Level I: Nodes within the submental and submandibular triangles.

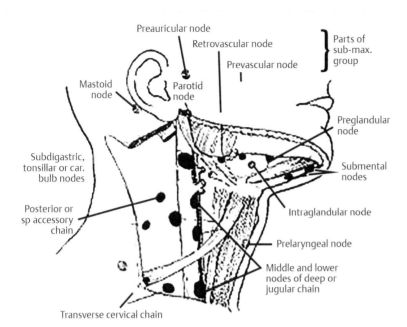

Fig. 2.3 Hayes Martin's nodal levels including divisions along the internal jugular vein.

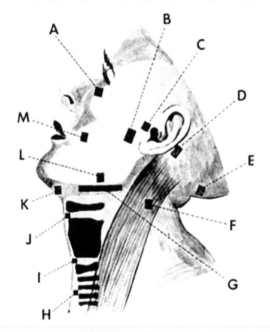

Fig. 2.4 Pack's circular chain lymph nodes. A, facial node; B, parotid lymph node; C, preauricular node; D, posterior auricular nodes; E, occipital nodes; F, superficial cervical node; G, submaxillary lymph nodes; H, pretracheal node; I, prelaryngeal node; J, infrahyoid node; K, submental node; L, facial node; M, facial node.

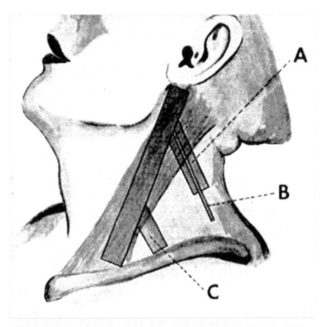

Fig. 2.5 Pack's vertical chain lymph nodes. Extensions of the vertical chain along the spinal accessory nerve and above the clavicle. A, the accessory chain; B, spinal accessory nerve; C, supraclavicular nodes.

- Levels II, III, IV: Nodes of the upper, middle, and lower thirds of the internal jugular chain, respectively, divided into equal thirds. The IJV and SCM are included in these levels.
- Level V: Nodes along the SAN and within the posterior cervical triangle.[39,40]

The topographical distribution of lymph nodes has been maintained in the classification of lymph node levels since that time.

The two modern-day systems include those from the American Academy of Otolaryngology – Head and Neck Surgery (AAO-HNS) and the Japanese Neck Dissection Study Group (JNDSG). The AAO-HNS system, which is now almost universally accepted, utilizes Roman numerals to designate groups of lymph nodes in different regions of the neck. In this system, six levels (I–VI) are used that encompass the complete topographic anatomy of the neck; sublevels have been introduced into some levels, to designate zones that may have clinical significance (▸ Fig. 2.7). Level VII is added to designate the upper mediastinal nodes (▸ Table 2.1).

13

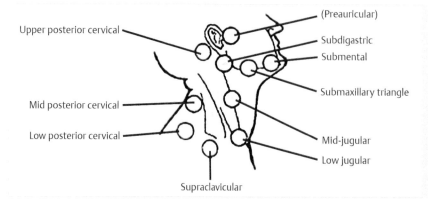

Fig. 2.6 Lindberg's nine nodal groups.

Upper posterior cervical

(Preauricular)

Subdigastric

Submental

Submaxillary triangle

Mid posterior cervical

Low posterior cervical

Mid-jugular

Low jugular

Supraclavicular

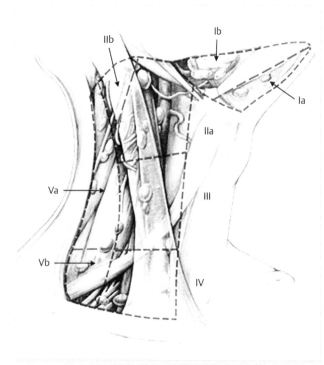

Fig. 2.7 Lymph node groups/levels of the neck.

The JNDSG system, created in 2005, divides the cervical lymph nodes into four basic regions (with several subregions) and four other regions. The four basic regions and two of the other regions lie within the neck. These regions include submental/submandibular (S), lateral deep cervical/internal jugular (J), lateral deep cervical/posterior triangle (P), anterior deep cervical/central compartment (C), retropharyngeal (rp), and superficial cervical (sc; ▶ Fig. 2.8).[41,42]

2.3 Classification of Neck Dissections

As a result of the evolution of neck dissections described earlier in this chapter, by the mid-1980s, the term "modified radical neck dissection" (MRND) was no longer adequate to refer to various operations that were being used for the surgical treatment of the neck in patients with head and neck tumor. Thus, in 1987, Suen and Goepfert[43] were among the first to suggest a

Table 2.1 Classifications of neck dissections

AAOHNS/ASHNS 2001 classification	2010 proposed classification
1. Radical neck dissection (ND)	1. ND (I–V, SCM, IJV, CNXI)
2. Modified radical ND	2. ND (I–V, SCM, IJV), ND (I–V, IJV, CNXI), (ND I–V, CNXI)
3. Selective neck dissection (SND):	3. ND (I, II, III/IV)
SND (I–III/IV)	ND (II, III, IV)
SND (II–IV)	ND (II, III, IV,V, postauricular, sub-occipital)
SND (II–V, postauricular, subocci-pital)	ND (VI)
SND (level VI)	4. ND (levels removed, additional nodes or structures removed)
4. Extended ND	

Abbreviations: AAOHNS, American Academy of Otolaryngology–Head and Neck Surgery; ASHNS, American Society for Head and Neck Surgery.

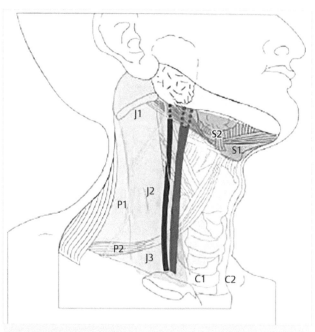

Fig. 2.8 Japanese Neck Dissection Study Group (JNDSG) nomenclature system for cervical lymph nodes.

classification of neck dissections, which was expanded by Medina in 1989.[10] The basic premise of these authors was that a rational classifications of neck dissections should take into account the lymph node groups that are removed (the nomenclature of which needed to be standardized) and the important anatomic structures (such as the SAN, the IJV, and the SCM) that are preserved. In essence, three broad categories of neck dissections were identified: (1) the comprehensive neck dissections, (2) the SNDs, and (3) the extended neck dissections.

Following the same premise, in 1991, the Committee for Head and Neck Surgery and Oncology created by the AAO-HNS, in conjunction with the Education Committee of the American Society for Head and Neck Surgery (ASHNS, now the AHNS) proposed a classification system that was revised in 2002 and updated in 2008.[44,45] The latter is outlined in ▶ Table 2.1. Levels VI and VII were introduced into the classification system at this time. Because of its simplicity, this classification is currently accepted worldwide. Analyzing neck dissections from the point of view of the lymph node levels removed and the structures that are preserved in a neck dissection, there are essentially four anatomic types of neck dissections:

- RND: In RND dissection, the lymph node levels I through V are removed along with the SCM, the IJV, and the spinal accessory nerve (XIN 2; ▶ Fig. 2.9).
- MRND: In this type of neck dissection, lymph node levels I through V are removed, as in the RND; however, one or more of the following structures are preserved: SCM, IJV, or the XIN (▶ Fig. 2.10, ▶ Fig. 2.11).
- Some clinicians refer to the RND and MRND as "comprehensive" neck dissections, since all five levels of the neck are removed.[10]
- SNDs: These neck dissections remove selected lymph nodes, based on their risk of containing metastases, which depends

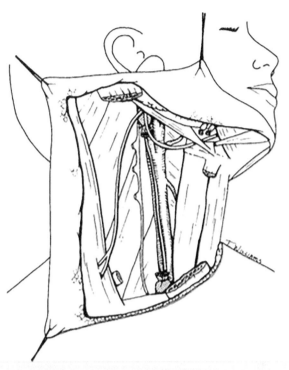

Fig. 2.10 Modified radical neck dissection with preservation of the spinal accessory nerve (ND I–V, cranial nerve [CN] XI).

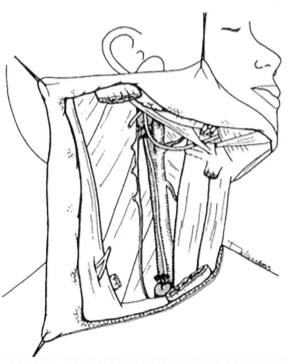

Fig. 2.9 Radical neck dissection (ND I–V, sternocleidomastoid muscle [SCM], internal jugular vein [IJV], cranial nerve [CN] XI).

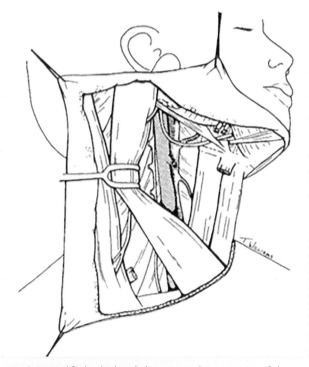

Fig. 2.11 Modified radical neck dissection with preservation of the spinal accessory nerve, the internal jugular vein (IJV), and the sternocleidomastoid muscle (ND I–V, SCM, IJV, cranial nerve [CN] XI).

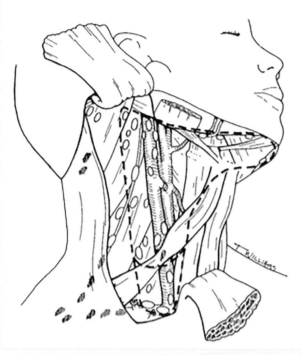

Fig. 2.12 Selective neck dissection of levels I–III/IV (ND I, II, III/IV).

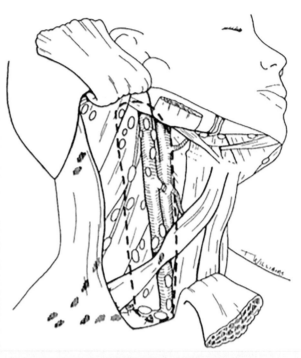

Fig. 2.13 Selective neck dissection of levels II–IV (ND II, II, IV).

on the location of the primary tumor. The SCM, IJV, and XIN are usually preserved.

- There are four main types of SNDs:
  - SND of levels I to III ("supraomohyoid" neck dissection) and SND of levels I to IV (also referred to as "extended supraomohyoid" neck dissection; ▶ Fig. 2.12). These are the neck dissections commonly used in the treatment of patients with squamous cell carcinoma of the oral cavity. The lymph nodes removed are those contained in levels I to III. The posterior limit of the dissection is marked by the cutaneous branches of the cervical plexus and the posterior border of the SCM. The inferior limit is the omohyoid muscle as it crosses the IJV. Some surgeons prefer to perform an SND of level I to IV in cases with cancer of the oral tongue.[46] For cancers of the oral cavity that are close to or involve the midline, either type of SND is done bilaterally, since the lymph nodes in both sides of the neck are at risk. These operations have been described in detail by Medina.[47]
  - SND of levels II to IV (lateral neck dissection). This neck dissection consists of the removal of the lymph nodes in levels II, III, and IV (▶ Fig. 2.13). It is commonly used in the treatment of patients with squamous cell carcinoma of the larynx, oropharynx, and hypopharynx. The superior limit of the dissection is the digastric muscle and the mastoid tip. The inferior limit is the clavicle. The anteromedial limit is the lateral border of the sternohyoid muscle. The posterior limit of the dissection is marked by the cutaneous branches of the cervical plexus and the posterior border of the SCM. For tumors of the supraglottic larynx and posterior pharyngeal walls, the dissection is often done bilaterally. A description of the technique for this operation has been provided by Medina[47] and Khafif.[48]

  - SND of level VI. This operation, also called "anterior" neck dissection or "central compartment" dissection, consists of the removal of the prelaryngeal, pretracheal lymph nodes, as well as the paratracheal lymph nodes on both sides. It is used in the treatment of patients with cancer of the midline structures of the anteroinferior aspect of the neck and thoracic inlet, such as the thyroid, the glottic and subglottic regions of the larynx, the pyriform sinus, and the cervical esophagus and trachea. It should be noted that using a single denomination (i.e., SND of level VI) to refer to any dissection of the lymph nodes in this region is confusing. For instance, if the surgeon choses to remove the prelaryngeal, pretracheal, and the right paratracheal lymph nodes, the operation would have the same designation as one in which only the left paratracheal nodes are removed. Therefore, until consensus is reached about grouping of the lymph nodes in this area (i.e., level VIA and VIB), it is best to describe the operation in terms of the specific lymph nodes removed (e.g., left thyroid lobectomy with dissection of level VI that included the pretracheal and left paratracheal nodes). These operations have been described by Weber and Holsinger[49] and Medina.[47]
  - SND of levels II to V, retroauricular, suboccipital (posterolateral neck dissection). This operation is done for skin cancers originating from the posterior scalp and the upper lateral aspect of the neck. The superior limit of this dissection is the posterior belly of the digastric muscle and the mastoid tip anterolaterally and the nuchal line/ridge posteriorly. The inferior limit is the clavicle. The anteromedial limit is the lateral border of the sternohyoid muscle. The posterolateral limit of the dissection is marked by the anterior border of the trapezius muscle inferiorly and the posterior midline of the neck superiorly[50] (▶ Fig. 2.14).

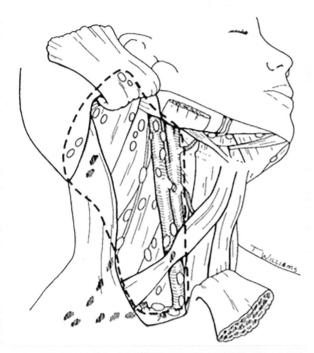

Fig. 2.14 Posterolateral neck dissection (ND II, III, IV, V, postauricular, suboccipital).

- Extended neck dissection. This designation is used to indicate that the neck dissection includes either nodal groups (such as the retropharyngeal or superior mediastinal) or nonlymphatic structures (such as skin of the neck, levator scapula muscle, hypoglossal nerve, carotid artery), which are not ordinarily removed in the other neck dissections.

2.3.1 Other Classifications

In 2005, the JNDSG proposed a classification of neck dissections,[41] based on the nomenclature of regional lymph nodes used in Japan.[42] This system divides the cervical lymph nodes into three basic regions that are designated by letters S (submental-submandibular), J (jugular), and P (posterior triangle). Subregions are identified by numbers after each letter (S1, S2, J1, J2, J3, P1, and P2). The two components of this classification categories are the dissected region (S, J, and P) and resected nonlymphatic tissue (N: SAN, V: IJV, and M: SCM). These are described with parentheses, and with a slash (/) to distinguish between them. For example, ND (SJP/VNM) denotes "v"; ND (J, P) denotes "selective neck dissection (II–IV, VI)."

Recently, clinicians from around the world have proposed a nomenclature for neck dissections that is advocated as "logical, unambiguous, precise, and easy to remember."[51]

In this classification, the following three descriptors are used to label a neck dissection:

- "ND" to represent neck dissection that is prefaced by either "L" or "R" for side. If bilateral, each side must be classified independently.
- The levels and sublevels of lymph nodes removed designated by Roman numerals I through VI in ascending order. For levels that contain sublevels (I, II, and V), listing

of the level without a sublevel indicates that the entire level (both A and B) was excised.

- The nonlymphatic structures removed designated by their internationally recognized initials, that is, SCM for sternocleidomastoid muscle, IJV for internal jugular vein, and XIN for the SAN.

The potential advantage of this classification is that it conveys precisely the groups of lymph nodes included as well as the nonlymphatic structures removed in a neck dissection. This will allow a standardized reporting and meaningful comparison of outcomes. However, it remains to be seen if it will be adopted widely.

It must be emphasized that, irrespective of the nomenclature used, it is the responsibility of the surgeon to divide or otherwise orient the neck dissection specimen, identifying the different groups of lymph nodes it contains immediately after surgery. Only then, can the pathologist be expected to render a report that is useful clinically and prognostically. Such a report describes the location and number of lymph nodes examined, the number of nodes that contain cancer, and the presence or absence of capsular extension of tumor.

References

[1] Martin H, Del Valle B, Ehrlich H, Cahan WG. Neck dissection. Cancer. 1951; 4(3):441–499

[2] Jawdynski F. Przypadek raka pierwotnego szyi. tz raka skrzelowego Volkmann'a. Wyciecie nowotworu wraz z rezekcyja teetnicy szyjówej wspólnej i zyły szyjowej wewnetrznej. Wyzdrowienie Gaz Lek. 1888; 8:530–537

[3] Crile G. Excision of cancer of the head and neck with special reference to the plan of dissection based on one hundred and thirty-two operations. J Am Med Assoc. 1906; XLVII:1780–1786

[4] Blair VP, Brown JB. The treatment of cancerous or potentially cancerous cervical lymph-nodes. Ann Surg. 1933; 98(4):650–661

[5] Dargent M, Papillon J. Les séquelles motrices de l'évidement ganglionnaire du cou, comment les éviter? Lyon Chir. 1945; 40:718–731

[6] Martin H. Surgery of Head and Neck Tumors. 1st ed. New York, NY: Hoeber-Harper Publishers; 1957

[7] Ward GE, Robben JO. A composite operation for radical neck dissection and removal of cancer of the mouth. Cancer. 1951; 4(1):98–109

[8] Suarez O. El problema de las metastasis linfaticas del cancer de laringe y de hipofaringe. Rev Otorrinolaringol. 1963; 23:83–99

[9] Jesse RH, Ballantyne AJ, Larson D. Radical or modified neck dissection: a therapeutic dilemma. Am J Surg. 1978; 136(4):516–519

[10] Medina JE. A rational classification of neck dissections. Otolaryngol Head Neck Surg. 1989; 100(3):169–176

[11] Fisch UP, Sigel ME. Cervical lymphatic system as visualized by lymphography. Ann Otol Rhinol Laryngol. 1964; 73:870–882

[12] Shah JP. Patterns of cervical lymph node metastasis from squamous carcinomas of the upper aerodigestive tract. Am J Surg. 1990; 160(4):405–409

[13] Shah JP, Candela FC, Poddar AK. The patterns of cervical lymph node metastases from squamous carcinoma of the oral cavity. Cancer. 1990; 66(1):109–113

[14] Lindberg R. Distribution of cervical lymph node metastases from squamous cell carcinoma of the upper respiratory and digestive tracts. Cancer. 1972; 29 (6):1446–1449

[15] Wong RJ, Rinaldo A, Ferlito A, Shah JP. Occult cervical metastasis in head and neck cancer and its impact on therapy. Acta Otolaryngol. 2002; 122(1):107–114

[16] Brazilian Head and Neck Cancer Study Group. End results of a prospective trial on elective lateral neck dissection vs type III modified radical neck dissection in the management of supraglottic and transglottic carcinomas. Head Neck. 1999; 21(8):694–702

[17] Buckley JG, Feber T. Surgical treatment of cervical node metastases from squamous carcinoma of the upper aerodigestive tract: evaluation of the evidence for modifications of neck dissection. Head Neck. 2001; 23(10):907–915

[18] Ferlito A, Partridge M, Brennan J, Hamakawa H. Lymph node micrometastases in head and neck cancer: a review. Acta Otolaryngol. 2001; 121(6):660–665

[19] Byers RM, Clayman GL, McGill D, et al. Selective neck dissections for squamous carcinoma of the upper aerodigestive tract: patterns of regional failure. Head Neck. 1999; 21(6):499–505

[20] Davidson J, Khan Y, Gilbert R, Birt BD, Balogh J, MacKenzie R. Is selective neck dissection sufficient treatment for the N0/Np+neck? J Otolaryngol. 1997; 26 (4):229–231

[21] Pitman KT, Johnson JT, Myers EN. Effectiveness of selective neck dissection for management of the clinically negative neck. Arch Otolaryngol Head Neck Surg. 1997; 123(9):917–922

[22] Spiro RH, Gallo O, Shah JP. Selective jugular node dissection in patients with squamous carcinoma of the larynx or pharynx. Am J Surg. 1993; 166 (4):399–402

[23] Zhang B, Xu ZG, Tang PZ. Lateral neck dissection vs radical neck dissection in the management of supraglottic carcinoma with pathologically negative nodes. Zhonghua Er Bi Yan Hou Ke Za Zhi. 2003; 38(6):426–429

[24] Caversaccio M, Negri S, Nolte LP, Zbären P. Neck dissection shoulder syndrome: quantification and three-dimensional evaluation with an optoelectronic tracking system. Ann Otol Rhinol Laryngol. 2003; 112(11):939–946

[25] Buckley JG, MacLennan K. Cervical node metastases in laryngeal and hypopharyngeal cancer: a prospective analysis of prevalence and distribution. Head Neck. 2000; 22(4):380–385

[26] Cheng PT, Hao SP, Lin YH, Yeh AR. Objective comparison of shoulder dysfunction after three neck dissection techniques. Ann Otol Rhinol Laryngol. 2000; 109(8, pt 1):761–766

[27] Laverick S, Lowe D, Brown JS, Vaughan ED, Rogers SN. The impact of neck dissection on health-related quality of life. Arch Otolaryngol Head Neck Surg. 2004; 130(2):149–154

[28] van Wilgen CP, Dijkstra PU, Nauta JM, Vermey A, Roodenburg JL. Shoulder pain and disability in daily life, following supraomohyoid neck dissection: a pilot study. J Craniomaxillofac Surg. 2003; 31(3):183–186

[29] van Wilgen CP, Dijkstra PU, van der Laan BF, Plukker JT, Roodenburg JL. Shoulder complaints after neck dissection; is the spinal accessory nerve involved? Br J Oral Maxillofac Surg. 2003; 41(1):7–11

[30] Zhang B, Tang PZ, Xu ZG, Qi YF, Wang XL. Functional evaluation of the selective neck dissection in patients with carcinoma of head and neck. Zhonghua Er Bi Yan Hou Ke Za Zhi. 2004; 39(1):28–31

[31] De Zinis LO, Bolzoni A, Piazza C, Nicolai P. Prevalence and localization of nodal metastases in squamous cell carcinoma of the oral cavity: role and extension of neck dissection. Eur Arch Otorhinolaryngol. 2006; 263 (12):1131–1135

[32] Woolgar JA, Rogers SN, Lowe D, Brown JS, Vaughan ED. Cervical lymph node metastasis in oral cancer: the importance of even microscopic extracapsular spread. Oral Oncol. 2003; 39(2):130–137

[33] Cooper JS, Pajak TF, Forastiere AA, et al. Radiation Therapy Oncology Group 9501/Intergroup. Postoperative concurrent radiotherapy and chemotherapy for high-risk squamous-cell carcinoma of the head and neck. N Engl J Med. 2004; 350(19):1937–1944

[34] Ferlito A, Buckley JG, Shaha AR, Rinaldo A. Rationale for selective neck dissection in tumors of the upper aerodigestive tract. Acta Otolaryngol. 2001; 121(5):548–555

[35] Ambrosch P, Freudenberg L, Kron M, Steiner W. Selective neck dissection in the management of squamous cell carcinoma of the upper digestive tract. Eur Arch Otorhinolaryngol. 1996; 253(6):329–335

[36] Rouviere H. Lymphatic system of the head and neck. In: Rouviere H, ed. Anatomy of the Human Lymphatic System. Tobias MJ, translator. Ann Arbor, MI: Edwords Brothers; 1938:5–28

[37] Rouvière H, Tobias MJ. Anatomy of the Human Lymphatic System. Ann Arbor, MI: Edwords Brothers; 1938

[38] Pack G, Ariel IM. The Lymph Node System. Treatment of Cancer and Allied Disease. 2nd ed. Tumors of the Head and Neck. New York, NY: Hoeber-Harper; 1962

[39] Barrie JR, Knapper WH, Strong EW. Cervical nodal metastases of unknown origin. Am J Surg. 1970; 120(4):466–470

[40] Spiro RH, Alfonso AE, Farr HW, Strong EW. Cervical node metastasis from epidermoid carcinoma of the oral cavity and oropharynx. A critical assessment of current staging. Am J Surg. 1974; 128(4):562–567

[41] Hasegawa Y, Saikawa M, Hayasaki K, et al. A new classification and nomenclature system for neck dissections: a proposal by the Japan Neck Dissection Study Group (JNDSG). Jpn J Head Neck Cancer. 2005; 31:71–78

[42] Committee on Classification of Regional Lymph Nodes of Japan Society of Clinical Oncology. Classification of regional lymph nodes in Japan. Int J Clin Oncol. 2003; 8(4):248–275

[43] Suen JY, Goepfert H. Standardization of neck dissection nomenclature. Head Neck Surg. 1987; 10(2):75–77

[44] Robbins KT, Medina JE, Wolfe GT, Levine PA, Sessions RB, Pruet CW. Standardizing neck dissection terminology. Official report of the Academy's Committee for Head and Neck Surgery and Oncology. Arch Otolaryngol Head Neck Surg. 1991; 117(6):601–605

[45] Robbins KT, Shaha AR, Medina JE, et al. Committee for Neck Dissection Classification, American Head and Neck Society. Consensus statement on the classification and terminology of neck dissection. Arch Otolaryngol Head Neck Surg. 2008; 134(5):536–538

[46] Byers RM, Weber RS, Andrews T, McGill D, Kare R, Wolf P. Frequency and therapeutic implications of "skip metastases" in the neck from squamous carcinoma of the oral tongue. Head Neck. 1997; 19(1):14–19

[47] Medina JEVN. Neck Dissections. Colour Atlas of Surgical Technique. New Delhi: Jaypee—The Health Sciences Publisher; 2017

[48] Khafif A. Lateral neck dissection. Oper Tech Otolaryngol Head Neck Surg. 2004; 15:160–167

[49] Weber RS, Holsinger FC. Central compartment dissection (of levels VI and VII) for carcinoma of the larynx, hypopharynx, cervical esophagus, and thyroid. Oper Tech Otolaryngol Head Neck Surg. 2004; 15:190–195

[50] Medina JE. Posterolateral neck dissection. Oper Tech Otolaryngol Head Neck Surg. 2004; 15:176–179

[51] Ferlito A, Robbins KT, Shah JP, et al. Proposal for a rational classification of neck dissections. Head Neck. 2011; 33(3):445–450

3 Surgical Anatomy of the Neck

Jumin Sunde and Mauricio A. Moreno

Abstract

The neck anatomy covered in this chapter is from the perspective of the surgeon. The organization is unique in that the anatomy is compartmentalized by neck level. Each level of the neck is approached with a discussion of pertinent boundaries followed by a detailed discussion of the anatomical contents highlighting critical relationships. Special effort has been taken to discuss important anatomical variations when present.

Keywords: neck anatomy, lateral neck, central neck, posterior neck, cervical fascia

3.1 Introduction

3.1.1 Division of the Neck by Triangles

In discussing anatomy of the neck, it is helpful to have some scheme of subdividing the neck. This has been traditionally accomplished by describing cervical triangles that topographically divide the neck by means of clinically identifiable muscles (▶ Fig. 3.1). This is a simple system that aids the clinician in communicating general locations more effectively.

Two muscles, the sternocleidomastoid muscle (SCM) and the trapezius (TPZ), divide the neck into anterior and posterior triangles. These muscles are clear by visual inspection and palpation. The anterior triangle is limited posteriorly by the anterior border of the SCM, anteriorly by the anatomic midline, superiorly by the lower aspect of the mandible, and a line connecting the angle of the mandible to the mastoid tip. The anterior triangle can further be subdivided into the following triangles:

- Submental triangle: It is the midline structure defined by the anterior belly of the digastric (ABD) bilaterally and the hyoid bone at its base. The mylohyoid muscles form its floor. It contains the submental lymph nodes and the distal aspect of the submental branch of the facial artery.
- Submandibular (digastric) triangle: It is defined between the anterior and posterior bellies of the digastric, and superiorly by the inferior border of the mandible, and a line that connects the mandibular angle to the mastoid. Its floor is defined by the mylohyoid, hyoglossus, and superior pharyngeal constrictor muscles. It contains the facial vessels and their branches, the submandibular gland (SMG), marginal mandibular and cervical branches of the facial nerve, and lymph nodes.
- Carotid triangle: It is bounded by the posterior belly of the digastric (PBD) superiorly, the SCM posteriorly, and the superior belly of the omohyoid anteriorly. Its floor is defined by the middle and inferior pharyngeal constrictors. It contains the carotid artery and its branches, jugular vein, cranial nerves (CN) X and XII, and lymph nodes.
- Muscular (visceral) triangle: Its boundaries are anatomical midline anteriorly, the superior belly of the omohyoid muscle superiorly, and anterior border of the SCM inferiorly. It contains the infrahyoid (strap) muscles: sternohyoid, sternothyroid, and thyrohyoid and viscera (thyroid, parathyroid).

The posterior triangle is bound anteriorly by the posterior edge of the SCM, posteriorly by the anterior edge of the TPZ, its apex in the occiput at the junction of the SCM and TPZ, and its base is the middle third of the clavicle.[1] The posterior triangle as illustrated can further be divided by the crossing of the posterior belly of the omohyoid into the occipital triangle superiorly, and the supraclavicular triangle anteriorly. As described, the critical area covered by the SCM is not technically a part of either triangle.

3.1.2 Division of the Neck by Levels

Another common method for subdividing the neck is the use of the level system. This was first described by the Sloan Kettering Group in 1981[2] and has since been adopted by the American Head and Neck Society (AHNS) for the classification of neck dissection with various modifications (▶ Fig. 3.2).[3] There are several obvious reasons to favor this classification as a template to describing neck anatomy systematically in a text devoted to neck dissection. As a major objective, this classification allows

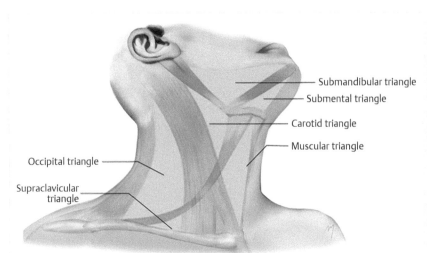

Occipital triangle

Supraclavicular triangle

Submandibular triangle

Submental triangle

Carotid triangle

Muscular triangle

Fig. 3.1 Regions of the neck divided into triangles. Anterior triangle is green and the posterior triangle is blue separated by the sternocleidomastoid muscle. These triangles are further subdivided in the image. (Reproduced with permission of Watanabe K, Shoja MM, Loukas M, Tubbs RS, eds. Anatomy of Plastic Surgery of the Face, Head, and Neck. 1st ed. New York, NY: Theime; 2016.)

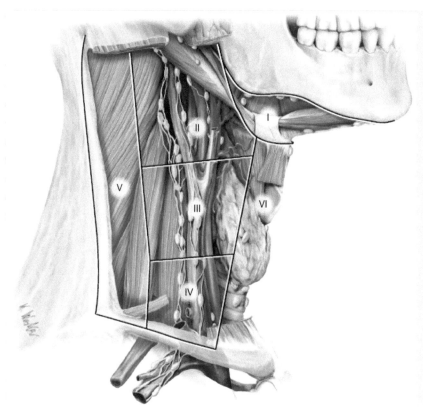

Fig. 3.2 Neck with the sternocleidomastoid muscle removed divided into cervical levels I to VI. (Adapted from THIEME Atlas of Anatomy: General Anatomy and Musculoskeletal System. Thieme 2005. Illustrations by Karl Wesker.)

for consistent communication of pathology radiographically and clinically, therefore providing a framework for conceptualizing the neck. It also serves as the foundation for describing various selective neck dissections as will be discussed in future chapters. Each level can be thought of as a compartment unto itself that may or may not be dissected. As such, it is beneficial for surgeons to be familiarized with the cervical anatomy as defined by the confines of each level.

The neck is divided in six main levels and additional sublevels. We will discuss each level in order with a description of relevant boundaries, followed by a detailed description of their contents. There are common boundaries to all neck levels; these include the prevertebral fascia—or deep layer of the deep cervical fascia (DLDCF)—which serves as the deep boundary, and the investing—or superficial—layer of the DCF, which serves as a superficial boundary. For this reason, we will begin with a description of cervical fascia layers.

3.2 Facial Layers of the Neck

3.2.1 Introduction

The facial layers of the neck are of critical importance to a fundamental understanding of surgical neck anatomy. They are utilized for surgical access, as they provide generally clean and avascular planes of dissection. They can also serve as natural barriers to the spread of disease processes within the neck, whether neoplastic or infectious. A keen understanding of these layers helps the surgeon to compartmentalize the neck anatomy.

The cervical facial layers, although simple in concept, have been varied in their description throughout history. A nice summary of

landmark historical descriptions highlighting this variability is provided by Natale et al.[4] Modern descriptions of cervical fascia typically organize the layers into a superficial cervical fascia (SCF) and a DCF, which is then further subdivided into three layers of muscular or visceral fascia.[5] Since the muscular and visceral fascial layers contained within the deep space are morphologically distinct, we will approach these separately, as in previous reports.[4] The fascial layers will be described from superficial to deep, in the same order as they would be encountered during a typical cervical approach. Of note, although debated, muscular layers are generally considered to form concentric layers that circumscribe the neck (▶ Fig. 3.3).

3.2.2 Superficial Cervical Fascia

Between the dermis and the deep fascia is a region of loose connective tissue joined to both layers known as the SCF. This layer is present in some form throughout the body.[1,4] In the anterior neck, this thin layer envelops the platysma, and is continuous with the superficial musculoaponeurotic system (SMAS) investing the muscles of facial expression anteriorly, and with the galea capitis posteriorly (▶ Fig. 3.4).

The platysma originates at the level of the upper thorax, anterior to the clavicle. It has attachments to the subcutaneous tissues of the subclavicular and acromial regions, as well as the pectoralis and deltoid fascia. It projects superiorly in an upward and medial direction, and has a variable midline dehiscence with decussating fibers submentally. The platysma has numerous insertions, all of which are above the neck including the skin of the cheek, perioral muscles and SMAS, parotid fascia, zygoma, and mandible. The platysma is most commonly innervated by

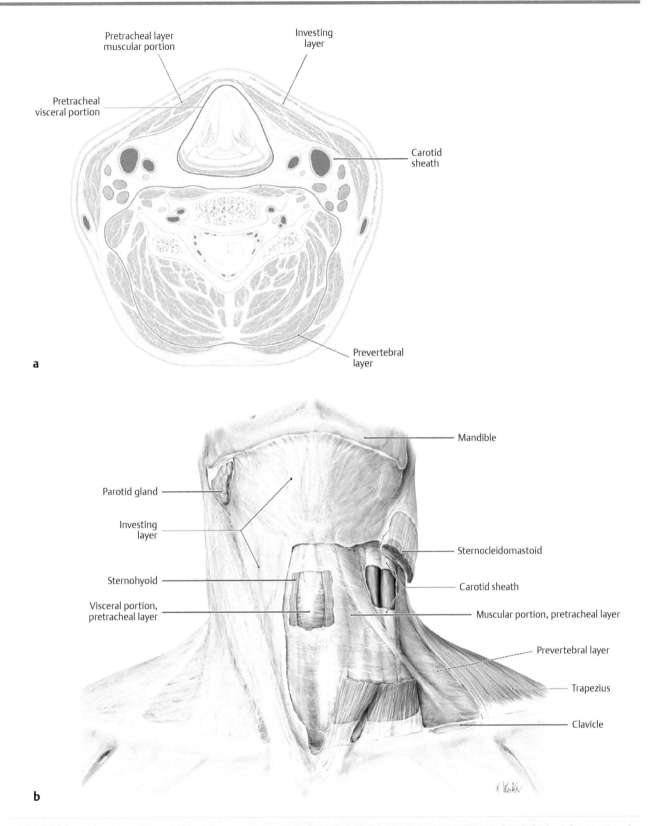

Fig. 3.3 Cervical fascia layers. **(a)** Transverse section taken at the level of the glottis larynx. **(b)** Anterior view of the neck with the fascia layers exposed. (Adapted from THIEME Atlas of Anatomy: General Anatomy and Musculoskeletal System. © Thieme 2005. Illustrations **(a)** by Markus Voll and **(b)** by Karl Wesker.)

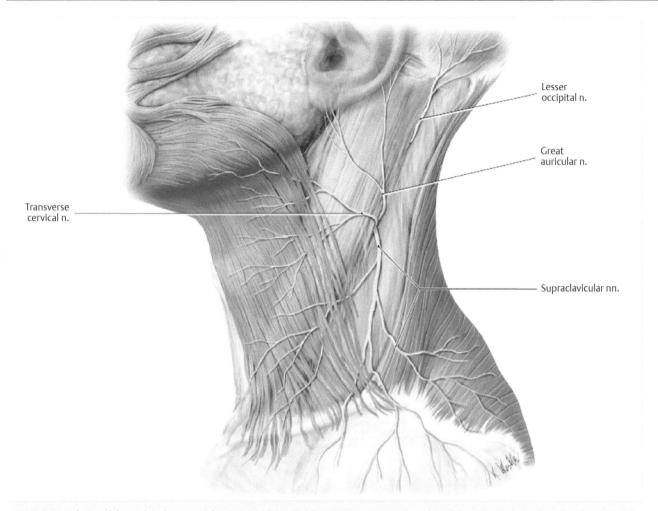

Fig. 3.4 Lateral view of the neck with investing fascia exposed showing the cutaneous sensory branches of the cervical plexus piercing posterior to the sternocleidomastoid muscle. The platysma is found superficial to this fascia layer. (Adapted from THIEME Atlas of Anatomy: General Anatomy and Musculoskeletal System. © Thieme 2005. Illustrations by Karl Wesker.)

the cervical branch of the facial nerve, which descends to enter the deep surface of the muscle near the angle of the mandible.[1,6]

There are several superficial veins with associated lymphatics that exist within the plane between the platysma and the DCF. The external jugular vein (EJV) is formed by the posterior branch of the retromandibular, and the postauricular vein in close association with the angle of the mandible, and drains portions of the face and scalp (▸ Fig. 3.5, ▸ Fig. 3.6). It courses in on oblique fashion crossing the SMC and transverse cervical nerves toward the midclavicle.[1] In the supraclavicular fossa, it pierces the deep fascia and drains into the subclavian, the jugulosubclavian confluence, or the internal jugular vein (IJV).[7] The course of the EJV is most commonly found either at the border, or posterior to the border of the platysma, and in its superior half it courses anterior to the great auricular nerve.[8]

The anterior jugular vein is formed from superficial submandibular vessels near the level of the hyoid, and descends in the neck typically as a bilateral structure between the midline and the anterior border of the SCM. It traverses laterally inferiorly piercing the superficial layer of the DCF (SLDCF) and courses deep to the SCM and superficial to the infrahyoid straps to confluence with the EJV or subclavian vein directly.[1] The anatomy of these superficial veins can be duplicate and quite variable in their course.[7]

3.2.3 Deep Cervical Fascia

Deep to the platysma and the SCF lies the three layers of muscular DCF and the visceral fascia (▸ Fig. 3.3, ▸ Fig. 3.7).[4] The first of these muscular fascial layers encountered is the SLDCF, also known as the investing layer of DCF, which invests the SCM and TPZ muscles, and is continuous posteriorly into the nuchal ligament. Anteriorly, it joins the opposing sheet as well as the hyoid. Superiorly, it has attachments to the superior nuchal line, mastoid, and the lower aspect of the mandible, extending deep to the parotid. Inferiorly, it merges with the periosteum of the manubrium, clavicle, and acromion.[1] Techniques utilizing plastination have recently brought into question the anatomic integrity of the SLDCF in the anterior cervical triangle, between the medial borders of the SCM, and in the posterior triangle between the lateral borders of the SCM and the TPZ.[9,10] These findings have not been widely accepted, and this layer is still considered the superficial boundary of cervical levels I to V.

In the anterior triangle, immediately deep to the SLDCF, lies the second muscular layer of DCF, referred to here as the middle layer of DCF (MLDCF), also referred to as the muscular pretracheal fascia.[5] This layer is composed of muscular fascia surrounding the infrahyoid strap muscles, as well as the mylohyoid

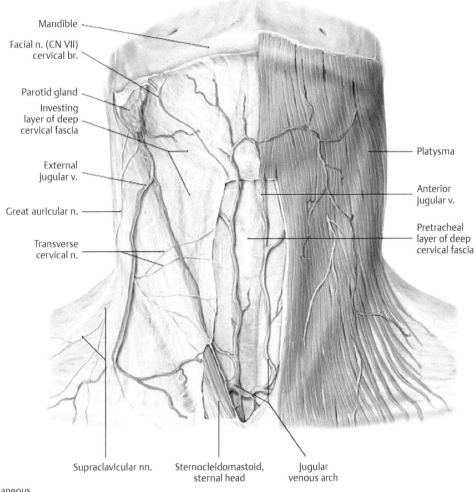

Mandible

Facial n. (CN VII) cervical br.

Parotid gland

Investing layer of deep cervical fascia

External jugular v.

Great auricular n.

Transverse cervical n.

Platysma

Anterior jugular v.

Pretracheal layer of deep cervical fascia

Supraclavicular nn.

Sternocleidomastoid, sternal head

Jugular venous arch

Superficial layer. *Removed:* Subcutaneous platysma (right side) and investing layer of deep cervical fascia (center).

Fig. 3.5 Neurovascular structures found between the superficial fascia and the deep cervical fascia. (Adapted from THIEME Atlas of Anatomy: General Anatomy and Musculoskeletal System. © Thieme 2005. Illustrations by Karl Wesker.)

and geniohyoid muscles above the hyoid bone (▶ Fig. 3.3, ▶ Fig. 3.7). There is evidence that this fascia communicates posteriorly with the levator scapula muscle, thus forming a concentric lamina with the DLDCF encircling the visceral space.[4] This fascial layer serves as the superficial boundary for the level VI (central neck) compartment and the deep boundary for level I.

The third muscular fascial layer is the DLDCF commonly known as the prevertebral fascia. This fascial layer is thickest near the midline covering the vertebral bodies and extends laterally to cover the longus muscles, the anterior and middle scalene muscles, and the levator scapulae. This fascia extends along the brachial plexus and subclavian artery, which emerges behind the anterior scalene and forms the axillary sheet. The superficial sensory branches of the C1–C4 ventral rami forming the cervical plexus, which will be discussed later, pierce this fascia, while the phrenic nerve remains posterior throughout its course in the neck (▶ Fig. 3.8, ▶ Fig. 3.9).[1] The superior attachment of the DLDCF is the skull base and continues into the superior mediastinum. Laterally there is a loose areolar attachment to the carotid sheath. The DLDCF serves as the floor, or deep boundary for cervical levels II to VI.

The final fascial layer of the neck is the visceral fascia, a very thin layer that envelops the viscera of the neck, which is analogous to the subperitoneal and subpleural fascia of the abdomen and thorax, respectively.[4] Visceral structures include the laryngotracheal complex, thyroid and parathyroids, and esophagus. The buccopharyngeal fascia is a condensation of the epimysium of the pharyngeal constrictors and esophagus and separates the visceral compartment from the DLDCF with an intervening loose alveolar space (▶ Fig. 3.7). Some authors consider the carotid sheath to be included in this visceral classification, while *Gray's Anatomy* describes the carotid sheath simply as a condensation of all surrounding DCF layers, one being the pretracheal or visceral fascia.[1,4] The carotid sheath houses the common and internal carotid artery, IJV, and the vagus nerve.

3.3 Levels of the Neck

The neck is divided in six levels (I–VI) with additional sublevels (A, B) in levels I, II, and V (▶ Fig. 3.2).

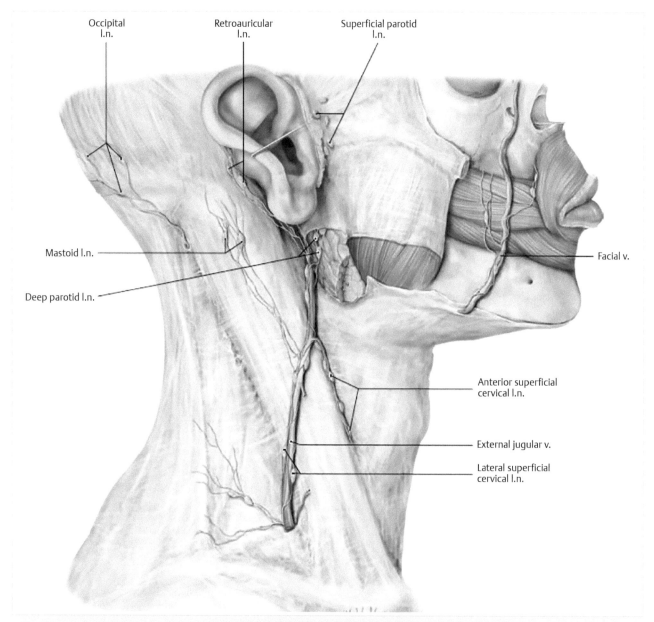

Occipital l.n.

Retroauricular l.n.

Superficial parotid l.n.

Mastoid l.n.

Deep parotid l.n.

Facial v.

Anterior superficial cervical l.n.

External jugular v.

Lateral superficial cervical l.n.

Fig. 3.6 Superficial lymphatics of the neck. (Adapted from THIEME Atlas of Anatomy: General Anatomy and Musculoskeletal System. © Thieme 2005. Illustrations by Karl Wesker.)

3.3.1 Level I

This level is subdivided into sublevels IA and IB, which correlate with the submental and digastric triangles, respectively. We will discuss these sublevels including their boundaries and contents separately (▸ Fig. 3.10).

Level IA

Level IA is an unpaired central triangle bound by the ABD and the body of the hyoid bone inferiorly. Its apex is the symphysis of the mandible superiorly. The roof of this triangle is the SLDCF immediately deep to the superficial fascia investing the platysma and the floor is the MLDCF, which is the muscular fascia investing the mylohyoid.

The ABD receives its blood supply from the submental artery. The course of this artery and associated vein has been well described in the literature as it pertains to the submental flap. It is a branch of the facial artery and courses along the inferior border of the mandible toward the lateral aspect of the ABD. It has a terminal but variable cutaneous perforator near the apex of the submental triangle on either side of the ABD.[11] The ABD is continuous with the PBD by an intermediate tendon attached to the hyoid via a fibrous sling. It is innervated by the nerve to the mylohyoid, a branch off the lingual distribution of V3.[1]

Level IB

The boundaries of this triangle are the ABD anteroinferiorly, the stylohyoid muscle posteroinferiorly, and the base of the

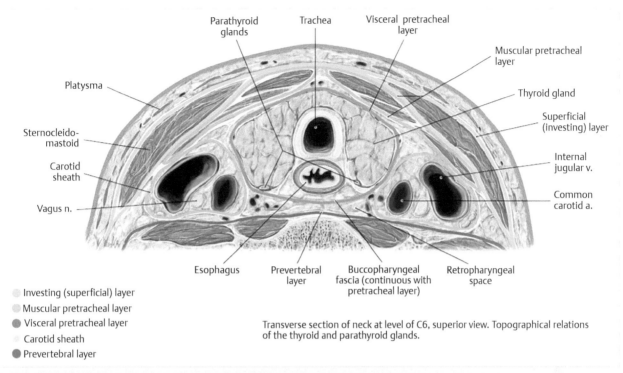

Parathyroid glands
Trachea
Visceral pretracheal layer
Muscular pretracheal layer
Platysma
Thyroid gland
Superficial (investing) layer
Sternocleido-mastoid
Internal jugular v.
Carotid sheath
Common carotid a.
Vagus n.
Esophagus
Prevertebral layer
Buccopharyngeal fascia (continuous with pretracheal layer)
Retropharyngeal space

○ Investing (superficial) layer
○ Muscular pretracheal layer
● Visceral pretracheal layer
○ Carotid sheath
● Prevertebral layer

Transverse section of neck at level of C6, superior view. Topographical relations of the thyroid and parathyroid glands.

Fig. 3.7 Cervical fascia layers transverse cut at the level of the thyroid. (Adapted from THIEME Atlas of Anatomy: General Anatomy and Musculoskeletal System. © Thieme 2005. Illustrations by Karl Wesker.)

mandible superiorly. To make the posterior boundary of level 1B more recognizable on clinical examination and radiographically, the AHNS modified the boundary to be the posterior plane of the posterior edge of the SMG rather than the stylohyoid muscle.[12] The floor of this triangle is the mylohyoid and hyoglossus muscles. The roof of this triangle is the SLDCF.

The contents of level IB will be discussed from superficial to deep as encountered beneath the platysma (▶ Fig. 3.11).[5] The marginal branch of the facial nerve (MBFN) and cervical branch of the facial nerve are encountered superficial to level IB on the SLDCF fascia, immediately deep to the platysma (▶ Fig. 3.12). The angle and base of the mandible have been the most common landmarks used to describe the location of the MBFN. The neck position affects the location of the nerve relative to the mandible. The nerve is most commonly described as having two branches, but it may have multiple. It has a downward trajectory after leaving the parotid parenchyma coursing over the angle of the mandible. In 78 neck dissections, the lowest branch of the nerve was found at average of 1.25 cm below the margin of the mandible in the location lateral to the facial vein overlying the fascia of the SMG with the neck extended.[13]

The facial vein and artery lie deep to the MBFN, with the vein consistently posterolateral to the artery. The vein is found in the fascia superficial to the SMG and courses in a posteroinferior trajectory as it descends lateral to the PBD as it leaves level IB. It is joined by the anterior division of retromandibular vein, sometimes referred to as the posterior facial vein, in this location and will be discussed later in level II (▶ Fig. 3.13).[5]

The facial artery enters level IB deep to the stylohyoid muscle and PBD after branching off the external carotid as will be discussed with the level II anatomy. The facial artery courses anterior and superior along the lateral surface of the hyoglossus muscle. It indents the posterior and lateral surfaces of the SMG

taking a inferolateral trajectory along the lingual surface of the mandible, exiting the triangle at the facial notch of the mandible. At the inferior mandible, it is immediately anterior to the facial vein. The artery is notable for its tortuous appearance throughout its course. The submental artery leaves the facial artery near the inferior border of the mandible.

The SMG is found immediately deep to the facial vein. It occupies much of the volume of level 1B and is partially cradled by support from myofascial attachments to the hyoid bone from the mylohyoid medially and SLDCF laterally, both extending from the hyoid to the mandible. It has an irregular shape imparted by straddling the posterior free edge of the mylohyoid dividing the gland into a deep and superficial lobe.

The superficial lobe constitutes the bulk of the gland and defines the posterior border of level IB. Superiorly, the gland extends medially to the body of the mandible and inferiorly the gland may drape the digastric tendon. It is found deep to the SLDCF, which courses deep to the tail of parotid. A condensation of SLDCF called the stylomandibular ligament separates the two glands posteriorly.[1]

The deep lobe lies in the space between the mylohyoid laterally and the hyoglossus muscle medially. It extends anteriorly deep to the floor of the mouth approximating the sublingual gland anterosuperiorly (▶ Fig. 3.11).[5] This space between the mylohyoid and hyoglossus muscles is traversed by the lingual nerve, the submandibular duct, and the hypoglossal nerve (HN; ▶ Fig. 3.14).[5]

The lingual nerve, which originates as a branch of V3 in the infratemporal fossa, is closely associated with the mandibular periosteum near the third molar. It descends into level IB lateral to the hyoglossus muscle, along the superior aspect of the floor of level 1B (▶ Fig. 3.15). As the lingual nerve travels anteriorly, it courses medial to the mylohyoid muscle superior to the HN. The lingual nerve descends lateral to the submandibular duct

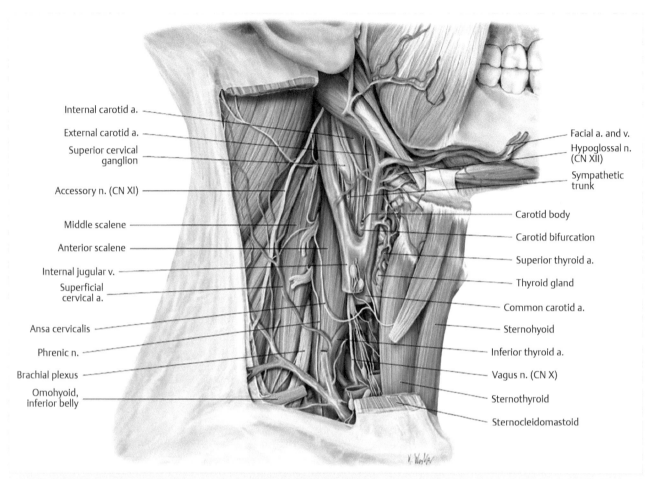

Internal carotid a.
External carotid a.
Superior cervical ganglion
Accessory n. (CN XI)
Middle scalene
Anterior scalene
Internal jugular v.
Superficial cervical a.
Ansa cervicalis
Phrenic n.
Brachial plexus
Omohyoid, inferior belly

Facial a. and v.
Hypoglossal n. (CN XII)
Sympathetic trunk
Carotid body
Carotid bifurcation
Superior thyroid a.
Thyroid gland
Common carotid a.
Sternohyoid
Inferior thyroid a.
Vagus n. (CN X)
Sternothyroid
Sternocleidomastoid

Fig. 3.8 Lateral view of the neck exposed to the level of the deep fascia and paraspinal muscles. (Adapted from THIEME Atlas of Anatomy: General Anatomy and Musculoskeletal System. © Thieme 2005. Illustrations by Karl Wesker.)

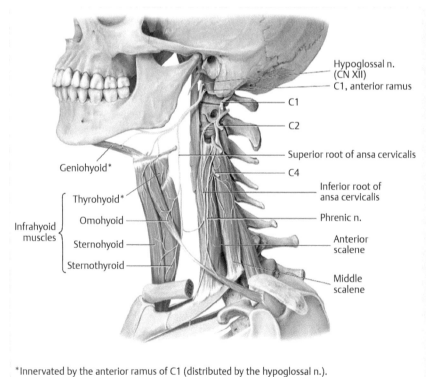

Fig. 3.9 Cervical plexus with superficial sensory branches transected. (Adapted from THIEME Atlas of Anatomy: General Anatomy and Musculoskeletal System. © Thieme 2005. Illustrations by Karl Wesker.)

Hypoglossal n. (CN XII)
C1, anterior ramus
C1
C2
Superior root of ansa cervicalis
C4
Inferior root of ansa cervicalis
Phrenic n.
Anterior scalene
Middle scalene

Geniohyoid*
Thyrohyoid*
Omohyoid
Sternohyoid
Sternothyroid
Infrahyoid muscles

*Innervated by the anterior ramus of C1 (distributed by the hypoglossal n.).

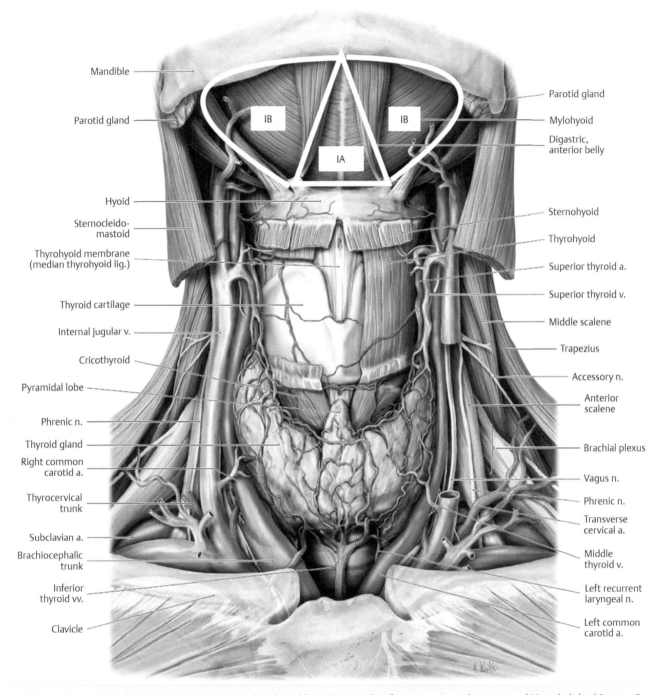

Fig. 3.10 Anterior view of the neck with level I outlined. (Adapted from THIEME Atlas of Anatomy: General Anatomy and Musculoskeletal System. © Thieme 2005. Illustrations by Karl Wesker.)

near the anterior border of the hyoglossus, and cradles the undersurface of the duct before projecting medially to innervate the anterior oral tongue.[1] The lingual nerve is immediately associated with the deep surface of the SMG and is in continuity with the submandibular ganglia; this is the site of postsynaptic parasympathetic fibers that innervate the gland (▶ Fig. 3.11).[5]

The HN enters the triangle deep to the stylohyoid muscle associated with the inferior and deep surfaces of the gland medial to the digastric tendon and lateral to the hyoglossus muscle (▶ Fig. 3.15). It courses anteriorly with associated vena

comitans, which drain into the lingual vein. The nerve courses deep to the mylohyoid and inferior to the lingual nerve and submandibular duct.

3.3.2 The Lateral Neck (Levels II–IV)

The lateral neck contains the upper, middle, and lower jugular chain of lymph nodes and correlates with levels II, III, and IV, respectively. The lateral neck extends form the skull base superiorly to the clavicle inferiorly (▶ Fig. 3.2). Its superficial boundary or roof

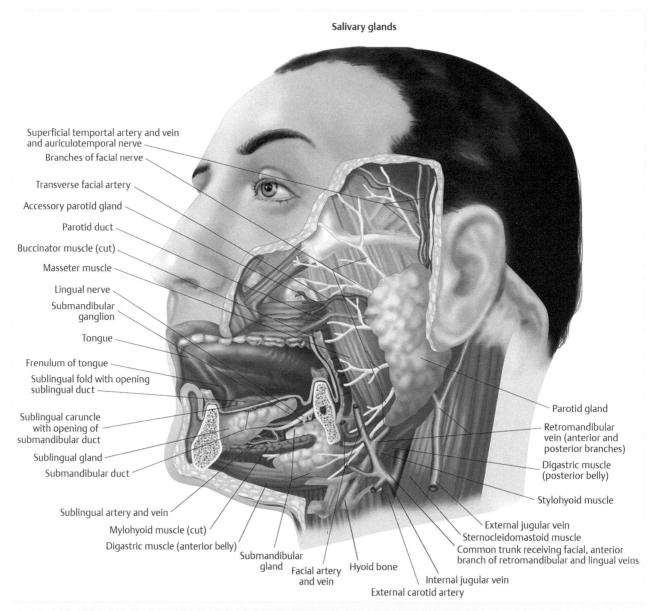

Salivary glands

Superficial temporal artery and vein
and auriculotemporal nerve

Branches of facial nerve

Transverse facial artery

Accessory parotid gland

Parotid duct

Buccinator muscle (cut)

Masseter muscle

Lingual nerve

Submandibular
ganglion

Tongue

Frenulum of tongue

Sublingual fold with opening
sublingual duct

Sublingual caruncle
with opening of
submandibular duct

Sublingual gland

Submandibular duct

Sublingual artery and vein

Mylohyoid muscle (cut)

Digastric muscle (anterior belly)

Submandibular
gland

Facial artery
and vein

Hyoid bone

Parotid gland

Retromandibular
vein (anterior and
posterior branches)

Digastric muscle
(posterior belly)

Stylohyoid muscle

External jugular vein

Sternocleidomastoid muscle

Common trunk receiving facial, anterior
branch of retromandibular and lingual veins

Internal jugular vein

External carotid artery

Fig. 3.11 Anterolateral view of submandibular triangle with the platysma and SLDCF (superficial layer of the deep cervical fascia) removed. The mandibulectomy defect allows visualization of the contents of the submandibular triangle deep to the mylohyoid muscle.

is the SLDCF, which invests the SCM (▶ Fig. 3.16). The deep boundary or floor is the DLDCF synonymous with the prevertebral fascia that covers the paraspinal muscles including the longus muscles, the anterior scalene, and levator scapulae, which contribute to the muscular floor of the lateral neck (▶ Fig. 3.3). The posterior boundary of these levels is defined by the posterior edge of the SCM as well and the superficial sensory branches of the cervical plexus, which is particularly useful intraoperatively.[3] This separates the lateral neck from level V posteriorly, which will be reviewed later. The anterior boundary of lateral neck at levels III and IV is defined by the lateral border of the sternohyoid superficially, and the medial aspect of the common carotid in the deep plane (▶ Fig. 3.8).[3,12] More superiorly, the anterior boundary of level II is the vertical plane of the posterior border of SMG, which approximates the stylohyoid muscle but is more clinically and

radiographically appreciated that muscle.[12] We will begin our review of the lateral neck by discussing the critical structures that form these boundaries and then proceed to discuss each level and its contents individually.

The Posterior Boundary of the Lateral Neck

Cervical Plexus

The superficial or sensory branches of the cervical plexus have a critical role in demarcating the division between the lateral (levels II–IV) and posterior (level V) neck and therefore the whole of the cervical plexus will be discussed here. This superficial plexus along with the posterior border of the SCM demarcates the posterior border of levels II to IV (▶ Fig. 3.16). The

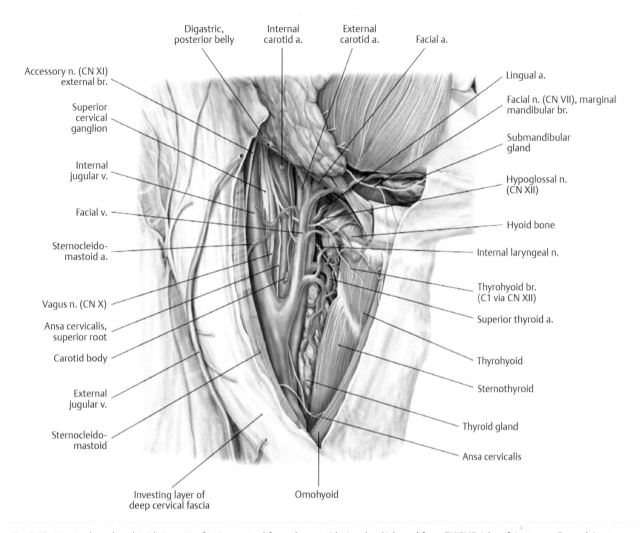

Fig. 3.12 Anterior lateral neck with investing fascia removed from the carotid triangle. (Adapted from THIEME Atlas of Anatomy: General Anatomy and Musculoskeletal System. © Thieme 2005. Illustrations by Karl Wesker.)

cervical plexus is formed by the ventral rami of C1–C4 (▶ Fig. 3.17).[5] These rami function to innervate muscles of the neck and diaphragm as well as provide sensory innervation to the skin of the neck and chest (▶ Fig. 3.9). In general, the cervical ventral rami are larger than dorsal rami except for the first and second, which are smaller than their dorsal counterparts (the cervical dorsal rami provide cutaneous cervical innervation to the posterior neck as well as paraspinal muscular innervation). The cervical plexus enters the neck piercing the DLDCF between the anterior and middle scalene except for the phrenic nerve, which remains deep to the fascia. There are ascending and descending branches from each level except for C1, and multiple communicating branches between levels. Additionally, there are superficial and deep branches; superficial branches have cutaneous sensory functions and pierce the SLDCF, while the deep branches innervate muscle.[14]

The superficial branches provide the anatomic demarcation between the lateral neck compartment and the posterior compartment (level V). They radiate laterally until they reach the posterior border of the SCM, at which point they take either an ascending or descending trajectory piercing the SLDCF. They are found immediately deep to the superficial fascia and platysma in this location (▶ Fig. 3.16).

The deep branches provide muscular innervation to the strap muscles, geniohyoid, diaphragm, and anterior paraspinal muscles (▶ Fig. 3.9). Additionally, via lateral muscular branches and contributions to the spinal accessory nerve (SAN), the cervical plexus innervates the SCM, TPZ, levator scapula, and scalene muscles. The ansa cervicalis is formed by a superior and inferior root supplied by cervical plexus contributions from C1 and C2–C4, respectively, which supplies all strap muscles with the exception of the thyrohyoid.[1] The superior root branches from the HN as it courses lateral the carotid sheath near the occipital artery. The superior root descends, coursing along or within the carotid sheath, to meet the descending inferior root in the mid neck on the lateral surface of the IJV.

The phrenic nerve innervates the diaphragm and is formed by contributions from C3–C5. It is formed in the floor of the lateral neck and descends on the surface of the anterior scalene and is unique in that it does not pierce the DLDCF.

Veins of oral and pharyngeal regions

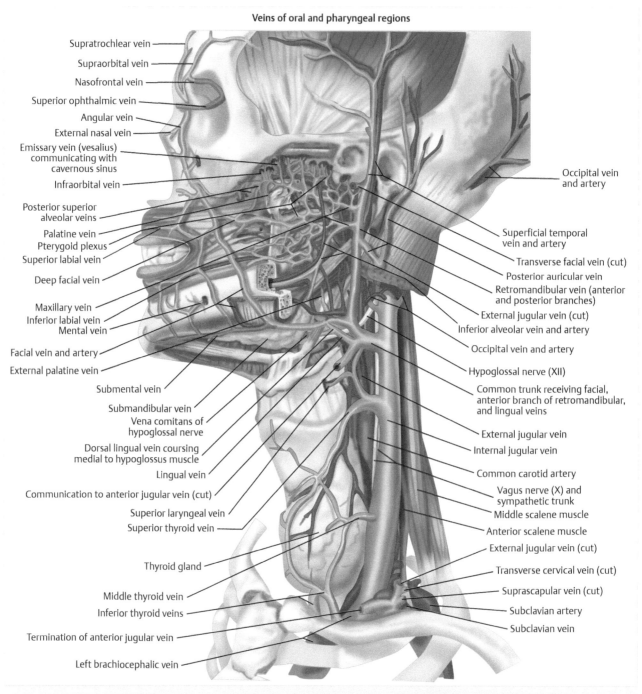

Supratrochlear vein
Supraorbital vein
Nasofrontal vein
Superior ophthalmic vein
Angular vein
External nasal vein
Emissary vein (vesalius) communicating with cavernous sinus
Infraorbital vein
Posterior superior alveolar veins
Palatine vein
Pterygoid plexus
Superior labial vein
Deep facial vein
Maxillary vein
Inferior labial vein
Mental vein
Facial vein and artery
External palatine vein
Submental vein
Submandibular vein
Vena comitans of hypoglossal nerve
Dorsal lingual vein coursing medial to hypoglossus muscle
Lingual vein
Communication to anterior jugular vein (cut)
Superior laryngeal vein
Superior thyroid vein
Thyroid gland
Middle thyroid vein
Inferior thyroid veins
Termination of anterior jugular vein
Left brachiocephalic vein

Occipital vein and artery
Superficial temporal vein and artery
Transverse facial vein (cut)
Posterior auricular vein
Retromandibular vein (anterior and posterior branches)
External jugular vein (cut)
Inferior alveolar vein and artery
Occipital vein and artery
Hypoglossal nerve (XII)
Common trunk receiving facial, anterior branch of retromandibular, and lingual veins
External jugular vein
Internal jugular vein
Common carotid artery
Vagus nerve (X) and sympathetic trunk
Middle scalene muscle
Anterior scalene muscle
External jugular vein (cut)
Transverse cervical vein (cut)
Suprascapular vein (cut)
Subclavian artery
Subclavian vein

Fig. 3.13 Lateral view of the neck with the straps and sternocleidomastoid muscle removed highlighting the venous system.

Sternocleidomastoid Muscle

The posterior border of the SCM is an additional landmark for the posterior boundary of the lateral neck. It is invested by the SLDCF and forms the roof over a large majority of the lateral neck (▶ Fig. 3.16). The muscle is formed by two heads inferiorly, the sternal anteriorly, and the clavicular posteriorly, with a slight depression between the two, which terminates as the muscle bellies merge. It has an oblique course in the neck as it ascends toward the mastoid process and lateral nuchal line superiorly. It is innervated by the SAN and contributions from the lateral muscular branches of the cervical plexus (C2–C3),

which descends obliquely to reach the muscle's deep surface near the junction of the upper and middle third.

The Medial Boundary of the Lateral Neck

The Carotid Sheath

The medial boundary of levels III to IV is defined by the medial wall of the common carotid inferiorly and internal carotid artery more superiorly (▶ Fig. 3.12). This landmark is generally more useful radiographically as surgically the lateral border of the sternohyoid is more commonly used. As the carotid is the

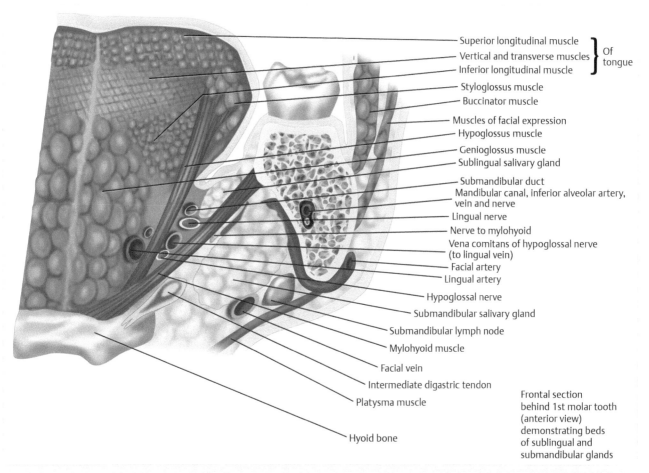

Superior longitudinal muscle ⎫
Vertical and transverse muscles ⎬ Of
Inferior longitudinal muscle ⎭ tongue
Styloglossus muscle
Buccinator muscle
Muscles of facial expression
Hypoglossus muscle
Genioglossus muscle
Sublingual salivary gland
Submandibular duct
Mandibular canal, inferior alveolar artery,
vein and nerve
Lingual nerve
Nerve to mylohyoid
Vena comitans of hypoglossal nerve
(to lingual vein)
Facial artery
Lingual artery
Hypoglossal nerve
Submandibular salivary gland
Submandibular lymph node
Mylohyoid muscle
Facial vein
Intermediate digastric tendon
Platysma muscle

Frontal section
behind 1st molar tooth
(anterior view)
demonstrating beds
of sublingual and
submandibular glands

Hyoid bone

Fig. 3.14 Cross section through level IB and the oral cavity allows demonstration of the neurovascular structures relative to the mylohyoid and hyoglossus muscles and the submandibular gland.

most medial structure within the carotid sheath, the contents of the sheath are in the domain of the lateral neck. The contents of the sheath are the common and internal carotid arteries, the IJV, the vagus nerve, and portions of the ansa cervicalis. Within the sheath, the carotid lies medial to the IJV, while the vagus nerve is situated between and posterior to both vessels.

The common carotid is derived from the aortic arch in the left neck, and the brachiocephalic artery on the right with rare exceptions. From the deep plane to the sternoclavicular joint, the course of both arteries is similar, diverging laterally and coursing more superficially until their bifurcation.[14] The bifurcation into external and internal carotids served as the demarcation between levels II and III prior to the revised classification, which adopted the inferior border of the hyoid bone (which approximates the carotid bifurcation). Above the level of the cricoid, the carotid is more superficial, emerging from the anterior medial border of the SCM. The common carotid generally does not branch prior to the bifurcation though rarely branches of the external carotid may arise from it (▶ Fig. 3.10).

The internal carotid continues within the carotid sheath to supply the anterior cerebral circulation, eye, nose, and portions of the forehead without branching in the neck. For a brief period, prior to ascending deep to the stylohyoid muscle, the internal carotid may serve as the anterior limit of level III below the plane of the hyoid bone.

3.3.3 Level IV

Level IV contains the lower jugular chain lymph nodes and occupies the space superior to the clavicle and inferior to the lower border of the cricoid cartilage (▶ Fig. 3.2). We will discuss the pertinent anatomy of this level relative to the major vascular structures.

The arterial supply to the head and neck enters through the root of the neck traversing level IV (▶ Fig. 3.8). These include the common carotid, and branches of the subclavian including the vertebral artery, and vessels classically associated with the thyrocervical trunk (TCT). The most medial of these vessels forms the medial boundary of level IV, the common carotid. Anterior to the common carotid artery are the sternohyoid and sternothyroid strap muscles as well as the SCM more superficially. The artery is crossed anteriorly by the middle thyroid vein and omohyoid muscle, both in proximity to the superior border of this level. The omohyoid approximates the position of the cricoid as it crosses the lateral surface of the carotid sheath, and was previously used as the distinction between levels III and IV (▶ Fig. 3.8).[3]

Medial to the artery lies level VI, which will be discussed in detail later. Laterally, the artery is bound by the IJV, which can rotate to a more anterior position low in the neck. The vagus nerve is posterolateral to the artery.

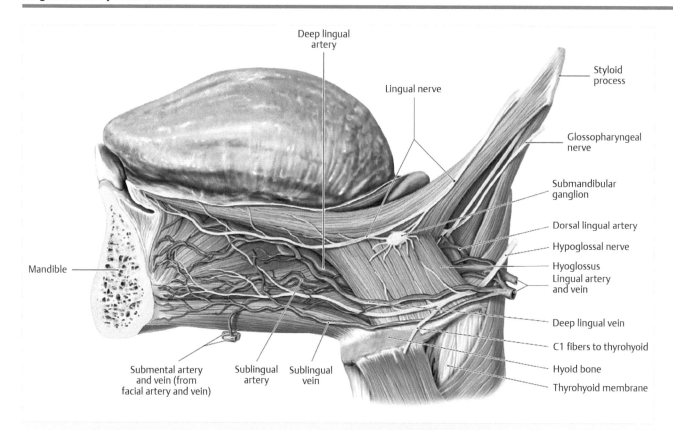

Deep lingual artery

Lingual nerve

Styloid process

Glossopharyngeal nerve

Submandibular ganglion

Dorsal lingual artery

Hypoglossal nerve

Hyoglossus

Lingual artery and vein

Deep lingual vein

C1 fibers to thyrohyoid

Hyoid bone

Thyrohyoid membrane

Mandible

Submental artery and vein (from facial artery and vein)

Sublingual artery

Sublingual vein

Fig. 3.15 Left lateral view of the floor of level IB. (Adapted from THIEME Head and Neck Anatomy for Dental Medicine. © Thieme 2010. Illustrations by Karl Wesker.)

Deep to the common carotid lies the muscular floor of the neck composed of paraspinal muscles covered by prevertebral fascia, otherwise known here as the DLDCF. In level IV, these muscles include the longus colli medially the anterior scalene laterally (▶ Fig. 3.19). The anterior scalene has attachments to the transverse processes of the lower cervical vertebra (C3–C6), which lie immediately posterior to the common carotid. The muscular fibers of the anterior scalene join in an oblique course leaving the neck to insert on the first rib. The phrenic nerve is a very critical structure that runs over the anterior surface of the muscle deep to the DLDCF. At the lateral border of the anterior scalene, the ventral rami of the cervical plexus (C2–C4) pierce the DLDCF demarcating the lateral extent of the lateral neck levels. As the lateral border of the anterior scalene is followed inferiorly, the brachial plexus is encountered emerging between the anterior and middle scalene muscle covered by an extension of the DLDCF. However, being posterior to the posterior border of the SCM, the brachial plexus lies deep to the floor of level V.

Deep to the common carotid and inferior to the transverse process of C6, an angle is formed as the anterior scalene diverges from the more medial longus colli muscle (▶ Fig. 3.18). In this angle, the vertebral artery, inferior thyroid artery (ITA), sympathetic trunk, and thoracic duct (on the left) can be found (▶ Fig. 3.19).[14]

The ITA is a terminal branch of the TCT. The vertebral artery and TCT originate from the first part of the subclavian artery, which is the segment lateral to the anterior scalene. These are consistently the first and second superior branches of the first part of the subclavian as demonstrated in 498 neck dissections (▶ Fig. 3.19).[15]

The vertebral artery ascends in a posterior and medial trajectory crossing behind the common carotid in a lateral to medial direction before piercing the angle between the longus colli and anterior scalene to ascend in the vertebral canal of the transverse process (C6–C1). The artery enters at C6 in more than 80% of cases (▶ Fig. 3.20).[16] The sympathetic truck is in proximity to the medial aspect of the vertebral artery below C6 and posterior to the common carotid in this location. The middle cervical ganglion of the sympathetic trunk may be found in this location, below C6, and anterior and inferior to the ITA (▶ Fig. 3.19).

The TCT, which originates from the subclavian artery lateral to the vertebral artery near the medial border of the anterior scalene, branches almost immediately into the inferior thyroid, the transverse cervical, and the suprascapular arteries in its classical description. However, as we will discuss, this anatomy can be quite variable. The ITA, which is considered the terminal branch of the TCT, initially ascends over the medial aspect of the anterior scalene before turning medially. The ascending cervical artery consistently branches superiorly from the ITA to supply the paraspinal muscles. In its medial trajectory, the ITA crosses over the vertebral artery and deep to the common carotid and sympathetic trunk before entering level VI.[14,15]

The other branches of the TCT include the transverse cervical (also referred to as the superficial cervical artery), the suprascapular, and dorsal scapular arteries. There is a high degree of variability in the origin of these vessels. The transverse cervical artery (TCA) originated from the TCT (75%) or the subclavian artery (21%), with the remaining cases originating from the internal thoracic artery in a series of 498 dissections.[15] The TCA originates from the TCT at a mean of 17 mm superior to the

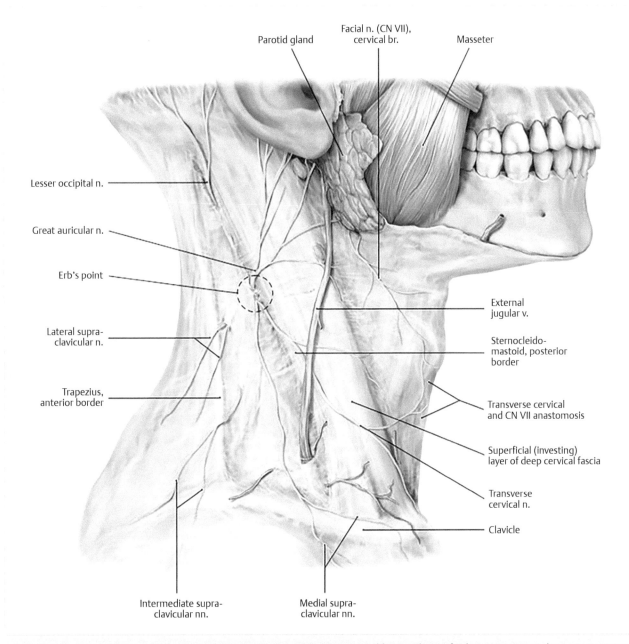

Parotid gland

Facial n. (CN VII), cervical br.

Masseter

Lesser occipital n.

Great auricular n.

Erb's point

Lateral supra-clavicular n.

Trapezius, anterior border

Intermediate supra-clavicular nn.

Medial supra-clavicular nn.

External jugular v.

Sternocleido-mastoid, posterior border

Transverse cervical and CN VII anastomosis

Superficial (investing) layer of deep cervical fascia

Transverse cervical n.

Clavicle

Fig. 3.16 Lateral view of the neck at the depth of the investing layer of the deep cervical fascia with superficial venous system and cutaneous sensory nerves depicted. (Adapted from THIEME Atlas of Anatomy: General Anatomy and Musculoskeletal System. © Thieme 2005. Illustrations by Karl Wesker.)

clavicle at the anterior border of the SCM.[17] The TCA traverses level IV deep to the IJV and SCM, coursing from medial to lateral superficial to the anterior scalene and DLDCF in level V. The suprascapular artery has a more inferior course descending posterolateral anterior to the subclavian artery paralleling the omohyoid toward the suprascapular notch.

The IJV is the major venous structure in level IV and is in the carotid sheath lateral and occasionally anterior to the common carotid inferiorly. Deep cervical nodes in this level are found anterior and lateral to the IJV. The IJV is crossed anteriorly by the intermediate tendon or superior belly of the omohyoid approximating the superior border of level IV. It is covered by the strap muscles, followed by the SCM more

superficially. Anteroinferiorly, it is crossed by the anterior jugular veins, which are superficial to the strap muscles. The anterior jugular and EJV may enter the IJV directly, but more commonly they join the subclavian vein. The subclavian vein joins the IJV posterior to the medial head of the clavicle and forms the brachiocephalic vein, anterior to the first part of the subclavian artery. The confluence of these great veins is a landmark for critical lymphatic drainage.

The lymphatic drainage and major lymphovenous connections are highly variable but of paramount importance in level IV neck anatomy. The lymphatic system, in addition to its immunologic role, is responsible for transporting lymph, a fluid produced from interstitial fluid that permeates the walls of

Cervical plexus in situ

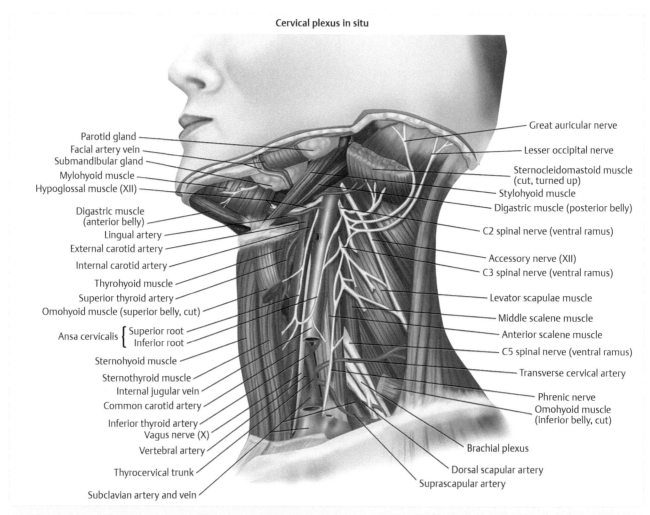

Parotid gland
Facial artery vein
Submandibular gland
Mylohyoid muscle
Hypoglossal muscle (XII)

Digastric muscle (anterior belly)
Lingual artery
External carotid artery
Internal carotid artery
Thyrohyoid muscle
Superior thyroid artery
Omohyoid muscle (superior belly, cut)

Ansa cervicalis { Superior root / Inferior root

Sternohyoid muscle
Sternothyroid muscle
Internal jugular vein
Common carotid artery
Inferior thyroid artery
Vagus nerve (X)
Vertebral artery
Thyrocervical trunk
Subclavian artery and vein

Great auricular nerve
Lesser occipital nerve
Sternocleidomastoid muscle (cut, turned up)
Stylohyoid muscle
Digastric muscle (posterior belly)
C2 spinal nerve (ventral ramus)
Accessory nerve (XII)
C3 spinal nerve (ventral ramus)
Levator scapulae muscle
Middle scalene muscle
Anterior scalene muscle
C5 spinal nerve (ventral ramus)
Transverse cervical artery
Phrenic nerve
Omohyoid muscle (inferior belly, cut)
Brachial plexus
Dorsal scapular artery
Suprascapular artery

Fig. 3.17 The sternocleidomastoid muscle reflected and contents of the lateral neck exposed to the level of the deep layer of the deep cervical fascia to better demonstrate the cervical plexus (*continued*).

lymph capillaries throughout the body, as well as lipids and proteins from the intestine known as chyle. The thoracic duct is the largest lymphatic vessel in the body, draining lymph from all areas except for the right upper extremity, right head and neck, and right upper hemithorax, which is the domain of the right lymphatic duct. The thoracic duct ascends from the thorax, anterior to the spine and medial to the aorta, to enter the base of the neck. The thoracic duct empties into the great veins in the left neck in up to 95% of cases, with the remaining cases having a right-sided or rarely bilateral drainage pattern.[18]

The thoracic duct enters the neck after its ascent through the superior mediastinum, along the left lateral aspect of the esophagus being crossed anteriorly by the aortic arch. Below C6, it is found posterior to the common carotid. In this location, it courses laterally, posterior to the carotid sheath, and arches 3 to 5 cm above the clavicle. Once lateral to the IJV, it courses anteroinferiorly to the subclavian artery on its way to the confluence of the IJV and subclavian vein, which is its most common point of drainage. The location immediately lateral to the inferior carotid sheath is the most likely site of injury. In this location, the thoracic duct is joined by lymphatic branches from the jugular and subclavian trunks, and terminates as one or multiple vessels. The termination is most commonly the venous angle of

the IJV and subclavian, or the IJV itself with termination usually occurring within 15 mm of this angle (▶ Fig. 3.19).[18,19]

The lymphatics in the right neck do not contain chyle except in the cases of right-sided or duplicate thoracic ducts, in which case chyle leaks have been reported. The lymphatic terminus in the right neck as in the left is centered around the confluence of the IJV and subclavian veins. It is formed by the confluence of jugular, subclavian, and bronchomediastinal lymphatic trunks. It is more common for these trunks to individually terminate into the venous circulation but on occasion they coalesce toward the right lymphatic trunk, which may approach a centimeter in length.[14,19]

Critical neural structures of level IV have been mentioned and include, from lateral to medial, the phrenic and vagus nerves as well as the cervical sympathetic trunk. These neural structures are protected by fascia: the phrenic below the DLDCF, the vagus housed within the carotid sheath, and the sympathetic trunk posterior to the carotid sheath on the surface of the prevertebral fascia. They all have a vertical course in the neck, and can be found immediately anterior to the first part of the subclavian artery when traced inferiorly. It is in this location in the right neck that the recurrent laryngeal nerve (RLN) branches from the vagus nerve. The RLN then loops

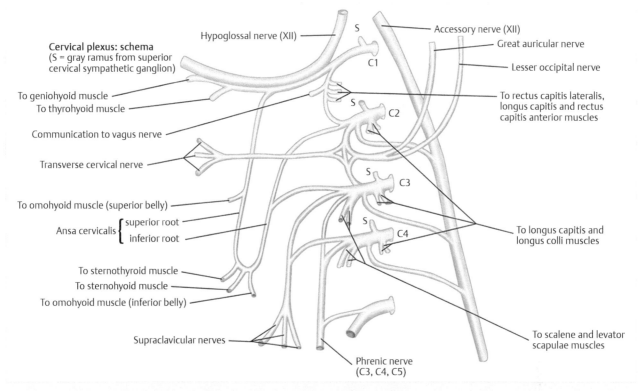

Cervical plexus: schema
(S = gray ramus from superior cervical sympathetic ganglion)

Hypoglossal nerve (XII)

Accessory nerve (XII)
Great auricular nerve
Lesser occipital nerve

To geniohyoid muscle
To thyrohyoid muscle

To rectus capitis lateralis, longus capitis and rectus capitis anterior muscles

Communication to vagus nerve

Transverse cervical nerve

To omohyoid muscle (superior belly)

Ansa cervicalis { superior root
inferior root

To longus capitis and longus colli muscles

To sternothyroid muscle
To sternohyoid muscle
To omohyoid muscle (inferior belly)

Supraclavicular nerves

To scalene and levator scapulae muscles

Phrenic nerve
(C3, C4, C5)

S
C1
S
C2
S
C3
S
C4

Fig. 3.17 (*Continued*) Schema of the cervical plexus.

around the subclavian artery inferiorly and ascends obliquely behind the common carotid to enter level VI. On the left, the RLN branches from the vagus near the anterior aortic arch, and ascends after looping under the arch to assume a more medial position in the tracheoesophageal (TE) groove without traversing the lateral neck.

3.3.4 Level III

Middle jugular lymph nodes are contained within level III, which extends form the inferior border of the cricoid cartilage to the inferior border of the hyoid bone (▶ Fig. 3.2). For the sake of organization, we will utilize the carotid bifurcation as the superior limit of this discussion and reserve our discussion of the external carotid artery (ECA) and its branches to level II.

The use of radiographically identifiable landmarks has served as a major driving force to modifications in cervical level boundaries.[3],[12] The initial work by Som et al was critical in the adoption of the revised superior, inferior, and medial borders of level III.[20] The superior and inferior borders were revised in 2002: the superior border changed to the inferior border of the hyoid rather than the carotid bifurcation, and the inferior border changed to the inferior cricoid cartilage rather than the omohyoid.[3] In 2008, the medial boundary of the common carotid was accepted by the AHNS as an alternate landmark to the sternohyoid muscle.[12]

The common carotid, with rare exceptions, is devoid of branches and bifurcates, in most instances, superior to the inferior aspect of the hyoid in level IIA. The IJV, which lies lateral to the artery within the carotid sheath, has the superior and middle thyroid vein as its only major tributaries at this level. The thyroid veins cross anterior to the common carotid. The vagus

nerve is found posterior to the carotid artery and IJV within the carotid sheath. In this location, the anterior aspect of the carotid sheath is draped by the ansa cervicalis, which innervates the strap muscles immediately adjacent to it. The lymphatics of the midjugular chain include the jugulo-omohyoid node, located immediately superior to the superior belly of the omohyoid, near its junction at the superficial of the carotid sheath.

The superficial boundary of level III is the SLDCF, which invests the SCM. It extends medially to the MLDCF investing the lateral aspect of the sternohyoid muscle. In the superior reaches of level III, near the hyoid bone, the carotid has a more superficial course emerging from behind the medial aspect of the SCM, immediately deep to the SLDCF (▶ Fig. 3.12).

The floor of level III is formed by the DLDCF. The muscles deep to the fascial floor of level III are the anterior scalene, lateral to the transverse process of the cervical spine, and the longus muscles medial to this structure (▶ Fig. 3.8, ▶ Fig. 3.18). To better understand the contents surrounding the floor of level III, it is helpful to know which cervical vertebrae are likely to be present deep to this level. Using superficial radiographically identifiable landmarks like those used in delineating cervical level boundaries, Shen et al have made critical correlations to deeper structures based on radiographic data from 108 patients in consistent anatomical position. Using the plane of the superior thyroid cartilage, which approximates the inferior hyoid bone, and therefore the superior plane of level III, the authors determined that in more than 90% of cases this fell in the C4–C5 level. The carotid bifurcated greater than 1 cm above the level of this plane in 81.5% of cases, and therefore in the inferior aspect of level IIA. The inferior cricoid plane, which delineates the inferior boundary of level III, was most commonly at C7 (41.5%) ranging from C5 to T1.[16] It is worthwhile noting that the reported location of the

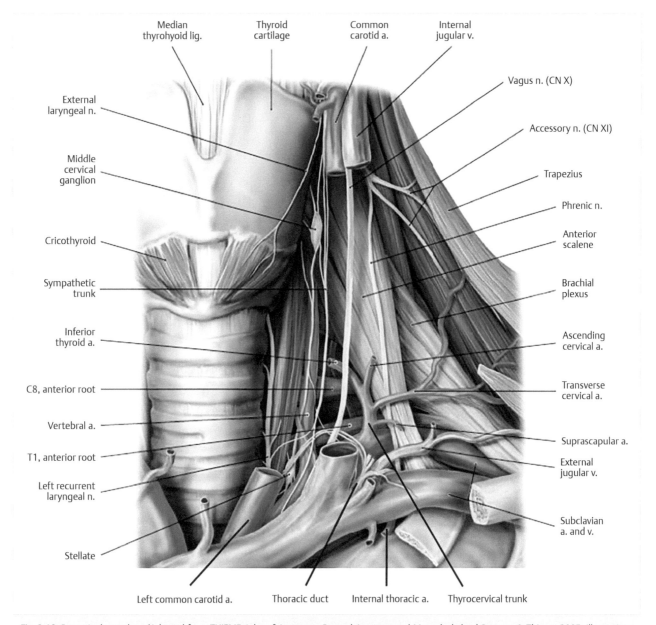

Median
thyrohyoid lig.

Thyroid
cartilage

Common
carotid a.

Internal
jugular v.

External
laryngeal n.

Vagus n. (CN X)

Accessory n. (CN XI)

Middle
cervical
ganglion

Trapezius

Phrenic n.

Cricothyroid

Anterior
scalene

Sympathetic
trunk

Brachial
plexus

Inferior
thyroid a.

Ascending
cervical a.

C8, anterior root

Transverse
cervical a.

Vertebral a.

T1, anterior root

Suprascapular a.

External
jugular v.

Left recurrent
laryngeal n.

Subclavian
a. and v.

Stellate

Left common carotid a.   Thoracic duct   Internal thoracic a.   Thyrocervical trunk

Fig. 3.18 Paraspinal muscles. (Adapted from THIEME Atlas of Anatomy: General Anatomy and Musculoskeletal System. © Thieme 2005. Illustrations by Karl Wesker.)

carotid bifurcation has been quite variable, with other prominent sources siting its location to be at the plane of the upper thyroid cartilage in the plane C3–C4 disc space.[14]

Based on these data, the contents of the floor of level III are estimated to be related to C4–C7. The critical structure deep to the floor of the neck below the DLDCF would be the phrenic nerve, over the anterior scalene posterior lateral to the carotid sheath. The sympathetic trunk is also found in the floor of the neck posteromedial to the carotid sheath. The sympathetic trunk is generally found on the DLDCF covering the longus muscles; however, this can be variable, with some sources describing it deep to the fascia, and yet others reporting it within the carotid sheath.[21] It takes a more medial course near the anterior tubercle of C6, which is recognized as the most prominent tubercle in the neck, and as previously mentioned, the

level at which the vertebral artery enters the transvers foramina. In 30 cadaver dissections, the sympathetic trunk was found just over 1 cm lateral to the medial border of the longus colli muscle at C6.[21] In the same study, the intermediate ganglia of the sympathetic trunk was found most commonly in the C5–C6 level. The critical structures found in proximity to C6, and discussed in detail in the preceding section on level IV, should be kept in mind when dissecting deep in the floor of level III.

3.3.5 Level II

The upper jugular chain lymph nodes are contained in level II, which extends from the skull base inferiorly to the plane of the inferior aspect of the hyoid bone (▶ Fig. 3.2). Its anterior margin is the stylohyoid muscle, or radiographically the vertical plane

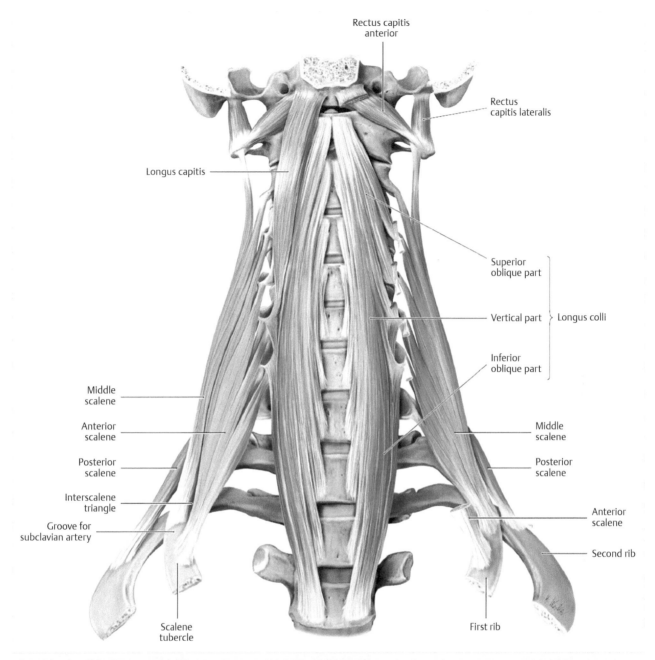

Fig. 3.19 Root of the neck. (Adapted from THIEME Atlas of Anatomy: General Anatomy and Musculoskeletal System. © Thieme 2005. Illustrations by Karl Wesker.)

posterior to the SMG, which was formally accepted by the AHNS as the anterior boundary in 2008.[3,12] Posteriorly, as with other lateral neck levels, the posterior border of the SCM demarcates this level from level V. Level II is further divided into sublevels IIA and IIB, with the latter being superior and posterior to the oblique plane of the SAN (CN XI). The floor of level II is formed by the DLDCF covering the paraspinal muscles including the superior extent of the anterior and middle scalene, splenius capitis, and the superior portion of the levator scapulae near its insertion on the lateral process of C1, which is a prominent palpable landmark. The SAN traverses superficial to the levator scapulae throughout its course in the neck. Anteriorly, the floor is formed by the buccopharyngeal fascia covering the middle pharyngeal

constrictor as well as muscular fascia over the posterior inferior hyoglossus muscle (▶ Fig. 3.8). The roof of level II is the SLDCF.

Arterial Anatomy

External Carotid System (Netter's Plate 30, 65)[5]

The ECA originates at the carotid bifurcation. As discussed previously, this is thought to occur within level IIA in the majority of cases based on radiographic data.[16] After bifurcating from the common carotid, the ECA is initially found anterior and medial to the internal carotid. As it ascends with the internal carotid, it takes a gentle spiraling course to an anterior and then lateral position relative to the internal carotid. The ECA exits

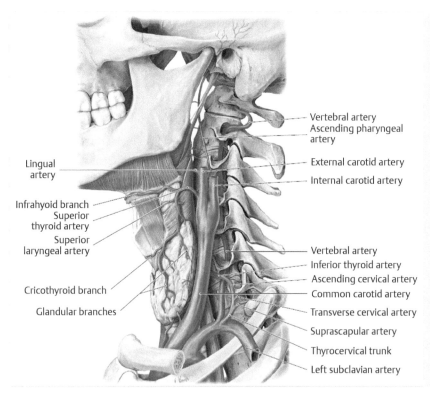

Fig. 3.20 Arterial anatomy of the root of the neck. (Adapted from THIEME Atlas of Anatomy: General Anatomy and Musculoskeletal System. © Thieme 2005. Illustrations by Karl Wesker.)

level IIA midway between the styloid process and the angle of the mandible as it courses deep to the stylohyoid and closely associated posterior digastric muscle. It is located lateral to the more superior stylopharyngeus and styloglossus muscles, and stylohyoid ligament, which separates the external carotid from the internal carotid, which lies medial to these styloid based structures (▶ Fig. 3.8).[14]

Reflecting on the embryology of the branchial apparatus provides a road map to critical relationships within level IIA. The third arch derivatives include the common and proximal internal carotid, the glossopharyngeal nerve, and the stylopharyngeus muscle. The styloid process and stylopharyngeus muscle, as well as the glossopharyngeal nerve, cross the immediate lateral surface of their third arch artery, the internal carotid, and intervene between it and the more lateral ECA.

Our discussion of ECA anatomy will be limited to branches found inferior to the stylohyoid muscle. Superior to this the artery enters the deep lobe of the parotid and travels superiorly in the parapharyngeal space before terminally branching into the internal maxillary and superficial temporal arteries. We will categorize ECA branches based on the orientation of branching: anterior, posterior, or medial.

The anterior branches found in level IIA include the superior thyroid, lingual, and facial arteries, which typically branch from the ECA in that order (▶ Fig. 3.21). The superior thyroid artery (STA) is the first branch of the external carotid. After branching from the anterior surface of the ECA, near the carotid bifurcation, it descends toward the superior pole of the ipsilateral thyroid lobe paralleling the lateral surface of the thyrohyoid muscle. In very rare cases, it may branch from the ECA as a common trunk with the lingual artery.[22] The STA has one branch of limited clinical significance in the lateral neck, the SCM artery, which transverses the carotid sheath laterally to

perfuse the midportion of the SCM. Beyond this, the STA is a central neck structure that has a critical relationship with the superior laryngeal nerve, and will be discussed further in level VI anatomy.[14]

The lingual artery is found above the STA, branching anteriorly from the ECA in proximity to the greater cornu of the hyoid[14] (▶ Fig. 3.12). As its name suggests, it provides the major blood supply to the tongue. According to data from 41 cadavers, the location of lingual artery branching is approximately 1 cm above the carotid bifurcation. In approximately 80% of cases, the artery arises an independent branch, while in approximately 20% of cases the artery arises as a common trunk, known as the linguofacial trunk with the facial artery (▶ Fig. 3.21). In such cases, the trunk has an average length of less than 1 cm prior to bifurcating into its respective arteries.[23] It has also been described in rare cases arising with the STA (thyrolingual trunk) or as a common trunk with all three vessels (thyrolingual facial trunk). After branching, the artery has an initially ascending course with an anterior and medial trajectory before descending parallel to the hyoid. The middle pharyngeal constrictor is found immediately deep to the artery at this level. The artery is more superficial in its initial trajectory through level IIA, on its path deep to level IB where it courses medial to the hyoglossus muscle. Rare variations have been described with the artery coursing lateral to the hyoglossus muscle.[24] The lingual artery is crossed laterally, in level IIA—at its most superior point—by the HN, which courses lateral to the external and internal carotid, and medial to the IJV and branches of the facial artery.[14]

The facial artery is the most superior of the anterior branches of the ECA in level IIA, and as described, has a variable pattern of origin not infrequently occurring from a common trunk particularly with the lingual artery. The artery is usually found immediately

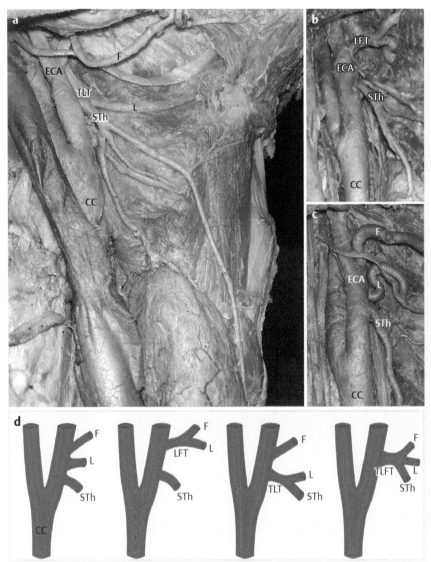

Fig. 3.21 Anterior branches of the external carotid artery. **(a)** Thyrolingual, **(b)** linguofacial, **(c)** separate branching pattern, **(d)** and a representation of various branching patterns. CC, common carotid artery; ECA, external carotid artery; F, facial artery; L, lingual artery; LFT, linguofacial trunk; TLFT, thyrolinguofacial trunk; TLT, thyrolingual trunk; STh, superior thyroid artery. (Reproduced with permission of Watanabe K, Shoja MM, Loukas M, Tubbs RS, eds. Anatomy of Plastic Surgery of the Face, Head, and Neck. 1st ed. New York, NY: Theime; 2016.)

above the superior cornu of the hyoid, although the distance from the carotid bifurcation can be quite variable (8–50 mm).[14,25] Like the lingual, the facial artery is superficial in level IIA, immediately deep to platysma and SLDCF and anterior to the SMC in the carotid triangle (▶ Fig. 3.12). It takes an anterosuperior course deep to the stylohyoid and posterior digastric muscle, entering level IB. On its deep surface is the middle pharyngeal constrictor, and on the lateral surface the HN. There are two branches of the facial artery, each with a vertical trajectory in this level: the ascending palatine and tonsillar arteries.

The ascending pharyngeal artery is the lone medial branch of the ECA arising from its deep surface (▶ Fig. 3.20). It originates near the STA close to the carotid bifurcation. It has a vertical trajectory and a deep course medial to the internal carotid and the stylopharyngeus and styloglossus muscles, supplying deep neuromuscular structures on its course to the skull base.[14]

The only posterior branch of the ECA within level IIA is the occipital artery (▶ Fig. 3.22).[5] The occipital artery branches from the ECA and courses posterosuperiorly, lateral to the contents of the carotid sheath and following the deep surface of the digastric muscle. Near its origin, it is crossed laterally by the HN. It courses

between the lateral process of C1 inferiorly and the mastoid process superiorly, exiting level IIB deep to the SCM and digastric muscles. Its two major branches are to the SCM. The superior branch follows the SAN.[14] The relationship between the superior branch and the accessory nerve was investigated by Rafferty et al in 33 neck dissections. The branch was consistently located inferior and lateral to the entry point of the nerve into the medial SCM with an average of 6.2 mm (1- to 11-mm range).[26]

The Internal Carotid

The internal carotid has a vertical trajectory from the carotid bifurcation to the skull base, except for rare cases in which it may take a medial and retropharyngeal course. It does not contribute branches in the neck. Many of the critical relationships of the internal carotid have been previously discussed. It leaves the carotid triangle deep to the digastric, and exits level IIA deep to the styloid process and its associated muscles: the stylohyoid, styloglossus, and stylopharyngeus. At its lateral surface is the IJV and vagus nerve more posteriorly. As the skull base is approached, the IJV takes a more posterior position with neural structures intervening

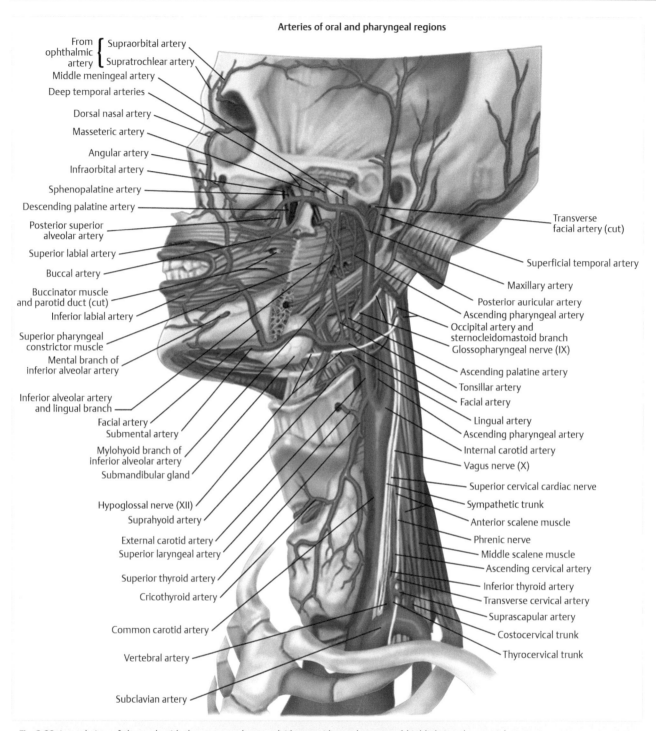

Arteries of oral and pharyngeal regions

From ophthalmic artery { Supraorbital artery / Supratrochlear artery
Middle meningeal artery
Deep temporal arteries
Dorsal nasal artery
Masseteric artery
Angular artery
Infraorbital artery
Sphenopalatine artery
Descending palatine artery
Posterior superior alveolar artery
Superior labial artery
Buccal artery
Buccinator muscle and parotid duct (cut)
Inferior labial artery
Superior pharyngeal constrictor muscle
Mental branch of inferior alveolar artery
Inferior alveolar artery and lingual branch
Facial artery
Submental artery
Mylohyoid branch of inferior alveolar artery
Submandibular gland
Hypoglossal nerve (XII)
Suprahyoid artery
External carotid artery
Superior laryngeal artery
Superior thyroid artery
Cricothyroid artery
Common carotid artery
Vertebral artery
Subclavian artery

Transverse facial artery (cut)
Superficial temporal artery
Maxillary artery
Posterior auricular artery
Ascending pharyngeal artery
Occipital artery and sternocleidomastoid branch
Glossopharyngeal nerve (IX)
Ascending palatine artery
Tonsillar artery
Facial artery
Lingual artery
Ascending pharyngeal artery
Internal carotid artery
Vagus nerve (X)
Superior cervical cardiac nerve
Sympathetic trunk
Anterior scalene muscle
Phrenic nerve
Middle scalene muscle
Ascending cervical artery
Inferior thyroid artery
Transverse cervical artery
Suprascapular artery
Costocervical trunk
Thyrocervical trunk

Fig. 3.22 Lateral view of the neck with the straps and sternocleidomastoid muscle removed highlighting the arterial system.

between the great vessels (CN IX–XII). It is bordered medially by the middle and superior pharyngeal constrictors, with the superior laryngeal nerve coursing between (▶ Fig. 3.22).[5] Posteriorly is the longus capitis muscle and the transverse processes of the upper cervical vertebrae, and as has been the case throughout the neck, the sympathetic chain can be found in this space between the deep fascial and the posterior surface of the artery. As the artery courses superiorly, it is crossed laterally in sequence by the lingual and facial veins, the HN (which contributes the superior root of the ansa in this location), the digastric muscle,

occipital artery, the glossopharyngeal nerve, the stylohyoid muscle, and the styloid process.

The Venous System of Level II

The IJV leaves the skull base as a continuation of the sigmoid sinus and jugular bulb, and it is found in the posterior aspect of the jugular foramen known as the pars vascularis (▶ Fig. 3.23). The IJV is closely associated with CNs IX through XI exiting the foramen as will be discussed in the following section. The IJV is

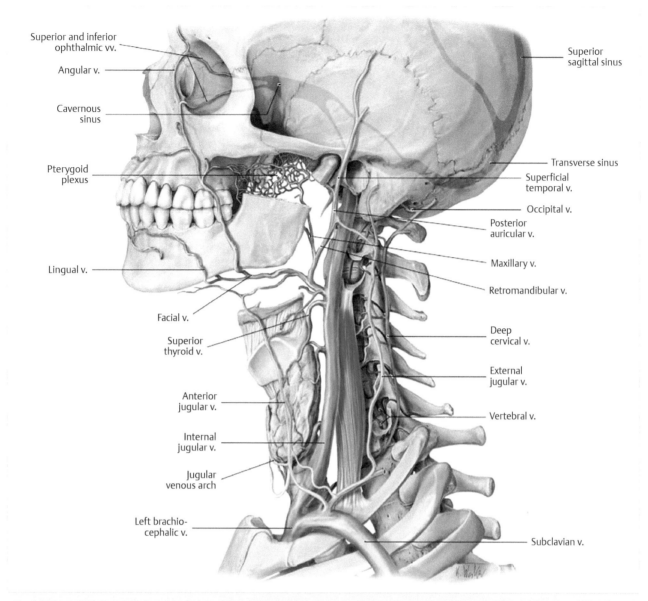

Fig. 3.23 Venous drainage of the neck. (Adapted from THIEME Atlas of Anatomy: General Anatomy and Musculoskeletal System. © Thieme 2005. Illustrations by Karl Wesker.)

found posterior to the internal carotid at the skull base, but assumes a lateral position in the carotid sheath as it descends. The IJV exits the skull base deep and posterior to the styloid and its associated muscles. In level II, it is crossed on its lateral surface in descending order by CN XI (this is a variable relationship), the occipital artery with its SCM branches, the digastric muscle, and the ansa cervicalis (▶ Fig. 3.13).[5] Medial to the vein, at this level, is the transverse processes of the upper cervical vertebra, the paraspinal muscles (splenius capitis, levator scapulae, and anterior and middle scalene muscles) with associated DLDCF, and the cervical plexus.

The major tributaries of the IJV include the superior thyroid and lingual and facial veins. The location of the confluence of these vessels with the IJV can be approximated by the greater cornu of the hyoid (▶ Fig. 3.23).[14] The distal lingual and facial veins were discussed in more detail with level IB, and the superior thyroid will be discussed with level VI. The facial vein

enters level IIA superficial to the digastric muscle traveling in a posterior trajectory. It is soon joined by the anterior division of the retromandibular vein, which descends through the parotid to enter level IIA traveling in the same plane as the facial vein (▶ Fig. 3.12). This confluence forms the common facial vein. The common facial vein is superficial to the HN, lingual artery, and external and internal carotid arteries on its posteroinferior course to the IJV.[14] The lingual vein enters level IIA in plane with the lingual artery, deep in the hyoglossus muscle traveling superficially in plane with the facial vein to confluence in the IJV. Additional venous drainage from the deep and sublingual territories coalesces to form the vena comitans of the HN, which also terminates into the IJV directly or indirectly (▶ Fig. 3.13).[5]

In 58 unilateral cadaver dissections, Shima et al described 5 variations in the pattern of confluence of the 3 major venous tributaries (facial, lingual and superior thyroid) with the IJV.

The thyrolinguofacial type, with all three vessels merging as a common trunk, was seen in 46.6% of dissections, followed by the linguofacial type in which the lingual and facial entered as a common trunk with the superior thyroid entering separately in 22.4% of dissections (▶ Fig. 3.23). In the least common variant (6.9%), the lingual and superior thyroid entered as a common trunk below the facial. In the remaining 24.1% of specimens, there were lingual and superior thyroid tributaries without a facial vein contribution to the IJV, but no further mention was made regarding the whereabouts of the facial drainage.[27] It is interesting to note that in a series of 178 unilateral cadaver dissections, 9% of facial veins drained superficially, directly into the EJV and did not pierce the SLDCF which could explain the finding from the above series. In these cases, the EJV was formed by the retromandibular vein, which did not divide into anterior and posterior divisions, joining the posterior auricular vein. The various branching patterns with the facial vein are described in detail by Gupta et al.[28]

Neural Anatomy of Level II

Taken in numerical order, we will discuss CN IX–XII, the sympathetic chain and pertinent branches of each. CN IX (glossopharyngeal nerve) exits the skull base in the pars nervosa of the jugular foramen anterior to the IJV, interposed between the internal carotid artery and the IJV. This is the common foramen for CN IX–XI with CN X and XI found just posterior to CN IX and associated with the medial wall of the IJV (pars vascularis). From here, CN IX descends medial to the styloid process and its associated muscles along the posterior border of the stylopharyngeus, which is the only muscle it innervates (▶ Fig. 3.15).[14] As mentioned, embryologically it is a third arch derivative, and as is courses along the stylopharyngeus it curves anteriorly along its lateral surface, and travels toward the superior constrictor dividing the internal and external carotid as does the stylopharyngeus. As the nerve continues anteriorly, it travels deep into the stylohyoid muscle and out of level IIA into the parapharyngeal space (▶ Fig. 3.24).[5]

CN X (vagus nerve) descends in the carotid sheath, between the carotid and IJV, as in lower levels in the neck. It originates from the medial aspect of the jugular foramen. It is medial to the styloid process, and may be found in a plane between the styloid anteriorly and the transverse process of C1 posteriorly, in close association with CN IX to XII near the skull base. There are two enlargements in this level of the vagus, the superior and larger inferior (nodose) ganglia, which contain cell bodies for sensory fibers.[14] The superior ganglia lie at the level of the jugular foramen, and the nodose lies just below it. The superior laryngeal nerve is a major branch from the vagus and originates at the inferior ganglia. It descends medial to the internal carotid, and lateral to the middle pharyngeal constrictor as it travels anteroinferiorly. It divides into internal and external branches near the medial aspect of the external carotid, as it continues its descent.[29] The anatomy of these terminal branches will be discussed with level VI.

CN XI (SAN) has a complicated intracranial origin with both cranial and spinal roots. For the purposes of level II neck anatomy, the main interest lies with the spinal root, as the cranial root joins the vagus nerve near the skull base above the inferior ganglion. The spinal root continues to provide motor innervation to the SCM and TPZ, and is the structure identified during neck dissection. The SAN descends from the jugular foramen near the medial wall of the IJV, deep and posterior to the plane of the styloid. It travels in a posterior and lateral trajectory with a variable relationship to the IJV, which it crosses near the superior border of the digastric (▶ Fig. 3.8). The literature is surprisingly varied on this topic, with the nerve most commonly reported lateral to the IJV (39.8–96%).[30,31] In very rare cases (< 3%), the nerve may pierce the artery. The nerve has a consistent relationship with the superior branch of the occipital artery, which is found inferior and lateral to the SAN. The occipital artery continues after the division of its superior branch to cross lateral to the nerve.

The SAN nerve traverses the contents of the lateral neck dividing the posterosuperior contents into level IIB and the anteroinferior contents into level IIA. Deep to the nerve, and below the DLDCF, is the levator scapulae muscle that the nerve travels superficial to through its course in levels II and V. The SAN is associated with the anteromedial surface of the SCM in its upper third. The nerve has been classified by Shiozaki et al as having three anatomical variants (types A, B, and C) at the SCM: not penetrating, partially penetrating, and completely penetrating, respectively.[32] The nonpenetrating variant (A) is less common than the combined penetrating subtypes (B + C), but have been observed as frequently as 45.9% in one series.[30] The cervical plexus has variable contributions to the SAN from the C2-C3 level, joining the nerve within the substance of the SCM. From the lateral margin of the SCM, the nerve enters level V and will be discussed later.

CN XII (HN) originates from the hypoglossal canal medial and anterior to the jugular foramen. In its descent, it initially courses laterally and is found posterior to the internal carotid and CN IX and is closely associated with the inferior vagal ganglia. From here, it assumes a vertical trajectory between the IJV and internal carotid.[14] At a location approximated by the vertical plane of the mandibular angle, the HN curves anteriorly to assume a horizontal trajectory, and in doing so it courses between the IJV laterally and the internal carotid medially. It is in this location that the ansa hypoglossi divides and descends along the internal carotid. In 46 cadaver dissections, this point was on average 2.8 cm posterior to the angle of the mandible. The HN passed superiorly above the carotid bifurcation at an average of 15 mm.[29] As the nerve coursed lateral to the external carotid, it crossed over the lingual artery in 72% of the cases, and it was inferior to its origin in the remaining 28%. The nerve continues anteriorly, superior to the hyoid, to enter level IB medial to the digastric and stylohyoid, and lateral to the hyoglossus muscles (▶ Fig. 3.8). The HN has a consistent relationship with the posterior course of the occipital artery, which courses lateral to the vertical segment of the nerve.[29]

The cervical sympathetic chain (CSC) has been discussed in lower levels of the neck, and its position is consistent at this level, medial to the carotid sheath and in close relationship with the DLDCF associated with the longus muscles, specifically the longus capitis. The superior cervical ganglia is the largest of the ganglia, and readily identified in the C2–C4 level (▶ Fig. 3.8).[21] From this ganglia, postganglionic fibers are distributed broadly throughout the head and neck as well as intracranially via the carotid.[14] Injury to the nerve produces Horner's syndrome with the triad of ipsilateral ptosis, miosis, and anhidrosis.

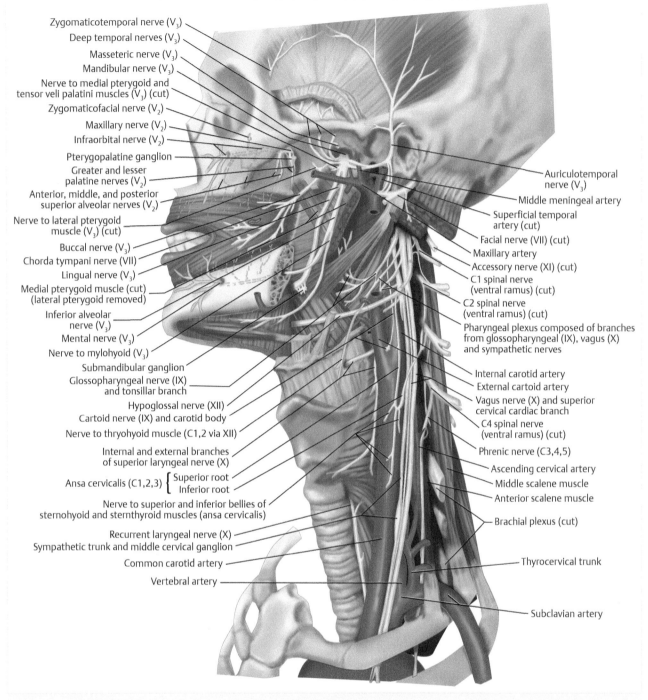

Zygomaticotemporal nerve (V₃)
Deep temporal nerves (V₃)
Masseteric nerve (V₃)
Mandibular nerve (V₃)
Nerve to medial pterygoid and
tensor veli palatini muscles (V₃) (cut)
Zygomaticofacial nerve (V₂)
Maxillary nerve (V₂)
Infraorbital nerve (V₂)
Pterygopalatine ganglion
Greater and lesser
palatine nerves (V₂)
Anterior, middle, and posterior
superior alveolar nerves (V₂)
Nerve to lateral pterygoid
muscle (V₃) (cut)
Buccal nerve (V₃)
Chorda tympani nerve (VII)
Lingual nerve (V₃)
Medial pterygoid muscle (cut)
(lateral pterygoid removed)
Inferior alveolar
nerve (V₃)
Mental nerve (V₃)
Nerve to mylohyoid (V₃)
Submandibular ganglion
Glossopharyngeal nerve (IX)
and tonsillar branch
Hypoglossal nerve (XII)
Cartoid nerve (IX) and carotid body
Nerve to thryohyoid muscle (C1,2 via XII)
Internal and external branches
of superior laryngeal nerve (X)
Ansa cervicalis (C1,2,3) { Superior root
                          Inferior root
Nerve to superior and inferior bellies of
sternohyoid and sternthyroid muscles (ansa cervicalis)
Recurrent laryngeal nerve (X)
Sympathetic trunk and middle cervical ganglion
Common carotid artery
Vertebral artery

Auriculotemporal
nerve (V₃)
Middle meningeal artery
Superficial temporal
artery (cut)
Facial nerve (VII) (cut)
Maxillary artery
Accessory nerve (XI) (cut)
C1 spinal nerve
(ventral ramus) (cut)
C2 spinal nerve
(ventral ramus) (cut)
Pharyngeal plexus composed of branches
from glossopharyngeal (IX), vagus (X)
and sympathetic nerves
Internal carotid artery
External cartoid artery
Vagus nerve (X) and superior
cervical cardiac branch
C4 spinal nerve
(ventral ramus) (cut)
Phrenic nerve (C3,4,5)
Ascending cervical artery
Middle scalene muscle
Anterior scalene muscle
Brachial plexus (cut)
Thyrocervical trunk
Subclavian artery

Fig. 3.24 Lateral view of the neck with the straps and sternocleidomastoid muscle removed highlighting the neural and arterial anatomy.

3.3.6 Level V: The Posterior Triangle

Otherwise referred to as the posterior neck or posterior triangle, level V boundaries are as follows: the posterior SCM border and cervical plexus sensory branches anteriorly, the anterior border of the TPZ posteriorly, the junction of the SCM and TPZ superiorly, and the clavicle inferiorly. This level is further subdivided into VA and VB by an imaginary plane extending from the inferior border of the cricoid, which also demarcates levels III from IV.

The contents of level V are bound superficially by the SLDCF—or investing fascia—which invests the SCM and TPZ muscles (▶ Fig. 3.25). This layer is immediately deep to the platysma, which is present superficially to the inferior aspect of level V (▶ Fig. 3.4). The SLDCF is more poorly defined over the posterior triangle than anterior to the SCM, and is described as an areolar layer in this location in *Gray's Anatomy*.[1] The deep boundary of level V is the DLDCF, which covers the surface of the paraspinal muscles making up the floor of this level (▶ Fig. 3.17).[5] This includes from superior to inferior the splenius capitis, levator

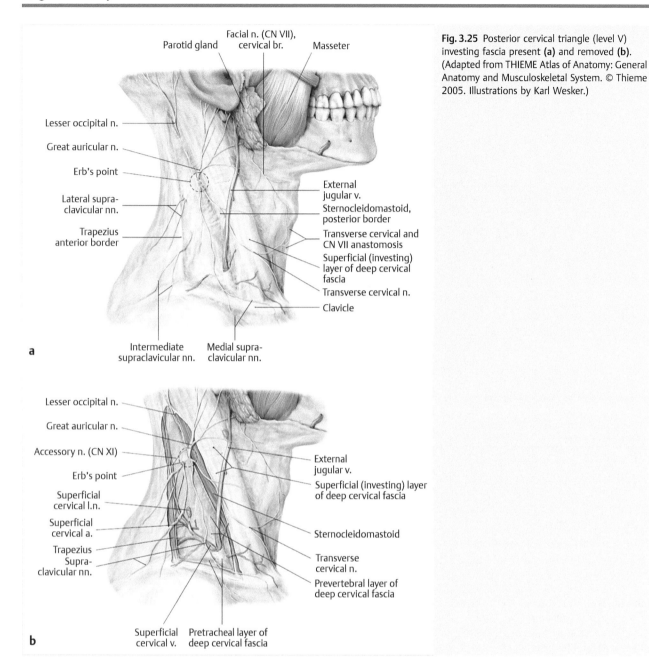

Fig. 3.25 Posterior cervical triangle (level V) investing fascia present **(a)** and removed **(b)**. (Adapted from THIEME Atlas of Anatomy: General Anatomy and Musculoskeletal System. © Thieme 2005. Illustrations by Karl Wesker.)

scapulae, and the middle and anterior scalene muscles (▶ Fig. 3.26).

Critical structures that traverse level V will be discussed from superior to inferior. The SAN previously discussed in level II is of high importance in level V, as it has a superficial course and is particularly prone to injury. It travels across level V in a posterior inferior trajectory superficial to the levator scapulae in the fibrofatty tissue of level V. It can be found entering level V at the posterior border of the SCM. In 50 ipsilateral dissections, this point was found 6.13 cm below the mastoid tip, near the junction of the upper and middle third of the SCM.[33] In a series of 80 ipsilateral dissections, the relationship of the SAN was found to be consistently superior to the nerve point (also referred to as Erb's point). The nerve point signifies the location of emerging superficial sensory branches of the cervical plexus near the midpoint of the SCM, and includes from superior to

inferior the lesser occipital, great auricular, transverse cervical, and supraclavicular nerves (▶ Fig. 3.25). The SAN was found within 2 cm superior to this point and at an average of 0.97 cm from it. This relationship has been supported by numerous authors, and is perhaps the most consistent means of locating CN XI in the posterior triangle.[34]

After traversing level V, CN XI reaches the anterior border of the TPZ and innervates the muscle on its deep surface. This point on the TPZ is approximately 4 cm from the clavicle.[1,33] CN XI frequently branches prior to reaching the TPZ, with up to five branches reported, with the majority having fewer than three (▶ Fig. 3.19).[32,33]

The TCA, also known as the superficial cervical artery, has a variable origin, but most commonly branches from the TCT, which originates from the first part of the subclavian artery in the base of level IV. The TCA has a posterolateral trajectory after

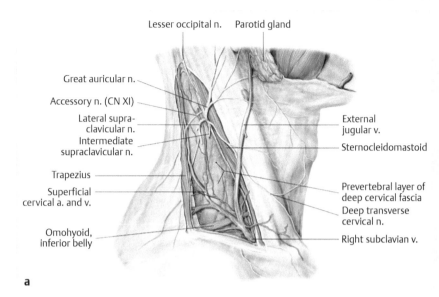

Lesser occipital n.   Parotid gland

Great auricular n.

Accessory n. (CN XI)

Lateral supra-
clavicular n.
Intermediate
supraclavicular n.

Trapezius

Superficial
cervical a. and v.

Omohyoid,
inferior belly

External
jugular v.

Sternocleidomastoid

Prevertebral layer of
deep cervical fascia
Deep transverse
cervical n.

Right subclavian v.

a

Fig. 3.26 Posterior cervical triangle (level V) muscular pretracheal fascia or middle layer of the deep cervical fascia removed (a) and prevertebral or deep layer of the deep cervical fascia removed (b). (Adapted from THIEME Atlas of Anatomy: General Anatomy and Musculoskeletal System. © Thieme 2005. Illustrations by Karl Wesker.)

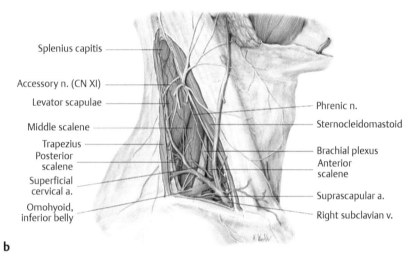

Splenius capitis

Accessory n. (CN XI)

Levator scapulae

Middle scalene

Trapezius
Posterior
scalene

Superficial
cervical a.

Omohyoid,
inferior belly

Phrenic n.

Sternocleidomastoid

Brachial plexus
Anterior
scalene

Suprascapular a.

Right subclavian v.

b

entering level V, at a point approximated by the lateral border of the anterior scalene (▶ Fig. 3.26). It is located within the fibrofatty tissue, superficial to the deep fascia and muscular floor of the neck and brachial plexus, and courses deep to the omohyoid and TPZ. The TCA can be found approximately 2 cm superior to the clavicle and is found paralleling the traverse cervical vein in a deep and superior plane. The vein drains into either the EJV or the subclavian vein, and has a variable course relative to the omohyoid with a deep position predominating (75%).[35]

The posterior belly of the omohyoid muscle is a prominent structure low in level V (▶ Fig. 3.26). It travels through the fibrofatty tissue of the level in a posteroinferior trajectory toward the scapular notch, in a plane superficial to the TCA. It runs superficial to the deep fascia covering the brachial plexus and muscular floor of the neck, and deep to the TPZ, and is covered by muscular pretracheal fascia.

The brachial plexus is derived from the ventral rami of C5–T1, and supplies motor and sensory innervation to the upper limb. It is found in the anterior-inferior-posterior triangle between with anterior and middle scalene and remains covered by deep fascia, forming the axillary sheath. It is associated with the third part of the subclavian artery, which emerges posterior to the lateral border

of the anterior scalene (▶ Fig. 3.26). The branchial plexus exits the posterior triangle in a plane posterior to the artery. The subclavian artery may extend partially above the clavicle, and can be up to 4 cm above the clavicle in the inferomedial aspect of level V, near the lateral border of the SCM.[1] The subclavian vein is anterior and inferior to the artery, and may also extend into the supraclavicular fossa and into the base of level V.

The suprascapular artery is mentioned because it may be encountered in the inferior reaches of level V, originating from the TCT in approximately 50% of cases, with the remaining cases originating from the subclavian or internal thoracic artery. It shares a common destination with the omohyoid, the suprascapular notch. It enters level V crossing anterior scalene, approximated by the lateral border of the SCM, and travels laterally parallel to the clavicle, superficial to the subclavian artery and brachial plexus (▶ Fig. 3.26).[1,15]

The dorsal scapular artery is found in the inferior aspect of level V, originating from the TCT in 76% of cases, with 16% of these cases arising as a common trunk with the TCA in a series of nearly 500 dissections. In most remaining cases, the origin was more lateral as a trunk from the third part of the subclavian artery. The dorsal scapular artery may pass either through the brachial plexus or superficial to it, as it courses posterolaterally toward the superior angle of the scapula, deep to the levator scapulae muscle.[15]

3.3.7 Level VI: The Central Neck

The boundaries of the central neck extend vertically from the hyoid bone to the sternal notch, and laterally to the common carotid arteries. The roof of level VI is formed by the muscular fascia investing the strap muscles, referred to as the MLDCF or muscular pretracheal fascia. The floor is formed by the DLDCF. The visceral structures enveloped by the fine visceral facial layer are critical to the intricate anatomy of the central neck, and include the laryngotracheal complex, hypopharynx, esophagus, thyroid, and parathyroid glands. We will discuss anatomy pertinent to central neck dissection for each of these structures in addition to discussing the neurovascular and muscular anatomy of level VI.

The laryngotracheal complex and hyoid form the central ridged framework of level VI anatomy (▸ Fig. 3.27). The hyoid bone is near the C3–C4 level and separates level I superiorly from level VI inferiorly.[1,16] It is a U-shaped bone with a central rectangular body attached laterally to the greater cornu bilaterally (▸ Fig. 3.28). Near this typically ossified junction is small superior projection, the lesser cornu. The hyoid is suspended superiorly by multiple muscles (▸ Fig. 3.15, ▸ Fig. 3.29). Those inserting into the body include the geniohyoid and mylohyoid. Near the junction of the body and greater cornu are the stylohyoid and digastric tendon, and along the length of the greater cornu is the hyoglossus. The lesser cornu is the insertion of the stylohyoid ligament.[1]

The middle pharyngeal constrictor is a fan-shaped muscle that attaches to the lesser cornu, and the upper aspect of the greater cornu of the hyoid (▸ Fig. 3.30).[5] Its transverse and inferior oblique fibers, which project deep to the inferior constrictor muscle,

meet at the posterior midline raphe and are within the confines of level VI. These form the superior portion of the muscular wall of the hypopharynx. The hypopharynx serves as a conduit between the oropharynx and cervical esophagus and extends from the plane of the hyoid bone to the inferior border of the cricoid. The hypopharyngeal wall is closely associated with both the middle and inferior pharyngeal constrictors, which are covered by buccopharyngeal fascia.

The hyoid serves as the superior attachment for numerous structures (▸ Fig. 3.27, ▸ Fig. 3.29). From medial to lateral, the sternohyoid and omohyoid are found inserting into the body of the hyoid bilaterally, with the thyrohyoid attaching laterally along the greater cornu. The sternohyoid originates from the posteromedial clavicle and superior manubrium with a near vertical course to the hyoid. The superior belly of the omohyoid courses vertically, adjacent to the lateral surface of the sternohyoid. It transitions from the posterior belly (discussed in levels III and V) and is at the intermediate tendon, which is formed by a condensation of deep fascia over the IJV near the level of the cricoid cartilage. The thyrohyoid has a short vertical course attaching to the oblique line of the thyroid cartilage.[1] These muscles are covered by muscular fascia referred to previously as the MLDCF. Deep to the strap muscles in the superior central neck is the thyrohyoid membrane. This fascial layer attaches the medial aspect of the body and greater cornu of the hyoid with the superior surface of the thyroid cartilage.

The thyroid cartilage is a prominent shield-shaped structure with a superior border approximated by the C4–C5 level in close proximity to the height of the carotid bifurcation.[16] Its two laminae are joined in the midline with an intervening superior thyroid notch. On the lateral aspect of the lamina is a ridge called the *oblique line*, which connects the superior and inferior thyroid tubercles and is directed from anterior to posterior in an oblique superolateral trajectory (▸ Fig. 3.27). As

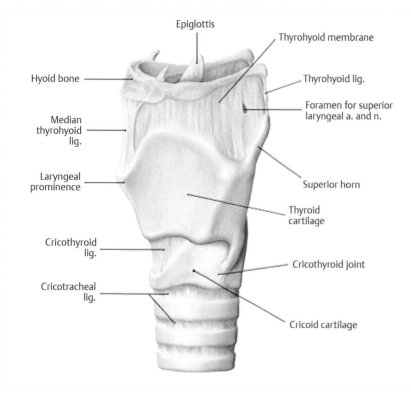

Epiglottis

Thyrohyoid membrane

Hyoid bone

Thyrohyoid lig.

Foramen for superior laryngeal a. and n.

Median thyrohyoid lig.

Laryngeal prominence

Superior horn

Thyroid cartilage

Cricothyroid lig.

Cricothyroid joint

Cricotracheal lig.

Cricoid cartilage

Fig. 3.27 Lateral view of the skeletal components for the laryngotracheal complex. (Adapted from THIEME Atlas of Anatomy: General Anatomy and Musculoskeletal System. © Thieme 2005. Illustrations by Karl Wesker.)

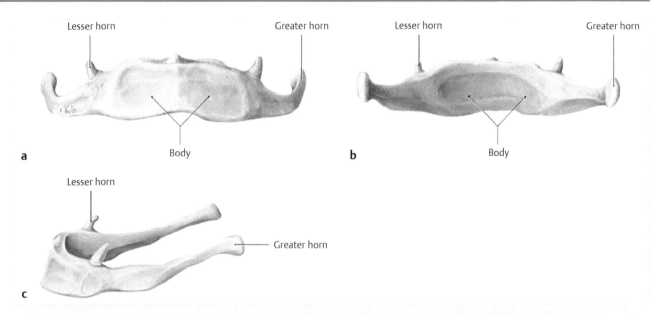

a

b

c

Fig. 3.28 Hyoid bone depicted from **(a)** anterior, **(b)** posterior, and **(c)** lateral oblique views. (Adapted from THIEME Atlas of Anatomy: General Anatomy and Musculoskeletal System. © Thieme 2005. Illustrations by Karl Wesker.)

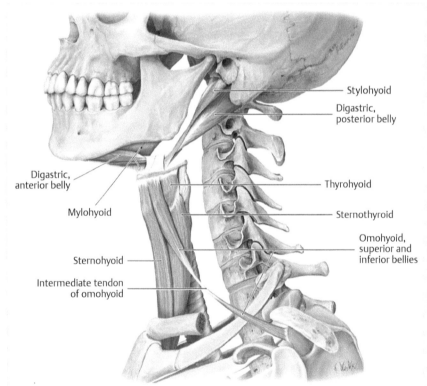

Fig. 3.29 Muscular attachments to the hyoid. (Adapted from THIEME Atlas of Anatomy: General Anatomy and Musculoskeletal System. © Thieme 2005. Illustrations by Karl Wesker.)

mentioned earlier, this is the attachment of the thyrohyoid muscle as well as its associated sternothyroid muscle, which originates from the manubrium and first rib below the sternohyoid. The *oblique line* also serves as the attachment of the thyropharyngeus, which is the upper portion of the inferior constrictor muscle, which attaches at the posterior midline raphe to the contralateral muscle. The superior and inferior cornua are located at the posterior aspect of thyroid cartilage. The superior cornu is attached to the greater cornu of the hyoid via a condensation of thyrohyoid membrane fascia. The shorter

inferior cornu articulates with the lateral aspect of the cricoid forming a synovial joint.[1]

The cricoid cartilage is found inferior to the thyroid cartilage with which it articulates. It is the only complete ring in the laryngotracheal complex (▶ Fig. 3.30).[5] The inferior plane of the cricoid is most commonly found at C7 in adults.[16] The cricoid is composed of an arch anteriorly that is narrow relative to the lamina posteriorly (▶ Fig. 3.27). The superior border is oblique, sloping superiorly to the wider posterior lamina, and the inferior border is horizontal attaching to the first tracheal ring via

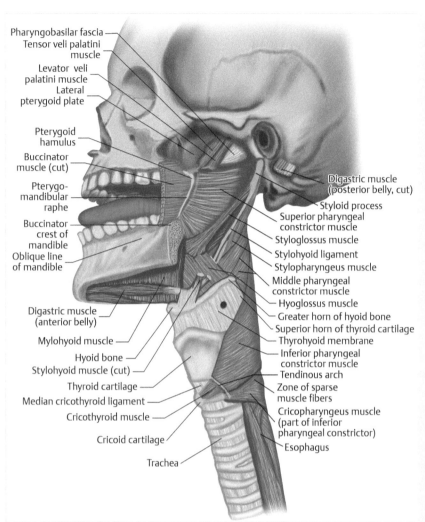

Pharyngobasilar fascia
Tensor veli palatini muscle
Levator veli palatini muscle
Lateral pterygoid plate
Pterygoid hamulus
Buccinator muscle (cut)
Pterygo-mandibular raphe
Buccinator crest of mandible
Oblique line of mandible
Digastric muscle (anterior belly)
Mylohyoid muscle
Hyoid bone
Stylohyoid muscle (cut)
Thyroid cartilage
Median cricothyroid ligament
Cricothyroid muscle
Cricoid cartilage
Trachea

Digastric muscle (posterior belly, cut)
Styloid process
Superior pharyngeal constrictor muscle
Styloglossus muscle
Stylohyoid ligament
Stylopharyngeus muscle
Middle pharyngeal constrictor muscle
Hyoglossus muscle
Greater horn of hyoid bone
Superior horn of thyroid cartilage
Thyrohyoid membrane
Inferior pharyngeal constrictor muscle
Tendinous arch
Zone of sparse muscle fibers
Cricopharyngeus muscle (part of inferior pharyngeal constrictor)
Esophagus

Fig. 3.30 Lateral view of the neck demonstrating the laryngotracheal anatomy with associated musculoskeletal structures (straps absent).

the cricotracheal ligament. The cricoid attaches to the thyroid cartilage via the previously mentioned joint, the cricothyroid ligament, the cricothyroid muscle, and the inferior constrictor muscle. The cricothyroid muscle attaches anteriorly to the arch of the cricoid, and posteriorly to the inferior tubercle and inferior cornu of the thyroid lamina. The inferior constrictor is the most robust of the constrictors, and has attachments to the thyroid (mentioned above) as well as the cricoid. There is a tendinous arch connecting the lesser thyroid tubercle and the posterior cricoid lamina that loops over the cricothyroid muscle and provides additional attachment for the thyropharyngeus, the superior contribution to the inferior constrictor. The cricopharyngeus muscle is the lower contribution to the inferior constrictor, and attaches to the cricoid arch, posterior to the cricothyroid muscle. This muscle serves as the transition between the hypopharynx and the cervical esophagus, and is the functional upper esophageal sphincter. The buccopharyngeal fascia, a thickening of epimysium, envelops the constrictor muscles. There is an intervening loose areolar space separating this fascia from the prevertebral fascia covering the vertebral bodies, and longus muscles.[1]

The esophagus and trachea continue inferiorly in the central neck before exiting posterior to the manubrium. The esophagus deviates toward the left of midline as it descends in the neck toward the superior mediastinum posterior to the trachea and anterior the prevertebral fascia.

The thyroid gland is composed of an isthmus, situated anterior to the cervical trachea approximating rings 2 through 4, and joining the right and left thyroid lobes. The lobes are roughly conical in shape, with a taped superior pole and rounded inferior pole (▶ Fig. 3.10). Medially, the thyroid lobes are related to the inferior constrictor, posterior cricothyroid muscle, larynx, trachea, esophagus, and the contents of the TE groove including the RLN. Posterolaterally, the thyroid is related to the carotid sheath and the common carotid artery. The anterior and lateral aspects of the gland are related to the deep surface of the strap muscles. These muscles include the sternohyoid medially, which joins its contralateral muscle pair at the midline linea alba (▶ Fig. 3.7). Laterally, it is associated with the sternothyroid, found deep to the omohyoid, inserting into the oblique line of the thyroid cartilage. This muscular insertion into the oblique line serves as an anterosuperior limit for the superior pole of the thyroid. The thyroid is tethered to the cricoid and upper two tracheal rings at the ligament of Berry. This is a condensation of thyroid capsule commonly referred to as the posterosuperior suspensory ligament and is responsible for the elevation of the thyroid with swallowing.

The embryology of thyroid formation results in common anatomic variations. The pyramidal lobe—a remnant of the thyroglossal tract—extends superiorly from the isthmus and can be identified in over half of patients. The tubercle of Zuckerkandl is a posterolateral projection of thyroid that may be variably positioned laterally, or rarely medial to the RLN near its laryngeal entry point. It is thought to represent a remnant of thyroid near the fusion of its median and lateral anlage. Thyroid rests may also be found below the inferior pole, with variable connection with the thyroid within the thyrothymic tract.[36]

The parathyroid glands are discrete organs located within the perithyroidal soft tissues, adjacent to the posterior thyroid capsule. They are approximately 5 mm in greatest dimension, and receive blood supply through a laterally based vascular pedicle. They are derivatives of the branchial pouches, which provide insight into their anatomical location. The superior glands originate from fourth pouch with the parafollicular C-cells, which form the lateral thyroid anlage and have a shorter path of migration relative to the inferior parathyroids. Their location is more consistent and generally found in proximity to the posterolateral aspect of the superior thyroid pole, within 1 cm of the cricothyroid joint posterior to the plane of the RLN. They are most commonly perfused by the ITA but may also receive contributions from the STA. The inferior parathyroid glands are derived from the third pouch with the thymus. It has a longer path of migration and notoriously more variable location. It is most commonly found within the loose perithyroidal fatty tissue, off the inferior or lateral aspect of the inferior thyroid pole, and superficial to the plane of the RLN. This can be highly variable with ectopic locations described from the mandible to the mediastinum. It is also perfused by the ITA.[37]

The RLN is a sixth arch derivative, branching from the vagus nerve to loop under the lowest persisting aortic arch derivative on each side (the fourth arch vessel). With the rare exception of a nonrecurrent right RLN (0.5–1%), in the case of an anomalous

right subclavian artery, the right RLN has a more lateral trajectory to the central neck as it loops under the subclavian artery, while the left RLN loops under the aortic arch below the ligamentum arteriosum (▶ Fig. 3.31). On the right, the RLN enters the central neck after passing posterior to the origin or the common carotid artery. The right RLN tends to take a more oblique course through the central neck en route to the laryngeal entry point. This distal segment of the nerve is the most anatomically consistent. The nerve enters the larynx deep to the lowest fibers of the inferior constrictor muscle posterior to the cricothyroid joint and muscle. The nerve commonly bifurcates, and rarely trifurcates prior to this point with approximately one quarter remaining unbranched.[38,39] Immediately proximal to the laryngeal entry point, the nerve is most commonly posterior to Berry's ligament but may be found within its posterior fibers.

The left RLN is more acute in trajectory than the right and can more commonly found in the TE groove. Shindo et al classified the RLN by its angle of approach in its distal segment, near the laryngeal entry point relative to the coronal plane of the TE groove, and found the majority of right nerves approach at 15 to 45 degrees, whereas left nerves approached most commonly at 0 to 30 degrees.[40] More proximally, in the midpolar location, the RLN has a close association with the ITA. The nerve is most commonly deep to the plane of the artery, but may also be found encompassed by distal branches, or less commonly anterior to the artery.[38]

The superior laryngeal nerve originates as one of the first branches of the vagus nerve at the inferior (nodose) ganglion, and its course within level II has been previously discussed (▶ Fig. 3.31). It enters the central neck after first descending posterolateral to the internal carotid, then crossing medial to

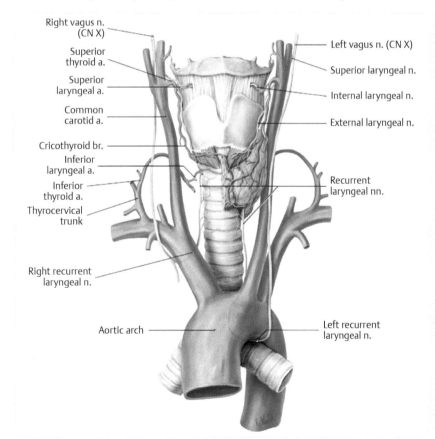

Fig. 3.31 The vagus, recurrent laryngeal, and superior laryngeal nerves depicted in relationship to vascular anatomy and visceral compartment of the neck and thorax. (Adapted from THIEME Atlas of Anatomy: General Anatomy and Musculoskeletal System. © Thieme 2005. Illustrations by Karl Wesker.)

Right vagus n. (CN X)
Superior thyroid a.
Superior laryngeal a.
Common carotid a.
Cricothyroid br.
Inferior laryngeal a.
Inferior thyroid a.
Thyrocervical trunk
Right recurrent laryngeal n.
Aortic arch

Left vagus n. (CN X)
Superior laryngeal n.
Internal laryngeal n.
External laryngeal n.
Recurrent laryngeal nn.
Left recurrent laryngeal n.

the internal and external carotid as it travels toward the larynx. It divides into external and internal branches approximately 1.5 cm inferior to the nodose ganglia.[41] This point of division is located variably in relationship to the superior pole of the thyroid, but is typically within 3 cm. The internal branch provides sensory function to the supraglottic larynx and pharynx. It travels in proximity to the superior laryngeal branch of the STA, penetrating the thyrohyoid membrane posterior to the thyrohyoid muscle after ramifying into multiple branches.[7] The external branch of the superior laryngeal nerve (EBSLN) provides the sole motor function to the cricothyroid muscle. It descends along the inferior constrictor muscle, and medial to the sternothyroid muscle, the STA, and occasionally the superior pole of the thyroid before reaching the cricothyroid muscle. The most widely used classification for this variable relationship with the superior pole of the thyroid was proposed by Cernea et al[42] and constitutes the following:

- Type 1: EBSLN crossing the STA greater than 1 cm above the plane of the superior pole.
- Type 2a: EBSLN crossing the STA less than 1 cm above the plane of the superior pole.
- Type 2b: EBSLN crossing the STA below the plane of the superior thyroid.

The frequency of each type varies within the different reports, but approximately 20% may be considered high risk for injury (type 2b) and 60% low risk (type 1).

The arterial anatomy of the central neck will be approached from superior to inferior, beginning with the STA (▸ Fig. 3.20, ▸ Fig. 3.31). Reference the section on level II anatomy for a discussion of its origin from the ECA. The STA takes an anterior and then inferior course from the ECA along the lateral aspect of the inferior constrictor muscle posterior to the thyrohyoid muscle. It has a close relationship to the superior laryngeal nerve as previously mentioned. As it approaches the superior pole of the thyroid, it arborizes into terminal branches supplying the thyroid parenchyma; the posterior branch may anastomose with the ITA supplying the superior parathyroid. The superior laryngeal artery is a larger branch of the STA that accompanies the internal branch of the superior laryngeal nerve piercing the thyrohyoid membrane.

ITA is a terminal branch of the TCT and the proximal course was discussed in level IV anatomy (▸ Fig. 3.8, ▸ Fig. 3.20, ▸ Fig. 3.31). The ITA enters the central neck deep to the internal carotid artery and sympathetic chain and superficial to the deep fascia covering the longus colli muscle. It arborizes prior to reaching the thyroid parenchyma near the midpolar level. As discussed, the artery has an intimate association with the RLN in this area. The ITA is the primary blood supply to the parathyroid glands via laterally based vascular pedicles.

The thyroid ima artery is a rare, unpaired artery, supplying the inferior pole of the thyroid and lying anterior to the trachea. It may originate for the brachiocephalic, common carotid, aortic arch, or internal thoracic artery, and is more commonly right sided. It may be associated with variable vascular anatomy including absent ITA.[43] Another consideration in midline vascular anatomy is a high riding innominate (brachiocephalic) artery, which is the first branch of the aortic arch. It is found anterior to the trachea and in rare cases may extend as high as the inferior pole of the thyroid gland.[44]

Venous drainage of the thyroid and central neck includes the superior thyroid vein, which accompanies the artery in a superior pole vascular pedicle and is a tributary to the IJV (▸ Fig. 3.10, ▸ Fig. 3.23).[5] The middle thyroid vein is unaccompanied, and drains the lateral aspect of the thyroid, traversing anterior to common carotid on its lateral course to the IJV. The inferior thyroid veins may be varied and numerous, forming a plexus below the isthmus and anterior to the trachea, draining into the brachiocephalic veins.

References

[1] Standring S. Gray's Anatomy: The Anatomical Basis of Clinical Practice. 39th ed. New York, NY: Elsevier Ltd; 2005

[2] Shah JP, Strong E, Spiro RH, Vikram B. Surgical grand rounds. Neck dissection: current status and future possibilities. Clin Bull. 1981; 11(1):25–33

[3] Society N, Surgery N. Neck dissection classification update. Head Neck. 2012; 128:751–758

[4] Natale G, Condino S, Stecco A, Soldani P, Belmonte MM, Gesi M. Is the cervical fascia an anatomical proteus? Surg Radiol Anat. 2015; 37(9):1119–1127

[5] Netter FH. Atlas of Human Anatomy. 3rd ed. Teterboro, NJ: ICON Learning Systems; 2003

[6] Hwang K, Kim JY, Lim JH. Anatomy of the platysma muscle. J Craniofac Surg. 2017; 28(2):539–542

[7] Paraskevas G, Natsis K, Ioannidis O, Kitsoulis P, Anastasopoulos N, Spyridakis I. Multiple variations of the superficial jugular veins: case report and clinical relevance. Acta Med (Hradec Kralove). 2014; 57(1):34–37

[8] Aboudib Júnior JH, de Castro CC. Anatomical variations analysis of the external jugular vein, great auricular nerve, and posterosuperior border of the platysma muscle. Aesthetic Plast Surg. 1997; 21(2):75–78

[9] Zhang M, Lee ASJ. The investing layer of the deep cervical fascia does not exist between the sternocleidomastoid and trapezius muscles. Otolaryngol Head Neck Surg. 2002; 127(5):452–454

[10] Nash L, Nicholson HD, Zhang M. Does the investing layer of the deep cervical fascia exist? Anesthesiology. 2005; 103(5):962–968

[11] Kim JT, Kim SK, Koshima I, Moriguchi T. An anatomic study and clinical applications of the reversed submental perforator-based island flap. Plast Reconstr Surg. 2002; 109(7):2204–2210

[12] Robbins KT, Shaha AR, Medina JE, et al. Committee for Neck Dissection Classification, American Head and Neck Society. Consensus statement on the classification and terminology of neck dissection. Arch Otolaryngol Head Neck Surg. 2008; 134(5):536–538

[13] Nason RW, Binahmed A, Torchia MG, Thliversis J. Clinical observations of the anatomy and function of the marginal mandibular nerve. Int J Oral Maxillofac Surg. 2007; 36(8):712–715

[14] Susan Standring P, Berkovitz B, Atkinson M, et al., eds. Gray's Anatomy. The Anatomical Basis of Clinical Practice. 99th ed. New York, NY: Elsevier Ltd; 2005

[15] Weiglein AH, Moriggl B, Schalk C, Künzel KH, Müller U. Arteries in the posterior cervical triangle in man. Clin Anat. 2005; 18(8):553–557

[16] Shen X-H, Xue H-D, Chen Y, et al. A reassessment of cervical surface anatomy via CT scan in an adult population. Clin Anat. 2017; 30(3):330–335

[17] Tessler O, Gilardino MS, Bartow MJ, et al. Transverse cervical artery: consistent anatomical landmarks and clinical experience with its use as a recipient artery in complex head and neck reconstruction. Plast Reconstr Surg. 2017; 139(3):745e–751e

[18] Hematti H, Mehran RJ. Anatomy of the thoracic duct. Thorac Surg Clin. 2011; 21(2):229–238, ix

[19] Smith ME, Riffat F, Jani P. The surgical anatomy and clinical relevance of the neglected right lymphatic duct: review. J Laryngol Otol. 2013; 127(2):128–133

[20] Som PM, Curtin HD, Mancuso AA. Imaging-based nodal classification for evaluation of neck metastatic adenopathy. AJR Am J Roentgenol. 2000; 174 (3):837–844

[21] Civelek E, Karasu A, Cansever T, et al. Surgical anatomy of the cervical sympathetic trunk during anterolateral approach to cervical spine. Eur Spine J. 2008; 17(8):991–995

[22] Hayashi N, Hori E, Ohtani Y, Ohtani O, Kuwayama N, Endo S. Surgical anatomy of the cervical carotid artery for carotid endarterectomy. Neurol Med Chir (Tokyo). 2005; 45(1):25–29, discussion 30

[23] Fazan VPS, da Silva JH, Borges CT, Ribeiro RA, Caetano AG, Filho OAR. An anatomical study on the lingual-facial trunk. Surg Radiol Anat. 2009; 31(4):267–270

[24] Seki S, Sumida K, Yamashita K, Baba O, Kitamura S. Gross anatomical classification of the courses of the human lingual artery. Surg Radiol Anat. 2017; 39 (2):195–203

[25] Lucev N, Bobinac D, Maric I, Drescik I. Variations of the great arteries in the carotid triangle. Otolaryngol Head Neck Surg. 2000; 122(4):590–591

[26] Rafferty MA, Goldstein DP, Brown DH, Irish JC. The sternomastoid branch of the occipital artery: a surgical landmark for the spinal accessory nerve in selective neck dissections. Otolaryngol Head Neck Surg. 2005; 133(6):874–876

[27] Shima H, von Luedinghausen M, Ohno K, Michi K. Anatomy of microvascular anastomosis in the neck. Plast Reconstr Surg. 1998; 101(1):33–41

[28] Gupta V, Tuli A, Choudhry R, Agarwal S, Mangal A. Facial vein draining into external jugular vein in humans: its variations, phylogenetic retention and clinical relevance. Surg Radiol Anat. 2003; 25(1):36–41

[29] Salame K, Masharawi Y, Rochkind S, Arensburg B. Surgical anatomy of the cervical segment of the hypoglossal nerve. Clin Anat. 2006; 19(1):37–43

[30] Lee SH, Lee JK, Jin SM, et al. Anatomical variations of the spinal accessory nerve and its relevance to level IIb lymph nodes. Otolaryngol Head Neck Surg. 2009; 141(5):639–644

[31] Hinsley ML, Hartig GK. Anatomic relationship between the spinal accessory nerve and internal jugular vein in the upper neck. Otolaryngol Head Neck Surg. 2010; 143(2):239–241

[32] Shiozaki K, Abe S, Agematsu H, et al. Anatomical study of accessory nerve innervation relating to functional neck dissection. J Oral Maxillofac Surg. 2007; 65(1):22–29

[33] Symes A, Ellis H. Variations in the surface anatomy of the spinal accessory nerve in the posterior triangle. Surg Radiol Anat. 2005; 27(5):404–408

[34] Durazzo MD, Furlan JC, Teixeira GV, et al. Anatomic landmarks for localization of the spinal accessory nerve. Clin Anat. 2009; 22(4):471–475

[35] Yu P. The transverse cervical vessels as recipient vessels for previously treated head and neck cancer patients. Plast Reconstr Surg. 2005; 115(5):1253–1258

[36] Agarwal A, Mishra A, Lambardi C, Raffaelli M. Surgery of the Thyroid and Parathyroid Glands. 2nd ed. In: Randolph G, ed. Philadelphia, PA: Saunders; 2013

[37] Randolph G, Orlo C. Surgery of the Thyroid and Parathyroid Glands. 2nd ed. Randolph G, ed. Philadelphia, PA: Saunders; 2013

[38] Ardito G, Revelli L, D'Alatri L, Lerro V, Guidi ML, Ardito F. Revisited anatomy of the recurrent laryngeal nerves. Am J Surg. 2004; 187(2):249–253

[39] Kulekci M, Batioglu-Karaaltin A, Saatci O, et al. Relationship between the recurrent laryngeal nerve and the inferior thyroid artery and its branches: an applied anatomical study. Ann Otol Rhinol Laryngol. 2012; 121(10):650–656

[40] Shindo ML, Wu JC, Park EE. Surgical anatomy of the recurrent laryngeal nerve revisited. Otolaryngol Head Neck Surg. 2005; 133(4):514–519

[41] Kambic V, Zargi M, Radsel Z. Topographic anatomy of the external branch of the superior laryngeal nerve. Its importance in head and neck surgery. J Laryngol Otol. 1984; 98(11):1121–1124

[42] Cernea CR, Ferraz AR, Nishio S, Dutra A, Jr, Hojaij FC, dos Santos LR. Surgical anatomy of the external branch of the superior laryngeal nerve. Head Neck. 1992; 14(5):380–383

[43] Lovasova K, Kachlik D, Santa M, Kluchova D. Unilateral occurrence of five different thyroid arteries-a need of terminological systematization: a case report. Surg Radiol Anat. 2017; 39(8):925–929

[44] Moubayed SP, Ayad T. High-riding innominate artery encountered during neck surgery. Otolaryngol Head Neck Surg. 2014; 151(5):888–889

4 Biological Mechanisms of Lymphatic Spread

Joseph Zenga, Patrik Pipkorn, and Brian Nussenbaum

Abstract

The biological mechanisms of lymphatic spread are intricate, highly regulated active processes involving the concert of trophic factors, lymphatic growth, and tumor chemotaxis. Dissemination of head and neck cancer beyond its primary site has a significant detrimental impact on treatment outcomes with clinical neck disease decreasing survival by 50%. For years, tumor spread was considered a passive process dependent on tumor volume and interstitial pressure leading to tumor shedding into regional lymphatics. During the last few decades, however, the discovery of specific lymphatic immunohistochemical markers has enabled researchers to study the mechanisms in lymphangiogenesis and lymphatic spread in greater detail. These investigations have revealed that lymphatic spread instead involves highly active and regulated mechanisms. Although much remains to be elucidated, several of the most critical steps have been identified. The process begins with tumor lymphangiogenesis and the epithelial-to-mesenchymal transition of malignant cells. Through specific chemotactic signaling and extracellular matrix degradation, tumor cells intravasate into peritumoral lymphatics to reach the draining nodal basin. Although multiple trophic factors influence this sequence, the vascular endothelial growth factor C (VEGF-C)/VEGF-D/VEGFR-3 signaling axis has been shown to play a central role in the regulation of lymphatic spread. Intervention through downregulation of this axis has been identified as an attractive target for pharmacotherapy, preventing or limiting lymphatic dissemination. Although many agents have held early promise in preclinical animal experiments, human studies are just beginning. The exact role of these agents in the future remains to be seen.

Keywords: lymphangiogenesis, lymphatic system, metastasis, vascular endothelial growth factor, epithelial-to-mesenchymal transition, chemotaxis

4.1 Introduction

For most cancer patients who succumb to their disease, it is not the result of an uncontrolled local tumor but from dissemination of cancer cells through lymphatic or hematogenous spread to regional nodes and distant organ systems. When these metastases have progressed far enough, they become resistant to conventional therapies. For certain tumors, including many sarcomas, renal cell carcinoma, and follicular thyroid carcinoma, early dissemination is typically hematogenous. For many others, however, including upper aerodigestive tract squamous cell carcinoma (SCC), initial spread is primarily to the regional lymphatics. While the reasons for these differences remain to be fully elucidated, the prognostic value of lymph node metastasis in head and neck cancer is substantial, decreasing survival probability by 50%.[1] Although distant metastasis is an even more ominous prognostic sign, less than 10% of patients with head and neck cancer demonstrate overt distant metastatic disease at initial presentation.

Given the propensity of head and neck cancer to develop lymphatic metastasis and the associated decrement in survival, a great deal of work has focused on the diagnosis and treatment of regional nodal disease. Patients who present with clinical regional metastasis are treated with conventional surgical or nonsurgical management paradigms. For patients who present with clinically negative regional nodes, however, management of the neck becomes more complicated. Neck dissection with pathological assessment of the resected nodal levels is the current "gold" standard staging tool for regional metastases in a clinically negative neck. This invasive procedure comes with risk, however, and is beneficial only if the probability of detecting occult regional disease is high enough. A significant proportion of clinically negative patients are also pathologically negative and will, therefore, undergo an unnecessary invasive staging procedure. Nonetheless, in the population of patients at approximately a 20% or greater risk of harboring occult metastasis, regional control and survival are overall improved in those undergoing lymphatic staging by neck dissection as compared to observation.[2]

There are no current widely accepted minimally invasive techniques to achieve accurate regional staging. Although sentinel lymph node biopsy has been used, it is limited in general to SCC of oral cavity subsites and is performed at specialized centers. It is still an invasive procedure, nonetheless, and comes with its own risks and challenges. Imaging techniques are limited in resolution, and positron emission tomography scanning can identify nodal involvement as low as 7 mm in diameter but cannot reliably detect occult micrometastatic disease.[3]

A predictive genetic or morphologic signature of a resected primary tumor would be ideal to determine the risk of occult metastasis and help better select patients for elective neck treatment or observation. Although molecular profiling of primary head and neck tumors has been investigated to identify genetic markers of lymphatic spread, none have been widely adopted or validated in large cohorts.[4] Examining the biological mechanism of lymphatic spread, including trophic factors, signaling pathways, and morphological changes, provides another possible method to identify primary tumors at high risk for regional metastasis. This requires a detailed knowledge of how tumors spread to the regional lymphatics and may provide an opportunity to develop therapeutic agents to block regional dissemination of disease. This, in turn, necessitates an understanding of the structure and function of the lymphatic system, methods for microscopic assessment, and an overview of the major molecular mechanisms driving lymphatic spread.

4.2 The Lymphatic System

4.2.1 Lymphatic Function

Nutrients in the bloodstream reach tissues by extravasation from capillary vessels under high pressures from the arterial system. This milieu of extravasated fluid and macromolecules makes up the interstitial fluid, allowing cells to take up these nutrients and dispose of waste products. Through both active and passive processes, this fluid and its components are recycled and returned to the circulation through the lymphatic system. Initial lymphatics are blind-ended channels composed of a single layer of endothelial cells with minimal basement membrane and large gap junctions to allow uptake of interstitial fluid. Anchoring filaments tether the initial lymphatics to the extracellular matrix to prevent vessels collapse under interstitial pressures. Lymph then proceeds into precollecting and larger collecting lymphatic vessels propelled by perivascular smooth muscle contraction along with extrinsic skeletal muscle pressure. These larger lymphatic vessels are less permeable, limiting extravasation, and one-way valves prevent lymphatic backflow. Lymph is first filtered through draining regional lymphatic basins, centers for antigen recognition, and initiation of any requisite immune response. From these lymphatics, lymph is ultimately returned to the venous circulation through the thoracic or right lymphatic ducts.

4.2.2 Lymphatic Origins and Development

An appreciation of lymphatic embryology can aid in understanding how tumor trophic factors may lead to lymphangiogenesis or invasion of existing host lymphatics. Due to difficulties with visualization and tracking of nascent lymphatics, development of the lymphatic system has been a subject of controversy for over 100 years. Although the exact origins of the lymphatic and venous systems have been debated, lymphatic development appears to begin through the formation of lymphatic sacs that sprout from the embryonic venous system as early as the fifth week of fetal development. These paired lymphatic sacs, which ultimately give rise to the thoracic and the right lymphatic ducts, expand and ramify into a lymphatic plexus. Lymph node formation follows as specialized myofibroblasts proliferate and form a scaffold for lymphoid tissue, through which immune cells are recruited. Although aspects of this process remain unclear, several key factors contributing to lymphatic development and proliferation have recently been identified.

An early and critical developmental step, determining the fate of lymphatic endothelial cells, is expression of the transcription factor, Prospero-related homeobox protein 1 (Prox1). Prox1 knockout mice are devoid of lymphatics and deletion at any point during development results in lymphatic regression. Although the exact mechanisms that leads to induction of Prox1 expression remain unclear, bone morphogenic protein and Notch signaling pathways have been identified as inhibitors of Prox1-induced lymphangiogenesis and drive venous cell differentiation, while Wnt signaling appears to increase Prox1 expression in lymphatic progenitor cells. Certain transcription factors, as well, have been associated with induction of Prox1 signaling, including Sox18 and Coup-TF2. Ultimately, the Prox1 molecular switch results in expression of requisite proteins for lymphatic endothelial cell growth and migration.[5]

A significant advance in understanding lymphangiogenesis came with the discovery that vascular endothelial growth factors (VEGF) played a central role in stimulating lymphatic proliferation. These growth factors are composed of a family of subtypes, with five described members in mammals, including VEGF-A through VEGF-D and placental growth factor (PlGF). Each exerts its effects through specific membrane receptors coupled to downstream intracellular pathways. VEGF-A, VEGF-B, and PlGF are primarily involved in vasculogenesis and angiogenesis. VEGF-A was the first-described growth factor of this group and represents the dominant trophic signal for blood vessel endothelial cell proliferation and migration. VEGF-A binds to vascular endothelial growth factor receptors 1 and 2 (VEGFR-1 and VEGFR-2), although the majority of angiogenic effects are mediated through VEGFR-2.

A third vascular endothelial growth factor receptor (VEGFR-3) was subsequently discovered, and its major ligands, VEGF-C and VEGF-D, were identified as a target of Prox1 activation and a key trophic axis for lymphatic proliferation. Early in embryogenesis, however, VEGFR-3 signaling is important for vascular development, and VEGFR-3 knockout mice die at an early embryonic stage of cardiovascular defects. Later in development, VEGFR-3 expression becomes restricted to lymphatics and is critical to lymphangiogenesis and lymphatic migration. VEGFR-3 heterozygous animals exhibit substantial lymphatic defects and similarly, the human condition Milroy's disease is associated with a VEGFR-3 mutation and results in congenital lymphedema. Further, lymphatic sprouting is at least in part a VEGF-C-dependent process, as endothelial cells have been shown to migrate toward a VEGF-C gradient and VEGF-C-deficient mice develop a hypoplastic lymphatic system. Although VEGF-D is also a VEGFR-3 ligand and a known lymphangiogenic trophic factor, lesser congenital defects in lymphatic migration are seen in VEGF-D-deficient mice, including smaller caliber and less functional superficial lymphatics.[5,6]

A second EGF system, the angiopoietin–Tie (Ang-Tie) axis, is involved in angiogenesis and lymphangiogenesis as well. Angiopoietin 1 (Ang1) and 2 (Ang2) along with their receptors Tie1 and Tie2 are the best characterized members of this signaling pathway. Ang1 is an obligate agonist of Tie2, while the inhibitory or stimulatory effects of Ang2 are context dependent. Although the Ang-Tie system is primarily known for its role in vascular and cardiac embryology, it has been shown to be critical to the stability and remodeling of lymphatic endothelial cells later in development.

As understanding of these pathways continues, the molecular picture becomes increasingly complex (▶ Fig. 4.1). There appears to be crossover between the function of VEGFR-2 and VEGFR-3, including both homodimer and heterodimer formation leading to specific angiogenic and lymphangiogenic effects. VEGF-C is also known to bind the receptor neuropilin2 (Nrp2). Nrp2 is seen in high levels in the developing lymphatic plexus, and Nrp2-deficient mice exhibit normal central lymphatics but absent superficial lymphatic networks.[7]

In addition, all these factors are closely regulated by extrinsic and intrinsic processes. VEGF-C is regulated by collagen and calcium-binding EGF domains 1 (CCBE-1), a protein necessary for normal lymphatic development in animal models, and mutations of which lead to lymphatic dysplasia in humans. CCBE-1 plays a role in proteolytic processing of VEGF-C to its most active form. Nrp-2 signaling, which results in lymphatic proliferation when binding VEGF-C, has been shown to be regulated by semaphorins, a family of signaling proteins. When binding Nrp2, class 3 semaphorins result in inhibition of lymphatic cell proliferation and induction of apoptosis. VEGFR-3 is also highly regulated by additional pathways independent of Prox1 signaling. Ephrin-B2, a transmembrane ligand for Eph receptor tyrosine kinases, promotes lymphatic sprouting through VEGFR-3 modulation. Similarly, T-box transcription factor 1 regulates

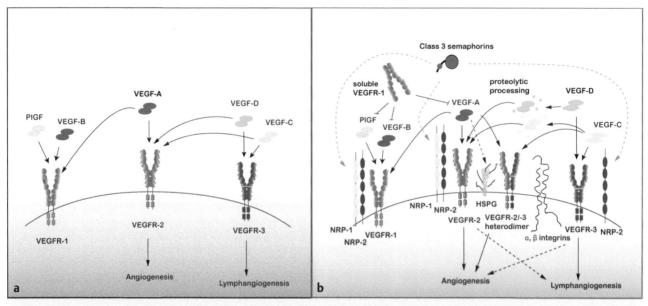

Fig. 4.1 Early understanding of a simplified relationship between the role of vascular endothelial growth factor receptor ligands and receptors with angiogenesis and lymphangiogenesis (**a**) gave way to an increasingly complex and highly regulated molecular cascade (**b**).

Table 4.1 Lymphatic markers

Marker	Type	Function	Advantage	Limitation
Podoplanin	Transmembrane glycoprotein	Implicated in development and wound healing	Strongly expressed on all lymphatics Not expressed on normal blood vessels	Expressed in some pathological conditions including malignancy
LYVE-1	Transmembrane hyaluronic acid receptor	Implicated in wound healing and cell migration	Strongly expressed on initial lymphatics	Expressed on some blood vessels and malignancies
VEGFR-3	Transmembrane tyrosine kinase receptor	Involved in lymphangiogenesis and lymphatic development	Strongly expressed on normal lymphatics	Upregulated in neoendothelium of malignancy and some vascular tumors
Prox-1	Transcription factor	Involved in lymphangiogenesis lymphatic development	Highly specific for lymphatics Not expressed on neoendothelium of malignancy	Expressed on some nonendothelial tissue

Abbreviations: LYVE-1, lymphatic vessel endothelial hyaluronan receptor 1; Prox-1, prospero-related homeobox protein 1; VEGFR-3, third vascular endothelial growth factor receptor.

VEGFR-3 expression and appears to be necessary for lymphatic endothelial cell growth and maintenance. Finally, VEGFR-3 may be activated independently of a VEGF ligand through binding of extracellular matrix components.[8]

4.2.3 Lymphatic Markers

The study of the lymphatic system and its interaction with malignancy is ultimately limited by the quality of lymphatic markers. Studies evaluating tumor lymphangiogenesis and lymphatic invasion must be interpreted in light of the specificity of the technique used to identify lymphatic vessels. With traditional hematoxylin and eosin staining, lymphatic endothelium cannot be reliably detected and quantified. Immunochemical staining, therefore, must be used to target specific lymphatic markers, each with its own drawbacks and advantages (▶ Table 4.1). There are multiple commercially available antibodies specific for the lymphatic markers examined below.[9]

Podoplanin

Podoplanin is a transmembrane glycoprotein expressed in multiple tissue types including bone, lung, kidney, and choroid plexus. Although its physiological role is unclear, it is important for normal pulmonary and lymphatic development and has been implicated in wound healing and cell migration. It is strongly expressed on all lymphatics but not blood vessel endothelium. It is upregulated in certain pathological conditions, including some skin carcinomas and vascular tumors, which may limit its specificity as a lymphatic marker.[10]

Lymphatic Vessel Endothelial Hyaluronan Receptor 1

Lymphatic vessel endothelial hyaluronan receptor 1 (LYVE-1) is a transmembrane hyaluronic acid receptor also implicated in cell migration and wound healing. It is expressed on initial lymphatics but less strongly on collecting vessels. Although it is found widely on both luminal and extraluminal surfaces of lymphatic channels, it is also found on select blood vessels including liver, spleen, and pulmonary capillaries, as well as certain activated tissue macrophages. It may also be expressed on a percentage of blood vessels in pathological conditions including some malignancies.[11]

Vascular Endothelial Growth Factor Receptor 3

As discussed earlier, VEGFR3 (also known as FLT4, fms-like tyrosine kinase receptor 4) is a transmembrane protein receptor involved in lymphangiogenesis and maintenance of lymphatic differentiation. Although it is a specific marker for normal lymphatics, VEGFR-3 may be upregulated in vascular endothelium when associated with malignancy. It can be seen in myoepithelial cells and is highly expressed in certain vascular tumors.

Prospero-Related Homeobox Protein 1

As discussed earlier, Prox1 is a homeobox transcription factor critical to lymphatic development. In contrast to other lymphatic markers, Prox1 immunofluorescence is nuclear rather than membrane bound. It is seen in all lymphatic endothelial cells, regardless of patient age, including lymphatic capillaries and lymphatic trunks. Prox1 is not seen in blood vessel endothelium or pericytes and does not appear to be expressed in vascular neoendothelium of carcinomas. It is seen in some nonendothelial tissue including the lens, heart, liver, pancreas, and nervous system.

4.3 Lymphatic Spread in Head and Neck Cancer

Early studies in head and neck SCC reported high rates of neck disease with low distant metastatic rates. This suggested that regional nodal involvement may be a prerequisite for distant spread

and perhaps a linear process of cancer dissemination. The early prevailing view held that cancer spreads passively to the cervical nodes, which served as a filter against distant metastasis.

This theory of passive tumor shedding was challenged by emerging clinical data in the latter 20th century. First, patients with head and neck SCC were found to occasionally have clinical distant metastasis without regional nodal involvement. Second, as experience grew with unknown primary carcinoma, it became clear that a microscopic primary tumor could lead to an aggressive cervical metastasis with evidently different pathobiology. Taken together, these clinical data suggested that lymphatic and hematogenous metastases may be separate and specific events, and further that lymphatic spread was an active process with associated fundamental pathobiological changes occurring in those cancer cells that progress to lymphatic metastases (▶ Fig. 4.2).[12]

Ultimately, dissemination to regional lymph nodes appears to require multiple active steps including modulation of intratumoral or peritumoral lymphatics, physical entry into lymphatic vessels, survival and transport in local and regional lymphatics, and finally deposition and proliferation in regional nodes (▶ Fig. 4.3). Although much of the work investigating these steps has been done in other organ systems, the underlying mechanisms appear largely conserved and can be applied to understanding lymphatic spread in head and neck cancer.

4.3.1 Tumor Lymphangiogenesis

Whether tumors use preexisting host lymphatic vessels or whether tumor-induced lymphangiogenesis was critical to regional spread has been long debated. Deciphering this process, however, is vital to the development of antineoplastic therapy. An agent that blocks lymphangiogenesis will be ineffective if tumors simply employ host lymphatics for regional dissemination.

In the early 2000s, evidence emerged from animal models that tumor lymphangiogenesis leads to lymphatic metastases by upregulating VEGF-C and VEGF-D production. Experimental

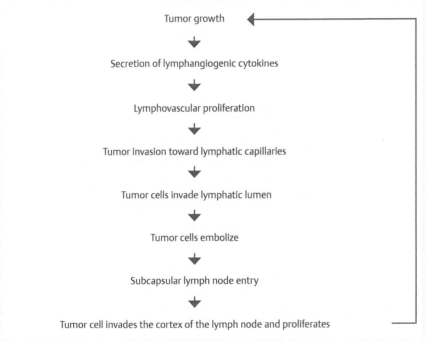

Fig. 4.2 Critical active steps in the process of lymphatic dissemination from the primary tumor to the regional nodal basin.

Tumor growth

Secretion of lymphangiogenic cytokines

Lymphovascular proliferation

Tumor invasion toward lymphatic capillaries

Tumor cells invade lymphatic lumen

Tumor cells embolize

Subcapsular lymph node entry

Tumor cell invades the cortex of the lymph node and proliferates

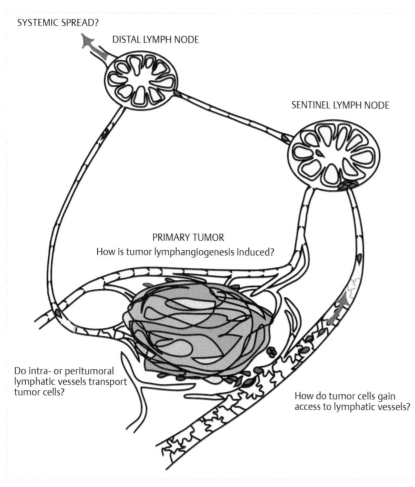

SYSTEMIC SPREAD?

DISTAL LYMPH NODE

SENTINEL LYMPH NODE

PRIMARY TUMOR
How is tumor lymphangiogenesis induced?

Do intra- or peritumoral lymphatic vessels transport tumor cells?

How do tumor cells gain access to lymphatic vessels?

Fig. 4.3 Schematic of lymphatic spread with critical questions that this review will address including the role of tumor lymphangiogenesis, intratumoral and peritumoral lymphatics, and tumor cell entry into functional lymphatic vessels.

overproduction of these growth factors significantly increased both tumor-associated lymphatics and regional metastases. The majority of subsequent clinical and bench investigation supported these findings in many different tumor types and suggested that regional metastases were at least partly regulated by the VEGF-C/VEGF-D/VEGFR-3 signaling axis and specifically related to tumor-associated lymphangiogenesis. This pathway also appeared restricted to lymphatic proliferation and distinctly separate from angiogenesis. VEGF-C overexpression in the skin of transgenic mice resulted in hyperplasia of the dermal lymphatics without significantly affected vascular endothelium. Further, when classically nonlymphangiogenic nonmetastatic tumors were induced in transgenic mice to overexpress VEGF-C, peritumoral lymphatic hyperplasia and regional metastases were seen. In other cancer models, when an anti-VEGFR-3 antibody was either systemically administered or secreted by tumors, decreased intratumoral lymphatics and decreased regional metastases were seen. In human studies, a correlation between VEGF-C and VEGF-D levels in primary tumors and regional metastases has been identified in multiple tumor types.[13]

Although clinical evidence in head and neck SCC is limited, several studies have identified an association between prolymphangiogenic factors and regional metastases. The majority of these data come from retrospective studies evaluating tissue levels of signaling molecules and their correlation with tumor stage and prognosis. Although many have found a significant association between upregulation of the VEGF-C/VEGF-D/VEGFR-3 signaling axis and regional metastases, others have found no such correlation.[14,15]

Other proteins involved in the lymphangiogenic cascade have also been implicated in head and neck cancer including Prox1, neuropilins, and semaphorins.[14,16] Ultimately, although prolymphangiogenic signals play a role in the development of regional metastasis, the process is more complex, requiring not only growth factors, but also changes in lymphatic vasculature, tumor invasion and migration, as well as survival in regional nodal basins to achieve clinical regional dissemination.

4.3.2 Significance of Lymphatic Vessel Density

If upregulation of lymphangiogenic signaling pathways plays a role in lymphatic metastasis, it becomes critical to understand where in the tumor environment lymphatic proliferation occurs, both for informing prognosis from surgical specimens and to identify therapeutic targets. Increases in both intratumoral and peritumoral lymphatic vessel density (LVD) have been correlated with lymphatic spread in multiple tumor types. Although the association of tumoral microvessel density with survival has been recognized since the early 1990s, in head and neck cancer it appears that LVD has even greater prognostic value. A recent meta-analysis identified intratumoral LVD as a more important predictive factor than blood vessel density, with a greater than twofold increased risk of death in patients with high intratumoral lymphatic counts.[17,18]

Although intratumoral LVD has significant prognostic value, peritumoral lymphatics may be more functionally important for lymphatic spread. In animal models, intratumoral lymphatics have been shown to be nonfunctional in many cases, either invaded or compressed by tumor, and do not provide an effective draining pathway to regional lymphatics. Peritumoral vessels, however, are often dilated and functional, particularly in the presence of VEGF-C overexpression. Further, regional metastases have been demonstrated in the absence of intratumoral lymphatics, suggesting that a peritumoral lymphatic network is sufficient for lymphatic spread. Additionally, meta-analyses in other tumor types, including breast cancer and melanoma, have identified a stronger correlation of regional metastases with peritumoral LVD than with intratumoral LVD.[14]

4.3.3 Tumor Entry into Lymphatics

Although dilation and functional drainage of peritumoral lymphatics may be associated with lymphatic spread, to enter the lymphatic system, tumor cells must make an epithelial-to-mesenchymal transition (EMT), migrate to nearby lymphatics, and intravasate. Although early theories proposed that this was a passive process, driven by changes in interstitial fluid pressure and volume, recently, EMT and intravasation have been recognized as complex and active processes involving the concert of multiple chemotactic factors and signaling pathways.

Epithelial cells are characterized by cell polarity and adhesion. Migration and metastases require cell detachment and cytoskeletal reorganization. Two fundamental cellular changes, downregulation of E-cadherin and upregulation of vimentin, have been associated with loss of cell-to-cell adhesion, increased cell motility, and an EMT phenotype. Head and neck cancers with this clinical signature have a nearly universal metastatic rate, while those without it have a metastatic rate of less than 50%. A large number of other signaling components, along with trophic stimuli from transforming growth factor-β (TGF-β) and epidermal growth factor (EGF) have been identified, all contributing to morphological and functional changes that lead to cell detachment and invasion.[19]

Once EMT is established, tumor cells must migrate toward functional lymphatics to achieve lymphatic spread. In nonpathological conditions, lymphatic vessels are an important source of chemotactic factors, including chemokine ligand 21 (CCL21) that binds to chemokine receptor 7 (CCR7) on immune cells, allowing them to migrate to and enter the lymphatic system to initiate a normal immune response. Upregulation of CCR7 in certain tumors has been associated with an increase in lymphatic metastases, suggesting that lymphatic chemotaxis plays an important role in the process of lymphatic spread.[13] In addition, effective tumor cell migration requires degradation of the extracellular matrix, mitigated by upregulation of certain proteases, particularly the matrix metalloproteinases (MMP). This family of endopeptidases play a critical role in tumor-associated basement membrane degradation including entry into lymphatics and extracapsular spread from lymph nodes.[20]

4.4 Clinical Applications

4.4.1 Importance of Head and Neck Subsites

It is well known that head and neck cancers at various subsites have different propensities and patterns for nodal metastasis.

In the oral cavity, it is widely known that the incidence of lymphatic metastasis is associated with subsite, T-stage, and depth of invasion. For the larynx, early on, glottic cancers were noted to have a low risk of nodal spread, while oral and pharyngeal sites were more likely to develop regional metastases. More recently, a dramatic increase in human papillomavirus (HPV) related oropharyngeal cancers have renewed interest in elucidating the mechanisms of lymphatic spread. These HPV-driven tumors are typically small at the primary site with early and sometimes extensive spread to regional nodes.

Several hypotheses have been suggested for the discrepancies observed in nodal spread between subsites. Earlier symptoms from vocal cord tumors may lead to earlier detection and therefore less nodal disease. Even advanced glottic cancer, however, appeared to have less lymphatic spread than similar supraglottic primaries, and it was hypothesized that the density of the lymphatic system in the submucosa may account for the different rate of lymphatic invasion. Beginning in the 1980s, dyes studies performed in cadaveric specimens as well as in vivo demonstrated sparse lymphatics in the glottic submucosa, particularly anteriorly, and a somewhat more developed network in the deeper connective tissue with few anastomotic connections. These studies also suggested that there were few lymphatic connections in a vertical axis between subglottis, glottis, and supraglottis. Although initial reports using different methodology often led to different conclusions, the use of electron microscopy combined with immunohistochemical lymphatic staining provided compelling evidence that the baseline density of lymphatics is intrinsically different between laryngeal subunits. This difference may, to some extent, explain the difference in nodal spread between glottic and supraglottic cancers.[21,22]

In addition to differences in metastatic rate, specific head and neck subsites appeared to drain to distinct nodal stations (▶ Fig. 4.4). Based on pathological nodal stage from large groups of patients undergoing comprehensive neck dissection for head and neck cancer, the most common drainage pathways for various head and neck subsites were determined.[23] This knowledge has allowed for more targeted treatment with selective neck dissection in N0 patients to limit morbidity. The predictability of the exact pathways of lymphatic drainage may be variable between patients and sites, particularly for cutaneous primary tumors.

A visual understanding of differential drainage from different head and neck primary sites was achieved with the development of lymphoscintigraphy. Peritumoral injection of radio-opaque dye revealed that distinct lymphatic channels existed specific to each patient and tumor location. This gave surgeons extensive information about the variability of the cervical lymphatic system and valuable clues to explain the existence of skip metastases and patients with involvement of multiple nodal stations. This concept was further adapted to intraoperative lymphatic mapping to identify the first echelon, or sentinel, node as a minimally invasive method to stage a clinically negative neck. This hypothesis, that lymphatic drainage from a given primary site would reliably drain to primary echelon nodes and the status of these nodes would be representative of the status of the neck basin, was confirmed and widely applied to cutaneous malignancy. The sentinel lymph node concept appears to be effective for staging N0 necks for mucosal primary sites as well.

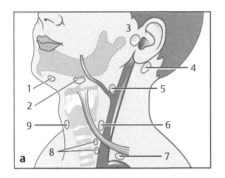 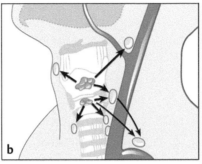

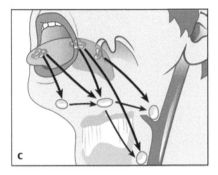 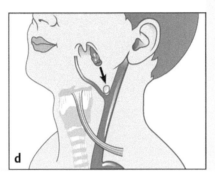

Fig. 4.4 (a) Typical sites for regional lymph node metastases. 1, submental; 2, submandibular; 3, parotid and preauricular; 4, retroauricular; 5, jugulodigastric; 6, deep cervical chain; 7, juguloomohyoid; 8, pretracheal and peritracheal; 9, prelaryngeal lymph nodes. **(b)** Laryngeal carcinoma. **(c)** Carcinoma of the tongue. **(d)** Tonsillar carcinoma.

4.4.2 Antilymphangiogenic Therapeutic Targets

As discussed earlier, the view that regional metastasis is a passive process has largely been replaced by evidence that lymphatic spread is an intricate active process involving the coordination of several events including multiple trophic factors and signaling cascades. Tumor lymphangiogenesis is an early critical step that provides an attractive target for pharmacologic intervention. Limiting lymphatic ingrowth in early-stage primary tumors may limit the development of lymphatic spread. By decreasing intratumoral and peritumoral lymphatic channels and their associated chemotactic factors, those tumor cells that have made the EMT may be less likely to achieve regional dissemination.

Although many of the mechanisms underlying lymphatic embryology, and the analogous process of tumor lymphangiogenesis, have been elucidated, development of antilymphangiogenic pharmacotherapy has been more limited. The majority of evidence comes from preclinical studies focusing largely on the VEGF-C/VEGF-D/VEGFR-3 signaling axis. In animal models, inhibitory antibodies or downregulation of this signaling cascade has been shown to reduce the rate of lymph node metastasis.

The first VEGF inhibitor approved for human use was bevacizumab, a humanized monoclonal antibody specific for VEGF-A. Used in several different solid tumors, including colorectal, lung, and renal cancers, its efficacy is primarily related to its antiangiogenic properties, although it has shown some antilymphangiogenic effects as well. VEGFR-2, the primary receptor for VEGF-A, has been identified on lymphatic endothelial cells and may lead directly to lymphatic proliferation. In addition, VEGF-A has been shown to be a chemotactic factor for immune cells, which in turn secrete VEGF-C and VEGF-D, leading to lymphangiogenesis. Many other multitargeted receptor tyrosine kinase inhibitors acting on VEGF pathways have been developed since, several with anti-VEGFR-3 activity, including sunitinib, pazopanib, and axitinib. In recent clinical trials, several of these inhibitors have shown some modest activity in head and neck SCC, particularly in the recurrent-metastatic setting. Despite the theoretical antilymphangiogenic activity of these inhibitors, the extent and clinical importance of their effect on lymphatic growth remains uncertain.

Along with multitargeted therapies, several agents specific to the VEGF-C/VEGF-D/VEGFR-3 axis are in development. IMC-3C5 and VGX-100, monoclonal antibodies specific for VEGFR-3 and VEGF-C, respectively, have undergone phase I trials in patients with advanced solid tumors. Although minimal direct antitumor activity was observed, these agents are relatively well tolerated, and require testing in larger-scale trials powered to detect changes in recurrence and metastasis to determine efficacy.[24] In addition to direct antibody-mediated inhibition, the proteolytic processing of VEGF-C and VEGF-D may be targeted, preventing the conversion of these growth factors into their most active form. Although this has shown promise in preclinical models, its in vivo effects remain unexplored.

In addition to the VEGF-C/VEGF-D/VEGFR-3 axis, other components of lymphangiogenic signaling may be targeted including VEGF-A/VEGFR-2, Ang/Tie, neuropilins, semaphorins, and the transcriptional control of lymphatic proliferation. Although several inhibitors if the VEGF-A/VEGFR-2 and Ang/Tie systems have been developed, their primary mechanism of action is thought to be through regulation of tumor angiogenesis and the extent and efficacy of their antilymphangiogenic effects are not well understood. Inhibitors of several other molecular targets of the lymphangiogenic signaling cascade are in development and have shown promise in preclinical reports. In addition, modulation of the transcriptional control of lymphatic proliferation, including Prox1 and its transcriptional inducer Sox-18, which are critical to normal lymphatic development as well as tumor lymphangiogenesis, may provide an essential complement to downstream molecular inhibitors. In vitro and in vivo knockout studies have shown that inhibition of lymphangiogenic transcription factors decreases lymphatic migration and proliferation.[25]

4.5 Conclusion

Lymphatic dissemination of head and neck cancer is the most common route of metastatic spread and is associated with a significantly worse prognosis along with the need for more intensive multimodality treatment. Recent molecular advances, including the development of lymphatic-specific markers, have improved understanding of the mechanisms of lymphatic dissemination. Contrary to early hypotheses, lymphatic spread is an active process with fundamental pathobiological changes in those metastatic cells enabling them to dissociate from the primary tumor mass, migrate toward intratumoral or peritumoral lymphatics, make lymphatic vessel entry and travel to the regional nodal basin while remaining viable. These steps are governed by multiple molecular pathways and chemotactic agents, with the vascular EGFs and receptors central among them. As understanding of these processes grows, the development and therapeutic role of specific antilymphangiogenic targets is likely to expand.

References

[1] Roberts TJ, Colevas AD, Hara W, Holsinger FC, Oakley-Girvan I, Divi V. Number of positive nodes is superior to the lymph node ratio and American Joint Committee on Cancer N staging for the prognosis of surgically treated head and neck squamous cell carcinomas. Cancer. 2016; 122(9):1388–1397

[2] D'Cruz AK, Vaish R, Kapre N, et al. Head and Neck Disease Management Group. Elective versus therapeutic neck dissection in node-negative oral cancer. N Engl J Med. 2015; 373(6):521–529

[3] Erdi YE. Limits of tumor detectability in nuclear medicine and PET. Mol Imaging Radionucl Ther. 2012; 21(1):23–28

[4] Lallemant B, Evrard A, Chambon G, et al. Gene expression profiling in head and neck squamous cell carcinoma: clinical perspectives. Head Neck. 2010; 32(12):1712–1719

[5] Semo J, Nicenboim J, Yaniv K. Development of the lymphatic system: new questions and paradigms. Development. 2016; 143(6):924–935

[6] Srinivasan RS, Escobedo N, Yang Y, et al. The Prox1-Vegfr3 feedback loop maintains the identity and the number of lymphatic endothelial cell progenitors. Genes Dev. 2014; 28(19):2175–2187

[7] Secker GA, Harvey NL. VEGFR signaling during lymphatic vascular development: From progenitor cells to functional vessels. Dev Dyn. 2015; 244(3):323–331

[8] Alitalo A, Detmar M. Interaction of tumor cells and lymphatic vessels in cancer progression. Oncogene. 2012; 31(42):4499–4508

[9] Ordóñez NG. Immunohistochemical endothelial markers: a review. Adv Anat Pathol. 2012; 19(5):281–295

[10] Ugorski M, Dziegiel P, Suchanski J. Podoplanin: a small glycoprotein with many faces. Am J Cancer Res. 2016; 6(2):370–386

[11] Baluk P, McDonald DM. Markers for microscopic imaging of lymphangiogenesis and angiogenesis. Ann N Y Acad Sci. 2008; 1131:1–12

[12] Allen CT, Law JH, Dunn GP, Uppaluri R. Emerging insights into head and neck cancer metastasis. Head Neck. 2013; 35(11):1669–1678

[13] Karaman S, Detmar M. Mechanisms of lymphatic metastasis. J Clin Invest. 2014; 124(3):922–928

[14] Zhang B, Gao Z, Sun M, et al. Prognostic significance of VEGF-C, semaphorin 3F, and neuropilin-2 expression in oral squamous cell carcinomas and their relationship with lymphangiogenesis. J Surg Oncol. 2015; 111(4):382–388

[15] de Sousa EA, Lourenço SV, de Moraes FP, et al. Head and neck squamous cell carcinoma lymphatic spread and survival: Relevance of vascular endothelial growth factor family for tumor evaluation. Head Neck. 2015; 37(10):1410–1416

[16] Sasahira T, Ueda N, Yamamoto K, et al. Prox1 and FOXC2 act as regulators of lymphangiogenesis and angiogenesis in oral squamous cell carcinoma. PLoS One. 2014; 9(3):e92534

[17] Weidner N, Semple JP, Welch WR, Folkman J. Tumor angiogenesis and metastasis: correlation in invasive breast carcinoma. N Engl J Med. 1991; 324(1):1–8

[18] Yu M, Liu L, Liang C, et al. Intratumoral vessel density as prognostic factors in head and neck squamous cell carcinoma: a meta-analysis of literature. Head Neck. 2014; 36(4):596–602

[19] Smith A, Teknos TN, Pan Q. Epithelial to mesenchymal transition in head and neck squamous cell carcinoma. Oral Oncol. 2013; 49(4):287–292

[20] Kim HS, Park YW. Metastasis via peritumoral lymphatic dilation in oral squamous cell carcinoma. Maxillofac Plast Reconstr Surg. 2014; 36(3):85–93

[21] Werner JA, Schünke M, Rudert H, Tillmann B. Description and clinical importance of the lymphatics of the vocal fold. Otolaryngol Head Neck Surg. 1990; 102(1):13–19

[22] Kirchner JA. Glottic-supraglottic barrier: fact or fantasy? Ann Otol Rhinol Laryngol. 1997; 106(8):700–704

[23] Shah JP. Patterns of cervical lymph node metastasis from squamous carcinomas of the upper aerodigestive tract. Am J Surg. 1990; 160(4):405–409

[24] Dieterich LC, Detmar M. Tumor lymphangiogenesis and new drug development. Adv Drug Deliv Rev. 2016; 99:148–160

[25] Rho CR, Choi JS, Seo M, Lee SK, Joo CK. Inhibition of lymphangiogenesis and hemangiogenesis in corneal inflammation by subconjunctival Prox1 siRNA injection in rats. Invest Ophthalmol Vis Sci. 2015; 56(10):5871–5879

5 Extracapsular Spread: Biology, Imaging, Surgical Management, Pathological Diagnosis, and Therapeutic Implications

Kathryn M. Vorwald and J. Trad Wadsworth

Abstract

This chapter is a comprehensive discussion of the most current knowledge of a familiar but ever-evolving topic in head and neck cancer. The recent addition of extracapsular spread (ECS) as a criterion used in the eighth edition of the American Joint Committee on Cancer (AJCC) TNM (*t*umor size, *n*ode involvement, and *m*etastasis status) staging system reflects the importance of ECS on prognosis and will undoubtedly produce an abundance of updated clinical data. This chapter encompasses everything from diagnosis to management and describes the current and future investigations that will continue to change the landscape in each of these areas.

Keywords: extracapsular spread, extracapsular extension, extranodal spread, extranodal extension, perinodal spread, perinodal extension, transnodal spread, transnodal extension, cervical nodal metastasis, high-risk head and neck cancer

5.1 Background of Extracapsular Spread

Extracapsular spread (ECS) of metastatic head and neck cancer (HNC) continues to capture the interest of professionals today just as it did for Rupert A. Willis, MD, back in 1928 when he encountered the impressive dissemination of "epidermoid carcinoma" of the head and neck during his postmortem examinations.[1] ECS refers to extension of malignant tumor from within a lymph node through the fibrous capsule and into the surrounding connective tissue. There are various terms that have been used to refer to ECS including extracapsular extension, extranodal spread/extension, perinodal spread/extension, transcapsular spread/extension, and capsular rupture. It also includes those soft-tissue deposits of carcinoma found in the tissues of the neck that lack evidence of lymphoid tissue but are not a direct extension of the primary tumor as these may represent extralymphatic deposits of carcinoma or simply lymph nodes that have been completely replaced by tumor.[2]

ECS eventually found its way into the forefront of HNC in 1971 when Bennett et al sought to identify additional prognostic factors. They found that the presence of ECS resulted in a decline in survival rates beyond that of regional metastasis alone.[2] Early investigators thus urged for its consideration as a prognostic criterion to place patients into a high-risk category.[3] As such, they recommended considering adjuvant therapies for those patients with ECS in hopes of achieving better local and regional control to improve cure rates.

An abundance of research has since been conducted in relation to ECS, confirming its profoundly negative effect on outcomes of HNC with a 5-year disease-specific survival (DSS) of a mere 25.0% in patients with ECS as compared to those without

at 57.8% (*p* < 0.001).[4] This remained statistically significant even in multivariate models that accounted for the effect of other prognostic factors. Furthermore, there was found to be over twice the risk of death from HNC in those with ECS present, based on a hazard ratio of 2.44. As a result of research such as this, ECS has now earned its place in the formal staging of HNCs. The eighth edition of the American Joint Committee on Cancer (AJCC) Staging Manual[5] now includes ECS in its nodal classification, which preliminary evidence demonstrates will more accurately reflect the true prognosis of HNCs.[6,7,8] This is due to the upstaging of many cancers as a direct result of the presence of ECS-producing N classifications of N2a or N3b, categorizing them as stage IV cancers.[5] This will also likely have the effect of increasing the use of adjuvant therapies, accordingly.

Inclusion of the ECS criterion applies to the majority of HNCs but does not apply to human papillomavirus (HPV) related oropharyngeal cancers or mucosal melanomas. The HPV-positive oropharyngeal cancers were recently separated due to insight into their biologic difference and subsequent improvement in prognosis, regardless of ECS status.[6] From this point forward, the chapter will refer to ECS as it pertains to HPV-negative squamous cell carcinoma, unless otherwise specified.

Even with this noteworthy progress, ECS is still in its infancy of discovery, and much of the historical data may be somewhat compromised. This can be partially attributed to the nonexistence of defined clinical and pathological diagnostic criteria, an absence of specific pathologic reporting, and a lack of HPV designation. The reported incidences of ECS can also vary due to compounding effects of other factors such as procedure performed, interpreting pathologist, primary site, lymph node size, disease stage, prior therapies, and tumor biology. Regardless of the variation, there is undoubtedly a high overall incidence of ECS. In a recent study of nearly 300 patients with oral cancer, there was found to be an overall incidence of ECS of 54.1% in patients with regional metastases,[8] which was similar to a large meta-analysis of 1,188 patients with an overall incidence of 50.5%.[7] Even in clinically negative (cN0) necks, ECS has been microscopically identified in 22.2% of patients.[9] With such a high prevalence and new role in nodal staging, there is certain to be continued growth surrounding this topic.

5.2 Biology of Extracapsular Spread

Despite a wealth of clinical data on the impact of ECS on patients with HNC, there seems to be a relative paucity of knowledge on the actual pathophysiologic mechanism behind it. The complex nature of cancer biology, in particular how cancer cells are able to migrate outside of the lymph node capsule, still riddles us today. It was initially thought to be simply due to the outgrowth of the enlarging metastatic tumor beyond the lymph node boundaries, and studies have, in fact, demonstrated an association between node size and ECS.[4,8] However, the fact that even subcentimeter nodes with tiny deposits of tumor also exhibit ECS[10] challenges this idea and calls for alternative theories.

Recently, Curry et al built off the foundation of the well-known monocarboxylate transporter 4 (MCT4) and its association with cellular motility and invasiveness in various cancer types including head and neck tumors.[11] They demonstrated its presence in the cancer-associated fibroblasts found in the extracellular matrix surrounding primary HNCs as well as those specific sites where tumor cells have broken through the lymph node capsule. Therefore, they believe that the MCT4 may have a significant role in HNC invasion, including that which occurs in ECS. However, further investigation is needed to determine causality. There has also been extensive work on the epithelial-mesenchymal transition of cells, which has been shown to allow for invasion and metastatic dissemination of cancer cells through increased motility and invasiveness by degradation of the extracellular matrix.[12] It can be postulated that these same mechanisms at work in the primary tumor cells are also present in those which have metastasized to lymph nodes and potentially permit ECS.[13]

These ideas and the rampant search for potential biomarkers to assist in predicting and identifying ECS require continued study but may, in the future, provide valuable information in determining the actual mechanism by which ECS portends a worse prognosis and potentially give insight into developing therapies. It may also aid in the diagnosis and study of other ECS characteristics such as distance of spread beyond the capsule, level of the neck where ECS is identified, total number of nodes with ECS, or the ratio of metastatic lymph nodes to ECS. As the pursuit of demystifying the science behind ECS continues, the clinical management of ECS must, however, carry on and adapt to rising evidence.

5.3 Diagnosing Extracapsular Spread with Imaging

The first step in managing ECS is identifying its presence, so studies have investigated clinicians' abilities to utilize various imaging modalities to detect ECS. There have been several characteristics reported for its radiological diagnosis, and they are similar in both contrast-enhanced computed tomography (CT) and magnetic resonance imaging (MRI). Fujita et al have described the "established criteria" for radiographic evidence of macroscopic ECS to include thick-walled enhancing nodal margins, loss of outer nodal margin definition, capsular contour irregularity, infiltration of adjacent fat planes around portions of the node, invasion of adjacent structures, and multiple nodes abutting one another with loss of an intervening fat plane.[14]

The use of contrast-enhanced CT has shown a lack of specificity and sensitivity in correctly identifying ECS through simple interpretation of the images alone. Therefore, attempts have been made to improve the accuracy of diagnosis by combining associated findings such as central nodal necrosis (▸ Fig. 5.1), which raised the sensitivity and specificity to 95 and 85%, respectively,[15] and has been found to be an independent radiologic predictor of ECS.[16,17] Specificity was improved to 94% with

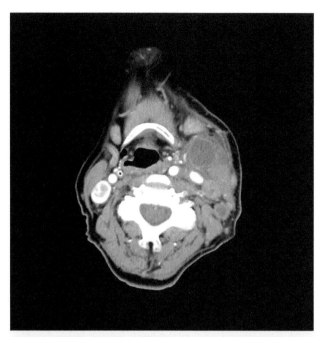

Fig. 5.1 Example of radiographic evidence of extracapsular spread on contrasted computed tomography scan, including central nodal necrosis. (This image is provided courtesy of John A. Arrington, MD.)

the identification of three or more nodes with radiographically suspicious characteristics including size greater than 2 cm in a single dimension, heterogeneous appearance, cystic change, and/or irregular borders.[18]

MRI is often touted as having better soft-tissue resolution, in general; however, this advantage has not been apparent in the diagnosis of ECS. In fact, the use of MRI to predict ECS was previously found to be no better than clinical palpation alone, both of which were inadequate as compared to the actual pathologic rate of ECS.[19] A recent systematic review and meta-analysis found that, although MRI may have a significantly higher sensitivity than CT, there was no difference in specificity and both had similar diagnostic efficacies.[20] One group identified a unique approach utilizing physiologic differences in lymph node blood flow and MRI signal, developing a pixel-based time-signal intensity curve profile within nodes 10 mm or larger and found a specificity of 100% and sensitivity of 96%, but this has not been studied further for application in the everyday clinical setting.[21]

Ultrasound examination is able to utilize additional characteristics such as marked internal echogenicity and the absence or narrowing of hilar echoes which, in combination with the known characteristics of ECS, further suggests its presence.[22] Despite this, no significant differences in the sensitivity and specificity have been found between ultrasound and CT.[23] In a comparison of ultrasound and MRI, they were found to have comparable accuracies, but ultrasound had a higher specificity than MRI.[24]

Given the shortcomings of standard imaging modalities, there was hope that the addition of metabolic information from fluorodeoxyglucose positron emission tomography (FDG PET) would enhance the ability to diagnose ECS. In fact, several retrospective studies from the same institution utilized FDG PET/CT images to deduct threshold SUV_{max} values ranging from 2.25

to 3.85 to identify ECS from various HNC primary subsites.[25] Unfortunately, sensitivities and specificities using these values ranged from a disappointing 80 to 85.7% and 74 to 88%, respectively. Others have actually demonstrated that ECS of HNC is more accurately detected by simply using contrast-enhanced CT alone rather than FDG PET/CT.[26]

Despite ever-improving technology and resolution, the AJCC Head and Neck Task Force determined that today's imaging modalities do not have the level of sensitivity and specificity to rely upon their ability to identify early or minor ECS and, therefore, cannot be the sole basis for diagnosing ECS when applying it to the AJCC clinical staging.[5] They do, however, allow for radiologic imaging as supportive evidence to physical examination in order to diagnose it, but the physical signs must then be unambiguous, such as with skin invasion, infiltration or dense tethering of musculature or adjacent structures, or dysfunction of a cranial nerve/brachial plexus/sympathetic trunk/phrenic nerve (▶ Fig. 5.2). This decision is further supported by the meta-analysis performed by Su et al[20] where they assessed the pooled data of 15 different studies and found a mean sensitivity/specificity for CT of 0.77/0.85, for MRI of 0.85/0.84, and for PET/CT of 0.86/0.86. Overall, this confirms that imaging modalities do not yet have the ability to provide routine, consistently accurate clinical diagnoses. This, in combination with the lack of standard diagnostic criteria, calls for the development of improved methods of detection since ECS has been shown to have a major role in prognosis and treatment decision-making. At the current time, it appears that the contrast-enhanced high-resolution thin-slice CT scan is the most valuable imaging modality for use as a routine study to predict ECS in a nonsurgical manner. Despite its shortcomings, it may provide additional information otherwise missed by physical examination alone.

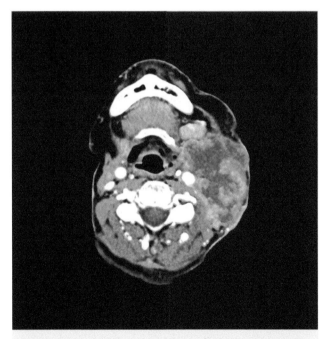

Fig. 5.2 Supportive radiographic evidence of extensive extracapsular spread involving adjacent structures on contrasted computed tomography scan. (This image is provided courtesy of John A. Arrington, MD.)

5.4 Surgical Management of the Neck

Since radiographic studies alone are not currently capable of reliably diagnosing ECS, surgical excision remains the only method to allow for histopathologic examination, which is the gold standard for diagnosis. The surgical management is the same for the clinically positive neck, namely, a modified radical neck dissection. However, the question that remains is how to address the cN0 neck, particularly in the new staging era of ECS inclusion. As with any surgical procedure, the decision relies upon assessment of the risks versus benefits. The general risk of performing a selective neck dissection (SND) is present and described elsewhere in this text but is of low morbidity in the hands of an experienced surgeon. The functional and esthetic results after an SND are also typically acceptable. This risk may be deemed worthwhile, if occult disease is identified; however, the ultimate risk would be in performing a neck dissection found to be pathologically negative (pN0), having then performed a truly nontherapeutic surgical intervention.

On the other hand, the benefit of having complete pathologic classification may be considered worthwhile, regardless of the findings. This would allow for proper staging upfront and avoid the potential of understaging, given the fact that minor ECS is equivalent to major ECS in the new system.[5] Even a pN0 classification is beneficial, particularly if it allows for de-escalation of adjuvant therapies. The additional benefit of identifying occult metastases, and especially occult ECS, is the ability to intervene early on in the process as compared to late where regional relapses in the undissected neck have been found to present at a more advanced stage and with higher rates of ECS.[27]

There is evidence to support the need to perform elective neck dissections based on the rate of occult ECS. In a 2002 study by Coatesworth and MacLennan,[9] 22.2% of all cN0 necks were found to have microscopic ECS and/or soft-tissue deposits present. Nearly 75% of the pathologically positive (pN+) necks had microscopic ECS and/or soft-tissue deposits present. In another study by the same group, 25% of cN0 necks examined and 44% of cN1 necks had ECS and/or soft-tissue deposits.[28] This is evidence that microscopic ECS and soft-tissue deposits are highly prevalent in patients with cN0 necks and that ECS can occur even at an early stage in metastasis. To highlight the influence of ECS, they also found no significant difference in the outcomes of patients with a pN0 neck and those with a pN+ neck but with completely encapsulated nodes (i.e., without ECS).[29]

More recently, D'Cruz et al[27] found that 74% of the cT1/T2 oral cavity node-negative patients in the nonelective neck dissection group eventually developed recurrent disease in the neck, and these patients had a significantly higher incidence of ECS ($p < 0.001$) with a more advanced nodal stage ($p = 0.005$) as compared to those treated with an elective neck dissection. Furthermore, the patients who were found to have pN+ neck disease in the upfront elective neck dissection had significantly better overall survival (OS) rates than those who had been carefully observed and later presented with nodal relapse.[30]

Similarly, in a retrospective chart review by Dik et al, management of the cN0 neck in patients with surgically resected early-stage (cT1/T2) oral squamous cell carcinoma were handled in either a "watchful waiting" approach or underwent an intentional upfront ipsilateral SND.[31] They found that a significantly larger number of positive lymph nodes with ECS were found in the watchful waiting group after they recurred than in those who were found to have nodal disease following upfront SND. This also produced a significantly worse DSS as compared to those who underwent upfront SND.

Additionally, a recent study found 66.7% of patients with salvage neck dissections had nodes with ECS present, and the 5-year salvage-specific survival for those patients was 32.0%, compared to 77.2% in those without ECS ($p = 0.0001$).[32] They noted that these patients with recurrent regional disease and ECS present had a 4.1 times higher risk of death as a consequence of the tumor as compared to those who did not have ECS present. The variable found to be most related to the presence of ECS in salvage neck dissections was the class of regional neck recurrence, with 19.2% of rpN1 necks with ECS, 75.9% of rpN2 necks, and 100% of rpN3 necks (classified according to the AJCC staging manual, seventh edition).

The evidence from these studies helps one to appreciate that an upfront neck dissection can have major implications on staging, prognosis, and adjuvant therapeutic options, especially if ECS is identified. On the same note, the risk of missing occult metastases and/or ECS seems to be worse than the risk of performing a neck dissection on a pN0 neck. Therefore, elective neck dissections should be strongly considered. Further study is needed regarding the prognostic effects of microscopic ECS and recurrent disease with ECS, now more than ever, for clarification on the surgical management of the cN0 neck.

In all cases of neck dissection, whether elective or therapeutic, and particularly when ECS is suspected, surgeons should be mindful of the fact that ECS may be present, and direct contact with tumor cells risks implantation/seeding. Respecting the fascial planes when possible also helps avoid direct contact with potential tumor cells present in the perinodal adipose tissue. Likewise, "node picking" or "node sampling" may miss microscopic metastases and soft-tissue deposits. Clinical suspicion for ECS pre- or intraoperatively should prompt the removal of any adjacent tissues that appear to potentially be involved such as the overlying skin or adjacent structures in the neck. Careful surgical technique with ECS in mind should help avoid the potential for leaving behind microscopic disease or inadvertently seeding tumor cells.

5.5 Pathological Diagnosis of Extracapsular Spread

Currently, histopathologic evaluation is the only method of definitively identifying ECS. Despite being the gold standard, there is a level of variability and subjectivity in its diagnosis, which has been demonstrated in several studies, even with experienced head and neck pathologists.[33] A low level of interobserver, and even intraobserver, agreement in the pathologic assessment of ECS has been contributed to the difficulties in evaluating lymph nodes that have been fully replaced by tumor and are surrounded by a desmoplastic reaction, mimicking a capsule, causing some pathologists to score lymph nodes negative for ECS.[34] Another debate occurs when tumor is present at the lymph node hilum, where there is naturally no true capsule present, requiring subjective determination as to whether this

should be considered a disruption in the capsule due to ECS or simply a deposit in the hilum. Juxtacapsular extension, where tumor tissue grows into the capsule but not outside of it, can also cause some disagreement among pathologists. This highlights the reality of the challenges in histopathologic diagnosis of ECS even though at first glance it seems straightforward. This may be partially due to the lack of a set of standardized diagnostic criteria; however, several common characteristics are reportedly used for its identification including perinodal fat involvement (▶ Fig. 5.3); skeletal muscle, nerve, and thick-walled vessel involvement; tumor beyond the nodal capsule; and desmoplastic stromal reaction outside the node.[33]

Once defined systems of diagnosis, classification, and reporting for ECS are in place, it will better enable associated information to be identified and collected, such as extent of disease beyond the lymph node capsule, which is an important topic of study. It is known that ECS is a poor prognostic factor, but, currently, both microscopic and macroscopic ECS have been lumped together. Some evidence shows there is a correlation between the level of extension of ECS and prognosis so microscopic ECS may play a role, but the exact threshold distance that is truly significant remains undefined.

In a study on 266 patients with oral cancer, Greenberg et al found no difference in survival when comparing the extent of ECS of ≤ 2 and > 2 mm from the capsule of the lymph node,[35] indicating there may be no difference in survival between microscopic and macroscopic ECS, allowing them to be grouped together. Jose et al likewise found that there was no significant difference in overall or recurrence-free survival between microscopic and macroscopic ECS.[29] A recent study on a cohort of pathologically node-positive oral cancer patients better defined the threshold when they found that the adverse prognosis of ECS was only clinically relevant when it extended more than 1.7 mm beyond the nodal capsule.[4]

For the eighth edition of the AJCC staging manual, minor ECS will be defined as extension ≤ 2 mm from the capsule and major ECS defined as either (1) extension apparent to the pathologist's

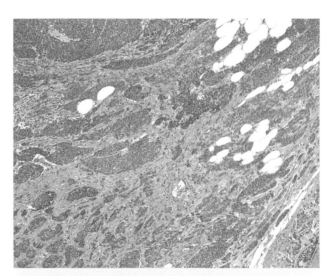

Fig. 5.3 Higher magnification showing carcinoma extending into perinodal soft tissues including mature adipose tissue, representing the presence of extranodal extension. (This image is provided courtesy of Bruce M. Wenig, MD.)

naked eye and/or to manual palpation when accessioning the surgical specimen or (2) greater than 2 mm of extension beyond the capsule microscopically.[6] Major ECS will also include those soft-tissue deposits of carcinoma that have no nodal architecture present. As of now, this measurement is little more than arbitrary given the minimal amount of supporting evidence. These two subdivisions of ECS were made for data collection purposes only, and either one is considered ECS positive for actual pathologic nodal staging.

With these recent staging changes, there has also been an update of the College of American Pathologists' (CAP) protocol.[36] There is now required reporting of ECS as "present," "not identified," or "cannot be determined" for all HNC except for HPV-positive oropharyngeal carcinomas for which ECS notation is not required as it is not used as a criterion in its nodal staging. For those that do require an ECS status designation, it may also include an optional notation of the extent of ECS, given in millimeters from the lymph node capsule with differentiation between major ECS or minor ECS. There is a comment by the CAP that some of the common pitfalls encountered when measuring ECS included occurrences of larger, matted nodes, nodes post fine-needle aspiration, and nodes with near total replacement of nodal architecture (▶ Fig. 5.4). They point out that doubt should arise if a large lymph node (> 3 cm) has been designated as ECS negative, in particular if there are fibrous bands traversing the tumor, as data have shown that a great majority of these exhibit ECS. The CAP also agrees that soft-tissue tumor deposits should be recorded as ECS. Moving forward with the AJCC staging updates and the paralleling recommendations of CAP to include a measurement of extent of tumor beyond the capsule, data collection for further investigations into the impact of ECS extent on prognostic endpoints should be less cumbersome.

Coatesworth and MacLennan pointed out that the technique used for assessing neck dissection specimens historically utilized a 3-mm cutoff for commenting on lymph nodes.[9] Therefore, micrometastases and, in particular, microscopic ECS or soft-tissue deposits would be missed or underreported. Thus,

they recommend dividing each of the neck levels grossly, then cutting these into 2-mm-thick blocks, embedding them in wax, and then sectioning them in their entirety at 6-μm-thick slices for microscopic evaluation. They later noted that this technique was able to assess microscopic ECS in lymph nodes as small as 0.5 mm, finding an average of 50.4 lymph nodes per neck dissection, making it appear labor intensive and time-consuming.[37] However, they state that the macroscopic assessment and block selection can be conducted quickly, generating an average number of 633 microscopic slides for a four-level neck dissection, and these slides are able to be screened in less than 30 minutes. This method avoids missing micrometastases and soft-tissue deposits, both of which may have a significant impact on patient prognosis and management.

To further highlight the need for comprehensive pathologic assessment, a study specifically looking at infracentimetric regional metastases found that 38% of cervical metastases were less than 1 cm, with 72% of those having ECS.[10] Even in the 2015 landmark study by D'Cruz et al, they noted that the difference in the incidences of nodal relapse (45.1%) compared to pathologic node positivity found in the elective neck dissections (29.6%) may indicate that their routine method of histopathological examination may have missed metastases.[27] Further clarifying studies can help find a balance in avoiding missed diagnoses but also keeping unnecessary efforts to a minimum. This will also translate into improved reporting of the specific ECS characteristics, including them only if they affect patient management and outcomes.

5.6 Therapeutic Implications of Extracapsular Spread

It is well known that the presence of regional metastasis to the cervical lymph nodes is one of the most important predictors of cancer outcomes[38] with regional and distant progression of disease accounting for the majority of treatment failures in HNC.[39] ECS is a characteristic of regional metastasis, which has been shown to be an independently significant factor on prognostic endpoints beyond that of regional disease alone. A meta-analysis on 1,620 patients to determine the impact of ECS on survival reported a 5-year OS rate of 58.1% in the group of patients with encapsulated lymph node metastasis.[40] In contrast, the survival rate of patients with ECS was a dismal 30.7%, concluding that ECS can be said to be associated with at least a 50% drop in the 5-year OS rate for any given TNM stage (AJCC manual, seventh edition) due to a summarized odds ratio of 2.7. Therefore, ECS serves as a major component in decision-making in patients with HNC.[41,42]

More recent evidence continues to confirm the significant and independent adverse effect of ECS on prognosis. Lydiatt et al conducted a retrospective analysis in order to internally validate the TNM classification changes for the AJCC manual and found that patients who were upstaged, as a result of their positive ECS status, had a worse OS.[6] Matos et al then performed an external validation study on their institution's data, which also reflected that the upstaged ECS patients had a worse disease-free survival (51.1 vs. 80.4%; $p = 0.007$) and worse OS (8.5 vs. 37.9%; $p < 0.001$).[8] Another meta-analysis confirmed the negative impact of ECS on distant metastasis with a summarized

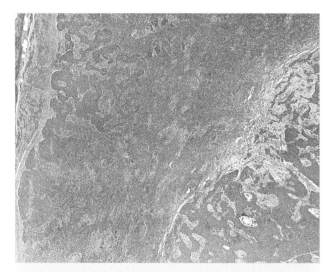

Fig. 5.4 Low magnification showing metastatic nonkeratinizing carcinoma to a cervical neck lymph node in which carcinoma effaces most of the nodal architecture. (This image is provided courtesy of Bruce M. Wenig, MD.)

odds ratio of 2.18.[25] This was again seen to be true in a recent article noting a significant association between the presence of ECS and the prevalence of distant metastasis (11.9% without ECS compared to 32.0% with ECS; $p = 0.001$).[43] Garzino-Demo et al retrospectively analyzed 525 patients with oral cancer and found that the differences in 5-year OS based on pathologic nodal status (pNx, pN0, pN+, or pN+with ECS) were statistically significant with ECS+patients being just a mere 15.15% compared to even pN+patients at 54.94%, both of which are much lower than the pN0 patient at 76.99%.[44]

There is evidence that reveals a difference in this adverse impact of ECS on oropharyngeal squamous cell carcinoma (OPSCC) apart from other head and neck sites, and it is well known that HPV-positive OPSCC patients have an overall better prognosis compared to HPV-negative HNC patients, in general. Most research has demonstrated the known adverse effect of ECS on HPV-negative OPSCC patient outcomes but has failed to identify the same effect on HPV-positive patients, although these are usually smaller, single-institution, and retrospective studies.[40, 45,46,47] Therefore, a larger study of 1,043 patients was conducted by An et al in order to further investigate the apparent lack of effect of ECS on prognosis in this subpopulation, and they did reveal a significance in survival statistics of OPSCC HPV-positive patients with ECS versus those without ECS, with 3-year OS rates of 89.3 versus 93.6%, respectively ($p = 0.010$).[48] There was no difference in OS for microscopic versus macroscopic ECS, but the mere presence of ECS revealed a hazard ratio of 1.89 on multivariable analysis, suggesting that ECS is independently associated with a nearly two times higher hazard of death. Furthermore, these OS data remained significant despite the fact that the ECS-positive patients also likely received concurrent chemoradiation therapy (CRT).

The changes in the updated staging manual now reflect the important revelations of the impact of both ECS and HPV positivity on prognostic endpoints.[5] The changes in nodal classification for the majority of HNCs, as stated previously, will cause upstaging to stage IV with the identification of any ECS. This will then place the patient into an advanced-stage cancer treatment protocol, which, at the current time, includes CRT based on recommendations for the addition of concurrent chemotherapy to postoperative irradiation. This comes from the level 1 evidence published in 2004 as a result of the two independent, randomized phase 3 trials: EORTC 22931[41] and RTOG 9501,[42] which were conducted from the mid-1990s to 2000. Just as some of the first investigators of ECS had proposed, these studies have since proven ECS as one of the high-risk adverse features in locally advanced HNC that benefits from the addition of cisplatin to adjuvant radiation therapy (RT). In a subsequent study on the pooled data, ECS and microscopically positive surgical margins were discovered to be the only two adverse features most likely to benefit from the addition of chemotherapy.[49] The addition of cisplatin to adjuvant RT in patients with these high-risk features produced a nearly 50% decrease in locoregional recurrence, a 38% increase in DSS, and a 33% improvement in OS. Therefore, these two features now serve as standard indications for concurrent adjuvant CRT. Interestingly, a recent study found that, of the 66.7% of salvage necks that had ECS present, the 5-year salvage-specific survival for patients with ECS who did not receive adjuvant treatment was only 15.2% compared to those

who received RT (36.4%) or CRT (47.1%).[32] This further supports the decision to add chemotherapy to the treatment plan for select patients with ECS.

Although abundant data support the use of concurrent CRT for the improvement of disease control and survival, this also comes with a cost in the form of increased rates of acute toxicity.[41,42] Cetuximab (Erbitux), an anti-endothelial growth factor receptor (anti-EGFR) monoclonal antibody, was studied as a replacement for cisplatin in an effort to reduce those toxicities. Bonner et al reported superior locoregional control and OS in a similar population of patients treated by concurrent cetuximab with RT as compared to RT alone.[50] They did find decreased rates of acute toxicities and improved OS with the addition of cetuximab, and this initially gave hope that it may serve as an alternative therapy to cisplatin in those patients who require adjuvant treatment but who are unable to tolerate platinum-based therapy. However, since then, there has been question as to whether this adjuvant therapy will truly improve outcomes or be a worthwhile treatment for these patients.[51] Additional studies are needed to clarify its use in patients with ECS, and the RTOG 1216 randomized phase II/III clinical trial is currently addressing this question; however, based on the currently available data, the use of postoperative concurrent cisplatin CRT for locally advanced HNC patients is the first-line adjuvant regimen for those with evidence of ECS.

In order to avoid unnecessary adverse effects of cisplatin-based CRT, clinical trials are still needed to confirm its indication in specific clinical settings. This is particularly true for HPV-positive OPSCC and is especially important since the two landmark trials indicating the benefits of concurrent CRT[41,42] were conducted in an era prior to the significant rise in HPV-associated OPSCC, so that subset likely made up only a small proportion of the patients studied. Newer studies are, however, in agreement that there are no significant differences between the outcomes of the HPV and ECS-positive OPSCC patients who received concurrent CRT versus those who received adjuvant RT alone.[45,52] An et al also showed that those OPSCC patients with the presence of ECS who received adjuvant CRT had similar 3-year OS rates of 89.3% compared to 89.6% for those that received RT alone ($p = 0.44$).[47] Another recent study demonstrated that, in a population of HPV-positive OPSCC with ECS and/or positive margins treated with postoperative CRT utilizing intensity-modulated RT with a dose reduction from 66 to 60 gray, there was no significant difference in locoregional recurrence-free survival (98.1 vs. 98.5%; $p = 0.421$).[53] Larger, prospective de-escalation trials are currently being conducted to study the subset of patients with HPV-positive OPSCC to investigate the possibility of reducing acute toxicity and impairment but, at the same time, maintaining the high survival rates.

Another group requiring future study are those patients who would have been classified pN1 under the seventh edition of the AJCC manual. Studies have found that there is no difference in survival in those patients with just one isolated node up to 3 cm regardless of the presence of ECS. However, many of these patients who were found to have ECS present were also subsequently treated with adjuvant CRT. Therefore, the apparent low impact of ECS in these patients may in fact be due to the efficacy of the intensification of adjuvant treatments due to the presence of their high-risk feature of ECS.[7] Along the same lines, Prabhu et al demonstrated that those with lower grades of ECS had no significant difference in failure-free survival as compared to those without ECS present.[54] However, this was again in the setting of postoperative concurrent CRT, suggesting that the adjuvant therapy intensification for ECS simply nullified the adverse prognosis typically associated with ECS. Highest-grade ECS maintained a poorer prognosis despite the same concurrent CRT, indicating the patients in this subgroup may require further intensification of treatment.

5.7 Conclusion

ECS has a large role in the treatment of HNC, and the new nodal classification scheme has incorporated it as well. This will be sure to draw additional attention to this developing topic, and the completion of the battery of clinical trials currently under way will provide additional insight into the management of patients with ECS in the future.

References

[1] Willis RA. Epidermoid carcinoma of the head and neck, with special reference to metastasis. J Pathol. 1930; 33:501–526

[2] Bennett SH, Futrell JW, Roth JA, Hoye RC, Ketcham AS. Prognostic significance of histologic host response in cancer of the larynx or hypopharynx. Cancer. 1971; 28(5):1255–1265

[3] Shah JP, Cendon RA, Farr HW, Strong EW. Carcinoma of the oral cavity. factors affecting treatment failure at the primary site and neck. Am J Surg. 1976; 132 (4):504–507

[4] Wreesmann VB, Katabi N, Palmer FL, et al. Influence of extracapsular nodal spread extent on prognosis of oral squamous cell carcinoma. Head Neck. 2016; 38 suppl 1:E1192–E1199

[5] American Joint Committee on Cancer. AJCC Cancer Staging Manual. 8th ed. New York, NY: Springer; 2017

[6] Lydiatt WM, Patel SG, O'Sullivan B, et al. Head and Neck cancers-major changes in the American Joint Committee on cancer eighth edition cancer staging manual. CA Cancer J Clin. 2017; 67(2):122–137

[7] Garcia J, Lopez M, Lopez L, et al. Validation of the pathological Gradeification of lymph node metastasis for head and neck tumors according to the 8th edition of the TNM Gradeification of Malignant Tumors. Oral Oncol. 2017; 70:29–33

[8] Matos LL, Dedivitis RA, Kulcsar MAV, de Mello ES, Alves VAF, Cernea CR. External validation of the AJCC Cancer Staging Manual, 8th edition, in an independent cohort of oral cancer patients. Oral Oncol. 2017; 71:47–53

[9] Coatesworth AP, MacLennan K. Squamous cell carcinoma of the upper aerodigestive tract: the prevalence of microscopic extracapsular spread and soft tissue deposits in the clinically N0 neck. Head Neck. 2002; 24(3):258–261

[10] Pauzie A, Gavid M, Dumollard JM, Timoshenko A, Peoc'h M, Prades JM. Infracentimetric cervical lymph node metastasis in head and neck squamous cell carcinoma: Incidence and prognostic value. Eur Ann Otorhinolaryngol Head Neck Dis. 2016; 133(5):307–311

[11] Curry J, Tassone P, Gill K, et al. Tumor metabolism in the microenvironment of nodal metastasis in oral squamous cell carcinoma. Otolaryngol Head Neck Surg. 2017; 157(5):798–807

[12] Lambert AW, Pattabiraman DR, Weinberg RA. Emerging biological principles of metastasis. Cell. 2017; 168(4):670–691

[13] Lee WY, Shin DY, Kim HJ, Ko YH, Kim S, Jeong HS. Prognostic significance of epithelial-mesenchymal transition of extracapsular spread tumors in lymph node metastases of head and neck cancer. Ann Surg Oncol. 2014; 21 (6):1904–1911

[14] Fujita A, Buch K, Truong MT, et al. Imaging characteristics of metastatic nodes and outcomes by HPV status in head and neck cancers. Laryngoscope. 2016; 126(2):392–398

[15] Zoumalan RA, Kleinberger AJ, Morris LG, et al. Lymph node central necrosis on computed tomography as predictor of extracapsular spread in metastatic head and neck squamous cell carcinoma: pilot study. J Laryngol Otol. 2010; 124(12):1284–1288

[16] Randall DR, Lysack JT, Hudon ME, et al. Diagnostic utility of central node necrosis in predicting extracapsular spread among oral cavity squamous cell carcinoma. Head Neck. 2015; 37(1):92–96

[17] Aiken AH, Poliashenko S, Beitler JJ, et al. Accuracy of preoperative imaging in detecting nodal extracapsular spread in oral cavity squamous cell carcinoma. AJNR Am J Neuroradiol. 2015; 36(9):1776–1781

[18] Geltzeiler M, Clayburgh D, Gleysteen J, et al. Predictors of extracapsular extension in HPV-associated oropharyngeal cancer treated surgically. Oral Oncol. 2017; 65:89–93

[19] Hao SP, Ng SH. Magnetic resonance imaging versus clinical palpation in evaluating cervical metastasis from head and neck cancer. Otolaryngol Head Neck Surg. 2000; 123(3):324–327

[20] Su Z, Duan Z, Pan W, et al. Predicting extracapsular spread of head and neck cancers using different imaging techniques: a systematic review and meta-analysis. Int J Oral Maxillofac Surg. 2016; 45(4):413–421

[21] Sumi M, Nakamura T. Extranodal spread in the neck: MRI detection on the basis of pixel-based time-signal intensity curve analysis. J Magn Reson Imaging. 2011; 33(4):830–838

[22] Yuasa K, Kawazu T, Kunitake N, et al. Sonography for the detection of cervical lymph node metastases among patients with tongue cancer: criteria for early detection and assessment of follow-up examination intervals. AJNR Am J Neuroradiol. 2000; 21(6):1127–1132

[23] Ishii J, Nagasawa H, Yamane M, et al. Ultrasonography and computed tomography of extracapsular invasion in cervical lymph nodes of squamous cell carcinoma in the oral cavity. J Med Ultrason (2001). 2004; 31(2):75–79

[24] Katayama I, Sasaki M, Kimura Y, et al. Comparison between ultrasonography and MR imaging for discriminating squamous cell carcinoma nodes with extranodal spread in the neck. Eur J Radiol. 2012; 81(11):3326–3331

[25] Mermod M, Tolstonog G, Simon C, Monnier Y. Extracapsular spread in head and neck squamous cell carcinoma: A systematic review and meta-analysis. Oral Oncol. 2016; 62:60–71

[26] Lee JR, Choi YJ, Roh JL, et al. Preoperative contrast-enhanced CT versus 18F-FDG PET/CT evaluation and the prognostic value of extranodal extension for surgical patients with head and neck squamous cell carcinoma. Ann Surg Oncol. 2015; 22 suppl 3:S1020–S1027

[27] D'Cruz AK, Vaish R, Kapre N, et al. Head and Neck Disease Management Group. Elective versus therapeutic neck dissection in node-negative oral cancer. N Engl J Med. 2015; 373(6):521–529

[28] Jose J, Coatesworth AP, MacLennan K. Cervical metastases in upper aerodigestive tract squamous cell carcinoma: histopathologic analysis and reporting. Head Neck. 2003; 25(3):194–197

[29] Jose J, Coatesworth AP, Johnston C, MacLennan K. Cervical node metastases in squamous cell carcinoma of the upper aerodigestive tract: the significance of extracapsular spread and soft tissue deposits. Head Neck. 2003; 25(6):451–456

[30] Deschamps DR, Spencer HJ, Kokoska MS, Spring PM, Vural EA, Stack BC, Jr. Implications of head and neck cancer treatment failure in the neck. Otolaryngol Head Neck Surg. 2010; 142(5):722–727

[31] Dik EA, Willems SM, Ipenburg NA, Rosenberg AJ, Van Cann EM, van Es RJ. Watchful waiting of the neck in early stage oral cancer is unfavourable for patients with occult nodal disease. Int J Oral Maxillofac Surg. 2016; 45 (8):945–950

[32] León X, Rigó A, Farré N, et al. Prognostic significance of extracapsular spread in isolated neck recurrences in head and neck squamous cell carcinoma patients. Eur Arch Otorhinolaryngol. 2017; 274(1):527–533

[33] Du E, Wenig BM, Su HK, et al. Inter-observer variation in the pathologic identification of extranodal extension in nodal metastasis from papillary thyroid carcinoma. Thyroid. 2016; 26(6):816–819

[34] van den Brekel MW, Lodder WL, Stel HV, Bloemena E, Leemans CR, van der Waal I. Observer variation in the histopathologic assessment of extranodal tumor spread in lymph node metastases in the neck. Head Neck. 2012; 34 (6):840–845

[35] Greenberg JS, Fowler R, Gomez J, et al. Extent of extracapsular spread: a critical prognosticator in oral tongue cancer. Cancer. 2003; 97(6):1464–1470

[36] Seethala RR, Bullock MJ, Carlson DL, et al. Protocol for the examination of specimens from patients with cancers of the lip and Oral Cavity, Version 4.0.0.0. Northfield, IL: College of American Pathologists; 2017

[37] Jose J, Coatesworth AP, MacLennan K. Cervical metastases in upper aerodigestive tract squamous cell carcinoma: histopathologic analysis and reporting. Head Neck. 2003; 25(3):194–197

[38] Marur S, Forastiere AA. Head and neck squamous cell carcinoma: update on epidemiology, diagnosis, and treatment. Mayo Clin Proc. 2016; 91(3):386–396

[39] Coatesworth AP, Tsikoudas A, MacLennan K. The cause of death in patients with head and neck squamous cell carcinoma. J Laryngol Otol. 2002; 116(4):269–271

[40] Dünne AA, Müller HH, Eisele DW, Kessel K, Moll R, Werner JA. Meta-analysis of the prognostic significance of perinodal spread in head and neck squamous cell carcinomas (HNSCC) patients. Eur J Cancer. 2006; 42(12):1863–1868

[41] Bernier J, Domenge C, Ozsahin M, et al. European Organization for Research and Treatment of Cancer Trial 22931. Postoperative irradiation with or without concomitant chemotherapy for locally advanced head and neck cancer. N Engl J Med. 2004; 350(19):1945–1952

[42] Cooper JS, Pajak TF, Forastiere AA, et al. Radiation Therapy Oncology Group 9501/Intergroup. Postoperative concurrent radiotherapy and chemotherapy for high-risk squamous-cell carcinoma of the head and neck. N Engl J Med. 2004; 350(19):1937–1944

[43] Duprez F, Berwouts D, De Neve W, et al. Distant metastases in head and neck cancer. Head Neck. 2017; 39(9):1733–1743

[44] Garzino-Demo P, Zavattero E, Franco P, et al. Parameters and outcomes in 525 patients operated on for oral squamous cell carcinoma. J Craniomaxillofac Surg. 2016; 44(9):1414–1421

[45] Sinha P, Lewis JS, Jr, Piccirillo JF, Kallogjeri D, Haughey BH. Extracapsular spread and adjuvant therapy in human papillomavirus-related, p16-positive oropharyngeal carcinoma. Cancer. 2012; 118(14):3519–3530

[46] Lewis JS, Jr, Carpenter DH, Thorstad WL, Zhang Q, Haughey BH. Extracapsular extension is a poor predictor of disease recurrence in surgically treated oropharyngeal squamous cell carcinoma. Mod Pathol. 2011; 24(11):1413–1420

[47] Kharytaniuk N, Molony P, Boyle S, et al. Association of extracapsular spread with survival according to human papillomavirus status in oropharynx squamous cell carcinoma and carcinoma of unknown primary site. JAMA Otolaryngol Head Neck Surg. 2016; 142(7):683–690

[48] An Y, Park HS, Kelly JR, et al. The prognostic value of extranodal extension in human papillomavirus-associated oropharyngeal squamous cell carcinoma. Cancer. 2017; 123(14):2762–2772

[49] Bernier J, Cooper JS, Pajak TF, et al. Defining risk levels in locally advanced head and neck cancers: a comparative analysis of concurrent postoperative radiation plus chemotherapy trials of the EORTC (# 22931) and RTOG (# 9501). Head Neck. 2005; 27(10):843–850

[50] Bonner JA, Harari PM, Giralt J, et al. Radiotherapy plus cetuximab for locoregionally advanced head and neck cancer: 5-year survival data from a phase 3 randomised trial, and relation between cetuximab-induced rash and survival. Lancet Oncol. 2010; 11(1):21–28

[51] Araki D, Redman MW, Martins R, et al. Concurrent cetuximab and postoperative radiation in resected high-risk squamous cell carcinomas of the head and neck: A single-institution experience. Head Neck. 2016; 38(9):1318–1323

[52] Amini A, Jasem J, Jones BL, et al. Predictors of overall survival in human papillomavirus-associated oropharyngeal cancer using the National Cancer Data Base. Oral Oncol. 2016; 56:1–7

[53] Chin RI, Spencer CR, DeWees T, et al. Reevaluation of postoperative radiation dose in the management of human papillomavirus-positive oropharyngeal cancer. Head Neck. 2016; 38(11):1643–1649

[54] Prabhu RS, Hanasoge S, Magliocca KR, et al. Extent of pathologic extracapsular extension and outcomes in patients with nonoropharyngeal head and neck cancer treated with initial surgical resection. Cancer. 2014; 120 (10):1499–1506

6 Radical Neck Dissection

Rachel Giese and Richard Wong

Abstract

Radical neck dissection was historically the standard of care for the management of cervical nodal metastases. A radical neck dissection includes the complete resection of all five levels of the cervical lymphatics, and additionally sacrifice of the spinal accessory nerve, sternocleidomastoid and the internal jugular vein. This procedure causes considerable morbidity, predominantly from shoulder dysfunction, and numerous studies have since demonstrated that the surgical preservation of non-invaded structures was oncologically sound. More recent modifications of neck dissection are now performed that selectively remove the lymph nodes in the anatomic levels that are at highest risk for harboring metastatic nodal disease while preserving key structures, and carry much less morbidity. The following chapter addresses the history, techniques, morbidity, post-operative considerations, and potential complications of a radical neck dissection.

Keywords: radical, neck, dissection

6.1 History

The initial concept of surgically removing cervical lymphatics en bloc represented a major conceptual advance in oncology. The first reports of removal of neck metastases came from independent efforts of four European surgeons: von Langenbeck, Billroth, von Volkmann, and Kocher.[1] Later, Sir Henry Butlin demonstrated that surgically removing metastases from the neck for oral cavity cancer improved survival. In 1888, a Polish surgeon, Franciszek Jawdynski, reported on a procedure similar to a radical neck dissection (RND). Early surgeries resulted in serious complications and morbidity. In 1906, George Crile popularized the systematic en bloc RND[2] that included the removal of all structures in the neck from the mandible to the clavicle, superficial to the deep muscles of the neck, except the carotid artery, brachial plexus and the vagal, lingual, and hypoglossal nerves. The specimen encompassed lymph nodes and fibrofatty tissue spanning levels I to V and includes the spinal accessory nerve (SAN), sternocleidomastoid muscle (SCM), and internal jugular vein (IJV). Recognizing that loss of these structures caused patients significant functional and cosmetic morbidity, Suarez modified the procedure in 1963 to preserve nonlymphatic structures when oncologically feasible. Bocca[3] and Martin et al[4] further refined the surgical procedure terming it a "functional neck dissection." The adapted procedure became widely adopted as it became clear that this modification was both oncologically safe and imparted less morbidity to the patient by preserving structures that were uninvolved by disease. Since then, many retrospective studies have repeatedly demonstrated the oncologic safety in preserving these structures. Knowledge of lymphatic drainage patterns specific to neck dissection has led to further evolution of this procedure into what is today referred to as the modified RND and selective neck dissection. Although Crile's neck dissection was initially the "gold standard neck dissection," with modifications in the subsequent four decades following the initial description, it is now referred to as the RND. This term is appropriate because it is a radical removal of sites of metastatic spread to the neck, sacrificing the SAN, SCM, and IJV. However, it is rarely required today, except in cases of extensive disease, and the evolution of the procedure to less aggressive resection has greatly improved the postoperative quality of life for patients.

6.2 Classification/Terminology

Surgeons at Memorial Hospital first classified the cervical lymph nodes into levels and later Byers et al described the levels most at risk for spread based on the primary tumor site in the head and neck.[5] When it became clear not all cervical lymphatics needed to be resected that an RND encompassed, surgeons modified the neck dissection to involve the lymphatics at highest risk for disease spread. Furthermore, the SAN, IJV, and SCM were preserved unless there was disease involvement. Because there were so many variations between lymphatic levels and structures sacrificed, the American Head and Neck Society (AHNS) standardized the terminology for classification of neck dissection in 1991 and there have been multiple revisions thereafter.[6] Most recently, the AHNS defined the RND as a cervical lymphadenectomy including en bloc removal levels I to V, the IJV, SCM, SAN, and the submandibular gland.[7] According to the AHNS classification, any neck dissection that preserves the three structures should be termed a "modified RND" and preserved structures should be stated when naming the procedure, an adaptation of Medina's terminology for structures preserved published in 1989. Ferlito et al proposed a further modification to this terminology suggesting that each level and structure resected should be clarified, with an RND termed ND (I–V, SCM, IJV, and cranial nerve [CN] XI).[8]

Due to the rarity of patients requiring an RND and sacrifice of the SAN, SCM, and IJV, the "modified" RND is now the standard of care for most patients with metastatic nodal disease where one or more of these structures can be preserved. RND imparts considerable comorbidity to the patients and should be avoided when oncologically possible. The term "modified RND" refers to preservation of nonlymphatic structures, whereas the term "selective neck dissection" refers to preservation of levels of lymphatics. The standardization of terminology is important to communicate to other practitioners which levels were dissected and which structures were resected for postoperative management. Stating that a patient had an RND accurately transmits the idea of extensive or invasive metastatic nodal disease in the neck.

6.3 Indications for Radical Neck Dissection

The goal of curative oncologic surgery should be the complete removal of all neoplastic tissue. Surgeons must balance the oncologic advantages of RND against the morbidity it brings to the patient. An RND is now performed only when necessary due to the extent and growth pattern of the disease. In most cases, this is due to disease invading the SCM, IJV, and SAN.

Uncommonly, an RND is performed due to direct spread of a primary tumor. Although neck dissections are not pathologically assessed for margins unless it is an en bloc resection of direct tumor spread, surgeons have applied the same reasoning that is used in tumor resection when resecting the lymphatics of the neck. That is, preferably, the disease will be surrounded by nondiseased (normal) tissue. In most dissections, this means the disease is within the capsule of the lymph node, but this is not typical of nodal disease in most cases requiring RND. However, in cases with extracapsular spread, the resection of adjacent structures such as SCM, IJV, and SAN may be required to get a "margin" around the disease, justifying the RND.

Some have suggested that RND is appropriate routinely for N3 disease of the upper neck, invasion of the SAN, and/or recurrent or persistent disease following definitive radiotherapy, chemoradiotherapy, or previous selective neck dissection.[9] Presumably, the recommendation of RND for all N3 diseases implies that a 6-cm metastasis would encompass the SAN and involve the SCM and IJV due to the confined anatomy of the neck and restricted space for spread. Such a global suggestion also likely stems from concerns that the posttreatment scarring may obscure tissue planes, making the clean removal of disease from the SAN, IJV, and SCM challenging. However, the specific relationships between disease and each anatomic structure in the neck should be better evaluated on a case-by-case basis, and adaptations and consideration of risks of involvement of each structure must be applied to each individual patient. It is possible that not all three structures (SAN, IJV, and SCM) implicit in RND need to be resected in every patient who has had a previous neck dissection or radiation.

Regarding indications for RND, some patients may have such extensive disease that more extended resection is needed than a traditional RND. Surgery may necessitate resection of structures outside the scope of a typical RND, including the strap muscles, digastric, omohyoid, cervical rootlets, brachial plexus, hypoglossal nerve, facial nerve, phrenic nerve, carotid artery, the skull base, or deep muscles of the neck. Involvement of these structures, especially the carotid artery, portends a very poor prognosis and thus may call into question the goals of the operation.

It is important to note not all cervical nodal disease may be surgically resectable. If disease may not be cleared even with extended RND, the morbidity of the surgery may not be justified. For example, if the carotid artery is involved and cannot be safely sacrificed or when sacrifice of the carotid is not guaranteed to remove all disease in the neck, it may be wiser to consider nonsurgical options including systemic therapy, radiation therapy, or entry into a clinical trial. Ultimately, the surgeon needs to discuss the options with the patients and tailor individualized treatment to each patient's particular clinical situation.

6.4 Preoperative Counseling and Evaluation

Documentation of arm and shoulder range of motion and strength should be made prior to surgery to assess SAN and brachial plexus function. Photos may aid in the preoperative counseling of the patient to set expectations for postoperative

neck, shoulder, and arm function (▶ Fig. 6.1). The patient should be counseled about potential postoperative morbidity and the need for rehabilitation prior to surgery. Expected contour changes to the neck, numbness, the expected incision line, and possible deficits of the particular CNs at risk should be reviewed. Other risks of surgery including bleeding, infection, chyle leak, carotid injury, stroke, nerve deficits, unresectable disease, and possible rapid recurrence despite surgery may be discussed. Postoperative morbidity intrinsic to the RND that is additional to the modified radial or selective neck dissection includes impaired shoulder and arm mobility, weakness, pain, cosmetic deformity, and lymphedema. In the rare case of bilateral IJV sacrifice, the patient must be counseled of the risk of potential facial and neck edema and decreased cerebral venous outflow. Counseling the patient preoperatively about the need for postoperative physical therapy may improve compliance with a postoperative rehabilitation program.

Patients should be counseled preoperatively about the possible morbidity of RND, but the decision to resect structures is sometimes made intraoperatively when assessment of resectability of the disease can be better assessed. As a general guideline, if a structure is not clearly involved by disease, and a clean resection can be achieved, then it should be structurally preserved. One example

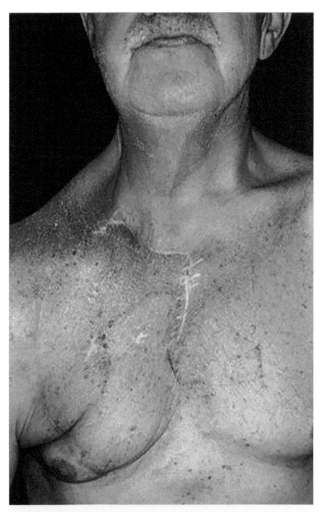

Fig. 6.1 Depressed right shoulder following radical neck dissection with resection of the spinal accessory nerve.

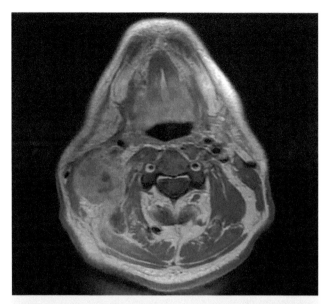

Fig. 6.2 Axial MRI showing metastatic carcinoma invading the internal jugular vein, sternocleidomastoid muscle, and deep neck musculature.

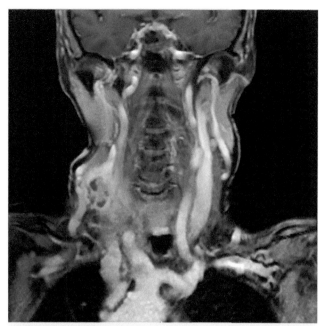

Fig. 6.4 Coronal MRI showing adenopathy in level 3 of the right neck involving the internal jugular vein.

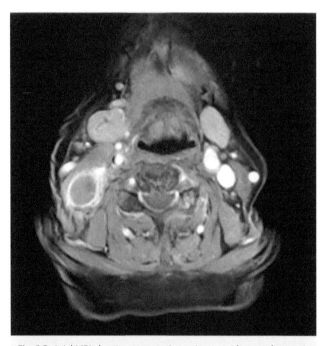

Fig. 6.3 Axial MRI showing metastatic carcinoma with central necrosis invading the sternocleidomastoid muscle.

may be a metastasis that is immobile in preoperative clinical evaluation because it is adherent to the SCM. Intraoperatively, after the skin and platysmal flaps are raised and superior and inferior SCM attachments are released, the tumor may become more mobile. Tumor fixation to the SCM may make it seem immobile, but there may be tissue planes between the IJV and SAN that facilitate its removal, and allow preservation of these structures. Conversely, some neck dissections may require removal of parapharyngeal and paraspinal lymphatics that are not included in the levels I to V of the RND. CT or MRI images with intravenous contrast should be carefully evaluated to assess relationships between nodal disease and normal structures (▶ Fig. 6.2, ▶ Fig. 6.3, ▶ Fig. 6.4).

Another important feature to note on preoperative imaging tumor is the relationship of the nodal disease with the carotid artery. If tumor is more than three quarters abutting the circumference of the carotid artery, there is a higher possibility that the common carotid may need to be sacrificed. In these cases, the pros and cons of carotid resection should be considered, and justification for performing a neck dissection should be made. Often neck dissection may not be indicated due to the extent of disease, the higher risks of surgery, and the low likelihood of disease eradication. In such a situation, conducting a detailed discussion with the patient, the patient's family, and the multidisciplinary medical team is essential to establish goals of care. If surgery is proposed, preoperative balloon occlusion angiography should be performed to assess the patency of the circle of Willis cerebral perfusion in the event of carotid resection. Vascular surgery should be on standby for possible carotid bypass and grafting if required. Regional or free tissue flap closure may be necessary to provide soft-tissue coverage of the exposed, dissected, or reconstructed carotid artery. Additional considerations of the carotid artery include thick atherosclerotic disease. In patients with atherosclerosis of the carotid, it is critical not to aggressively manipulate the carotid artery because it can cause embolus of atherosclerotic plaque material to the cerebral circulation.

6.5 Surgical Technique and Anatomic Considerations

A variety of skin incisions may be used to perform an RND, including those described by Martin[4] (double Y), Crile[2] (trifurcate), MacFee[10] (double transverse) incision, Schobinger,[11] and Babcock and Conley.[12] A trifurcate incision offers the advantage of optimal exposure, easier posterior flap elevation, and dissection of the posterior triangle of the neck. The disadvantage is

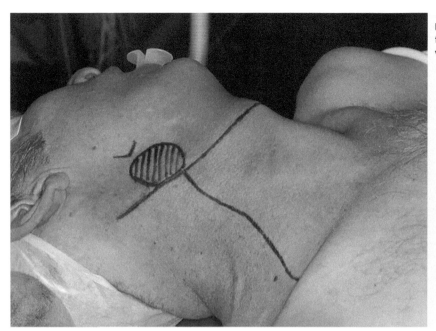

Fig. 6.5 A trifurcation incision in the neck allows for wide exposure. Alternatively, a single transverse incision may provide adequate exposure.

wound dehiscence at the union of the three flaps because the blood supply is divided between three flaps, especially in the irradiated neck.[13] If the trifurcate incision is used, it is important to make sure the vertical point of the "T" incision is at least 2 cm posterior to the common carotid artery to reduce the risk of carotid exposure (▸ Fig. 6.5).

After the skin incision, subplatysmal skin flaps are raised. If the tumor extends to the platysma, skin flap should be raised superficial to the platysma. Raising supraplatysmal a flap leads to a thinner skin flap that has less vascularity and offers less protection for underlying structures, particularly in the event that postoperative radiation is necessary. If the tumor is fixed to the dermis, resecting skin with the rest of the specimen is necessary to achieve clear margins (▸ Fig. 6.6). In these scenarios, local or free tissue transfer may be needed to achieve appropriate skin closure and protection of underlying neck structures.

6.5.1 Internal Jugular Vein

Dissection of the IJV both above and below the level of the disease will achieve proximal and distal control. It may be advisable to use vessel loops to apply compression to the IJV for vascular control during the dissection (▸ Fig. 6.7). Ligation of the IJV may be secured using a modified Halsted transfixation ligature (also known as a "stick tie"). With this approach, the vessel is clamped and a simple 2–0 silk ligature is placed. Next, before the clamp is released, a 2–0 silk with a needle is used to place a Halsted transfixation ligature (▸ Fig. 6.8). The other end of the IJV can be ligated in a similar fashion.

6.5.2 Spinal Accessory Nerve

Resection of the SAN is arguably the most morbid effect of RND. The SAN contains both sensory and motor fibers. It connects to the cervical rootlets C2–C4 and some suggest it is better described as the SAN plexus.[14] Three anatomic patterns of the SAN

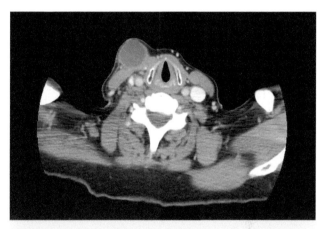

Fig. 6.6 A right neck metastasis invades the sternocleidomastoid muscle (SCM) and dermis, necessitating resection of skin, platysma and SCM.

have been described.[15] With the most common variation present in 66% of patients, the nerve courses into the SCM before dividing into branches to the trapezius and SCM. With the second most common variation, present in 22% of patients, the nerve divides before entering the SCM. This configuration facilitates preservation of the branch to the trapezius even when the branch to the SCM must be sacrificed. In every case, a meticulous attempt should be made to preserve the SAN.

Intraoperatively, the SAN may be reliably identified with retraction of the SCM laterally. The SAN descends from the skull base adjacent to the jugular vein and courses obliquely and posteriorly into the SCM. However, visualization of the SAN may not be feasible if there is bulky disease at level II. The SAN may also be identified posterior to the SCM near Erb's point where the cutaneous nerves and cervical rootlets course. If the SAN is being traced and preserved, care must be taken to avoid confusing the branch to the trapezius with sensory nerves at Erb's point

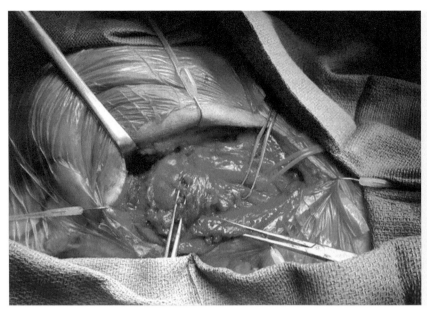

Fig. 6.7 Vessel loops around internal jugular vein and carotid prior to dissection allow for vascular control.

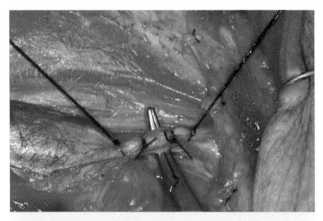

Fig. 6.8 Double suture ligation of the internal jugular vein using Halsted's transfixation technique.

(▶ Fig. 6.9). Finally, the SAN may also be reliably identified at its entry deep to the trapezius muscle in the posterior triangle. Intraoperative nerve monitoring of trapezius function may have utility in facilitating the identification and preservation of the SAN, particularly in cases with high-volume disease in the neck. If the SAN requires resection, a nerve graft (e.g., sural nerve) may help decrease atrophy of the trapezius and preserve muscle tone.[16,17] Nerve grafting is optimally performed at the time of SAN resection. Other experimental techniques have applied a bioabsorbable conduit to incorporate the two cut ends of the nerves.[18]

6.5.3 Other Structures

Although much attention is paid to the SCM, SAN, and IJV in discussions of the radical neck, it is important to acknowledge other structures that are at risk with neck dissection for aggressive or high-volume disease in the neck. Importantly, the vagus nerve, hypoglossal nerve, phrenic nerve, brachial plexus, cervical sympathetic chain, thoracic duct, deep neck musculature,

and other structures may require resection depending on the extent of disease. Intraoperative nerve monitoring may have significant utility for monitoring motor nerves when disease is known to be in proximity to these structures, and aids in nerve identification, dissection, and prognostication of nerve function. Lymphatics should be carefully ligated with silk suture to avoid chylous fistula, and Valsalva maneuvers help identify lymphatic leaks.

6.5.4 Coverage of Carotid Artery

Regional flap closure or free tissue transfer may be necessary in situations with significant skin and soft-tissue resection, carotid exposure, and particularly in the setting of previously radiated tissues. Prior radiation leads to diminished vascular perfusion to the skin flaps. In addition, most patients undergoing a neck dissection will require postoperative radiation and well-perfused tissue coverage of the carotid artery will afford better protection against carotid rupture.

When the IJV is sacrificed in the RND, the transverse cervical and external jugular veins are often the only ipsilateral remaining veins to which a free tissue transfer donor vein can be anastomosed. Preservation of the external jugular vein is prudent for use in reconstructive vascular anastomosis. However, the external jugular vein is superficial and susceptible to compression, and oriented in a superoinferior direction susceptible to rotation and occlusion. The transverse cervical vein may be used, but is located very inferior in the neck and therefore a longer flap vascular pedicle may be required to reach this recipient vein.

If a portion of the SCM can be preserved, the remnant may sometimes be rotated over the carotid sheath and sutured to the strap muscles to achieve coverage. The segmental blood supply of the SCM is an important consideration when using it for a rotational flap. Another option is a local tissue transfer using the pectoralis, or deltopectoral flaps, which are good alternatives for patients in whom a free tissue transfer may not be an option due to patient comorbidity, poor recipient vessels, or inadequate donor tissue.

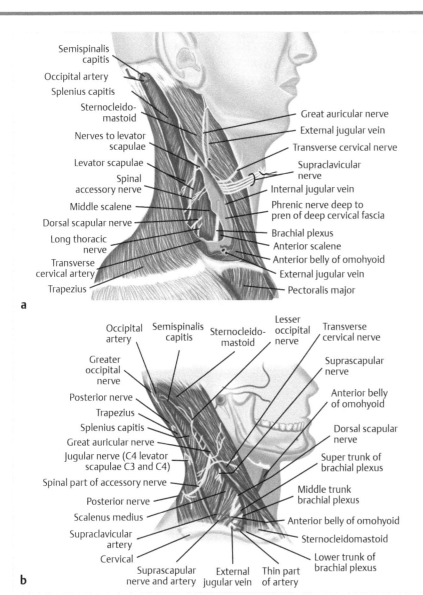

Semispinalis capitis

Occipital artery

Splenius capitis

Sternocleido-mastoid

Nerves to levator scapulae

Levator scapulae

Spinal accessory nerve

Middle scalene

Dorsal scapular nerve

Long thoracic nerve

Transverse cervical artery

Trapezius

Great auricular nerve

External jugular vein

Transverse cervical nerve

Supraclavicular nerve

Internal jugular vein

Phrenic nerve deep to pren of deep cervical fascia

Brachial plexus

Anterior scalene

Anterior belly of omohyoid

External jugular vein

Pectoralis major

a

Fig. 6.9 (a,b) The branch of the spinal accessory nerve (SAN) to the trapezius runs should be identified, traced, and preserved if oncologically feasible. Care must be taken to distinguish the SAN from the cervical plexus.

Occipital artery

Semispinalis capitis

Sternocleido-mastoid

Lesser occipital nerve

Transverse cervical nerve

Greater occipital nerve

Suprascapular nerve

Posterior nerve

Anterior belly of omohyoid

Trapezius

Splenius capitis

Dorsal scapular nerve

Great auricular nerve

Jugular nerve (C4 levator scapulae C3 and C4)

Super trunk of brachial plexus

Spinal part of accessory nerve

Posterior nerve

Middle trunk brachial plexus

Scalenus medius

Anterior belly of omohyoid

Supraclavicular artery

Sternocleidomastoid

Cervical

Lower trunk of brachial plexus

Suprascapular nerve and artery

External jugular vein

Thin part of artery

b

6.6 Postoperative Complications and Management

The simultaneous resection of bilateral IJVs should be avoided, as this may lead to severe facial edema and rarely even cerebral edema. Angiography after bilateral IJV ligation has shown the sigmoid sinus and brain drain through the vertebral venous (Batson's) plexus deep in the neck and empty into the subclavian vein at the cervicothoracic junction.[19] Although Ahn et al reported that staging the procedures by doing one RND at a time does not decrease the risk of cerebral edema,[20] anecdotal reports suggest that staged procedures are preferred and result in less severe facial edema, allowing for the interval development of vertebral venous plexus collaterals.

Sacrifice of the SAN, including the motor branch to the trapezius, motor branch to the SCM, and the sensory nerve plexus, is the most functionally devastating aspect of an RND. Selective neck dissection can also cause SAN palsy due to traction, demyelination, or devascularization, even when the nerve is not transected. The trapezius stabilizes the shoulder girdle, neck, back, and chest. It inserts on the occiput, the spinous process of the cervical and thoracic vertebrae, the acromion, and the clavicle. Accordingly, trapezius denervation affects shoulder abduction and can cause internal rotation ("winging") of the scapula, and drooping of the shoulder. Trapezius denervation is not an isolated muscle weakness. Because the scapula is destabilized, muscles that insert on the scapula have decreased strength as well. These include the serratus anterior, deltoid, supraspinatus, teres, and infraspinatus muscles. Impairment of this complex of muscles further exacerbates the shoulder destabilization from the trapezius denervation. The resulting inability to abduct the shoulder against gravity is termed "shoulder syndrome," first described by Ewing and Martin in 1952.[21] Functionally, this is manifested as diminished ability to don and doff a jacket sleeve, to style one's hair, or to lift objects.

All patients should be assessed for SAN palsy after any type of neck dissection and physicians should remember SAN palsy is not obvious in all patients immediately after RND surgery. While pain is almost always present, shoulder weakness may be a delayed finding.[17] Pain may be due to cut afferent fibers in the SAN or due to traction on the shoulder from the weight of the unsupported arm.[21] Often the patient has normal immediate postoperative shoulder function in the hospital because the trapezius has not yet atrophied and the shoulder girdle muscles are able to compensate for short term after injury. In addition, there is axoplasmic flow in the distal end of the nerve for weeks.[22] Patients receiving adjuvant chemotherapy and radiation exhibit worse shoulder function than those treated with neck dissection alone, even in cases in which the SAN is spared.[23]

A reliable sign of SAN palsy is the scapular flip test[24] in which the patient stands with arms by their sides and elbows bent 90 degrees. The patient attempts to externally rotate the shoulder, while the examiner resists at the distal forearm. If the patient has SAN palsy, the medial scapula will flip or lift from the thoracic wall. This maneuver distinguishes the SAN injury from long thoracic nerve injury. Interestingly, trapezius denervation may result in increased FDG activity on postoperative PET scan due to increased glucose utilization in denervated muscle.[25]

Occupational or physical therapy for SAN palsy after RND has been shown to improve patients' postoperative function.[22] Passive and active range of motion exercises are used to rehabilitate the shoulder. Therapy should be initiated within 8 weeks and most therapy lasts for up to 3 months.[22,26] In addition to improving shoulder function, therapy can also help patients who may have resting pain due to muscle spasm of the "surviving muscles," that is, muscle fibers of the trapezius with innervation from C2, C3, and C4 roots.[27] In some patients, denervation is more painful and functionally disruptive than others. Sacrifice of the SAN can result in a range of impaired shoulder abduction, from as low as 35 degrees to as high as 80 degrees (with 180 being normal).[27] These variations may be due to anatomic variations although the exact cause is not understood.[14]

SCM resection or denervation due to nerve resection does not cause as many functional complications as trapezius denervation. Cosmetically, however, loss of the soft tissue in a unilateral resection of the SCM can be very distressing to the patient. Furthermore, the brachial plexus and scalene muscles may be more evident just beneath the skin flap. There may be hollowing of the supraclavicular fossa as well. Accordingly, preoperative counseling of cosmetic as well as functional complications is critical.

Another complication of RND is chyle leak that results from inadvertent injury during dissection in level IV to the thoracic duct or its tributaries. Ideally a chyle leak will be identified intraoperatively and the duct and its branches will be ligated with suture or metal clips. Some surgeons have reported success with use of omohyoid rotational flaps and cyanoacrylate or fibrin glue to seal the area.[28]

Postoperative management is conservative at first with pressure dressings and a medium chain triglyceride and low fat diet. Somatostatin analogs (octreotide) or pancreatic lipase inhibitors (etilefrine) may be added. If high drain output fails to resolve, embolization or surgical ligation is necessary to resolve the leak. Although not a common complication, there are case reports of patients undergoing bilateral RND experiencing operative hypertension due to baroreflex dysfunction.[29] This is attributed to dissection of the nerve to the carotid sinus during dissection along the carotid sheath (▶ Fig. 6.10). The literature shows varying long-term sequelae: some patients have persistent hypertension, others become normotensive, and some have labile blood pressure. Risk factors include advanced age and preoperative radiation, and it usually happens in the immediate postoperative period when the vasodilatory effects of anesthesia have subsided. The best treatment for baroreflex failure is clonidine to stimulate the alpha-2 receptors centrally and decrease sympathetic tone.[30] In summary, the RND can impart severe postoperative morbidity to the patient, which underscores the need for meticulous attention during surgery toward the preservation of noninvolved structures, as well as detailed preoperative patient counseling to appropriately set expectations.

6.7 Conclusion

Although the RND was the historical standard of cervical lymphadenectomy, it has appropriately evolved such that it is only required currently in a select group of patients with aggressive nodal disease who require removal of the IJV, SAN, and SCM. Sacrifice of these structures, in particular the SAN, imparts functional and cosmetic morbidity to the patient. Careful preoperative image review is necessary to plan a neck dissection to achieve optimal clearance of disease, functional outcome, and appropriate coverage of the carotid artery. Patients should be counseled preoperatively about potential functional impairments and enrolled in rehabilitation programs postoperatively.

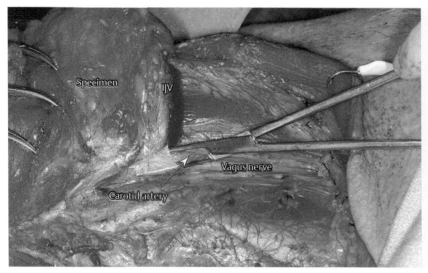

Fig. 6.10 Dissection along the carotid artery separates the internal jugular vein with the specimen.

References

[1] Rinaldo A, Ferlito A, Silver CE. Early history of neck dissection. Eur Arch Oto-rhinolaryngol. 2008; 265(12):1535–1538

[2] Crile G. Landmark article Dec 1, 1906: excision of cancer of the head and neck. With special reference to the plan of dissection based on one hundred and thirty-two operations. By George Crile. JAMA. 1987; 258(22):3286–3293

[3] Bocca E. Supraglottic laryngectomy and functional neck dissection. J Laryngol Otol. 1966; 80(8):831–838

[4] Martin H, Del Valle B, Ehrlich H, Cahan WG. Neck dissection. Cancer. 1951; 4(3):441–499

[5] Byers RM, Wolf PF, Ballantyne AJ. Rationale for elective modified neck dissection. Head Neck Surg. 1988; 10(3):160–167

[6] Robbins KT, Medina JE, Wolfe GT, Levine PA, Sessions RB, Pruet CW. Standardizing neck dissection terminology. Official report of the Academy's Committee for Head and Neck Surgery and Oncology. Arch Otolaryngol Head Neck Surg. 1991; 117(6):601–605

[7] Robbins KT, Shaha AR, Medina JE, et al. Committee for Neck Dissection Classification, American Head and Neck Society. Consensus statement on the classification and terminology of neck dissection. Arch Otolaryngol Head Neck Surg. 2008; 134(5):536–538

[8] Ferlito A, Robbins KT, Shah JP, et al. Proposal for a rational classification of neck dissections. Head Neck. 2011; 33(3):445–450

[9] McCammon SD, Shah JP. Radical neck dissection. Oper Tech Otolaryngol. 2004; 15(3):152–159

[10] MacFee WF. Transverse incisions for neck dissections. Ann Surg. 1960; 151(2):279–284

[11] Schobinger R. The use of a long anterior skin flap in radical neck resections. Ann Surg. 1957; 146(2):221–223

[12] Babcock WW, Jr, Conley J. Neck incision in block dissection. Experiences with the long anterior cervical flap incision. Arch Otolaryngol. 1966; 84(5):554–557

[13] Yii NW, Patel SG, Williamson P, Breach NM. Use of apron flap incision for neck dissection. Plast Reconstr Surg. 1999; 103(6):1655–1660

[14] Brown H, Burns S, Kaiser CW. The spinal accessory nerve plexus, the trapezius muscle, and shoulder stabilization after radical neck cancer surgery. Ann Surg. 1988; 208(5):654–661

[15] Lanisnik B, Zargi M, Rodi Z. Identification of three anatomical patterns of the spinal accessory nerve in the neck by neurophysiological mapping. Radiol Oncol. 2014; 48(4):387–392

[16] Göransson H, Leppänen OV, Vastamäki M. Patient outcome after surgical management of the spinal accessory nerve injury: a long-term follow-up study. SAGE Open Med. 2016; 4:2050312116645731

[17] Chandawarkar RY, Cervino AL, Pennington GA. Management of iatrogenic injury to the spinal accessory nerve. Plast Reconstr Surg. 2003; 111(2):611–617, discussion 618–619

[18] Ducic I, Maloney CT, Jr, Dellon AL. Reconstruction of the spinal accessory nerve with autograft or neurotube? Two case reports. J Reconstr Microsurg. 2005; 21(1):29–33, discussion 34

[19] Ensari S, Kaptanoğlu E, Tun K, et al. Venous outflow of the brain after bilateral complete jugular ligation. Turk Neurosurg. 2008; 18(1):56–60

[20] Ahn C, Sindelar WF. Bilateral radical neck dissection: report of results in 55 patients. J Surg Oncol. 1989; 40(4):252–255

[21] Ewing MR, Martin H. Disability following radical neck dissection; an assessment based on the postoperative evaluation of 100 patients. Cancer. 1952; 5(5):873–883

[22] McGarvey AC, Chiarelli PE, Osmotherly PG, Hoffman GR. Physiotherapy for accessory nerve shoulder dysfunction following neck dissection surgery: a literature review. Head Neck. 2011; 33(2):274–280

[23] Gallagher KK, Sacco AG, Lee JS, et al. Association between multimodality neck treatment and work and leisure impairment: a disease-specific measure to assess both impairment and rehabilitation after neck dissection. JAMA Otolaryngol Head Neck Surg. 2015; 141(10):888–893

[24] Kelley MJ, Kane TE, Leggin BG. Spinal accessory nerve palsy: associated signs and symptoms. J Orthop Sports Phys Ther. 2008; 38(2):78–86

[25] Lee SH, Seo HG, Oh BM, Choi H, Cheon GJ, Lee SU. Increased (18)F-FDG uptake in the trapezius muscle in patients with spinal accessory neuropathy. J Neurol Sci. 2016; 362:127–130

[26] McGarvey AC, Hoffman GR, Osmotherly PG, Chiarelli PE. Maximizing shoulder function after accessory nerve injury and neck dissection surgery: a multicenter randomized controlled trial. Head Neck. 2015; 37(7):1022–1031

[27] Chida S, Shimada Y, Matsunaga T, Sato M, Hatakeyama K, Mizoi K. Occupational therapy for accessory nerve palsy after radical neck dissection. Tohoku J Exp Med. 2002; 196(3):157–165

[28] Brennan PA, Blythe JN, Herd MK, Habib A, Anand R. The contemporary management of chyle leak following cervical thoracic duct damage. Br J Oral Maxillofac Surg. 2012; 50(3):197–201

[29] Prakash S, Rapsang A, Kumar SS, Bhatia PS, Gogia AR. Postoperative hypertension following radical neck dissection. J Anaesthesiol Clin Pharmacol. 2012; 28(1):121–123

[30] Wijeysundera DN, Naik JS, Beattie WS. Alpha-2 adrenergic agonists to prevent perioperative cardiovascular complications: a meta-analysis. Am J Med. 2003; 114(9):742–752

7 Modified Radical Neck Dissection

Mauricio A. Moreno

Abstract

A modified radical neck dissection is defined as functional resection of the lymphatic levels I to V in the neck. This procedure was pioneered by Suarez and Bocca, who were the first to understand the concept of nodal groups defined by fascial places during the second half of the last century. This operation revolutionized the practice of head and neck oncology, and laid the foundation for the development of ever less invasive approaches, even decades after its inception. In this chapter, critical aspects of the surgical anatomy of the neck are reviewed, and the reader is presented with strategies to avoid common pitfalls in the execution of the procedure.

Keywords: neck dissection, modified, functional, technique, complications.

7.1 Introduction

The concept of neck dissection refers to systematic resection of lymph nodes from well-defined fascial compartments in the neck. These will be, the vast majority of times, performed in the context of mucosal aerodigestive tract, salivary, cutaneous, or endocrine malignancies. The oncologic rationale for the procedure involves resecting lymph nodes that show clinical or radiological evidence of involvement (clinically positive necks or cN +) or are at risk of harboring microscopic disease (clinically negative necks or cN0). As such, depending on the clinical neck status, neck dissections are classified as therapeutic for patients with cN + and as elective or prophylactic in patients with cN0. Throughout its more than 100 years of history, neck dissection has continuously evolved from a mutilating radical surgery to an elegant, anatomically bound ablation with minimal functional impact. Similarly, as it relates to the nomenclature and indications, the last decades have seen a significant degree of consolidation that has laid the foundation for a common understanding of its oncological and technical aspects.

The current nomenclature for the boundaries and contents of the nodal groups in the neck is summarized in ▶ Table 7.1 and illustrated in ▶ Fig. 7.1. A modified radical neck dissection, which is the most comprehensive form of functional neck dissection, entails the resection of the nodal groups I through V, and is still considered the standard of care for management of the cN + neck. The width and scope of this surgery mandate a polished surgical technique and thorough knowledge of the anatomy. While this surgery can be analyzed from multiple perspectives, this chapter will primarily focus on its anatomical and technical aspects, which are essential to perform this surgery safely, effectively, and efficiently. As such, it is strongly recommended that the reader reviews Chapter 3 to get intimately familiar with the surgical anatomy of the neck.

Table 7.1 Contents and boundaries of the lymphatic levels of the neck.[23]

Level	Content and boundaries
Level I (submental and submandibular)	The lymph nodes between the mandible and hyoid bone. The posterior (lateral) boundary is the vertical plane defined by the posterior edge of the submandibular gland. This level is divided into two sublevels.
Sublevel IA (submental)	The lymph nodes within the triangular boundary of the anterior belly of the digastric muscles and the hyoid bone.
Sublevel IB (submandibular)	The lymph nodes within the boundaries of the anterior belly of the digastric muscle, the stylohyoid muscle, and the body of the mandible. The submandibular gland is usually included within the specimen when the lymph nodes of this triangle are removed.
Level II (upper jugular)	The lymph nodes located around the upper third of the internal jugular vein and spinal accessory nerve, extending from skull base to the level of the inferior border of the hyoid bone. The anterior (medial) boundary is the vertical plane defined by the posterior edge of the submandibular gland and the posterior (lateral) boundary is the posterior border of the sternocleidomastoid muscle.
Sublevel IIA	The lymph nodes located anterior (medial) to the spinal accessory nerve.
Sublevel IIB	The lymph nodes located posterior (lateral) to the spinal accessory nerve.
Level III (middle jugular)	The lymph nodes located around the middle third of the internal jugular vein extending from the inferior border of the hyoid bone (above) to the inferior border of the cricoid cartilage (below). The anterior (medial) boundary is the lateral border of the sternohyoid muscle, and the posterior (lateral) boundary is the posterior border of the sternocleidomastoid muscle.
Level IV (lower jugular)	The lymph nodes located around the lower third of the internal jugular vein extending form the inferior border of the cricoid cartilage (above) to the clavicle below. The anterior (medial) boundary is the lateral border of the sternohyoid muscle and the posterior (lateral) boundary is the posterior border of the sternocleidomastoid muscle.

Continued

Table 7.1 continued

Level	Content and boundaries
Level V (posterior triangle group)	The lymph nodes located along the lower half of the spinal accessory nerve and the transverse cervical artery. The supraclavicular nodes are also included in the posterior triangle group. The superior boundary is formed by the sternocleidomastoid and trapezius muscles, the inferior boundary is the clavicle, the anterior (medial) boundary is the posterior border of the sternocleidomastoid muscle, and the posterior (lateral) boundary is the anterior border of the trapezius muscle. This level is also divided at the level of anterior cricoid arch into sublevels VA and VB.
Sublevel VA	Contents of level V above the level of anterior cricoid arch.
Sublevel VB	Contents of level V below the level of anterior cricoid arch.
Level VI (anterior compartment group or central group)	The pretracheal and paratracheal nodes, precricoid (Delphian) node, and the perithyroidal nodes, including the lymph nodes along the recurrent laryngeal nerves. The superior boundary is the hyoid bone, the inferior boundary is the suprasternal notch, and the lateral boundaries are the common carotid arteries.
Level VII (upper mediastinal group)	Contains the paratracheal lymph nodes and fibrofatty tissue located between the suprasternal notch and the innominate artery.

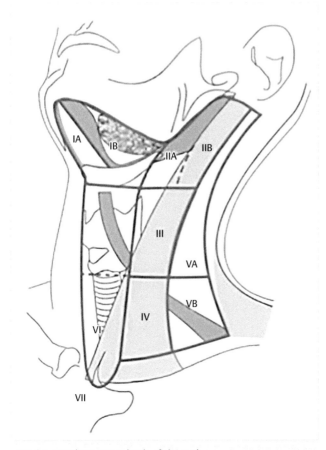

Fig. 7.1 Lymphatic group levels of the neck.

7.1.1 History and Classification

Historically, the first accounts of nodal resection for treatment of cancers date back to the 19th century, with Kocher and Packard describing the removal of cervical lymph nodes as treatment of oral cavity cancers. Franciszek Jawdyński is credited with the first description of a radical neck dissection in the Polish literature in 1888. However, George Crile was the surgeon who popularized the technique and established its oncologic rationale and indications.[1] In his description of radical neck dissection, Crile advocated for en bloc resection of cervical nodes and the internal jugular vein (IJV), sternocleidomastoid muscle (SCM), and spinal accessory nerve (SAN). The procedure was widely adopted and endorsed by prominent head and neck surgeons such as Vilray Blair and Hayes Martin and became the standard of care for neck management through the first half of the 20th century. In the second half of the 20th century, most of the modifications to the procedure were aimed at limiting morbidity, ushered by Ward, who described a SAN-sparing approach to neck dissection in 1951. This trend toward less radical procedures was fueled by further understanding of the fascial boundaries of the neck compartments, which led to the description of a comprehensive neck dissection sparing the SAN, IJV, and SCM by Suarez in 1963, which he named functional neck dissection.[2] It was Bocca and Pignataro,[3] however, who was largely responsible for disseminating and promoting the technique in the United States and Europe. The next incremental steps in the evolution of this procedure became possible thorough a more thorough understanding of the patterns for nodal spread depending on the location of the primary tumor.[4] This ushered in the concept of selective neck dissections, which only address the nodal basins at risk and spare other lymphatic groups, and largely reducing perioperative morbidity. Although these were initially implemented in the context of the cN0 neck, they are more commonly being used for treatment of cN +. As it relates to the classification of the procedure, the current nomenclature has not changed since 2002 (▶ Table 7.2) and modified radical neck dissection formally entails the resection of all lymphatic groups in the neck (I–V) with preservation of the IJV, SAN, and SCM. This procedure is still the standard of care in the management of the cN + neck, although there is growing evidence supporting the role of selective approaches in this setting as well. Given the low rate of involvement of level V, this level is commonly spared, yielding to the common practice among head and neck surgeons of colloquially calling a selective neck dissection of levels I to IV, a modified radical neck dissection. The history and the evolution of the procedure are reviewed in detail in Chapter 2.

7.2 Surgical Technique

The following section describes a step-by-step approach for the dissection of neck levels I to V in a sequential fashion. Decision points and critical aspects of the surgical anatomy will be addressed as the process is described, with the intention of contextualizing the information within the flow of the operation. For the same reason, intraoperative images were preferred over diagrams whenever possible. From the perspective of a practicing head and neck surgeon, the importance of having a systematic

approach to the neck cannot be overemphasized, and this chapter has been written with that goal in mind. In this author's experience, this consistency will reward practitioners with a level of confidence, and familiarity with the anatomy, that will prove essential when clinical judgment calls for an alternative surgical approach.

As it relates to the decision-making process before and during the operation, there are countless valid variations in planning and execution that truly epitomize the art of surgery. A such, the information presented by no means represents an exclusive view of this operation, but rather a compendium of collective knowledge and personal experience, validated over years of academic practice.

7.2.1 Patient Positioning

Once the airway is secured, the bed is routinely turned 90 to 180 degrees. Before placing a shoulder roll, the neck is inspected in the supine position under gently anterior flexion to identify and mark the location of skin creases. A shoulder roll is then placed at the level of the scapulas in order to gently lift the superior chest and neck. Care must be taken to ensure the head is not hanging, especially in older patients. The head must be supported with a soft device that holds it in position, such as a donut-shaped gel cushion. While the procedure can be performed in straight supine position, the best exposure is achieved in beach chair position, elevating the back of the table about 30 degrees, and gently lowering the legs. The head is extended and rotated to the opposite side; this maneuver not only provides the best exposure, but also brings the relevant anatomical structures to a more horizontal plane, significantly facilitating the dissection (▶ Fig. 7.2).

At this point, inspection and palpation are used to identify landmarks in surface anatomy such as the angle of the mandible, suprasternal notch, and mastoid tip. The neck can be gently flexed to identify natural skin creases, which should also be marked.

Table 7.2 Past and current classifications of neck dissection[24]

1991 classification	2002 classification	2008 update
Radical neck dissection	Radical neck dissection	Classification and terminology of neck dissection *has not changed.* New recommendations:
Modified radical neck dissection	Modified radical neck dissection	
Selective neck dissection • Supraomohyoid • Lateral • Posterolateral • Anterior	Selective neck dissection: each variation is depicted by "SND" and the use of parentheses to denote the levels or sublevels removed	• Boundaries between levels I and II, and levels III/IV and VI • Terminology of the superior mediastinal nodes (level VII) • The method of submitting surgical specimens for pathologic analysis
Extended neck dissection	Extended neck dissection	
(Committee for Head and Neck Surgery and Oncology of the American Academy of Otolaryngology–Head and Neck Surgery)	(American Head and Neck Society and Committee for Head and Neck Surgery and Oncology, American Academy of Otolaryngology–Head and Neck Surgery)	(American Head and Neck Society and Committee for Head and Neck Surgery and Oncology, American Academy of Otolaryngology–Head and Neck Surgery)

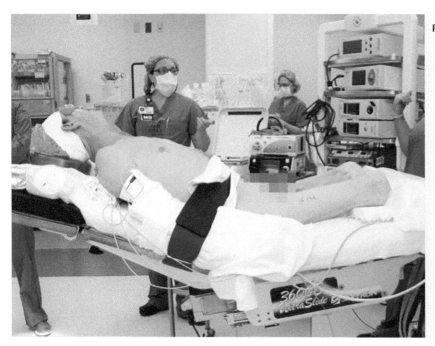

Fig. 7.2 Patient positioning.

7.2.2 Incision Placement

The placement of the surgical incisions for a neck dissection can have a profound impact on access, perioperative morbidity, and reconstructive considerations. During the evolution of neck dissection, many surgical approaches have been described (▶ Fig. 7.3) and are associated with the pioneers of the procedure. Nowadays, most of these approaches are seldom performed. As the collective knowledge has matured, a more utilitarian approach is overwhelmingly favored by most surgeons; as such, modern-day incisions are usually apron-type or transversal incisions at a skin crease.

The factors that must be considered for surgical planning are the following:
- Skin flap viability.
- Appropriate access to nodal groups of interest.
- Cosmetic outcome.
- Reconstructive needs (need for skin resection/rotational flaps).
- Reoperative exposure (risk of ipsilateral or contralateral neck recurrence).

Of these, skin flap viability is perhaps the most important consideration, and is affected by many factors, most of them outside the control of the surgeon (previous neck radiation or surgery, malignant cutaneous extension, vasculopathy). Regardless of the chosen approach, some common considerations are helpful in minimizing the risk of flap failure:
- Skin flaps must be broad based to maximize blood supply.
- Flap elevation should be in the subplatysmal plane and limited to the areas of oncologic interest.
- Trifurcate incisions should be avoided whenever possible.
- Placement of secondary limb incisions should consider the risk of carotid exposure.
- Preoperative planning is essential when performing cervical-based rotational flaps for reconstruction (i.e., platysma or submental flaps).

In terms of flap viability, the platysma plays an important role in neck dissections. The muscle covers the vast majority of the anterior neck, and it has a rich blood supply that originates primarily from the submental artery, with tributaries from the superior thyroid, occipital, and posterior auricular arteries.[5] For this reason, incorporating this muscle in the flaps maximizes blood supply to the overlying skin, thus significantly decreasing the risk of flap loss. This muscle is also important as it defines the appropriate fascial layers of the procedure. The platysma is enveloped by the superficial cervical fascia; elevating the skin flaps in the plane immediately deep to it will preserve the integrity of the superficial layer of the deep cervical fascia (SLDCF; considered the superficial boundary of the dissection).

There are some situations that mandate flap elevation in a supraplatysmal plane. These include cases where there is concern for involvement of the muscle by the disease process, such as extracapsular nodal extension, or when a myocutaneous platysma flap is considered for reconstructive purposes. While it has been largely replaced by other reconstructive options, the myocutaneous platysma flap should be part of the armamentarium of every head and neck surgeon, as it provides an elegant alternative for closure of small to medium sized intraoral defects, especially in patients with significant comorbidities. In a recent literature review, Eckard reported a flap success rate ranging from 71 to 100%[6] and concluded that most failures were related to history of previous radiation or ligation of the facial artery. From the technical standpoint, patient selection and surgical planning are of outmost importance if this flap is to be attempted. The flap can be harvested as a superiorly or posteriorly based island flap (▶ Fig. 7.4). Superiorly based flaps have the advantages of an increased arc of rotation, robust arterial supply, and capability of sparing the cervical branch of the facial nerve, while posteriorly based flaps have better venous drainage. Regardless of the chosen approach, these flaps must be marked preoperatively, and they dictate the location of the rest of the incisions for the neck dissection. In a similar fashion,

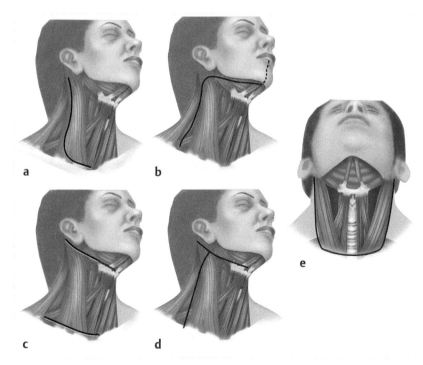

Fig. 7.3 Neck incisions for modified radical neck dissection. **(a)** Hockey stick or half-apron. **(b)** Boomerang. **(c)** MacFee. **(d)** Modified Schobinger. **(e)** Apron or bilateral hockey stick.

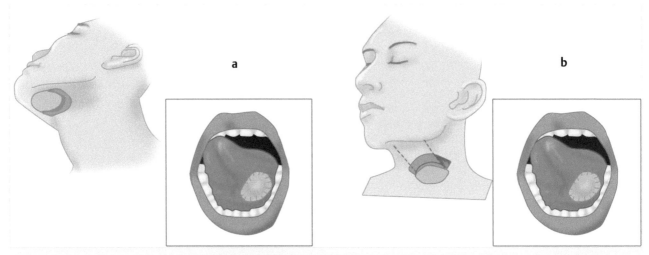

Fig. 7.4 (a) Superiorly based platysma flap. **(b)** Inferiorly based platysma flap.

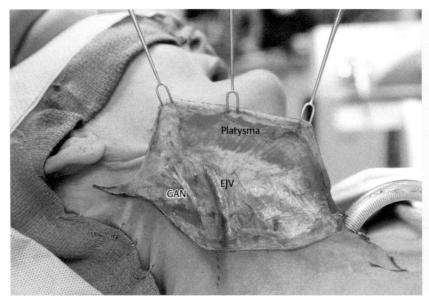

Fig. 7.5 Initial elevation of the subplatysmal flap. EJV, external jugular vein; GAN, greater auricular nerve.

submental rotational flap and cervicofacial flaps require thoughtful preoperative consideration when planning for incision placement.

7.2.3 Exposure: Skin Flap Elevation

Anatomically, a modified radical neck dissection requires wide exposure of the anterior and posterior neck triangles, so the boundaries for skin flap elevation are the mandibular margin and tail of parotid superiorly, the clavicle inferiorly, the strap muscles medially, and the anterior border of the trapezius muscle posteriorly.

Once the incision placement has been decided, the skin is incised with Bovie electrocautery and the incision is taken through the subcutaneous tissue and platysma, carefully avoiding violating the fascial layer below. Alternatively, the skin incisions may be performed with scalpel, prior injection with diluted lidocaine and epinephrine. At this point, skin flaps are elevated in the subplatysmal plane wide enough to expose all the anatomical landmarks and provide access to the nodal

groups of interest. This is a relatively avascular plane that is only intermittently pierced by cutaneous perforators, so flaps can be raised with sharp instrumentation or with Bovie electrocautery (▶ Fig. 7.5). For this reason, the rate of bleeding can be used as a surrogate for appropriateness of the surgical plane: if bleeding is significant, the skin flaps are likely being raised in the wrong plane (usually too deep).

In the midline, the platysma has a variable degree of dehiscence, and fibers that decussate in the submental area. For this reason, it is recommended that for patients undergoing bilateral neck dissection, lateral flaps are elevated first and subsequently addressing the anterior neck, once the correct plane has been established. If an apron skin flap is used for access, the superior elevation should not go above the level of the mandible, as there is risk to damage the lower branches of the facial nerve. Inferiorly, the skin flaps should be elevated to the level of the clavicles, although this plane can be extended into the anterior chest for reconstructive purposes, such as a cervicothoracic flap. This maneuver completes the skin flap elevation over the anterior triangle (▶ Fig. 7.6).

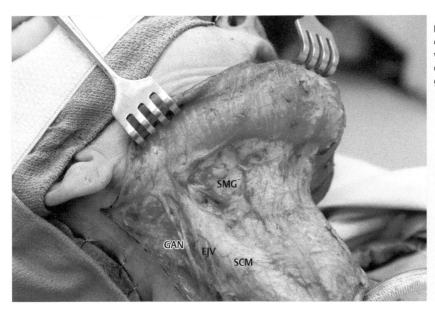

Fig. 7.6 Completed elevation of the skin flaps over the anterior triangle. EJV, elevated jugular vein; GAN, greater auricular nerve; SCM, sternocleidomastoid muscle; SMG, submandibular gland.

Posteriorly, the platysma extends roughly to the level of the external jugular vein or slightly beyond it, so elevating the skin flaps beyond this boundary is significantly more challenging. The external jugular vein can also be used as a landmark; since the SLDCF invests the SCM and the vein, the plane of dissection is immediately superficial to the vessel. The same is true for other veins of the superficial plexus, such as the anterior jugular veins. On a technical point, if the external jugular vein is injured to the point that requires ligation, the stumps must be maintained in the same anatomical plane (i.e., attached to the SCM) and not elevated with the skin flaps, a common mistake among neophyte surgeons.

Similarly, posterior to the platysma, cranial sensory nerves (greater auricular, lesser occipital, and transverse cervical) traverse over the SCM and are invested in the SLDCF, so they are reliable points of reference as the surgical plane is immediately superficial to them. This same surgical plane must be maintained as flap elevation proceeds over the posterior triangle. This is significantly more challenging in this area as there no consistent points of reference, so it is recommended to frequently compare the skin flap thickness to the anterior flaps. In terms of elevation of skin flaps, in the posterior triangle there is also risk of injury of the SAN. The nerve is exposed to injury along its entire course in this area as it has a very superficial location and it is only protected by a thin fascial layer. Flap elevation with electrocautery may lead to abrupt nerve stimulation (especially in the coagulation setting), causing a violent trapezius contraction that brings the tissue toward the instrument, posing an exceptional risk. Furthermore, this may happen even if the patient is fully paralyzed. As such, it is recommended that this portion is performed with scalpel or with the electrocautery in a low intensity, pure cut setting.

To fully expose the contents of level V, it is often necessary to drop an accessory limb from the main incision; ideally, this limb must merge with the main incision at a 90-degree angle to minimize the risk of tip necrosis. When planning a trifurcation incision, acute angles (< 45 degrees) should always be avoided. Most importantly, the point of trifurcation must be placed over the SCM when possible. This is the most likely area for wound

complications, so placing the trifurcation point over a critical structure, such as the carotid or the brachial plexus, can lead to significant morbidity in this event. If there is significant risk of carotid exposure (such as history of radiation or radical neck dissection), consider an elective interposition of myofascial pectoralis flap to protect these critical structures. This posterior limb can usually be placed within a dominant skin crease and may be extended to the posterior midline (or beyond) when performing a posterolateral neck dissection, which also encompasses the suboccipital and postauricular lymphatic groups.

Taking these points into consideration, the posterior elevation of skin flaps proceeds until the anterior border of the trapezius muscle is widely exposed (▸ Fig. 7.7).

7.2.4 Preservation of the Marginal Mandibular Branch of the Facial Nerve

A thorough understanding of the anatomy of the facial nerve and its relationships with neck structures is critical to preserve the function of its marginal mandibular branch (marginal nerve) and consequently perioral musculature. The marginal nerve is the fourth most inferior branch of the facial nerve, and after it has originated from its lower division, it exits the anteroinferior portion of the parotid near the angle of the mandible and remains deep to the investing cervical fascia. Near the mandibular midbody, the nerve swings upward and perforates the DCF near the mandibular border to continue within the fibroareolar tissue between the deep fascia and platysma. It continues anteriorly at this plane to innervate the depressor labii inferioris, depressor anguli oris, and mentalis muscles (▸ Fig. 7.8). The effects of each of these muscles are as follows:

- Depressor labii inferioris draws the lower lip downward (depresses) and laterally (irony).
- Depressor anguli oris depresses the oral commissure (frown).
- Mentalis raises and protrudes lower lip and wrinkles skin of chin (pout).

On the other hand, the cervical branch of the facial nerve further divides into an upper and a lower branch (▸ Fig. 7.9); these

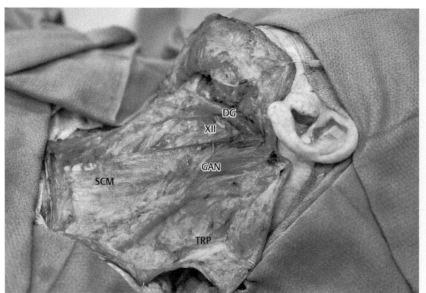

Fig. 7.7 Completed neck elevation over the posterior neck triangle. DG, digastric muscle; GAN, greater auricular nerve; SCM, sternocleidomastoid muscle; TRP, trapezius muscle; XII, hypoglossal nerve.

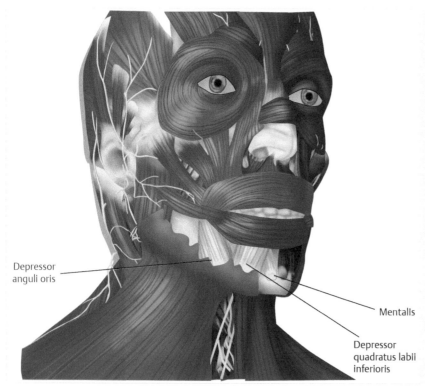

Fig. 7.8 Anatomical disposition of the muscles innervated by the marginal nerve.

Depressor anguli oris

Mentalis

Depressor quadratus labii inferioris

will innervate the platysma muscle and may have an effect on preserving lip symmetry. Distally, the marginal nerve can anastomose with other branches of the facial nerve (most commonly buccal) to create a plexus that will innervate the perioral musculature. The location of the nerve in relationship to the lower border of the mandible is variable; furthermore, this relationship may change depending on the segment of the nerve analyzed (anterior vs. posterior to the facial artery), as

shown in ▶ Table 7.3. This anatomical variability was also demonstrated by Al-Qahtani et al,[7] who showed that the nerve has a sinuous pattern in three-fourths of the cases, and in 15% it loops posteriorly beyond its point of origin (▶ Fig. 7.10). The nerve almost invariably (90%) courses as a single branch as it exits the parotid and throughout its course. However, distally, as it approaches the effector musculature, it expresses a branching pattern in more than 80% of the cases.[8]

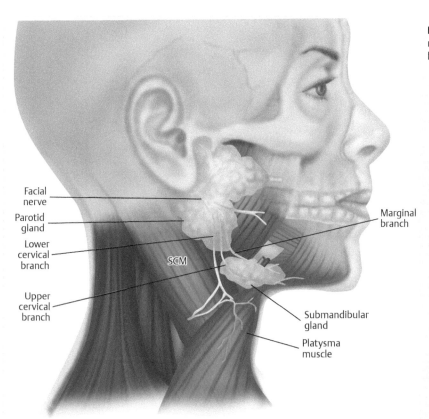

Fig. 7.9 Illustration showing the anatomical relationship of the marginal and cervical branches of the facial nerve.

Table 7.3 Summary of studies reviewing the anatomical relationship of the marginal nerve with the lower border of the mandible

Study	Subjects	Reference to facial artery	Reference to lower border mandible	
			Above	Below
Dingman and Grabb 1962	Cadaver	Anterior to Posterior to	100% 81%	0 19%
Wang et al 1991	Cadaver	Anterior to Posterior to	90% 67%	10% 33%
Savary et al 1997	Cadaver	Anterior to	27%	27%
Nelson and Gingrass 1979	Cadaver			100%
Woltmann et al 2006	Cadaver		57%	43%
Ziarah and Atkinson 1981	Cadaver		47%	53%
Nason et al 2007	Patient			64%
Baker and Conley 1979	Patient			Almost 100%

Source: Adapted from Al-Qahtani et al.[7]

From the surgical standpoint, there are two ways to spare the nerve function:

- The Hayes Martin maneuver, which entails the ligation of the facial vein two fingerbreadths below the lower border of the mandible, and subsequent cephalad retraction of the superior stump (▶ Fig. 7.11). Since the anatomy is constant in the sense that the marginal nerve is always superficial to the facial vessels at the mandibular edge, retracting the stump assures that the nerve will be contained within these fasciae. This is a time-tested approach that works well for most cases, but it has some limitations such as in cases where there is direct disease extension to the submental triangle, or significant nodal disease level lb or in facial lymph nodes.

- Exploration of the marginal nerve. In this approach, the fascia overlying the submandibular gland is incised horizontally, about 2 cm below the midpoint of the mandibular body, which closely correlates with the location of the facial artery notch. Meticulous subfascial dissection is performed in a caudal-to-cephalad direction while maintaining a bloodless surgical field and minimizing the use of electrocautery. The facial vessels—and more specifically the facial artery—may be used as landmarks to identify the nerve, which will always be in a

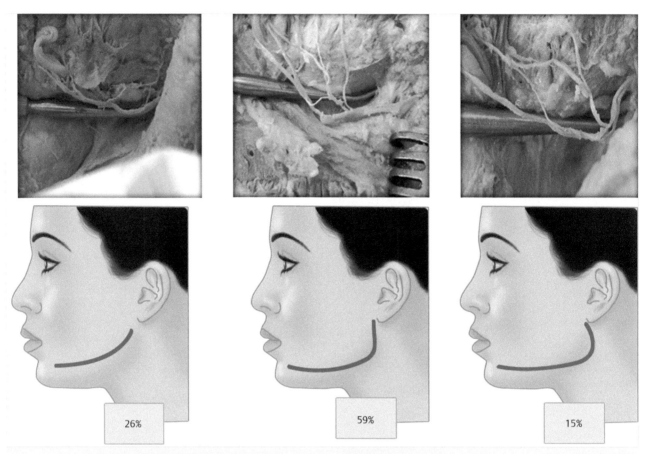

26%   59%   15%

Fig. 7.10 Anatomical variations of the course of the marginal nerve and their relative frequency.

plane immediately superficial to the vessels and appear as a structure parallel to the mandible (▶ Fig. 7.12). Once the nerve is identified, antegrade and retrograde dissections are performed until it is released from underlying attachments, and it can safely be reflected cephalad. Posteriorly, this dissection may course through the tail of the parotid gland, which in this case is reflected inferiorly and kept in continuity with the contents of level II. The level of the dissection must be continued until the posterosuperior boundaries of level IB (the lower border of the mandible and the stylohyoid muscles) are exposed. This approach is particularly useful if the anatomy is distorted or if there are facial lymphadenopathies.

7.2.5 Level Ia

This is usually the first level to be addressed, as it helps establish early anatomical points of reference and has a low potential for complications. In cases where a unilateral neck incision is performed, it is important to elevate skin flaps contralaterally (usually 2–3 cm) to expose the entire submental triangle. The fascia overlying the anterior belly of the digastric muscle is incised bilaterally in an anterior-to-posterior fashion with the Bovie electrocautery. If anterior jugular veins are identified over the boundaries of this level, it is safer to ligate them or control them with the harmonic scalpel, as the intraoperative combination of head elevation and relative hypotension may provide a false sense of hemostasis. Close to the anterior insertion of the

muscle, medial branches of the submental artery may have to be controlled. Once the lateral boundaries of the dissection have been established, the anterior bellies of the muscles are reflected laterally, and the fibrofatty contents of level Ia are dissected off the mylohyoid muscle, in an anterior-to-posterior fashion. This proceeds until the body of the hyoid bone is encountered (▶ Fig. 7.13). At this point, the specimen is transected at its base with the harmonic scalpel and sent for pathological analysis.

7.2.6 Level Ib

Once the marginal nerve has been addressed, attention is turned to defining the boundaries of the dissection. This triangular-shaped level defined by the anterior and posterior bellies of the digastric muscle, the lower border of the mandible, and the stylohyoid muscle. If the tail of the parotid gland extends over this compartment, it may be reflected superiorly, or transected and included in the specimen (after the continuity of the mandibular nerve has been established posteriorly). Depending on the drainage pattern of the superficial venous plexus, the retromandibular vein may need to be ligated to allow for adequate exposure. The submandibular glands may be ptotic, and extend below the boundaries of the digastric muscle, especially in elderly patients. In these cases, blunt dissection under hemostat exposure in the avascular plane immediately superficial to the muscle will help establish the boundaries while minimizing bleeding. This maneuver may be performed following the muscle in an anterior-to-posterior fashion or vice versa, all while the submandibular gland is retracted upward. The facial vein (and sometimes its branches) will course superficial to the gland, and must be ligated at this point (▶ Fig. 7.14).

Once the boundaries of the level are exposed, the next step is to ligate the facial vein as it emerges superiorly to the posterior belly of the digastric. While this step can be performed later in the dissection, most of the structures in this level receive their blood supply from this vessel, so ligating it earlier helps minimize bleeding. To achieve this, the submandibular gland is grasped and reflected anterosuperiorly, the posterior belly of the digastric is reflected inferiorly, and a Kittner blunt dissector is used to gently explore the space between these two structures.

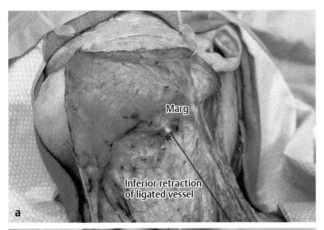

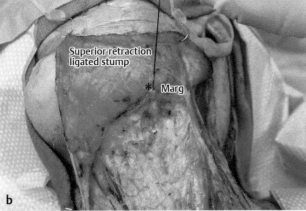

Fig. 7.11 Hayes Martin's maneuver for preservation of the marginal nerve. **(a)** Ligation of the facial vein 2 cm below the mandibular border (* denotes transected facial vein). **(b)** Superior retraction of the stump over the marginal nerve. Marg, marginal mandibular branch of the facial nerve.

The facial artery, which will appear coursing superiorly in a plane perpendicular to the muscle, may be then be clipped or ligated at this level (▶ Fig. 7.15).

Then, attention is turned to the anterior aspect of the dissection. The electrocautery is used to skeletonize the anterior belly of the digastric muscle, and the lower border of the mandible, carefully avoiding injuring the periosteum. Anteriorly, toward the angle created by the junction of these structures, the submental vessels appear in close relationship to the mandible, where they should be ligated. Then the anterior belly of the digastric is reflected inferiorly, and the fibrofatty contents of the space are dissected off the mylohyoid muscle in an anterior-to-posterior fashion with the electrocautery (▶ Fig. 7.16). This maneuver must be performed in a slow, continuous fashion, always maintaining a plane of dissection perpendicular to the mandible, until the free (posterior) edge of the mylohyoid is encountered. There are some technical points to be noted about this part of the procedure:

- This is not an avascular plane, and vessels traversing the mylohyoid muscle in a deep to superficial plane will have to be controlled (ideally with clips or bipolar), as slow bleeding from these vessels may lead to postoperative hematoma.
- A dehiscence of the mylohyoid muscle (or *mylohyoid boutonniere*) has been reported in 36 to 41% of cadaver dissections,[9,10] and as high as 77% of the population on imaging studies (▶ Fig. 7.17).[11] The difference is explained by the high sensibility of current imaging, which may detect clinically inapparent presentations. These cases are notorious for the protrusion of sublingual salivary tissue or fat—or both—into the submandibular space, putting these structures at risk during the dissection. While these anatomical variations may be identified in preoperative imaging, the surgeon must always carry a high index of suspicion during this portion of the dissection, as this condition may be quite confusing for the neophytes.
- Zealous resection of all the fibrofatty contents must be ensured. Upon completion of this portion, the digastric muscle, mylohyoid muscle, and the mandible should be devoid of any apparent soft tissue.

At this point, the detached components of the anterior level Ib and the submandibular gland are grasped together. A Green loop retractor is gently placed under the mylohyoid muscle and used to reflect the muscle anteriorly. The gland is then reflected superiorly to expose the hypoglossal nerve, which will be found deep and slightly superior to the digastric tendon (▶ Fig. 7.18a). The gland is then reflected inferiorly to expose the lingual nerve and the submandibular ganglion, which lies in close proximity to the gland (▶ Fig. 7.18b). The submandibular gland duct is located parallel to the lingual nerve, in a position immediately inferior to

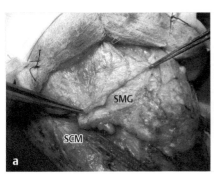

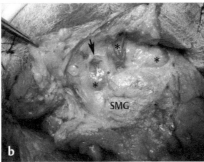

Fig. 7.12 Identification of the marginal branch by direct exploration. **(a)** Horizontal incision of the fascia over the right submandibular gland. **(b)** Superior elevation in the subfascial plane to expose the marginal nerve (*arrow*); * denote level Ib lymph nodes. SCM, sternocleidomastoid muscle; SMG, submandibular gland.

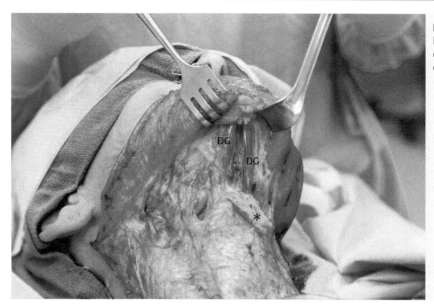

Fig. 7.13 Dissection of level Ia. The specimen (*) has been dissected off the anterior bellies of the digastric muscles, and the mylohyoid muscle. DG, digastric muscle.

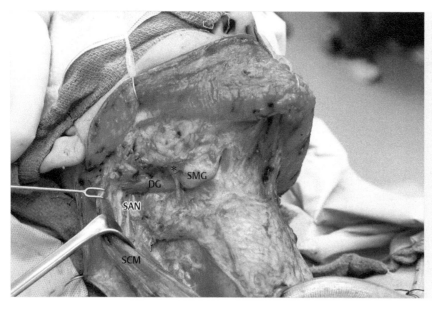

Fig. 7.14 Dissection of level Ib: facial vein (*) and submandibular gland. DG, digastric muscle; SAN, spinal accessory nerve; SCM, sternocleidomastoid muscle; SMG, submandibular gland.

it. The duct is thin walled and surrounded by salivary gland parenchyma, so under normal circumstances it may be difficult to identify, but the opposite is true if it is obstructed distally (such as floor of mouth tumors). In these cases, the duct is widely dilated and filled with mucopurulent content, markedly facilitating its identification.

Once all of these structures are identified, any soft tissue connections to the specimen or the submandibular gland are transected, leaving the gland attached anteriorly only by the lingual nerve and submandibular duct. The duct and submandibular ganglion are then clamped together, and the specimen is transected over the clamp and sent to pathological analysis. During this maneuver, especial care must be taken to avoid grasping the trunk of the lingual nerve with the clamp, and it is recommended that cold instrumentation be used to release the specimen in order to avoid electrocautery-related neuropraxia.

Alternatively, the specimen may be kept in continuity with the contents of the lateral neck by preserving the fascia overlying the posterior belly of the digastric muscle. This approach is technically more challenging and has questionable oncological benefits, so it is not routinely recommended.

7.2.7 Level II

The jugular lymph nodes (levels II–IV) are part of a continuum of lymphoid tissue that in the context of a modified radical neck dissection is routinely addressed as a single specimen. The boundaries between these levels are not anatomical, but arbitrarily established to help conceptualize the degree of nodal extension in the neck. In the following section, the critical aspects of the dissection of levels II to IV will be addressed separately; however, it is important to highlight that in reality there is significant overlap between these surgical steps.

To expose the jugular lymph nodes, the first step is to widely expose the SCM from its sternoclavicular insertion to the mastoid. In this regard, if the skin flap elevation was insufficient, it

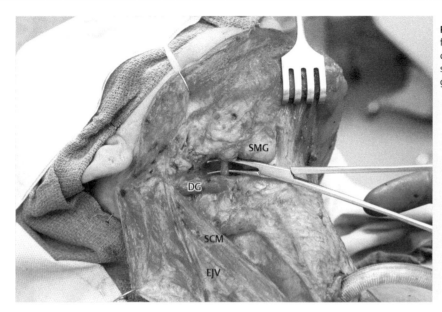

Fig. 7.15 Dissection of level Ib: ligation of the facial artery exposed by the instrument. DG, digastric muscle; EJV, external jugular vein; SCM, sternocleidomastoid muscle; SMG, submandibular gland.

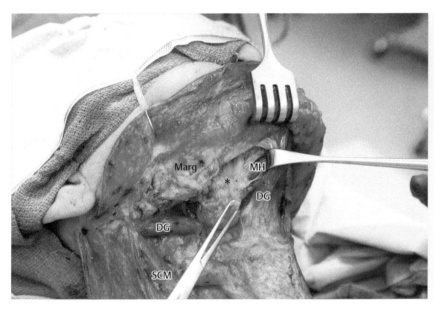

Fig. 7.16 Dissection of level Ib. As the anterior belly of the digastric muscle is retracted anteriorly, the specimen (*) which contains the submandibular gland and fibrofatty contents of level Ib is dissected off the mylohyoid muscle. DG, digastric muscle; Marg, marginal mandibular branch of the facial nerve; MH, mylohyoid muscle; SCM, sternocleidomastoid muscle.

must be expanded accordingly using the same principles previously described. A thorough understanding of the fascial compartments of the neck is particularly important for this portion of the procedure, and this topic is addressed in detail in Chapter 3. The SLDCF (or investing layer) wraps around the SCM covering its internal and external aspects (Chapter 3; ▶ Fig. 3.7). The fascia is incised along the anterior border of the SCM from the mastoid to its sternal insertion. The muscle is then reflected laterally, and the dissection proceeds on its internal aspect, in a superior-to-inferior fashion, while aiming to preserve its fascial envelope (▶ Fig. 7.19). During this process, the segmental blood supply to the muscle, which originates from the occipital, superior thyroid, and transverse cervical arteries,[12] is controlled with the harmonic scalpel as it enters the muscle. This maneuver proceeds continuously, aiming toward the posterior aspect of the muscle as it is gently released and reflected.

7.2.8 External Jugular Nodes

The external jugular lymph nodes are located on the lateral aspect of the SCM, along the course of this vessel, and deep to the investing fascia of the muscle. Routinely, this group is not electively included when the procedure is indicated for aerodigestive tract malignancies, but it should be addressed in other circumstances, such as in the presence of positive lymph nodes or for cutaneous malignancies. To address these, the fascia overlying the SCM is incised along the posterior border of the muscle, transecting the greater auricular and related sensory branches. The fascia (containing this nodal group) is then reflected anteriorly, and detached from the lateral surface of the SCM in a posterior-to-anterior fashion. The external jugular vein is transected on its superior aspect—as it merges with the retromandibular vein—and inferiorly as it leaves the confines of the SCM muscle. As soon as the dissection reaches the anterior edge of the SCM,

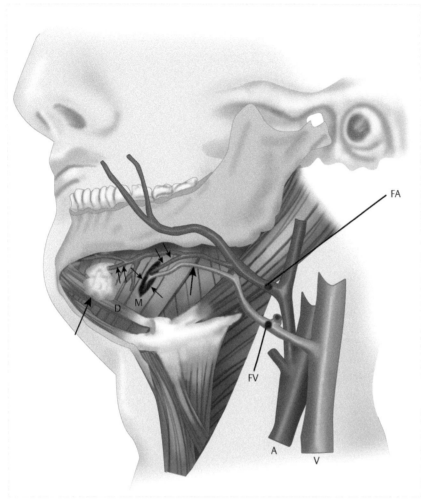

Fig. 7.17 Diagram of a mylohyoid muscle dehiscence.

the specimen may be amputated and sent for pathologic analysis, or maintained in continuity with the contents of levels II to IV.

7.2.9 Identification of the Spinal Accessory Nerve

Roughly midpoint through the dissection on the internal aspect of the SCM, and on the upper third of the muscle (level II), the SAN should be actively searched for. The nerve is usually surrounded by blood vessels, and care must be taken to avoid mistaking it for a vascular structure. The main trunk of the nerve (or the branch to the SCM) consistently enters the muscle on its internal aspect at this level, but other aspects of the anatomical relationship between the SAN and the SCM are significantly more variable. In an anatomical study aimed at documenting the anatomy of the SCM branch, Shiozaki at al[13] described three patterns for innervation of this muscle, which are presented in ▸ Table 7.4. In all the assessed specimens, either the trunk of the nerve or a major motor branch was confirmed to enter the SCM at its anticipated location, thus confirming the notion that the proximal portion of the nerve has a relatively constant anatomy.

On the other hand, distal arborization, specifically as it relates to the trapezius branch and cervical contributions, varies greatly. Recent studies have relied on electrophysiological analysis to provide further insight into these variations. Gavid et al[14] used this technique to assess the contributions of cervical nerves to the motor innervation of the trapezius muscle in cadavers. They found that while anatomical communications between the SAN cervical nerves were common (78% for C2, 48% for C3, and 52% for C4), in only 32% of the cases did they elicit a motor event in the trapezius. These findings suggest that the majority of cervical anastomoses could be sensory in nature. Similarly, Lanišnik recently described a functional classification of the anatomical variations of the trapezius branch by using electromyography in patients undergoing neck dissections[15] (▸ Table 7.5). This study highlights the complexity of the neural connections at this level, and helps explain why patients in whom the main trunk of the nerve was spared may present with shoulder impingement syndrome in the postoperative period. There is also anatomical variability of the nerve beyond its major motor branches to the SCM and trapezius muscles. Tubbs et al[16] describe that in 1.8% of the cases the nerve is duplicated (intracranially or extracranially) and that the nerve is communicated with—or gives origin to—the lesser occipital nerve in 5.4% of the cases. While these findings have little implication in terms of surgical technique, they should serve as a reminder of the variability and complexity of the SAN anatomy.

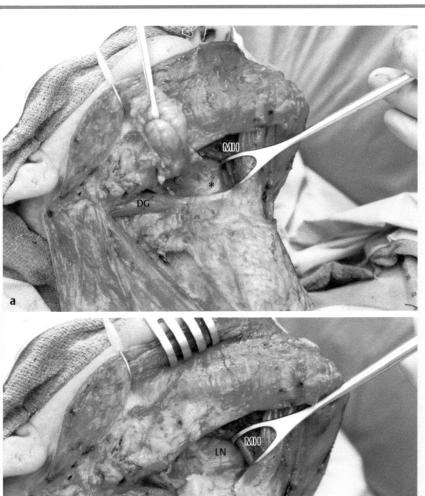

Fig. 7.18 (a) Superior retraction of the specimen to expose the hypoglossal nerve (*). (b) Inferior retraction of the specimen to expose the lingual nerve. DG, digastric muscle; LN, lingual nerve; MH, mylohyoid muscle.

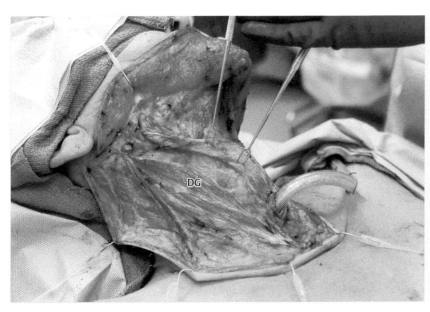

Fig. 7.19 Incision of the fascia over the anterior border of the sternocleidomastoid muscle, and initial retraction of the muscle. DG, digastric muscle.

Table 7.4 Patterns for spinal accessory nerve (SAN) innervation of the sternocleidomastoid muscle (SCM)[13]

Type	Description	Frequency (%)
A	A branch of the SAN innervates the SCM, but the main trunk of the nerve courses posteriorly along its inner surface without penetrating the muscle.	45.9
B	The main trunk of the SAN penetrates SCM and then reappears posteriorly as the branch to the trapezius muscle.	50.8
C	The main trunk of the SAN penetrates the SCM and emerges on its lateral surface as the branch to the trapezius muscle.	3.3

Table 7.5 Anatomical patterns of spinal accessory nerve (SAN) for innervation of the trapezius muscle, description and frequency according to Lanišnik[15]

Type 1	Type 2	Type 3
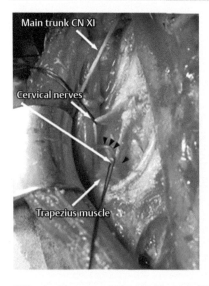	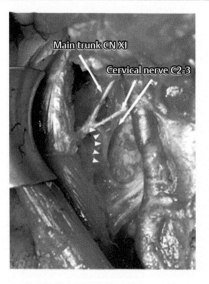	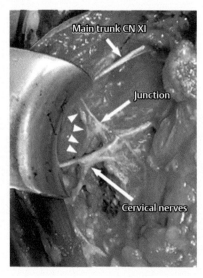
SAN enters the sternocleidomastoid muscle (SCM) and a single trapezius muscle branch exits from the posterior border of the muscle. This nerve receives communications from the cervical nerves, especially C2 and C3.	The motor branch for trapezius muscle separates from the main trunk at level II, before the SAN enters SCM. There are communicating branches with cervical nerves C2 and C3.	SAN enters the SCM in the same way as described in type 1, and the trapezius branch exits the muscle on its posterior border; *however*, it does not immediately travel to level V and the trapezius muscle, but instead takes a more medial course and mixes with cervical rootlets.
66%	22%	12%

Note: Arrowheads depict the location of the motor branch to the trapezius muscle.

As illustrated by these studies, meticulous and conservative dissection of the nerve, and all its branches and anastomoses, is paramount to achieve the best functional results. From the technique standpoint, this may be achieved by focusing on the more constant part of the nerve anatomy (identifying it as it enters the SCM) and subsequently utilizing meticulous retrograde dissection to expand on these findings. Special care must be taken to identify and spare the cervical contributions. These are commonly located at the posterior edge of the SCM, and consistently reach the trunk of the nerve from its caudal aspect. It is strongly recommended to use fine instrumentation, and limit electrocautery use to the bipolar, while actively dissecting this neural plexus.

7.2.10 Defining the Anatomy of the Superior Boundary of the Dissection

At this point, the posterior belly of the digastric should be completely exposed and dissected posteriorly until its junction with the SCM is widely exposed. As described earlier, the main trunk of the SAN should have been identified and isolated on the internal aspect of the SCM muscle. Then, the posterior belly is reflected superiorly and the SCM laterally to create a triangular working space. Weitlaner autostatic retractors may be used to facilitate exposure, but care must be taken to avoid placing them close to neurovascular structures. The trunk of the SAN is dissected cephalad aiming for the posterior

Table 7.6 Anatomical relationship between the spinal accessory nerve (SAN) and the internal jugular vein (IJV)

Study (year)	Subject type	Number of dissections	Lateral crossing (%)	Medial crossing (%)	Through IJV (%)
Taylor et al (2013)	Surgical Anatomy	207	95.6	2.8	0.9
Saman et al (2011)	Cadaver	84	80	19	1
Hinsley and Hartig (2010)	Surgical Anatomy	116	96	3	1
Lee et al (2009)	Surgical Anatomy	181	39.8	57.4	2.8
Kierner et al (2000)	Cadaver	92	56	44	
Krause et al (1991)	Cadaver	94	72.5	26.4	

Source: Adapted from Taylor et al.[25]
Note: Illustrations depict the posterior belly of the digastric muscle, the superior aspect of the internal jugular vein, and the main trunk of the SAN.

belly of the digastric. At this point, establishing the anatomical relationship between the nerve and the superior aspect of the IJV becomes the main objective. In this regard, there are three possible relationships between the structures: the nerve may be lateral to the IJV, medial to the IJV, or go through it (also known as IJV duplication). As presented in ▶ Table 7.6, the relative frequencies of these anatomical dispositions vary widely in the medical literature, yet from this author's observations, at this level the nerve is almost always lateral to the vein. In addition to this relationship, the surgeon must be aware of two anatomical considerations that warrant meticulous surgical technique:

- Commonly, the IJV will have small branches that course anteriorly or posteriorly, at or below the plane of the posterior belly of the digastric muscle. These may be a source of bleeding that is difficult to control given the limited exposure.
- The occipital artery can be consistently found in this region, as it courses posterosuperiorly in a plane superficial to the IJV and the SAN. In terms of the cephalocaudal location, in most patients the vessel has a course that is parallel and immediately deep to the posterior belly of the digastric muscle, but it may also be caudal to the muscle, and well within the boundaries of level II. When visualized, the occipital artery commonly interjects with the trunk of the SAN at a 45- to 90-degree angle. If the vessel is within the confines of level II, it may be ligated without apparent deficit (▶ Fig. 7.20).

7.2.11 Sublevel IIb

In the recent medical literature, there is growing evidence supporting conservative management of this level in multiple clinical scenarios, unless there is Frank's disease in level IIa.[17,18] There is a well-established rationale for this, as dissection of this level has been associated with a significant increase in shoulder dysfunction on multiple accounts.[19] There is also an anatomical component adding to the variability, as in some patients the trunk of the SAN enters the SCM muscle very close to its mastoid insertion, leaving little—if any—lymphoid tissue in this level.

From the standpoint of technique, this sublevel may be resected as a separate specimen, or in continuity with the rest of the lateral neck, which is this author's preference. Proper exposure is paramount to achieve an oncologically sound resection of the contents of the submuscular triangle. An autostatic retractor is used to separate the posterior belly of the digastric and the upper aspect of the SCM, and a small Richardson retractor placed in the junction of these two muscles. Then, the trunk of the SAN (which at this point has been dissected) is gently retracted anteroinferiorly with a nerve hook. This four-point retraction technique provides the best possible exposure of this sublevel. Then, using the Bovie electrocautery, the specimen is first detached from the undersurface of the SCM (aiming at its posterior boundary) and from the posterior belly of the digastric muscle. This can be a swift maneuver as there are no cervical rootlets above the level of the SAN in this region. It is recommended that the assistant use an Andrews–Pynchon suction, as the liquefied fats of the specimen reduce the efficiency of the electrocautery. Once the posterior and superior boundaries of the resection are defined, the specimen is gently grasped and dissected off the floor of the neck musculature, which at this level is constituted by the splenius capitis and the levator

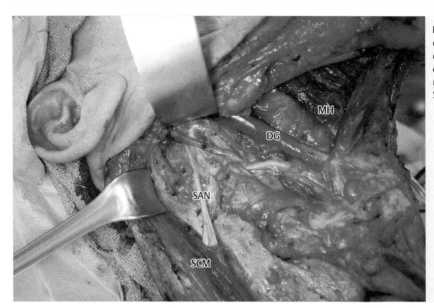

Fig. 7.20 Dissection of level II. The posterior belly of the digastric muscle is retracted, and the occipital artery (*) is seen coursing posterolaterally though level II. DG, digastric muscle; MH, mylohyoid muscle; SAN, spinal accessory nerve; SCM, sternocleidomastoid muscle.

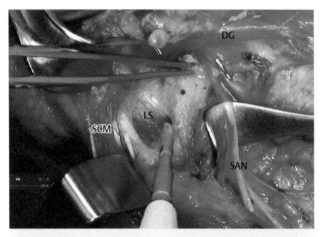

Fig. 7.21 Dissection of submuscular recess (level IIb). As the spinal accessory nerve is retracted anteriorly, the specimen (*) is dissected off the digastric, SCM and floor of the neck musculature. DG, digastric muscle; LS, levator scapulae muscle; SAN, spinal accessory nerve; SCM, sternocleidomastoid muscle.

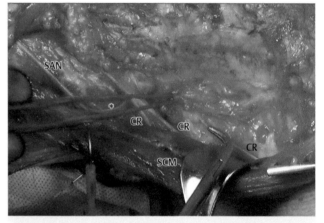

Fig. 7.22 Dissection of the cervical rootlets in level III. Note the branch to the trapezius muscle from the spinal accessory nerve (*). CR, transected cervical rootlets; SAN, spinal accessory nerve; SCM, sternocleidomastoid muscle.

scapula muscle (▶ Fig. 7.21). This maneuver is performed in a posterior-to-anterior fashion until the level of the SAN and the lateral aspect of the IJV are reached. It is important to note that, at this level, the lateral aspect of the IJV should have been previously dissected and exposed prior to addressing level IIb. Otherwise, there is risk for a high vascular injury of the vein, which is notoriously difficult to control. The specimen is then translocated under the trunk of the SAN and kept in continuity with the contents of level IIa.

It must be noted that the occipital artery may be visualized in this sublevel and be a source of intraoperative bleeding. If this is the case, it must be transected and partially included with the specimen.

7.2.12 Level III

The dissection proceeds along the internal aspect of the SCM muscle in a cephalad-to-caudal fashion. At this level, the main focus is to identify and dissect cervical rootlets, and most importantly, spare the contributions they may have to the trapezius branch of the SAN. It is recommended that the surgeon be very familiar with the variations in the neural anatomy in this region, as presented in ▶ Table 7.5. The specimen involving levels II and III (and subsequently IV) is grasped with Allis clamps and reflected medially by the assistant in an even fashion. Once the rootlets are visualized on the undersurface of the posterior edge of the SCM, they are dissected toward their point of emergence in the floor of the neck. There is a natural plane of dissection immediately superficial to each rootlet, so from this author's perspective this is better achieved with the blunt dissection technique under hemostat exposure. As each rootlet is dissected, the specimen is sequentially released, opening the surgical field to proceed to the next (caudal) nerve (▶ Fig. 7.22). From the anatomical standpoint, the plane of the rootlets marks the posterior boundary of levels III and IV, so there is no need to proceed deep to these structures at this stage. However, it must be noted that the fibrofatty tissue superficial to virtual plane that connects the rootlets should be included with the specimen. This is a common point of confusion, and a potential pitfall from the oncologic perspective, among other reasons, because there are no anatomical landmarks other than the rootlets. When two consecutive rootlets are exposed, a helpful maneuver is to dissect the most caudal one and open the fascia overlying it while reflecting the soft tissues located in between the rootlets, over the instrument. This assures an even plane of dissection while minimizing the risk of an incomplete removal of lymphatic tissues.

The rest of the dissection of level III involves detaching the specimen off the floor of the neck musculature, which is performed with level IV and will be discussed in the following section.

7.2.13 Level IV

This is an important level, as it carries significant risk to neurovascular structures and potential for significant complications. Thorough knowledge of the anatomy of the region is essential to reduce the risk of complications.

Normally, this level will be performed sequentially after level III, proceeding with the continuum, that is, the dissection of the lateral neck. At this point, the anterior fascia of the SCM has been opened, and the rootlets of level III identified and dissected. The next step is to provide ample exposure of this region, which is achieved by aggressive lateral retraction of the lower third of the SCM, and medial countertraction of the visceral compartment by the assistant. This maneuver exposes the omohyoid muscle, which serves not only as an intraoperative boundary between levels III and IV, but also as a landmark to identify the caudal aspect of the IJV, which lies immediately deep to its tendon. The muscle is transected at the level of its tendon, which allows for further exposure of the caudal jugular vein (▶ Fig. 7.23). At this point, it is recommended to palpate and acknowledge the location of the clavicle, the inferior boundary for the dissection. Since the procedure is being performed on a deeper plane, it is easy to lose perspective and transect the specimen too high on the neck, or too low toward the mediastinum.

Once the stage has been set, the first step is to continue the dissection on the undersurface of the SCM, as carried along from level III. The surgeon must actively look for lower cervical rootlets in this area, which will have the same anatomical disposition as in levels above and should be addressed likewise. Once the most caudal rootlet has been dissected, the junction where it intersects the posterior edge of the SCM (as seen from its undersurface) becomes

the pivotal point where the dissection turns medially to define the caudal boundary of level IV. This should roughly correlate with the level of the clavicle on surface anatomy.

At this stage, the specimen is still attached medially to the IJV, and to the floor of the neck, which at this level is constituted primarily by the anterior and middle scalene muscles. The transverse cervical vessels have a medial-to-lateral course in a plane immediately superficial to the prevertebral fascia. The phrenic nerve courses in an oblique plane over the surface of the anterior scalene, protected by this fascia. It is good practice to keep these constant anatomical relationships in mind, because if at any time the fibers of the anterior scalene become visible, the plane of dissection is too deep and it must be corrected immediately.

The surgeon must also be familiar with the lymphatic anatomy of the region, which is significantly more variable. At a rate of 1 to 2.5% of all modified radical neck dissections, the risk of postoperative chyle leak is low. This incidence, however, may be underreporting, as prospective studies have documented it as high as 8.3%.[20] The most important vessel in this regard is the thoracic duct, which measures about 45 cm in length, but only 2 to 3 mm in diameter. It courses superiorly on the left side, through the mediastinum, to drain on the posterior aspect of the junction between the internal jugular and the subclavian veins (▶ Fig. 7.24). However, there is significant variation of the course and termination of the duct, and it can drain higher (directly to the IJV) placing the patient at considerable risk for a chylous fistula.

Anatomically, on the right side there are three major lymphatic trunks (jugular, subclavian, and bronchomediastinal), which most commonly drain independently to the posterior aspect of the subclavian. However, in one-third of the cases, these trunks converge to form a larger vessel known as the right lymphatic duct, which has a short course (1–2 cm) to drain in the same location as the contralateral thoracic duct[21] (▶ Fig. 7.25). In the event of an injury to the right-sided duct, the patient presents with a lymphatic fistula, but no chyle, as this fluid will lack the enteric component. A common misconception is to attribute the risk of chyle leaks only to left-sided neck dissections. This is not true, as in 1 to 5% of the cases, the thoracic duct will drain on the right side, and there are also accounts of bilateral thoracic ducts. For these reasons, it is recommended that the surgeon have the same careful approach as to the lower neck, regardless of the side of the dissection.

Traditionally, to establish the lower boundary for the dissection in level IV, a lateral-to-medial approach has been advocated. In

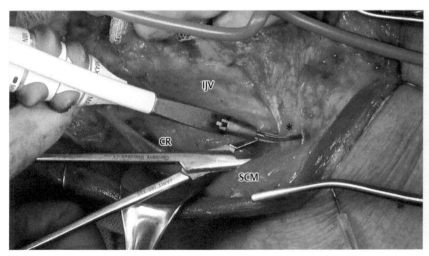

Fig. 7.23 Transection of the tendon of the omohyoid muscle (*) to expose level IV. CR, transected cervical rootlets; IJV, internal jugular vein; SCM, sternocleidomastoid muscle.

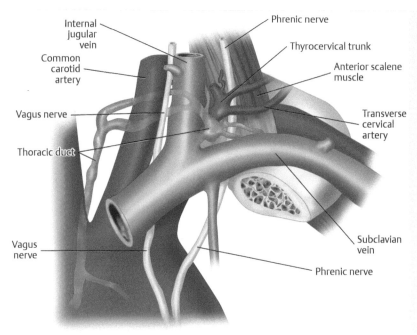

Fig. 7.24 Illustration of the anatomy of the thoracic duct, as it drains to the left jugulo-subclavian junction.

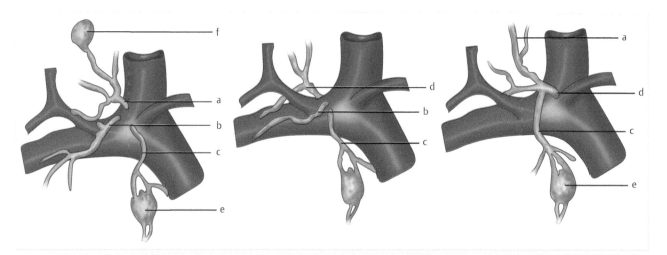

Fig. 7.25 Illustration of the variations in drainage patterns of the right neck lymphatics. a = jugular trunk, b = subclavian trunk, c = bronchomediastinal trunk, d = right lymphatic trunk, e = gland of internal mammary chain, f = gland of deep cervical chain.

this setting, the specimen is retracted medially, and the dissection proceeds medially from the posterior border of the SCM muscle (below the level of the lowest rootlet), over the prevertebral fascia and toward the IJV. While this is feasible and usually safe, it can be challenging, as the angle for dissection is not comfortable for the surgeon, and the plane transitions from deep to superficial (as the prominence of the anterior scalene muscle is encountered from the side). Also, the fascial planes are not as well defined laterally, close to the posterior border of the SCM muscle.

An alternative maneuver to define the lower boundary of level IV is a medial-to-lateral approach; based on this author's experience, this is easier to execute, more consistent, and proceeds as follows: when the lowest rootlet has been dissected on the medial aspect of the SCM, this point is marked with an instrument. Then the IJV is exposed at the level of the clavicle, and the fascia on its lateral aspect opened vertically over 3 to 4 cm, thus creating a "pocket" immediately lateral to the vein. Then, as the IJV is reflected medially and the rest of the specimen laterally, this pocket is expanded using a Kittner dissector for atraumatic blunt dissection. To establish a reference point, the surgeon must palpate the convexity of the anterior scalene muscle, and the dissection is oriented toward this structure. This is usually a relatively avascular plane, but if any bleeding is encountered it must be controlled immediately. Once the plane of the anterior scalene muscle is reached, the specimen is reflected upward (i.e., lifted off the neck) and blunt dissection with a Kittner dissector ensues over the anterior aspect in a medial-to-lateral fashion. At this point, the phrenic nerve will usually become apparent in the anterior surface of the muscle, behind a layer of prevertebral fascia. The main trunk of the transverse cervical vessels can usually be seen heading laterally over the plane of the nerve; these vessels may be dissected laterally and spared (▶ Fig. 7.26).

The dissection continues laterally in the same plane (over the scalene muscles) directed toward the point where the last rootlet intersects with the SCM, all while continuously gently lifting the specimen off the neck. When this point is reached, there is effectively a tunnel separating critical structures (deep), from the fibrofatty contents of level IV (superficial). At this stage, the caudal attachments of the specimen are transected and ligated in multiple sections, under direct visualization of the phrenic nerve. The thoracic duct—or major lymphatics vessels—can usually be visualized with this maneuver, located in a plane immediately lateral and posterior to the IJV (▶ Fig. 7.27). Most commonly, they can be spared, but if there is nodal disease in the area—or if located within the boundaries of level IV—they should be ligated.

At this point, the specimen encompassing levels II to IV has been released superiorly, laterally, and inferiorly, and remains partially attached to the floor of the neck, and medially to the IJV. The next step is to detach these levels off the floor of the neck musculature. Any incompletely dissected rootlets are addressed,

further releasing the specimen medially. As it relates to the floor of the neck, the prevertebral facial planes are more clearly defined on its lower third than in the superior two-thirds, among other reasons because of the course of the cervical rootlets. As such, one of the most significant risks during this stage is an injury to the phrenic nerve close to its origin, or to its contributions from C3–C5. In this regard, there are a couple of predisposing factors that should be pointed out, one being excessive traction of the specimen, which distorts the surgical planes and elevates the plane of the prevertebral fascia, and the other being the convexity of the anterior scalene muscle. It is important to conceptualize that, as the dissection proceeds medially and approaches the IJV, it should transition to a more superficial plane (and merge to the lateral aspect of the vein, which is roughly 2 cm superficial to the prevertebral fascia). Failing to do so (i.e., following the prevertebral fascia medially) leads to dissection underneath the IJV, posing significant risk to the carotid artery, vagus nerve, and cervical sympathetic chain. A helpful maneuver to properly address this surgical plane transition is to dissect with a hemostat on the lateral aspect of the IJV in a caudal-to-cephalad fashion, and reflect the specimen medially over the instrument (▶ Fig. 7.28). This all

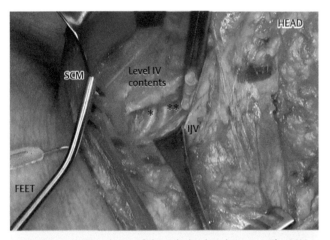

Fig. 7.26 Contralateral view of the right level IV dissection. The SCM and IJV are retracted. A medial-to-lateral approach has been used to expose the transverse cervical artery (**) and the phrenic nerve (*) over the anterior scalene muscle. IJV, internal jugular vein; SCM, sternocleidomastoid muscle.

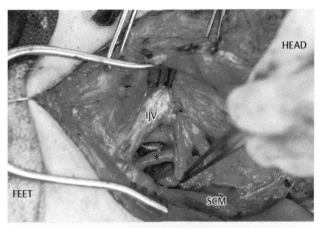

Fig. 7.27 Thoracic duct (*) identified during the dissection of left level IV. IJV, internal jugular vein; SCM, sternocleidomastoid muscle.

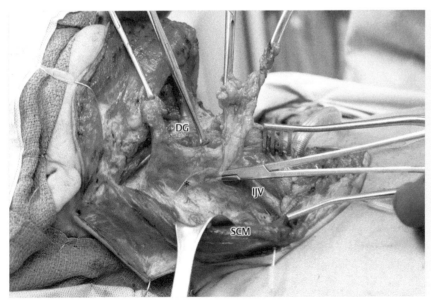

Fig. 7.28 Detaching the specimen off the prevertebral plane while dissecting on the lateral surface of the internal jugular vein; ansa cervicalis (*) can be seen crossing over the IJV. DG, digastric muscle; IJV, internal jugular vein; SCM, sternocleidomastoid muscle.

but guarantees the indemnity of the deep fascial planes and the neural structures within it. Roughly at the midpoint of the IJV, the surgeon will encounter the cervical contributions from C2–C3 forming the inferior root of the ansa cervicalis. This nerve can be identified coursing anteromedially from floor of the neck and looping over the vein, where it can be safely transected.

A tortuous internal carotid artery is an innocuous anatomical variation that can pose a risk in this part of the procedure. While releasing the specimen superiorly, close to the posterior belly of the digastric muscle, this vessel can appear like a level II lymphadenopathy adjacent to the floor of the neck; the surgeon must have a high index of suspicion to avoid a major vascular injury in these cases.

Once the specimen has been released from the floor, the IJV should appear widely exposed from the clavicle to the digastric. At this stage, the specimen is reflected superomedially over the vein, and the vessel is skeletonized in the subadventitial plane with a scalpel in a lateral-to-medial fashion. Appropriate tension is essential to safely perform this maneuver. It is recommended that the specimen is grasped with four Allis clamps and retracted in an even fashion, while the surgeon uses a sponge on his or her nondominant hand to provide even countertraction to the vessel (▶ Fig. 7.29). There are few branches on the lateral aspect of the vein, but they appear as the dissection proceeds medially and all these branches must be identified (prior to transection) and sequentially ligated. The common facial vein is usually the largest branch, and it may be ligated or dissected medially to minimize the functional impact of the procedure. Small injuries to the vein can usually be addressed with a clip (if there is a stump present) or by using two clips in a "V" disposition over the lateral wall of the vessel (if there is no stump). Larger injuries to the vein should be repaired with a Satinsky clamp with proper vascular technique. The dissection proceeds until the IJV is freed on its medial aspect, leaving the specimen attached to the carotid artery and strap muscles.

The next step is to identify the hypoglossal nerve on the carotid triangle. The nerve is deep to the tendon of the digastric muscle, and courses over the internal and external carotid arteries. To expose it, the posterior belly of the digastric muscle is reflected superiorly, and blunt dissection is performed a couple of centimeters caudal to the muscle, in a plane parallel to the hyoid bone; the nerve should become apparent as it loops anteriorly heading toward the submandibular triangle. The hypoglossal venous plexus (or ranine veins) consistently crosses over the nerve at this level. These vessels (which drain to the common facial vein) can be quite large and may represent a source for postoperative bleeding. Blunt dissection is performed over the hypoglossal nerve to expose and either ligate or transect these veins with the harmonic scalpel.

At this level, the superior branch of the ansa cervicalis (C1) should be visualized as it detaches from the hypoglossal nerve with a caudal direction over the carotid, heading to the strap muscles. When possible, this nerve should be preserved, as it may provide a useful landmark for the medial dissection of the specimen (▶ Fig. 7.30). When the anatomy of the upper neck is challenging (such as reoperative cases, or severe actinic damage), the ansa cervicalis can be retrogradely dissected to safely identify the hypoglossal nerve.

The final step in the dissection of levels II to IV is the medial release of the specimen from its boundary, defined as the lateral border of the sternohyoid muscle. On the superior part of the neck, the omohyoid muscle (which has been transected) may serve as a surrogate structure to establish this plane, while inferiorly the sternohyoid must be exposed. The lateral aspect of the strap muscles is skeletonized with the Bovie electrocautery, and the fascia lateral to it grasped with Allis clamps. Retrograde dissection (in a medial-to-lateral fashion) ensues proceeding toward rest of the specimen that is over the carotid artery (▶ Fig. 7.31). During the anterior approach to the carotid triangle, prominent perforating venous branches that connect the superficial and deep venous systems (from the superior thyroid to the anterior jugular) will be encountered. These must be ligated or transected with the harmonic scalpel, and care must be taken not to injure the superior thyroid artery during this process. Similarly, it is good practice to confirm the location of the hypoglossal nerve to avoid a distal injury. Finally, under direct visualization of all the critical structures, the specimen is detached from the carotid artery with the harmonic scalpel, divided into levels, and sent for pathological analysis.

7.2.14 Level V

As previously described, an accessory limb may be required to fully expose the boundaries of this level. The skin flaps must be elevated over the trapezius muscle (which should have its

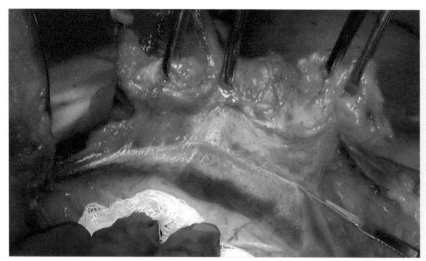

Fig. 7.29 Sharp dissection to release the contents of levels II to IV from the internal jugular vein.

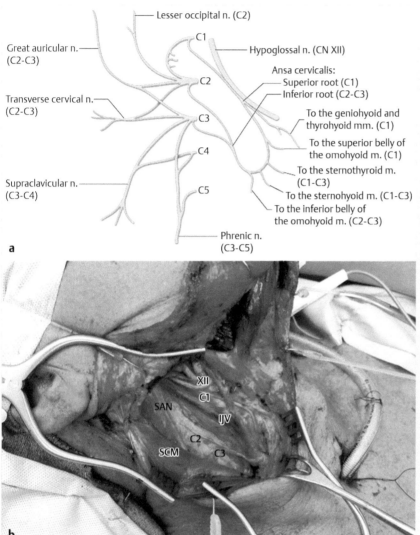

a

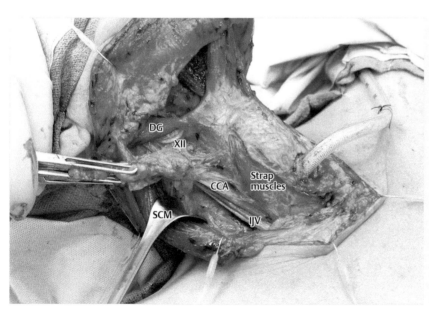

b

Fig. 7.30 (a) Illustration of the cervical contributions to the ansa cervicalis.
(b) Intraoperative image of a neck dissection where the entire loop of the ansa was dissected. The inferior root (C2–C3) and the superior root (C1) can be seen looping over the internal jugular vein. The hypoglossal nerve is also visualized. IJV, internal jugular vein; SAN, spinal accessory nerve; SCM, sternocleidomastoid muscle; XII, hypoglossal nerve.

Fig. 7.31 Dissection of the lateral border of the strap muscles, and release of the specimen over the carotid artery. CCA, carotid artery; DG, digastric muscle; IJV, internal jugular vein; SCM, sternocleidmastoid muscle; XII, hypoglossal nerve.

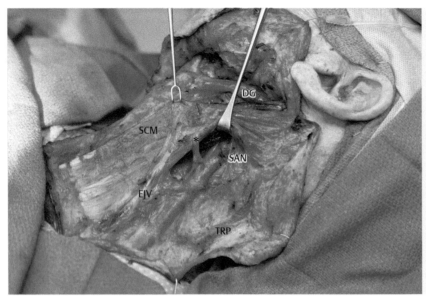

Fig. 7.32 Erb's point (*) being used as a reference to identify the spinal accessory nerve in the posterior triangle of the neck. DG, digastric muscle; EJV, external jugular vein; SAN, spinal accessory nerve; SCM, sternocleidomastoid muscle; TRP, trapezius muscle.

anterior border completely exposed) and inferiorly over the clavicle. Given the low rate of nodal involvement in this level, in contemporary oncological practice this level is commonly spared, unless Frank's disease is present or there are specific indications such as a cutaneous or a nasopharyngeal cancer.

The most important structure to preserve in this level is the trapezius branch of the SAN, which will emerge from the posterior border of the SCM and head posteroinferiorly, entering the trapezius muscle at the junction between its inferior third and its superior two-thirds. Another consideration is that the nerve enters the muscle from its undersurface, so during the dissection it will be perceived as "diving" under the muscle. This relationship is not consistently documented in the literature, and can be a source of confusion for neophyte practitioners. Because of its superficial location, and lack of clear anatomical boundaries, the nerve is at imminent risk during its entire course through the posterior triangle. As discussed earlier in this chapter, this is especially true when raising the skin flaps.

On their anatomical study, Shiozaki et al[13] describe five different branching patterns of the trapezius branch as it enters the anterior border of the muscle in the posterior neck triangle. In type 0 (3.8%), the main trunk of the CN XI did not exhibit any branching; in type 1 (50%), the main trunk produced one branch; in type 2 (26.9%), two branches were observed separating from the main trunk; in type 3 (11.5%), the main trunk produced three branches; and, finally, in type 4 (7.9%), the main trunk produced four branches.

There are several strategies to identify the nerve in the posterior triangle, and the surgeon must be familiar will all of them:

- *Using Erb's point.* The nerve can be identified on the posterior border of the SCM muscle, 1 to 2 cm above Erb's point—or nerve point—defined as the location where the four superficial branches of the cervical plexus (greater auricular, lesser occipital, transverse cervical, and supraclavicular) emerge from behind the muscle (Chapter 3; ▶ Fig. 7.16). Once this point has been localized, the SCM is grasped and reflected anteriorly over a short segment, and the fascia along its posterior border is incised vertically and explored with atraumatic technique. The nerve will appear as a structure forming an

acute angle with the SCM that will be located in a plane slightly deeper than the cervical nerves (▶ Fig. 7.32).

- *Dissection from an anterior approach.* If the trapezius branch of the SAN is visualized during the dissection of the jugular chain, it can be further dissected through the same approach as it enters level V. Alternatively, the position of the nerve can be marked with an instrument to use as a reference point during the exploration of the posterior triangle.
- *The nerve can also be identified as it reaches the trapezius muscle.* The fascia is opened in the posterior triangle, and atraumatic dissection proceeds over the anterior aspect of the trapezius, focusing on the junction between its lower third and its superior two-thirds. The limitation of this technique is that the nerve commonly expresses a branching pattern, making retrograde dissection technically more challenging and riskier from the perspective of branch injury.

Regardless of the technique chosen, the next step is to completely dissect the nerve, and all of its branches, through its entire course in level V. This is better achieved by a combination of sharp instrumentation and bipolar electrocautery, which prevents unexpected nerve stimulation (▶ Fig. 7.33).

The next step is dissection of the sublevel Va. The posterior border of the SCM (above the nerve) and the anterior border of the trapezius are skeletonized with the Bovie electrocautery. During this process, the lesser occipital nerve, which will originate from Erb's point and will have a posterosuperior orientation, will have to be transected. The specimen is detached from the floor of the neck musculature in a cephalad-to-caudal fashion, carefully preserving the fascia over these muscles. This is an important technical point, as the nerve (or nerves) to the levator scapulae originate from C4–C5 and travel on the surface of the muscle, protected only by its fascial layer. Any injury to the nerve will result in a functional deficit characterized by inability to raise the scapula and shoulder superomedially. As the specimen is detached, the muscles encountered will be the splenius capitis, levator scapula, and the posterior scalene, while the middle and anterior scalene muscles will be exposed during the dissection of level Vb. Once the specimen is released,

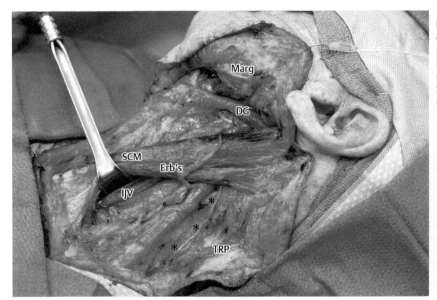

Fig. 7.33 The spinal accessory nerve has been completely dissected throughout its course in the posterior neck triangle (*). DG, digastric muscle; Erb's, Erb's point; IJV, internal jugular vein; Marg, marginal mandibular branch of the facial nerve; SCM, sternocleidomastoid muscle; TRP, trapezius muscle.

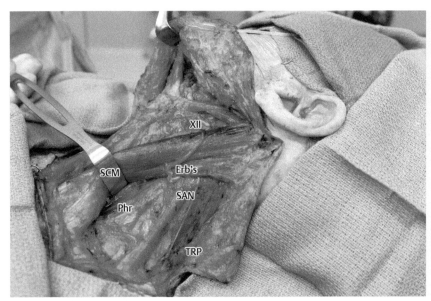

Fig. 7.34 The posterior neck dissection has been completed. Erb's, Erb's point; Phr, phrenic nerve; SAN, spinal accessory nerve; SCM, sternocleido-mastoid muscle; TRP, trapezius muscle; XII, hypoglossal nerve.

it is translocated under the SAN and kept in continuity with the contents of level Vb.

Then we turn our attention to level Vb. The SAN and its branches are reflected cephalad, and the boundaries of this sublevel are defined. Anteriorly, the posterior border of the SCM (below the nerve) is skeletonized. At this stage, the surgeon will encounter the supraclavicular nerve with its medial, intermediate, and lateral branches, which will originate from Erb's point and course inferolaterally in a superficial plane. These sensory rootlets must be sacrificed to address this sublevel, but when transecting them, it is important to leave a short stump at their point of origin to prevent injury to a cervical contribution of the phrenic nerve.

Inferiorly, the clavicle is exposed and the external jugular vein is transected at this level. Posteriorly, the omohyoid muscle will be identified and can be used as a surrogate for the inferior boundary of the resection. At this stage, the posterior border of the SCM muscle is reflected anteriorly, which should expose the previously dissected IJV, anterior scalene, and

phrenic nerve. The brachial plexus is covered by a thick fascial layer, and upon palpation it feels like a thick, noncompressible cord. The location of the brachial plexus is established, usually by palpation first. Once this structure has been identified, blunt dissection from medial to lateral is performed on a plane immediately superficial to the prevertebral fascia, releasing the specimen inferiorly. Anatomically, the contents of the supraclavicular fossa are continuous with the axillary fat, so as the dissection proceeds laterally, an arbitrary transection point is defined using the clavicle as a point of reference. In other words, the surgeon must avoid "pulling up" fat from below the clavicular plane. The harmonic scalpel works well in this situation, as there will be blood vessels and lymphatics in the area. The specimen is then sent for pathologic analysis, leaving the posterior neck triangle devoid of any lymphatic tissues, and the dissected SAN anatomically intact (▶ Fig. 7.34).

At this point, the neck is irrigated and hemostasis is confirmed under a Valsalva maneuver. Areas that should be directly explored are the undersurface of the SCM, branches of the transverse cervical vessels, hypoglossus venous plexus, and anterior jugular veins. The indemnity of the lymphatic system is confirmed by exploring level IV. While performing continuous abdominal compression,[22] any lymphatic leak should be promptly repaired. Closed suction drains are placed, and the incisions are closed in two layers according to the surgeon's preference.

7.3 Conclusion

The modified radical neck dissection is a comprehensive functional lymphadenectomy of the neck that only spares the groups in the central neck compartment. In this approach, the IJV, SAN, and SCM are spared, as well as all other significant neurovascular structures. This highly technical intervention demands for surgeons to master the anatomy of the neck, and to be familiarized with surgical strategies aimed at avoiding common intraoperative pitfalls. A systematic approach to this operation will help surgeons in training quickly to internalize the key elements necessary to perform this procedure safely and effectively.

References

[1] Crile G. Landmark article Dec 1, 1906: excision of cancer of the head and neck. With special reference to the plan of dissection based on one hundred and thirty-two operations. By George Crile. JAMA. 1987; 258(22):3286–3293

[2] Ferlito A, Rinaldo A. Osvaldo Suárez: often-forgotten father of functional neck dissection (in the non-Spanish-speaking literature). Laryngoscope. 2004; 114 (7):1177–1178

[3] Bocca E, Pignataro O. A conservation technique in radical neck dissection. Ann Otol Rhinol Laryngol. 1967; 76(5):975–987

[4] Byers RM, Clayman GL, McGill D, et al. Selective neck dissections for squamous carcinoma of the upper aerodigestive tract: patterns of regional failure. Head Neck. 1999; 21(6):499–505

[5] Uehara M, Helman JI, Lillie JH, Brooks SL. Blood supply to the platysma muscle flap: an anatomic study with clinical correlation. J Oral Maxillofac Surg. 2001; 59(6):642–646

[6] Eckardt AM. Platysma myocutaneous flap: its current role in reconstructive surgery of oral soft tissue defects. J Korean Assoc Oral Maxillofac Surg. 2013; 39(1):3–8

[7] Al-Qahtani K, Mlynarek A, Adamis J, Harris J, Seikaly H, Islam T. Intraoperative localization of the marginal mandibular nerve: a landmark study. BMC Res Notes. 2015; 8:382

[8] Batra AP, Mahajan A, Gupta K. Marginal mandibular branch of the facial nerve: an anatomical study. Indian J Plast Surg. 2010; 43(1):60–64

[9] Gaughran GR. Mylohyoid Boutonni'ere and sublingual bouton. J Anat. 1963; 97:565–568

[10] Nathan H, Luchansky E. Sublingual gland herniation through the mylohyoid muscle. Oral Surg Oral Med Oral Pathol. 1985; 59(1):21–23

[11] White DK, Davidson HC, Harnsberger HR, Haller J, Kamya A. Accessory salivary tissue in the mylohyoid boutonnière: a clinical and radiologic pseudolesion of the oral cavity. AJNR Am J Neuroradiol. 2001; 22(2):406–412

[12] Leclère FM, Vacher C, Benchaa T. Blood supply to the human sternocleidomastoid muscle and its clinical implications for mandible reconstruction. Laryngoscope. 2012; 122(11):2402–2406

[13] Shiozaki K, Abe S, Agematsu H, et al. Anatomical study of accessory nerve innervation relating to functional neck dissection. J Oral Maxillofac Surg. 2007; 65(1):22–29

[14] Gavid M, Mayaud A, Timochenko A, Asanau A, Prades JM. Topographical and functional anatomy of trapezius muscle innervation by spinal accessory nerve and C2 to C4 nerves of cervical plexus. Surg Radiol Anat. 2016; 38 (8):917–922

[15] Lanišnik B. Different branching patterns of the spinal accessory nerve: impact on neck dissection technique and postoperative shoulder function. Curr Opin Otolaryngol Head Neck Surg. 2017; 25(2):113–118

[16] Tubbs RS, Ajayi OO, Fries FN, Spinner RJ, Oskouian RJ. Variations of the accessory nerve: anatomical study including previously undocumented findings-expanding our misunderstanding of this nerve. Br J Neurosurg. 2017; 31 (1):113–115

[17] Lea J, Bachar G, Sawka AM, et al. Metastases to level IIb in squamous cell carcinoma of the oral cavity: a systematic review and meta-analysis. Head Neck. 2010; 32(2):184–190

[18] Vayisoglu Y, Ozcan C. Involvement of level IIb lymph node metastasis and dissection in thyroid cancer. Gland Surg. 2013; 2(4):180–185

[19] Roger V, Hitier M, Robard L, Babin E. Morbidity of neck dissection submuscular recess (sublevel IIb) in head and neck cancer. Rev Laryngol Otol Rhinol (Bord). 2014; 135(3):135–140

[20] Roh JL, Kim DH, Park CI. Prospective identification of chyle leakage in patients undergoing lateral neck dissection for metastatic thyroid cancer. Ann Surg Oncol. 2008; 15(2):424–429

[21] Smith ME, Riffat F, Jani P. The surgical anatomy and clinical relevance of the neglected right lymphatic duct: review. J Laryngol Otol. 2013; 127 (2):128–133

[22] Cernea CR, Hojaij FC, De Carlucci D, Jr., et al. Abdominal compression: a new intraoperative maneuver to detect chyle fistulas during left neck dissections that include level IV. Head Neck. 2012; 34(11):1570–1573

[23] Robbins KT, Shaha AR, Medina JE, et al. Committee for Neck Dissection Classification, American Head and Neck Society. Consensus statement on the classification and terminology of neck dissection. Arch Otolaryngol Head Neck Surg. 2008; 134(5):536–538

[24] Coskun HH, Medina JE, Robbins KT, et al. Current philosophy in the surgical management of neck metastases for head and neck squamous cell carcinoma. Head Neck. 2015; 37(6):915–926

[25] Taylor CB, Boone JL, Schmalbach CE, Miller FR. Intraoperative relationship of the spinal accessory nerve to the internal jugular vein: variation from cadaver studies. Am J Otolaryngol. 2013; 34(5):527–529

8 Selective Neck Dissection

Marcelo F. Figari

Abstract

In this chapter, we analyze the path followed since the beginning of the 20th century, when Crile conceived radical dissection to tackle regional spread of squamous carcinoma of the upper aerodigestive tract, until present, when selective neck dissections have become established, for elective treatment as well as for some curative indications in the neck. Based on the best available evidence, we analyze the indications and techniques of supraomohyoid, lateral, posterolateral, superselective, and extended dissections, pondering their advantages and disadvantages. We also address the role of the various sources of energy available to facilitate these procedures, as well as the potential for a progressive adoption of minimally invasive techniques today and in the near future.

Keywords: head and neck, squamous cell carcinoma, elective neck dissection, therapeutic neck dissection, selective neck dissection, minimally invasive surgery

8.1 Introduction

Neck dissection is a very valuable procedure in the battle against cancer of the upper aerodigestive tract. First performed in the beginning of the 20th century, during the 1960s, the technique evolved to less aggressive variants, which were more respectful of normal anatomy and physiology, while maintaining oncological radicality.

In this chapter, we will describe the historical evolution, the rationale of oncologic spread to preferred lymph nodes, indications and technique of selective dissections, the best available evidence, and potential future developments.

8.2 Brief History

Resection of cervical lymph nodes as part of the treatment of head and neck cancer began at the end of the 19th century and beginning of the 20th century, at a time when radiotherapy still had not become established as an ancillary or alternative treatment strategy. The original description of radical neck dissection, performed by Crile in 1906 and later made popular by Hayes Martin, required the functional sacrifice of soft tissues, vessels, and nerves, given the lack of options available at the time.[1,2] However, it is worth mentioning that, even before the radical procedure was conceived, multiple procedures that aimed at resecting selected lymph node groups had been described.[3] Such developments were pioneered by von Langenbeck, Kocher, von Volkmann, Butlin, and others. Butlin is also credited with the original idea of elective cervical dissection in necks without macroscopic involvement.[3] It is also worth mentioning that, among the first 132 cervical procedures reported by Crile in 1906, only 36 were radical. He then reported that 3-year survival achieved with the radical procedure was 75%, compared to 19% in the case of selective procedures. Such data were key to the acceptance of the radical neck dissection procedure.[3]

At the beginning of the 1960s, a more conservative therapeutic attitude was adopted. The possibilities of performing function-preserving surgeries or medical treatments for laryngeal or breast cancer are good examples of such attitude. By then, many ENT (ear, nose, and throat) surgeons worldwide had addressed the concept of cervical micrometastases without clinical findings in head and neck cancer, to justify potential prophylactic radical dissections (Agra and del Sel, Buenos Aires, 1947; Ogura, Washington University, St. Louis, MO, 1952; Alonso, Montevideo, 1952). That led professor Osvaldo Suárez, an otolaryngologist from Córdoba, Argentina, to describe in 1963 the functional radical neck dissection and to coin that name for the procedure.[3,4] This intervention combined the oncologic concept of complete resection of potentially involved lymph nodes with the preservation of certain structures. The proposal was to excise lymph nodes and lymphatic collectors, together with the aponeurosis and cellular tissue, while preserving the sternocleidomastoid muscle (SCM), the internal jugular vein, the accessory spinal nerve, and as many vascular and nervous structures as possible, without compromising the goal of a radical resection.

Although undoubtedly Osvaldo Suárez was the first to conceive this functional concept in radical neck dissection, his publications were in local journals and in Spanish. Other authors disseminated the technique in English-language publications, and hence they have been credited with its development. Interestingly, Bocca and Pignataro[5] made popular the following statement: "Radicality must be directed against the cancer rather than against the neck."

8.3 Classification of Neck Dissections

Based on the classification of cervical lymph node groups proposed by investigators at the Memorial Sloan Kettering Cancer Center (MSKCC),[2] mentioned in another section of this chapter and depicted in ▶ Table 8.1, in 1988 the Committee on Head and Neck Surgery and Oncology of the American Academy of Otolaryngology–Head and Neck Surgery met to establish a classification that would allow harmonizing definitions and nomenclature regarding neck dissections, thus improving communication among professionals and the reporting of strategies and results.[1] The modification introduced in 2002 by the Committee for Neck Dissection Classification of the American Head and Neck Society (AHNS) is depicted in ▶ Table 8.2.[6]

The first step was to define radical neck dissection as the standard procedure, considering the remaining procedures as modifications of the standard. The consensus decision was to call modified radical neck dissection those procedures that preserve some of the nonnodal structures that were excised during the classic procedure. Selective neck dissection (SND) was that in which one or more of the nodal groups that were excised during radical procedures were preserved.

Table 8.1 Cervical lymph node levels: modified Memorial Sloan Kettering Cancer Center classification[1,2,6]

Level	Clinical location	Surgical boundaries
Ia	Submental triangle	S: symphysis of mandible I: hyoid bone A (M): left anterior belly of digastric muscle P (L): right anterior belly of digastric muscle
Ib	Submandibular triangle	S: body of mandible I: posterior belly of digastric muscle A (M): anterior belly of digastric muscle P (L): stylohyoid muscle
IIa	Upper jugular	S: lower level of bony margin of jugular fossa I: level of lower body of hyoid bone A (M): stylohyoid muscle P (L): vertical plane defined by accessory nerve
IIb	Upper jugular	S: lower level of bony margin of jugular fossa I: level of lower body of hyoid bone A (M): vertical plane defined by accessory nerve P (L): posterior border of sternomastoid muscle
III	Mid jugular	S: level of lower body of hyoid bone I: horizontal plane along inferior border of anterior cricoid arch A (M): lateral border of sternohyoid muscle P (L): posterior border of sternocleidomastoid muscle or sensory branches of the cervical plexus
IV	Lower jugular	S: horizontal plane along inferior border of anterior cricoid arch I: clavicle A (M): lateral border of sternohyoid muscle P (L): posterior border of sternocleidomastoid muscle or sensory branches of the cervical plexus
Va	Posterior triangle	S: convergence of sternocleidomastoid and trapezius muscles I: horizontal plane along inferior border of anterior cricoid arch A (M): posterior border of sternocleidomastoid muscle or sensory branches of the cervical plexus P (L): anterior border of trapezius muscle
Vb	Posterior triangle (supraclavicular)	S: horizontal plane along inferior border of anterior cricoid arch I: clavicle A (M): posterior border of sternocleidomastoid muscle or sensory branches of the cervical plexus P (L): anterior border of trapezius muscle
VI	Anterior compartment	S: hyoid bone I: sternal notch A (M): common carotid artery P (L): common carotid artery

Table 8.1 continued

Level	Clinical location	Surgical boundaries
VII	Superior mediastinum	S: sternal notch I: innominate artery A (M): common carotid artery P (L): common carotid artery

Abbreviations: S, superior; I, inferior; A (M), anterior (medial); P (L), posterior (lateral).

Table 8.2 Neck dissection techniques classification[1,6]

Type of neck dissection	Description
Radical neck dissection (RND)	Removal of levels I–V, accessory nerve, internal jugular vein, and sternomastoid muscle
Modified radical neck dissection	Removal of levels I–V; preservation of one or more of the accessory nerve, internal jugular vein, or sternomastoid muscle (types I, II, III, respectively)
Selective neck dissection	Preservation of one or more levels of lymph nodes
Extended radical neck dissection	Removal of one or more additional lymphatic and/or nonlymphatic structure(s) relative to an RND, e.g., level VII, retropharyngeal lymph nodes, and hypoglossal nerve

Finally, extended radical neck dissection was defined as that which involves at least one additional nodal group or a nonnodal structure, compared to the radical procedure. We will review and define the various types of SNDs.

8.4 Types of Selective Neck Dissections

Four types of selective cervical dissections have been defined[1]:
- Supraomohyoid dissection (▶ Fig. 8.1). This entails resecting the following groups: submental, submandibular (group I, excising the submaxillary gland), high jugular (group II), and mid jugular (group III). The deep limit of resection consists of the branches of the cervical plexus and the posterior limit is the lateral border of the SCM. Since nodes are present medially and laterally to the accessory spinal nerve, node group II is divided into IIa (anterior and inferior to the nerve) and IIb (posterosuperior to the nerve).
- Lateral dissection (▶ Fig. 8.2). It involves the excision of levels II, III, and IV (upper, middle, and lower jugular lymph nodes).
- Posterolateral dissection (▶ Fig. 8.3). Mostly employed in skin diseases of the occipital region, it entails removing the suboccipital and retroauricular nodes together with node levels II, III, IV, and V.
- Anterior dissection (▶ Fig. 8.4). Mostly employed in the management of thyroid cancer, it involves the prelaryngeal (Delphian node), pretracheal and paratracheal chains (recurrent laryngeal nodes), and perithyroidal nodes in general.

Any variation different from these four types should be defined clarifying the node groups involved, for example, "selective dissection with resection of levels I and II," as may occur in the

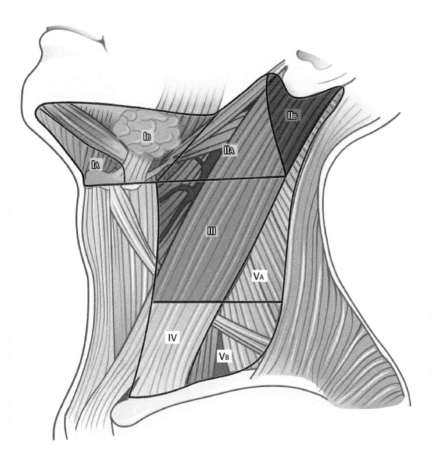

Fig. 8.1 Supraomohyoid neck dissection. Level IIb removed when necessary (see indications).

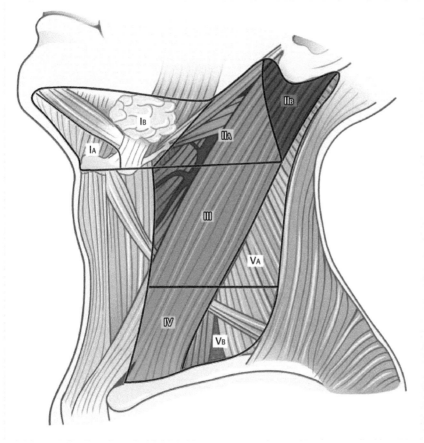

Fig. 8.2 Lateral neck dissection. Level IIb removed when necessary (see indications).

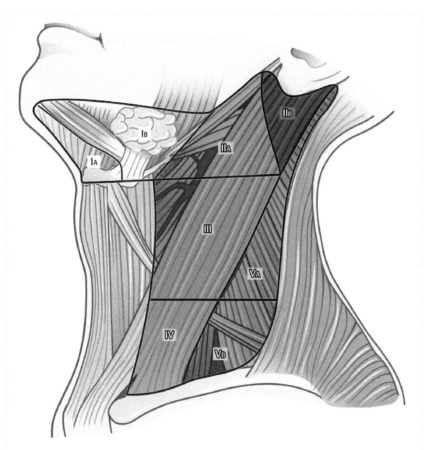

Fig. 8.3 Posterolateral neck dissection. Also includes occipital node level.

treatment of parotid gland cancer. In these selective dissections, the internal jugular vein, the spinal accessory nerve, and SCM are routinely preserved. Should it be necessary to sacrifice one of them, the dissection must be defined by the node groups resected, listing the structure or structures that have been sacrificed.

In 1994, Spiro et al, from the group of the MSKCC, reported on their 10-year experience with 10,650 patients. Considering only the 1,143 dissections performed on 1,035 patients, not previously treated, 420 were radical dissections, 263 were modified dissections, and 460 were selective dissections. During those years, there was a clear change in practice, since from 1984 to 1988 a total of 44% of radical dissections were performed, whereas the rate for the same procedure was 27%, during the period from 1989 to 1993.[2] The MSKCC group agrees in stating that thanks to Robbins et al the classification and nomenclature of dissections were established in an orderly manner. However, they suggest the name *selective* for those dissections involving less than four, but at least three groups of lymph nodes, reserving the name *limited* dissections to those involving only one or two groups of lymph nodes.[2]

In the United Kingdom National Multidisciplinary Guidelines addressing the management of lymph node metastases in head and neck cancer, the authors summarize the concept saying that there is a growing trend to divide dissections into two large groups: radical dissections (comprehensive, removing levels I–V) and selective dissections (excising < 5 node levels).[6]

8.5 Indications for Selective Neck Dissections and Reported Clinical Experiences

8.5.1 N0 Neck: Elective Dissection

Involvement of cervical lymph nodes is the single most ominous prognostic factor for carcinomas of the upper aerodigestive tract.[2,6] For primary tumors with an N0 neck by clinical assessment and tomography, there are three possible therapeutic options: elective cervical dissection, elective neck radiotherapy, or clinical surveillance, leaving the surgical option for cases with development of clinical metastases.[7]

Patients with primary tumors that will be treated surgically and with a greater than 20% risk of having microscopic cervical node metastases are candidates for elective neck dissection. Such conduct was already standard since the 1970s, when modified radical dissection became general practice, but became fully accepted in the 1990s, when the concept of selective dissection was reinforced.[7] Based on the fact that lymphatic drainage to the neck is predictable from the various primary sites, the concept of selective dissection implied not only removing the groups of lymph nodes with a higher risk of micrometastases, but also preserving others with a lower risk.[3] The surgical group at MD Anderson Cancer Center was probably the first to report a positive experience with selective dissection in

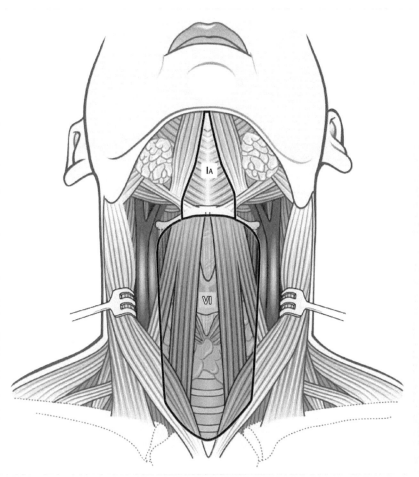

Fig. 8.4 Central neck dissection (levels VI, VII, and Delphian lymph nodes).

1978; recurrence rates were similar in selective and radical procedures performed for cancers of the oral cavity.[3]

In 1997, Pitman et al published a comparative study of modified radical dissection versus selective dissection as a staging strategy and treatment in primary tumors of the upper aerodigestive tract with N0 neck. Although the study has methodological limitations because it is retrospective and assessed heterogeneous populations, it clearly provides support to selective dissection as a diagnostic and therapeutic resource. Patients included had primary tumors in the oral cavity, oropharynx, hypopharynx, and larynx, and an N0 neck staged clinically and, since 1980, by computed tomography (CT); nodes were considered metastatic when they were larger than 1 cm. A group of 288 patients treated between 1974 and 1989 (modified radical dissection) and another group of 99 patients treated between 1990 and 1994 (selective dissection) fulfilled the following eligibility criteria: no prior treatment of the primary tumor or the neck (surgery or radiation), minimum follow-up of 24 months, free margins in the resected specimen of the primary tumor, complete pathology report describing the nodes' characteristics, surgical report describing in detail the dissected node levels, and complete report of adjuvant treatments. Conclusions of the study were that selective dissection was as effective as the radical procedure for cervical staging and that regional recurrence rates were similar for both procedures. Accuracy of selective dissection for the detection of occult metastases was 90% (superior to that of imaging techniques).[7] The

authors believed that further studies are required to determine the potential therapeutic value of selective dissection in N1 necks. Prospective and randomized studies that could provide an evidence base for selective procedures are scarce.

In 1998, the Brazilian Head and Neck Cancer Study Group published the first prospective randomized study on 148 patients with primary tumors of the oral cavity (T2–T4), located in the oral tongue ($n = 62$), floor of the mouth ($n = 49$), gums ($n = 12$), and retromolar trigone ($n = 25$). Patient groups were homogeneous, without previous treatment, and had negative necks. Lymph node levels most frequently involved were II and III. Local recurrence rate was similar, as was actuarial survival at 60 months (63% in the radical dissection group and 67% in the selective dissection group).[8] One year later, that same group of investigators published a similar experience, but prospectively comparing modified radical dissection with lateral neck dissection (LND) for the initial treatment of supraglottic and transglottic carcinomas staged as T2–T4, N0 M0.

A total of 71 patients underwent radical dissections (13 bilateral) and 61 underwent selective lateral dissections (18 bilateral). Again, most node groups involved were levels II and III; there were four ipsilateral recurrences in the radical group and two recurrences in the selective group. Actuarial 5-year survival was 72.3% in the group with radical dissection and 62.4% in the group with lateral selective dissection.[9]

Given the very low current morbidity of selective dissections, today there is good reason to propose the elective treatment of the neck in patients whose risk of micrometastases is lower than 20%. Paleri et al propose it for primary tumors with a greater than 15% risk of occult metastases, which would encompass almost all primary tumors, except for glottic T1 and T2 tumors, and some selected T1 tumors of the oral cavity.[6]

In 2015, a group of investigators at the University of Belgrade, in Serbia, published a prospective, observational experience of cases and controls. They compared the historical experience of patients with supraglottic carcinomas treated surgically between 1988 and 1996 to patients with the same disorder treated between 1996 and 2005 (period in which they standardized performance of lateral elective dissections in N0 necks). Patients in the control group ($n = 51$) were operated for their primary tumor and subsequently watched and followed. Patients in the study group ($n = 193$) underwent surgery for their primary tumor and bilateral elective lateral dissection. Patients who recurred after selective dissection underwent a radical neck dissection. Patients with occult metastases received postoperative radiotherapy. In the study group, 18% had occult metastases (most of them at node level II) and 20% had extracapsular spread. The most relevant finding was that the control group had an 11.8% rate of lymph node recurrence, whereas that rate was 4.15% in the group that underwent selective dissection. Overall 5-year survival was not significantly different between both groups. The study concluded that elective and selective treatment of the neck was useful in primary supraglottic tumors to reduce regional recurrence rates.[10]

8.5.2 Selective Dissections in Melanoma

The role of selective dissection in the elective treatment of an N0 neck in cases of melanoma of intermediate thickness has progressively been replaced by sentinel node biopsy, in spite of the greater hurdles that this procedure entails in cases of head and neck cancer compared to other regions of the body. However, when the sentinel node biopsy cannot be performed or is nondiagnostic, melanomas of intermediate thickness, after excising the margins of the primary tumor, should undergo SND according to the following recommendations based on the type of drainage.[11]

- Melanomas of the anterior region of the scalp, forehead, face, and pinna: selective dissection of levels I to IV. The actual value of resecting level IV has been questioned. Additionally, depending on the location, several authors have recommended performing a superficial parotidectomy.
- Melanomas of the scalp posterior to the coronal line could be amenable to a posterolateral dissection, including the occipital nodes and cervical levels II to V.

Undoubtedly, selective dissections offer a great opportunity to detect occult metastases with a minimum of morbidity, thus allowing the surgeons to offer patients adjuvant therapeutic options at an early stage of treatment. Also, detection of extracapsular spread in these occult metastases is a good predictor in high-risk patients.[7]

8.5.3 N + Neck: Therapeutic Dissection

Although selective cervical dissection was devised with the rationale of minimizing morbidity to electively treat negative

necks at risk, many groups have provided sufficient evidence showing that selective dissection may be curative in cases of positive necks that are not advanced.[3] In 2002, with the goal of assessing the role of the sentinel node, Andersen, Warren, and Spiro evaluated the oncological adequacy of selective dissection in a group of 106 patients. Although 54.7% of patients were N1, 4.7% were N2a, 26.4% were N2b, 13.2% were N2c, and 0.9% were N3, 34% had extracapsular spread and 71.7% of patients required postoperative radiotherapy; regional control achieved with selective dissection was 94.3%. Clearly, extracapsular spread was the most negative factor with regard to recurrence and disease-related survival.[3]

In 2010, Weinstein et al, from Pennsylvania, published their experience with oropharyngeal carcinomas and a positive neck, treated with a combination of TORS (transoral robotic surgery) and SND, and subsequently followed and treated with radiotherapy or chemotherapy. The study was a prospective, phase I trial. The investigation was designed to assess the possibility of controlling cervical disease with selective dissection and adjuvant therapies, since

- Cases were oropharyngeal carcinomas treated with TORS with free margins; hence, the potential indication of chemotherapy or radiotherapy would be due to cervical disease.
- In the selective dissection, levels IIa, IIb, III, and IV were excised.
- Since the study was prospective, with a single population arm, the decision of follow-up or adjuvant therapy was made at the beginning of treatment.

The primary outcome of the study was regional control and the secondary outcome was the assessment of complications. In 31 patients (29 men), 33 SNDs were performed (2 were bilateral). Primary oropharyngeal tumors treated with TORS: T1 in 29%, T2 in 48.4%, and T3 in 22.6% (as mentioned, all were resected with free margins). Results that attest to the usefulness of selective dissection show that staging increased by 33% in N0 necks and by 43% in N1 necks; extracapsular invasion could be detected in 70% of N2b necks and staging could be decreased to N0 in 4 of 14 N1 necks. Regarding adjuvant therapy, seven patients did not receive radiotherapy (four with N0, two with N1, and one with N2b). As to the remaining patients (24 patients), 50% received only adjuvant radiotherapy and another 50% received adjuvant chemoradiotherapy. Minimum follow-up was 3 years; only one patient had a contralateral recurrence and one patient had distant disease and was alive at the time of study closure. Investigators emphasized the high rate of local and regional control and the possibility of using selective dissection as an instrument to adapt and eventually decrease the intensity of adjuvant therapy.[12]

Another recent study of interest is that of Young Soo Rho et al, from Hallym University in South Korea. This was a prospective study in 44 patients with primary carcinomas of the oral cavity. Twenty-nine patients underwent SND (levels I–III: 12 patients; levels I–IV: 6 patients; and levels II–IV: 11 patients), and in 15 patients, due to the intraoperative finding of lymphatic metastases, the procedure was converted to a modified radical dissection (involving levels I–V). Extracapsular invasion was found in 8 cases of the selective group and in 6 cases of the radical group. In 20 cases of the selective group and in 11 cases of the radical group, adjuvant therapy was administered (chemoradiotherapy for stages T3 and T4, insufficient margins, extracapsular nodal or multiple nodal metastases, and radiotherapy only for early stages with limited extracapsular spread). There was no significant difference among the two groups in locoregional control, nor in overall or disease-related survival.[13] These findings show that in selected cases a selective dissection may be enough to achieve effective regional control, as well as to help decide the type of adjuvant therapy needed to achieve such control.

8.5.4 SND in Patients with HPV + Squamous Oropharyngeal Carcinoma

A recent multicenter study (Washington University – Mayo Clinic), although retrospective, has shed light on the value of selective dissection for the treatment of N+ necks in human papillomavirus–positive (HPV +) patients. All patients treated were included, according to the following criteria: carcinomas of the oropharynx, treated transorally, p16+, neck staged as N1 to N3, and selective dissection (levels II–IV ± levels I and V, depending on the case). On occasions, the dissection had to be extended to nonnodal vital structures (spinal accessory nerve in 7% of cases, internal jugular vein in 13%, and SCM in 8% of cases). A total of 324 patients were followed for a mean of 49 months, and 83% of them (270 patients) received adjuvant radiotherapy. Regional recurrences occurred in 4% of patients and distant metastases in 6%, with a regional control rate after rescue of 98%. On univariate analysis, the absence of radiotherapy was associated with recurrence. On multivariate analysis, the use of adjuvant radiotherapy had a positive impact on disease-free survival (DFS), but was not significant in the case of overall survival (OS) or disease-specific survival (DSS). Five-year survival rates by Kaplan–Meier's method for OS, DSS, and DFS were 88% (95% confidence interval [CI]: 84–92%), 93% (95% CI: 89–96%), and 83% (95% CI: 78–87%), respectively. These results support the notion that in cases of HPV + oropharyngeal carcinomas with clinical evidence of neck node metastases, selective dissection including levels II, III, and IV (occasionally extended to additional involved tissue), together with adjuvant radiotherapy, offers excellent regional control.[4]

8.5.5 Selective Dissection as Adjuvant Therapy

In addition to its role in the primary treatment of head and neck cancer, during this last decade its role has increasingly been explored as adjuvant therapy for tumors initially treated with nonsurgical therapies, mainly chemoradiotherapy.[3] The classic approach in patients initially treated with chemoradiotherapy for head and neck cancer was to perform, after treatment, a scheduled dissection (either radical or modified radical) in all patients whose initial stage was N2 or N3. Robbins, back in 1990, already postulated the use of selective dissections in patients treated with organ-preserving protocols. In a population of 171 patients, of which 130 had an N2 or N3 neck before beginning treatment, Robbins analyzed 84 patients who underwent neck dissections after chemoradiotherapy. Of the 106 dissections, 92 were selective. Of note, the regional recurrence rate for radical procedures was 16%, whereas it was 4%

for selective procedures. This could be partly attributed to a selection bias in this markedly heterogeneous population, but clearly, the low recurrence rate in selective procedures showed a change in therapeutic decision-making.

A more recent study also supports the role of selective dissections after chemoradiotherapy to treat persistent nodal disease. A population of 62 patients treated with chemoradiotherapy underwent 69 selective dissections, a mean period of 10 weeks after completing therapy. Residual tumor was found in 46% of the specimens. Mean follow-up was 33 months, and 65% of patients were disease free. Among the 22 patients who recurred, only 4 had a regional recurrence and of them, 3 recurred in the contralateral neck. Therefore, using selective dissection as a complement to nonsurgical treatment, only 1 of 62 patients had an ipsilateral regional neck recurrence.[14]

In recent years, the use of positron emission tomography-computed tomography (PET-CT) has become an established tool for decision-making in potential residual neck disease, once chemoradiotherapy has been completed. According to the United Kingdom National Multidisciplinary Guidelines, if at 10 to 12 weeks after completing treatment there is no evidence of disease by PET-CT, the patient does not require elective treatment of the neck. Dissection should be considered in patients in whom the evidence of disease by PET-CT is inconclusive or questionable.[6]

8.5.6 Superselective Dissection

The definition of superselective neck dissection (SSND) involves the removal of lymph nodes of two adjacent neck levels. In the cases of dissection performed as part of a primary treatment, the most typical example is that of supraglottic carcinomas, which rarely involve microscopically levels other than IIa and III. In a large retrospective series published by Ambrosch et al, superselective dissection was performed in almost all laryngeal carcinomas treated with laser, electively and with very good local control rates. The finding of metastases in those levels generally results in the subsequent use of adjuvant radiotherapy.[15] Superselective dissection also has a role in the treatment of residual node disease after chemoradiotherapy, since it is well known that in these cases persistence of nodes is usually limited to one or two levels.

In 2010, Goguen et al, from the Dana Farber Institute, proposed the use of superselective dissection in patients with residual nodes after chemoradiotherapy, when the disease was confined to a single node level. The authors reported that SSND was useful in 51 of 55 patients with disease limited to one node level and in 61 of 67 patients with disease limited to two levels.[3] In 2012, Robbins et al published a retrospective series from two institutions, analyzing 35 SSNDs performed in 30 patients. In 23 cases, the SSND had been planned and in 12 cases it was performed as a salvage procedure. Mean follow-up was 33 months (range: 8–72 months); 3 patients had a recurrence of their primary tumor and 5 patients had distant metastases, but none had a neck recurrence. The group had a 60% 5-year DSS.[16]

To date, there are no prospective studies that can provide evidence for the use of superselective dissection in the case of residual nodes after implementing organ-preserving protocols. However, the advantage of a lower morbidity seems justified by the acceptable regional control rates.

8.5.7 Extended Selective Dissections

The concept of extended selective neck dissections (ESND) applies to cases in which, in addition to the nodes of one or two neck levels, the disease extends to other nonnodal contiguous structures (sternocleidomastoid or prethyroid muscles, spinal accessory nerve, internal jugular vein). In the study by Dhiwakar et al, 39 patients received 43 of these procedures; 18 were performed as part of the primary treatment and 25 as a surgical salvage following chemoradiotherapy. Even in this case of extended procedures, the regional recurrence rate observed in the first group was 0% and DFS at 5 years was 40%. In the second group, the result was quite different; extended selective dissection was performed as a rescue procedure, in which neck recurrence was 40% and DFS decreased to 30%.[14]

8.6 Contribution of the Sentinel Lymph Node Biopsy

The concept of sentinel node states that the tumor will spread from the primary site to one or several first echelon lymph nodes, of which the selective biopsy will allow predicting the status of the remaining nodes. The sentinel lymph node biopsy (SLNB) is well established for the treatment of melanoma and breast cancer; the concept is attractive in the case of head and neck cancer, for the possibility of assessing, with minimum morbidity, which patients may benefit with the elective treatment of the neck. Undoubtedly, the sentinel node biopsy is a reliable procedure.

The American College of Surgeons (ACS) conducted a prospective multicenter trial involving 25 institutions during a 3-year period. They studied a total of 140 patients with T1 and T2 tumors of the oral cavity (95: oral tongue; 26: floor of the mouth; and 19: other locations). Among the 106 SLNB that were clinically and pathologically (hematoxylin and eosin) negative, no other positive nodes were found; hence, negative predictive value (NPV) was 94%. With additional sections and immunohistochemistry techniques, NPV improved to 96%. For T1 lesions of the oral cavity, metastases were correctly identified in 100% of cases.[17]

In 2015, Schilling et al reported the results of the EORTC 24021 protocol (Sentinel European Node Trial [SENT]) on the study of the sentinel node in oral cancer. Fourteen European centers prospectively recruited 415 patients with cancer of the oral cavity staged as T1 and T2 N0. They found an average of 3.2 sentinel nodes per patient. If the sentinel node was positive, a cervical dissection was performed 3 weeks later. Duration of follow-up was 3 years. The sentinel node was located in 99.5% of cases, and 23% of them were found to be positive for metastases. There were 14% of false-negative cases, which subsequently required rescue. The procedure had a sensitivity of 86% and an NPV of 95%. DSS was 94%.[18]

The studies described, as well as many others, show that sentinel node biopsy is a reliable procedure for the staging of initial oral cancer. However, there is still controversy regarding the need to subject patients to a second procedure when a positive result is found. Perhaps, optimization of the procedure, with the addition of fast, safe, and standardized techniques that will allow analysis of the sentinel node in the operating room will

contribute to its generalized acceptance for this group of patients in the future.[17]

8.7 Surgical Strategy According to Node Groups at Risk

The rationale of selective dissection is based on the fact that there are predictable patterns of lymphatic spread from the various mucosal sites of the upper aerodigestive tract. Many publications in the medical literature refer to this, although the first description was made by Lindberg, a radiotherapist, and later revisited by Byers, who in 1985 confirmed such patterns in the dissection specimens of 967 patients. The observation was relevant, but not perfect as a proof, since many of Byers' dissections were selective and hence not all the node groups were available for analysis.[3]

In 1990, Shah et al published the findings of a pathology study of 192 radical dissections performed electively due to oral cavity cancers. They confirmed very relevant data: the groups that were usually affected when the primary tumor was in the oral tongue, floor of the mouth, gums, retromolar trigone, or the buccal mucosa were levels I, II, and III. Group V was never affected, except in 2% of gum carcinomas. Group IV was considered to be very low risk, since it was involved in 0% of primary tumors of the buccal mucosa and in 6% of cases of the retromolar trigone.[19] Another important finding, in Byers' as well as in Shah's studies, is that primary tumors located in the visceral structures of the midline (oropharynx, hypopharynx, and larynx) generally do not involve level I.

In 2014, Pantvaidya et al,[20] from the Tata Memorial Center in Mumbai, India, published a prospective study on the dissection specimens obtained from 470 patients with primary tumors of the oral cavity. At that institution, patients with stage N0 undergo SND (levels I–III or I–IV) and patients with N + undergo radical dissection (levels I–V), either the classic or modified procedure, depending on the presentation. Dissection specimens obtained from patients with stage N3 or patients who had received prior treatment of the neck were excluded from the study. The goal was to study the frequency of involvement of the various node levels, and to assess the involvement of levels IIb and V, aiming at their potential preservation. The authors verified that 95.7% of metastases were located in levels I to IV. With the exception of lip tumors, cases in which the greatest involvement was level Ia, for the remaining sites of the oral cavity, levels Ib and IIa were the most frequently involved.

Level IV was affected from 0% (lip ad hard palate) to 9% (floor of the mouth). On average, involvement of levels IIb and V was 3.8 and 3.3%, respectively. Multivariate analysis showed that involvement of level IIa is an independent predictive factor of the involvement of levels IIb and V; hence, it suggests the need for their excision. But the general conclusion is that in most cases, SND of levels I to IV may be adequate for treatment of the neck in oral cancer.[20]

Another study from India, a country where oral cancer is the most frequent in its population, was conducted by Chheda et al, from Ahmedabad, and published in 2017. In a population of 210 patients with oral cancer (more than 70% originated in the tongue), operated between 2010 and 2012, and excluding patients treated with neoadjuvant chemotherapy, they prospectively studied specimens from 120 modified radical dissections,

40 extended supraomohyoid dissections, and 50 supraomohyoid classic dissections. Of the 210 dissections, only 2 (0.95%) showed involvement of level IIb, and in such cases, level IIa was also involved. There was no evidence of isolated involvement of level IIb. The authors suggested performing frozen biopsy of level IIa to determine the need for excision of level IIb, since sensitivity of the clinical judgment is extremely low. The goal was to minimize the aggression of the spinal accessory nerve.[21]

Another important prospective study, also from India, is that of Agarwal et al, which was published in 2018. From 2011, they studied the dissection specimens of 231 patients with primary carcinomas of the oral cavity, and a neck staged clinically and with imaging (magnetic resonance and CT) as N0 in the preoperative assessment. The most frequent primary sites were the oral tongue and the buccal mucosa. Of the 231 cases, 71 showed microscopic metastases (30.73%). Again, levels affected most often were Ib and IIa. Level IIb was involved in 0.86% of cases and no patient had metastases in level IV. As in the study by Chheda et al, whenever there was involvement of level IIb, level IIa was also involved. The authors concluded that classic supraomohyoid dissection (levels I–III) is sufficient to treat patients with a primary tumor of the oral cavity and a neck staged as N0, and that level IIb should only be excised when there is proven involvement of level IIa.[22]

Another interesting study is the one published in 2016 by Agarwal et al, in the same population previously studied, but looking at the involvement of another node group, that of perifacial nodes. Their dissection and excision also implies the need to selectively dissect the marginal mandibular branch of the facial nerve, in order to preserve it. Agarwal et al found perifacial involvement in 8.22% of the dissections performed in the 231 patients previously mentioned. Primary sites most frequently affected (oral tongue and buccal mucosa) had similar involvement of the perifacial group (7.14 and 7.75%, respectively); hence, the authors recommend including them in N0 neck dissections for tumors in those locations, especially in cases of patients younger than 25 years, with an advanced T stage or infiltration greater than 5 mm.[23]

8.8 Technical Aspects of Selective Neck Dissection

In this section, we describe the removal of node compartments that are part of the following selective dissections:
- Supraomohyoid neck dissection (SOHND): levels I, II, and III (▶ Fig. 8.1).
- LND: levels II, III, and IV (▶ Fig. 8.2).
- Posterolateral dissection: occipital level and levels II, III, IV, and V (▶ Fig. 8.3).

Indications are described in the appropriate sections. We will not discuss central neck dissection nor modified radical dissection, since both procedures are described elsewhere.

8.8.1 Perioperative Aspects

We shall not dwell on the general organizational aspects of head and neck surgical procedures, but we will underscore some issues relevant to SNDs. Preoperative informed consent should include the type of surgery, the functional preservation intent of the procedure, and also the potential functional sacrifices that could derive from changes in surgical conduct due to intraoperative findings. The preoperative history and physical examination should include information on past therapies that could influence certain steps of the dissection, such as neck biopsies, origin of neck scars, radiotherapy, etc. For the surgery, the patient is placed in supine position, with the thorax elevated approximately 30 degrees, or in inverted Trendelenburg position, to decrease venous congestion and bleeding. The type of airway control (orotracheal, nasotracheal, or tracheostomy) will depend mostly on the simultaneous treatment of the primary tumor. When the patient requires a tracheostomy, or if he or she already has one, we try not to include it in the incision planned for the dissection.

8.8.2 Skin Incisions

The incision employed should fulfill the following requirements:
- Allow for the best possible exposure.
- Include previous scars if they are located in the surgical path.
- Try to preserve skin flaps' blood supply, particularly in patients who have received previous radiotherapy.
- Protect the trajectory of large vessels (a relative issue in case of selective dissections, where vessels do not lose the muscle protection, which does occur in classic radical dissections).
- Facilitate the performance of reconstructive procedures, when necessary.
- Offer patients the best esthetic result possible.

Although there are many possible incisions, our first recommendation is that of transverse incisions, which comply with most of the requirements mentioned. For supraomohyoid and lateral dissections, a transverse incision performed on a preexisting skin fold is usually adequate. (▶ Fig. 8.5). For supraomohyoid dissections, the incision is located one or two fingerbreadths below the

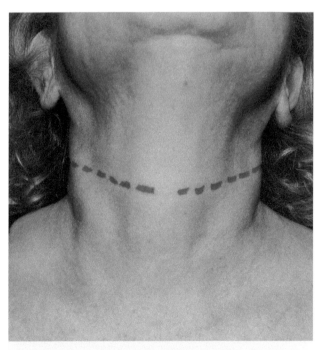

Fig. 8.5 Transverse incision performed on a preexisting skin fold, apt for supraomohyoid or lateral neck dissection. In case of bilateral dissection, separate or joined incision may be used.

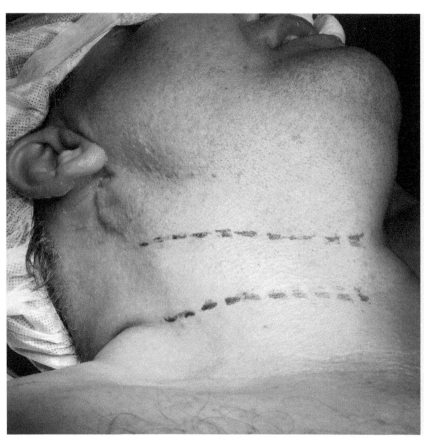

Fig. 8.6 MacFee incision (case of selective neck dissection for salivary gland cancer).

mandibular border, and for the lateral dissection, it is located in the midpoint of the area of dissection. If the patient is tall and slim, or if the dissection needs to be extended to the posterior triangle, or to reach the suboccipital region, a MacFee type of incision can be very helpful. It consists of two transverse incisions located on preexisting skin folds, approximately two fingerbreadths below the mandibular border and two fingerbreadths above the clavicle, respectively (▶ Fig. 8.6). In cases of bilateral dissections, two separate or joined incisions are indicated, if that is helpful for the treatment of the primary tumor (▶ Fig. 8.5).

In patients with laryngeal disease, who will require external primary surgery (partial or total laryngectomy), we occasionally use the Gluck Sorensen incision, which, from the cricoid level is extended laterally following the edge of the SCM. Since this incision crosses the skin tension lines, the esthetic result is suboptimal. In selective dissections, other classic incisions such as Hayes Martin, Crile, and Schöbinger are used less frequently.

8.8.3 Supraomohyoid Neck Dissection

In the case of SOHND, since we will be working near the marginal mandibular nerve, the ipsilateral commissure of the mouth should be observed directly through a clear sterile dressing.

Once the mentioned transverse incision is performed, the skin flaps are dissected; they need to reach the mandibular border in the cephalic direction and the level of the omohyoid muscle caudally. The flaps include skin and the platysma muscle, thus ensuring a good blood supply to the skin (▶ Fig. 8.7). The cutaneous borders of the flaps must be protected during the whole procedure, especially from marks or pressure if self-retaining retractors are used, or from thermal damage caused by the sources of energy.

There is no evidence that resecting the anterior fascia covering the SCM will add oncological radicality to the procedure. The initial approach follows the anterior border of the SCM muscle, throughout its extent. In some cases, it can be useful to ligate and cut the external jugular vein at the exit of the parotid tail, to allow for complete exposure, from the parotid tail to the omohyoid muscle. Sectioning the parotid tail also facilitates access to node compartment IIb.

Exposure of the Spinal Accessory Nerve

The procedure continues with the elevation and progressive retraction of the SCM, leaving its internal fascia intact with the tissue to be resected. A critical point, when advancing in cephalic direction, is to expose the entry of the spinal accessory nerve (cranial nerve XI) to the SCM, which occurs between the upper third and the lower two-thirds of the muscle belly (▶ Fig. 8.8). Neurostimulation can be very helpful to initially locate the nerve. Then, the surface of the nerve can be released in an atraumatic manner, exposing its trajectory between the internal jugular vein and the SCM. It is worth remembering that in most cases the nerve runs anterior to the internal jugular vein (70% of cases). The small vessels crossing anterior to the nerve surface should be carefully identified and cauterized with low-intensity bipolar coagulation or clipped and sectioned. By no means should monopolar coagulation be used near the nerve, since it significantly increases the possibility of postoperative functional limitation. Further, we shall discuss the advantages

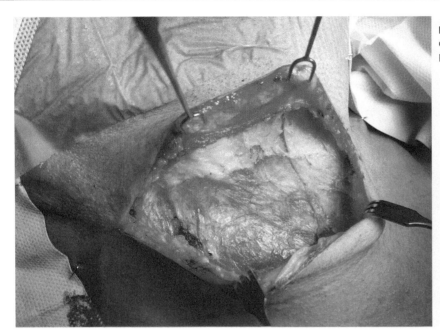

Fig. 8.7 Transverse incision for a selective neck dissection: flap dissection, including skin and platysma muscle.

of the harmonic scalpel in neck dissection. Despite the fact that it is less deleterious for nerves compared with other energy sources, caution applies regarding the use of harmonic scalpel in the close vicinity of the spinal nerve, due to the heat released. Also, care should be taken not to pull excessively on the spinal accessory nerve while retracting the SCM.

Submaxillary Triangle: Dissection of Level I

The next step is dissection of lymph node level I. As mentioned, its resection is not indicated in the treatment of thyroid carcinoma nor in lesions of the larynx and hypopharynx. Several authors have suggested preserving the submaxillary gland when dissecting level I. It is generally accepted that preserving the gland is justified only when such nodes do not warrant dissection. If dissection of level I were necessary, the submaxillary gland is resected together with the lymph nodes.

The extent of the dissection goes from the midline to the parotid tail. The first maneuver is to identify the marginal mandibular nerve, to prevent its injury. Given the marked anatomical variability of this nerve, there is no standardized technique to search for it. Formerly, the procedure suggested was to open the aponeurosis covering the submaxillary gland, and subsequently ligate and cut the facial vein; after retracting the vein, the nerve was protected. However, in oncological surgery, the perifacial nodes have to be removed, since they may be involved in certain tumors of the oral cavity, such as in carcinoma of the buccal mucosa. Hence, the current recommendation is to actively search for the nerve, a few millimeters below the mandibular edge (▶ Fig. 8.9), or to identify the nerve branch that descends toward the platysma and follow it in the cephalic direction.

The use of magnification and neurostimulation contributes to the localization, dissection, and mobilization of the marginal mandibular nerve, moving it away from the surgical field.

Subsequently, it is important to remove level Ia, which implies dissecting the fat and nodes located between the midline and the anterior belly of the digastric muscle. This must be performed carefully, since it is a well-known site for regional recurrence.

The specimen obtained from level Ia can be removed and submitted separately for histopathological examination. In general, to make their individual examination easier, lymph node groups resected may be labeled and shipped separately to the pathology laboratory.

The next step is to reflect the anterior pole of the submaxillary gland, exposing the anterior aspect of the mylohyoid muscle. After bipolar coagulation, vascular pedicles are sectioned above that muscle, helping release the submaxillary gland (▶ Fig. 8.10). Then, advancing over the gland's superior border, the facial artery (previously dissected) is ligated and sectioned. Occasionally, the artery does not penetrate inside the gland; vessels that enter the gland tissue can be dissected and, thus, facial artery integrity can be preserved. Once the submaxillary gland has been mobilized, a retractor allows moving the mylohyoid muscle medially and exposing the lingual nerve, Wharton's duct, occasionally an anterior prolongation of the submaxillary gland and, below it, the hypoglossal nerve surrounded by lingual veins. The lingual nerve should be exposed along its complete path, since it has one descending section and another ascending section, which together form the shape of a "V." From the apex of that "V" emerge the parasympathetic nerve branches (coming from the facial nerve through the chorda tympani) that constitute the submandibular ganglion and then enter the gland tissue (▶ Fig. 8.11). They have to be sectioned after bipolar coagulation.

Wharton's duct is ligated and sectioned as distally as possible. That allows us to completely retract the gland, with the accompanying fat and lymphatic tissue (level Ib). The gland, together with the fat and lymph nodes, remains suspended from the proximal facial artery (if it was sectioned in the mandibular edge), which is subsequently ligated and sectioned. Ligature and careful section of the lingual veins allow one to expose the hypoglossal nerve and release the block completely.

Dissection of Level II

The objective of this step is the systematic removal of the lymph nodes of level IIa and, if needed, of level IIb. The spinal

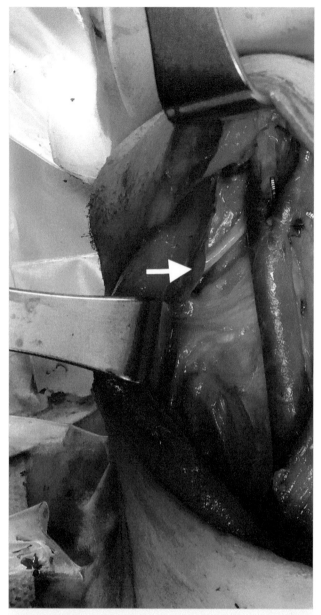

Fig. 8.8 Entry of the spinal accessory nerve to the sternocleidomastoid muscle (*arrow*).

accessory nerve, exposed during the first stages of dissection, from where it crosses the internal jugular vein until it enters the SCM, must be released from the fat and lymphatic tissue of level IIa (limited by the spinal nerve, the stylohyoid muscle, and the hyoid bone level). This maneuver must be performed without trauma or stretching of the nerve and without diffusing heat (using serial ligatures or clips or bipolar coagulation). Once lymphatic tissue has been separated from the spinal nerve and the anterior aspect of the internal jugular vein has been dissected, the deep limit of the dissection consists of the muscles of the back of the neck (levator scapulae). Once the level of the hyoid bone has been reached, level IIa can be separated from level III. If there is suspicion of involvement, the specimen can be sent for histopathological examination, because an intraoperative examination by frozen section can allow one to decide how to proceed with level IIb.

If removal of level IIb is necessary, the fat and lymphatic tissue found between the spinal nerve and the posterior border of the SCM are excised and separated from the muscle plane (▶ Fig. 8.12); precautions with the XI cranial nerve have already been mentioned.

Traditionally, it has been confirmed that, even preserving the spinal accessory nerve completely, functional consequences in the shoulder are often seen. The use of active neuromonitoring systems during surgery, with electrodes placed in the sternocleidomastoid and trapezius muscles, may help prevent aggressive maneuvers on the nerve, thus limiting the mentioned consequences. In a recent multicenter experience in Taiwan, the authors could avoid motor limitations of the shoulder in 25 consecutive patients who underwent selective or modified radical dissections, with the systematic use of intraoperative neuromonitoring.[24] Recently, Rastogi et al reported a prospective, randomized trial in 20 patients with primary T1 to T3 tumors of the oral cavity, 10 of whom underwent a classic supraomohyoid dissection (levels I–III) and another 10 patients underwent a superselective dissection, sparing level IIb. In the postoperative period, they performed the shoulder abduction test, a quality-of-life test, and assessed the regional recurrence rate; all showed a statistically significant advantage for the superselective group.[25]

Dissection of Level III

The goal of dissection is to remove the fat and lymph nodes of the midjugular space, located between the level of the hyoid bone and the cricoid cartilage, limited anteriorly by the prethyroid muscles, posteriorly by the posterior border of the SCM, and inferiorly by the omohyoid muscle. If the dissection is initiated medially, it begins with the elevation of the jugular and carotid fascia, facilitated by traction, which can be performed with a scalpel, scissors, or monopolar coagulation. The ansa of the hypoglossal nerve is preserved when possible. Once this fascia has been stripped from the main carotid and internal jugular vessels, and the vagus nerve exposed, the prescalene muscle plane is approached and the fat plane is separated from important nervous elements that must be preserved, that is, the branches of C2, C3, and C4, which usually anastomose with the spinal accessory nerve and contribute to the skin sensation of the neck, and mobility of the shoulder, and the origin of the phrenic nerve (in C3, C4, and C5) and its path on the anterior scalene muscle. The dissection proceeds above these structures, until it reaches the posterior border of the SCM, where the fat plane is interrupted in the case of a selective dissection (▶ Fig. 8.13).

8.8.4 SOHND including Level IV, Lateral Neck Dissections, and Posterolateral Neck Dissection

Dissection of Level IV

Level IV, which is less frequently involved in tumors of the aerodigestive tract, may be dissected in selective dissections in the following cases:
- An SOHND, extended to level IV because a higher risk of node involvement is suspected (carcinoma of the floor of the mouth or the retromolar trigone).
- A classic LND, for the treatment of a laryngeal or hypopharyngeal tumor.

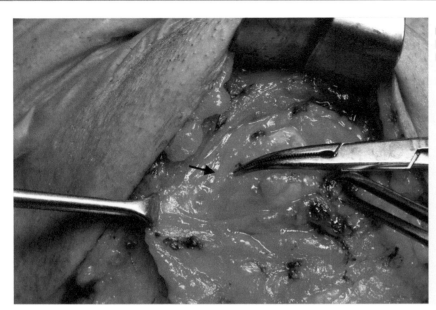

Fig. 8.9 Identification of the marginal mandibular nerve (visible between the *arrow* and the Halsted clamp).

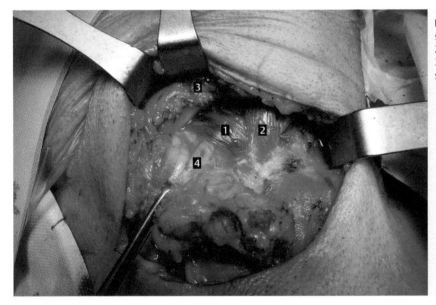

Fig. 8.10 Release of the anterior pole of the submaxillary gland. 1: mylohyoid muscle; 2: anterior belly of the digastric muscle; 3: sectioned facial vessels; 4: retracted submaxillary gland.

The goal is to remove the fat and lymphatic components with the same anterior and posterior limits from the omohyoid muscle, cephalad, to the clavicle, caudally. After elevating the jugular and carotid fascia, the dissection plane exposes the lower aspect of the vagus and phrenic nerves, the caudal trajectory of the low cervical branches, and the origin of the brachial plexus. Transverse cervical vessels are usually preserved (▶ Fig. 8.14). Extreme care must be taken to identify and preserve the thoracic duct on the left and the great lymphatic duct on the right.

An overlooked injury of those structures may complicate the postoperative period with a long-lasting lymphatic fistula. If there is any doubt about the integrity of these ducts, it is best to seal them with ligatures or metal clips.

Dissection of Level V

Level V dissection is only necessary when previously unsuspected involvement is found at that level (resulting in a change of procedure to a modified radical dissection), or in the case of a selective posterolateral dissection due to skin disease behind the coronal line (melanoma with a positive sentinel node biopsy, advanced nonmelanoma skin cancer, etc.). Generally, treatment of the posterior triangle implies extending the incision used to the anterior border of the trapezius muscle. When the posterior segment of the spinal accessory nerve has been located, between the SCM and trapezius muscle, it is released from the fat and lymphatic block, using the same maneuvers described for the treatment of level II. The dissection progresses in anteroposterior direction, preserving the distal portions of cervical branches C2, C3, and C4, as well as the branches of the brachial plexus (▶ Fig. 8.15). Finally, the block is transferred below the omohyoid muscle and the excision concludes with the ligature and distal section of the external jugular vein.

Usually, silicone-coated drains are used; they can be removed earlier, depending on the drainage volume, when level IV is not resected, and they are maintained during 4 or 5 days when level IV has been included in the dissection, due to the possibility of a late lymphatic fistula.

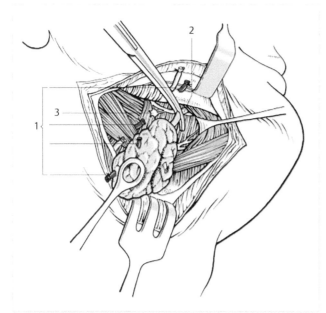

Fig. 8.11 Excision of the submandibular gland. 1: stumps of the transected facial artery; 2: division of Wharton's duct; 3: submandibular ganglion.

8.9 When is an Elective Neck Dissection Oncologically Sufficient?

Evidence suggests that for the treatment of a squamous carcinoma of the upper aerodigestive tract, resection of a minimum of 18 nodes is oncologically sufficient in an elective neck dissection. To prove that, the International Consortium for Outcome Research (ICOR) in Head and Neck Cancer analyzed data of 1,567 patients treated from 1970 to 2011 at nine centers of the Unite States, Brazil, Taiwan, Germany, Australia, Italy, and Israel. After a complex statistical procedure performed to homogenize the populations, a multivariate analysis showed that a number of nodes less than 18 in the specimen was associated with lower OS and DSS, and a higher regional recurrence rate. Thus, the finding confirmed that the number of lymph nodes (*nodal yield*) is a strong independent prognostic factor, applicable to all institutions and populations, and establishes 18 as the minimum acceptable number of nodes for analysis.[26]

8.10 Use of the Harmonic Scalpel in Neck Dissections

The harmonic scalpel is a device that converts electric energy into mechanical energy, with a handpiece that vibrates at 55,000 cycles/s and causes the following four effects in tissues: coaptation, coagulation, section, and cavitation. Specifically, the mechanism is a rupture in proteins' hydrogen bonds that seal small vessels, and the secondary heat causes protein denaturation.[27] By changing the velocity, cutting can be performed faster with less coagulation, and vice versa. The tension applied to the tissue also plays a role. The harmonic scalpel is a useful tool to coagulate and effectively seal medium-sized vessels, also cutting in the same surgical maneuver. Since the handpiece releases heat, it must be carefully used in the close vicinity of vessels and nerves to be preserved. Several groups have attempted to measure its effectiveness in neck dissection, in terms of the decrease in bleeding and reduction of surgical time. From 2004 to 2008, the group at the University of Córdoba, in Spain, performed a prospective and randomized study with 63 patients with primary tumors of the upper aerodigestive tract who underwent initial neck dissection (76.2% were selective and 23.8% were radical procedures). A conventional procedure was performed in 50.8% of patients, while 49.2% of patients were operated with a harmonic scalpel. The harmonic scalpel reduced 64 minutes of operating time in the selective dissection group and 7.5 minutes in the radical group, compared to the conventional technique. Additionally, bleeding volume decreased 80.5 and 76.6 mL, respectively. The use of the harmonic scalpel also significantly reduced drainage volumes and the time during which drains remained in place.[27]

In 2016, Mathialagan et al published a prospective study of 40 patients with neck dissection, comparing the use of a harmonic scalpel near the spinal nerve versus the use of conventional monopolar energy. Regarding postoperative shoulder pain and muscle function, the harmonic scalpel had a statistically better performance than the monopolar device.[28] More recently, the same group published the results in the same population analyzing intraoperative bleeding, drainage, and postoperative hospital stay, and only found a statistically significant difference in favor of the harmonic scalpel in the amount of bleeding.[29] Other investigators have not found significant differences in operative time or blood loss, when comparing neck dissection using the harmonic scalpel versus the conventional procedure (36 patients, prospective, randomized study).[30]

Summarizing, the harmonic scalpel is a useful tool in the surgeon's armamentarium, making many of the stages of neck dissection easier.

8.11 Complications

Evidence shows that selective dissections entail less morbidity than radical dissections.[6] Preservation of muscle structures, protection of large vessels, and preservation of nervous structures are all factors that contribute to minimizing the occurrence of complications.

As to the use of selective dissection as an adjuvant after chemoradiotherapy protocols, speculation has been that it might worsen the functional consequences of prior treatment. In a recent study, investigators at the MD Anderson Cancer Center analyzed a population of 347 patients previously treated with intensity-modulated radiotherapy (IMRT); they identified 75 patients (21%) who received a selective dissection post-IMRT. Overall, 12% of patients had chronic dysphagia, but addition of the dissection significantly increase neither the development of dysphagia nor the duration of the use of gastrostomy.[31]

8.12 New Horizons

SND has become established for the treatment of primary tumors of the upper aerodigestive tract. Numerous recent studies aim at further minimizing the esthetic impact of this surgical approach, maintaining the radicality of the procedure. In a recent review by Shen et al, the authors analyzed the potential

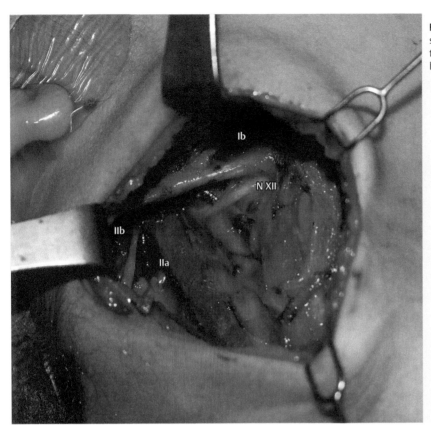

Fig. 8.12 Dissection of levels IIa and IIb on both sides of the spinal accessory nerve. See the trajectory of the hypoglossal nerve, crossing below the posterior belly of the digastric muscle.

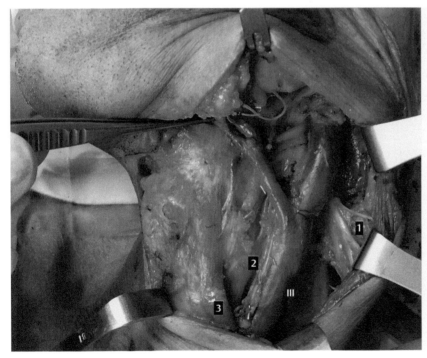

Fig. 8.13 Dissection of level III. 1: branches of the cervical plexus; 2: preserved ansa hypoglossi; 3: omohyoid muscle.

advantages and disadvantages of selective dissection, assisted with endoscopy and robotics. In both cases, the approach employed most often is the retroauricular approach (facelift approach). Although robotics adds the advantage of a three-dimensional view, its cost–benefit is questionable. Prospective and randomized studies will be needed to establish the value of these new technologies more definitively.[32]

Very recently, a group of investigators from China and Brazil compared in a prospective randomized trial with 60 patients the inflammatory response and surgical stress with conventional dissection and endoscopically assisted dissection. In the group that underwent an endoscopically assisted dissection, interleukin-6 (IL-6), IL-10, CRP (C-reactive protein), and cortisol levels were significantly lower, which confirms the hypothesis

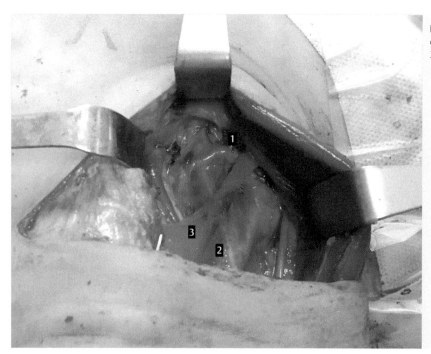

Fig. 8.14 Dissection of level IV. 1: transverse cervical artery (*blue mark*); 2: phrenic nerve; 3: omohyoid muscle.

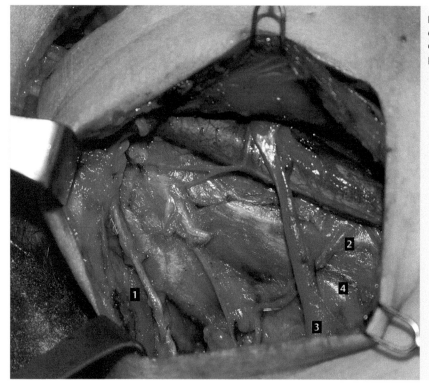

Fig. 8.15 Dissection of level V. 1: lower trajectory of the spinal accessory nerve; 2: transverse cervical artery; 3: omohyoid muscle; 4: brachial plexus.

of a lower inflammatory response and greater tolerance to stress with that procedure.[33]

8.13 Good Clinical Practices: Consensus Statements

Among the most recent consensus statements issued by various scientific societies, we wish to underscore those published by the United Kingdom National Multidisciplinary Guidelines on the Management of Neck Metastases in Head and Neck Cancer.[6] Its main recommendations regarding selective and elective dissections propose the following:

- Patients with a clinically N0 neck, with more than 15 to 20% risk of occult nodal metastases, should be offered prophylactic treatment of the neck (R).
- All patients with T1 and T2 oral cavity cancer and N0 neck should receive prophylactic neck treatment (R).
- SND is as effective as modified radical neck dissection for controlling regional disease in N0 necks for all primary sites (R).

- SND alone is adequate treatment for pN1 neck disease without adverse histological features (R).
- Postoperative radiation for adverse histologic features following SND confers control rates comparable with more extensive procedures (R).
- Postoperative chemoradiation improves regional control in patients with extracapsular spread and/or microscopically involved surgical margins (R).
- Following chemoradiation therapy, complete responders who do not show evidence of active disease on co-registered PET-CT scans performed at 10 to 12 weeks do not need salvage neck dissection (R).
- Salvage surgery should be considered for those with incomplete or equivocal response of nodal disease on PET-CT (R).

8.14 Acknowledgments

The author thanks Eduardo L. Mazzaro, MD, Juan J. Larrañaga, MD, and Pedro I. Picco, MD, for their contribution with surgical pictures.

References

[1] Robbins KT, Medina JE, Wolfe GT, Levine PA, Sessions RB, Pruet CW. Standardizing neck dissection terminology. Official report of the Academy's Committee for Head and Neck Surgery and Oncology. Arch Otolaryngol Head Neck Surg. 1991; 117(6):601–605

[2] Spiro RH, Strong EW, Shah JP, York N. Classification of neck dissection: variations on a new theme. Am J Surg. 1994; 168(5):415–418

[3] Robbins KT, Ferlito A, Shah JP, et al. The evolving role of selective neck dissection for head and neck squamous cell carcinoma. Eur Arch Otorhinolaryngol. 2013; 270(4):1195–1202

[4] Zenga J, Jackson RS, Graboyes EM, et al. Oncologic outcomes of selective neck dissection in HPV-related oropharyngeal squamous cell carcinoma. Laryngoscope. 2017; 127(3):623–630

[5] Bocca E, Pignataro O. A conservation technique in radical neck dissection. Ann Otol Rhinol Laryngol. 1967; 76(5):975–987

[6] Paleri V, Urbano TG, Mehanna H, et al. Management of neck metastases in head and neck cancer: United Kingdom National Multidisciplinary Guidelines. J Laryngol Otol. 2016; 130 S2:S161–S169

[7] Pitman KT, Johnson JT, Myers EN. Effectiveness of selective neck dissection for management of the clinically negative neck. Arch Otolaryngol Head Neck Surg. 1997; 123(9):917–922

[8] Brazilian Head and Neck Cancer Study Group. Results of a prospective trial on elective modified radical classical versus supraomohyoid neck dissection in the management of oral squamous carcinoma. Am J Surg. 1998; 176(5):422–427

[9] Brazilian Head and Neck Cancer Study Group. End results of a prospective trial on elective lateral neck dissection vs type III modified radical neck dissection in the management of supraglottic and transglottic carcinomas. Head Neck. 1999; 21(8):694–702

[10] Djordjevic V, Bukurov B, Arsovic N, et al. Prospective case–control study of efficacy of bilateral selective neck dissection in primary surgical treatment of supraglottic laryngeal cancers with clinically negative cervical findings (N0). Clin Otolaryngol. 2015

[11] O'Brien CJ, Petersen-Schaefer K, Ruark D, Coates AS, Menzie SJ, Harrison RI. Radical, modified, and selective neck dissection for cutaneous malignant melanoma. Head Neck. 1995; 17(3):232–241

[12] Weinstein GS, Quon H, O'Malley BW, Jr, Kim GG, Cohen MA. Selective neck dissection and deintensified postoperative radiation and chemotherapy for oropharyngeal cancer: a subset analysis of the University of Pennsylvania transoral robotic surgery trial. Laryngoscope. 2010; 120(9):1749–1755

[13] Park SM, Lee DJ, Chung EJ, et al. Conversion from selective to comprehensive neck dissection: is it necessary for occult nodal metastasis? 5-year observational study. Clin Exp Otorhinolaryngol. 2013; 6(2):94–98

[14] Dhiwakar M, Robbins KT, Vieira F, Rao K, Malone J. Selective neck dissection as an early salvage intervention for clinically persistent nodal disease following chemoradiation. Head Neck. 2012; 34(2):188–193

[15] Ambrosch P, Kron M, Pradier O, Steiner W. Efficacy of selective neck dissection: a review of 503 cases of elective and therapeutic treatment of the neck in squamous cell carcinoma of the upper aerodigestive tract. Otolaryngol Head Neck Surg. 2001; 124(2):180–187

[16] Robbins KT, Dhiwakar M, Vieira F, Rao K, Malone J. Efficacy of super-selective neck dissection following chemoradiation for advanced head and neck cancer. Oral Oncol. 2012; 48(11):1185–1189

[17] Ferris RL, Kraus DH. Sentinel lymph node biopsy versus selective neck dissection for detection of metastatic oral squamous cell carcinoma. Clin Exp Metastasis. 2012; 29(7):693–698

[18] Schilling C, Stoeckli SJ, Haerle SK, et al. Sentinel European Node Trial (SENT): 3-year results of sentinel node biopsy in oral cancer. Eur J Cancer. 2015; 51 (18):2777–2784

[19] Shah JP, Candela FC, Poddar AK. The patterns of cervical lymph node metastases from squamous carcinoma of the oral cavity. Cancer. 1990; 66 (1):109–113

[20] Pantvaidya GH, Pal P, Vaidya AD, Pai PS, D'Cruz AK. Prospective study of 583 neck dissections in oral cancers: implications for clinical practice. Head Neck. 2014; 36(10):1503–1507

[21] Chheda YP, Pillai SK, Parikh DG, Dipayan N, Shah SV, Alaknanda G. A prospective study of level IIB nodal metastasis (supraretrospinal) in clinically N0 oral squamous cell carcinoma in Indian population. Indian J Surg Oncol. 2017

[22] Agarwal SK, Akali NR, Sarin D. Prospective analysis of 231 elective neck dissections in oral squamous cell carcinoma with node negative neck: to decide the extent of neck dissection. Auris Nasus Larynx. 2018

[23] Agarwal SK, Arora SK, Kumar G, Sarin D. Isolated perifacial lymph node metastasis in oral squamous cell carcinoma with clinically node-negative neck. Laryngoscope. 2016; 126(10):2252–2256

[24] Lee C-H, Huang N-C, Chen H-C, Chen M-K. Minimizing shoulder syndrome with intra-operative spinal accessory nerve monitoring for neck dissection. Acta Otorhinolaryngol Ital. 2013; 33(2):93–96

[25] Rastogi S, Sharma A, Choudhury R, et al. Is superselective neck dissection safer than supraomohyoid neck dissection for oral carcinoma patients with N0 neck in terms of shoulder morbidity and recurrence rate? J Oral Maxillofac Surg. 2018; 76(3):647–655

[26] Ebrahimi A, Clark JR, Amit M, et al. Minimum nodal yield in oral squamous cell carcinoma: defining the standard of care in a multicenter international pooled validation study. Ann Surg Oncol. 2014; 21(9):3049–3055

[27] Dean A, Alamillos F, Centella I, García-Álvarez S. Neck dissection with the harmonic scalpel in patients with squamous cell carcinoma of the oral cavity. J Craniomaxillofac Surg. 2014; 42(1):84–87

[28] Mathialagan A, Verma RK, Panda NK. Comparison of spinal accessory dysfunction following neck dissection with harmonic scalpel and electrocautery: a randomized study. Oral Oncol. 2016; 61:142–145

[29] Verma RK, Mathiazhagan A, Panda NK. Neck dissection with harmonic scalpel and electrocautery? A randomised study. Auris Nasus Larynx. 2017; 44 (5):590–595

[30] Fritz DK, Matthews TW, Chandarana SP, Nakoneshny SC, Dort JC. Harmonic scalpel impact on blood loss and operating time in major head and neck surgery: a randomized clinical trial. J Otolaryngol Head Neck Surg. 2016; 45(1):58

[31] Hutcheson KA, Abualsamh AR, Sosa A, et al. Impact of selective neck dissection on chronic dysphagia after chemo-intensity-modulated radiotherapy for oropharyngeal carcinoma. Head Neck. 2016; 38(6):886–893

[32] Shen ZS, Li JS, Chen WL, Fan S. The latest advancements in selective neck dissection for early stage oral squamous cell carcinoma. Curr Treat Options Oncol. 2017; 18(5):31

[33] Fan S, Zhong JL, Chen WX, et al. Postoperative immune response and surgical stress in selective neck dissection: comparison between endoscopically assisted dissection and open techniques in cT1–2N0 oral squamous cell carcinoma. J Craniomaxillofac Surg. 2017; 45(8):1112–1116

9 Supraomohyoid Neck Dissection

Kristen Pytynia

Abstract

The presence of regional metastatic lymphadenopathy from mucosal squamous cell carcinoma decreases survival by 50%. The management and control of regional metastasis is paramount to both oncological and functional long-term outcomes. The supraomohyoid neck dissection gained popularity in the 1970s and 1980s as an alternative to the functionally debilitating radical neck dissection. Supraomohyoid neck dissection consists of removing lymph nodes in levels Ia, Ib, II, and III, while preserving the sternocleidomastoid muscle, the internal jugular vein, and the spinal accessory nerve. The omohyoid muscle is the lower limit of dissection. Level IIb can be included in the resection based on whether there is disease present in level IIa. A supraomohyoid neck dissection is indicated for patients with a clinically N0 neck, or with low-volume neck disease from a primary tumor that typically drains into levels I, II, or III. Most commonly, this procedure is performed for the management of oral cavity cancers.

Keywords: supraomohyoid neck dissection, occult disease, radical neck dissection, oral cavity, functional outcome

9.1 History and Rationale

The evolution of the surgical management of the neck is a fascinating tale, one which we briefly summarize here and note that avid historians have written more extensively on the topic.[1] In 1906, Crile proposed radical resection of all of the lymph nodes of the neck, including the sternocleidomastoid muscle, internal jugular vein, and spinal accessory nerve, and the lymph nodes from the mastoid to the clavicle to ensure an oncological sound procedure.[2] The sternocleidomastoid muscle, the internal jugular vein, and the accessory nerve were considered the anatomical borders of the fat packet containing the lymph nodes of the neck. Resection of the muscle, vein, and nerve improved access to the lymph nodes and ensured oncological removal. This procedure, which became known as radical neck dissection, was in line with the then contemporary surgical practice—championed by Halstead, who theorized that cancer recurrences were the product of too conservative surgical resections. To give Crile credit, he apparently did question the need for the resection of uninvolved structures, but continued to recommend a more radical approach. Radical neck dissection has mortality and morbidity associated with it: carotid blowout syndrome, skin flap necrosis, severe facial edema due to bilateral internal jugular vein sacrifice, shoulder dysfunction, neck fibrosis, and chronic pain syndrome are some of the known risks and sequelae associated with the procedure.

During the first half of the 20th century, chemotherapy agents were discovered, and radiation was found to be effective against cancer cells. With these additions to the treatment armamentarium, as well as the recurrence of some cancers despite aggressive resection, surgeons questioned the efficacy and necessity of an overtly aggressive surgery. In 1951, Ward and Robben suggested that shoulder dysfunction could be avoided while maintaining oncological principles by preserving the spinal accessory nerve.[3] They did recommend en bloc (contiguous) resection of the primary and cervical lymph nodes, as well as the sternocleidomastoid muscle and internal jugular vein, in order to remove the lymphatic vessels draining into the nodes. While preservation of the spinal accessory nerve improved some aspects of shoulder function, patients with large en bloc resections still had significant functional morbidity such as chronic pain, facial edema, and fibrosis. Furthermore, shoulder dysfunction was still a problem due to stretching of the accessory nerve. These debilitating morbidities associated with the procedure drove surgeons to consider other techniques.

Suarez and Bocca were two early champions of functional neck dissection, each publishing their experiences in the 1960s. There is some dispute over who originated the idea, as they had observed each other's techniques. Suarez published his experience in the South American literature, and Bocca in the European literature. Bocca's technique relied on the anatomical knowledge of the fascial planes of the neck, which allowed removing the fat packet containing the cervical lymphatics while preserving the internal jugular vein, sternocleidomastoid muscle, and accessory nerve.[4] He argued that it would be difficult for occult disease to cross these fascial barriers, and resection beyond those fascial barriers would not improve oncological outcome. Further, he advocated for this technique to be used on clinically positive lymph nodes, as long as they were not fixed to adjacent structures. Suarez's original article was published in Spanish, and was not widely recognized in the non-Spanish-speaking literature.[5] The original Suarez article is difficult to find translated into English; therefore, Ferlito et al offer a passionate defense of Suarez's role in the development or functional neck dissection.[6] He highlights Suarez's view that preservation of the sternocleidomastoid muscle protects the carotid artery from fatal rupture and the skin from necrosis. Their publications began a slow trend toward less radical surgery, in conjunction with the use of postoperative radiation. The modified radical neck dissection (MRND) was therefore any level I to IV or I to V neck dissection that preserved at least one structure: sternocleidomastoid muscle, internal jugular vein, or spinal accessory nerve.

In 1972, Lindberg characterized the location of positive nodes from upper aerodigestive tract of different sites of 2,044 previously untreated patients, essentially mapping the drainage patterns of various mucosal locations.[7] This study showed that there are reliable and predictable patterns of lymphatic drainage and involvement of first echelon nodes. In particular, oral cavity cancer was noted to most frequently drain to nodes in levels I, II, and III, and the likelihood of lymph node involvement was noted to increase with primary tumor size (thickness for oral tongue). Understanding of the predicted pattern of nodal metastasis allowed for a more targeted surgical approach, and ushered in the era of selective neck dissections. The supraomohyoid neck dissection is a type of selective neck dissection that consists of removal of nodes in levels I, II, and III. The lower limit is the omohyoid muscle, and the sternocleidomastoid muscle, internal jugular vein, and accessory nerve are preserved.

In 1988, after years of attempting to standardize the approach for selective neck dissection, Byers et al published one of the larger series of selective neck dissections, 428 patients with primary cancers at different sites.[8] This retrospective study examined the efficacy of supraomohyoid, MRND, and other selective neck dissections in patients with clinically negative (cN0) necks. Byers' classic article examined the drainage patterns of different sites in the upper aerodigestive tract, and mapped where occult metastases were found in clinically node-negative necks. Focusing on oral cavity primary sites, he showed that disease from the oral cavity primarily spreads to levels I, II, or III, in concordance with Lindberg but focusing on microscopic (occult), and not clinically positive disease. Patients with different types of selective neck dissection fared well, with 15% neck failure rate, many on the contralateral undissected side. Therefore, Byers recommended that with careful patient selection, selective neck dissection can be both diagnostic (by identifying occult nodal disease) and therapeutic. Patients with multiple histopathologically positive nodes benefited from postoperative radiation.

In a subsequent study, Medina and Byers noted similar recurrence rates for patient with oral cavity cancer undergoing supraomohyoid neck dissection versus those receiving radical neck dissection.[9] Spiro et al emphasized the importance of using the supraomohyoid neck dissection for low-volume disease, as well as postoperative radiation to decrease regional recurrence rates.[10] Surgeons across the world continued to turn away from radical resections, resecting only those structures with direct tumor invasion. These classic studies were often retrospective, and many authors have attempted to study the question of effectiveness of supraomohyoid neck dissection in a prospective manner. Certainly, the gold standard for a prospective study is performed in a randomized, controlled setting. The Brazilian Head and Neck Cancer Group published a study with these characteristics in 1998, comparing 148 patients with T2–T4, N0 squamous cell carcinoma of the oral cavity, randomized to either MRND with accessory nerve preservation or supraomohyoid dissection.[11] They found no differences in locoregional recurrence or survival, but the modified radical neck group had a significantly higher complication rate (41% MRND vs. 25% supraomohyoid). Complications observed included flap necrosis, wound infection, fistula, vascular rupture, hematoma, seroma, chyle leak, and postoperative death. All patients with positive nodes received postoperative radiation, and four patients with clinically positive nodes were converted to MRND at the time of the initial surgery, but were still included in the cohort. This study has often been cited to confirm the oncological equivalence of supraomohyoid neck dissection to MRND in the treatment of oral cavity cancer.

9.2 Functional Outcomes

Supraomohyoid neck dissection anatomically preserves the sternocleidomastoid muscle, internal jugular vein, and the spinal accessory nerve, and significantly limits the caudal extent of the dissection. The benefits of this approach may appear obvious to the surgeon, but systematic measurement has been difficult, as the preservation of these structures may not have a direct correlate in function, or quality of life (QOL). In these regards, Goldstein et al performed a review on articles looking at shoulder dysfunction after neck dissection. Their exhaustive review highlights the difficulty in characterizing and measuring shoulder dysfunction and surgical extent. Most articles agree, though, that there is an improvement in shoulder dysfunction in selective (compared to radical) neck dissections and that any manipulation of the accessory nerve can result in a degree of dysfunction.[12] Similarly, the benefits of supraomohyoid neck dissection on QOL were confirmed in a large European study including patients from Sweden, Germany, Austria, and Switzerland.[13] This retrospective study involved 1,652 patients with oral squamous cell carcinoma, who completed a QOL questionnaire at least 6 months after surgery. Overall, patients with supraomohyoid neck dissection had significantly improved scores for neck mobility and shoulder and arm movement when compared to those who underwent a modified or radical neck dissection.

9.3 Indications

Oral cavity cancer is unique in the head and neck area due to its high incidence of occult nodal metastases, defined as a cN0 but microscopically positive lymph nodes. That is to say, physical examination of the neck does not reveal any concerning lymphadenopathy, and nor does imaging, but histopathologic assessment reveals metastatic carcinoma in at least one lymph node. Given the lymphatic drainage pattern of the oral cavity, a supraomohyoid neck dissection will address the neck levels at highest risk of harboring occult nodal disease. Therefore, a supraomohyoid neck dissection for N0 oral cavity disease is considered both diagnostic and therapeutic. Some have posited if observation of N0 necks may be substituted for supraomohyoid neck dissection, and multiple studies have attempted to address this question. In this regard, a recent meta-analysis from Abu-Ghanem concluded that patients undergoing elective neck dissection had better regional- and disease-specific survival compared to those who were observed.[14] While oral cavity cancers constitute the most common indication for the procedure, its indications encompass any primary location where levels I to II or III are the primary echelon for lymphatic drainage, including oropharynx, sinonasal, salivary glands, and some cutaneous malignancies. Furthermore, it is important to keep in mind that low-volume nodal disease can also be addressed with a supraomohyoid neck dissection.

9.4 Surgical Technique

The dissection begins with an incision in the neck. The incision should be designed such that it allows access to the areas of interest, but is also cosmetically acceptable. If it is possible to hide a scar in an existing skin crease, the patient will have an improved cosmetic outcome. Anteriorly, in order to reach the submental triangle, the incision can be curved upward or extended across the midline (▶ Fig. 9.1). Remember that most radiation oncologists will radiate the entire incision as part of the postoperative radiation field; therefore, it is important to make an incision large enough to allow adequate access, but not larger than necessary. This author has not seen significant cosmetic differences in scarring in patients incised with a knife compared to the Bovie on the cut setting, particularly for those who

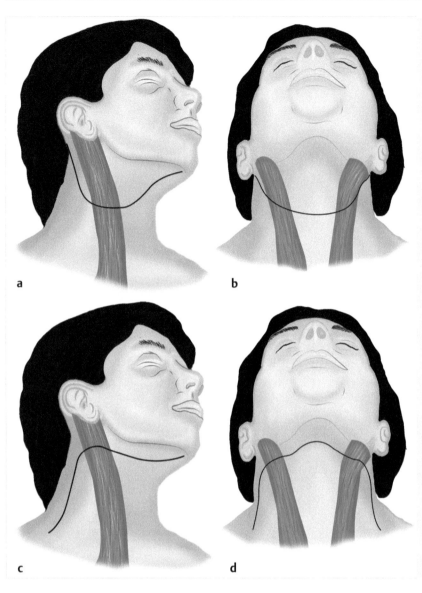

Fig. 9.1 Diagram of the most commonly used cervical incisions for a supraomohyoid neck dissection. **(a)** Unilateral apron approach extending to the submental area. **(b)** Bilateral apron incision extending across the midline. **(c)** Unilateral modified Schobinger incision. **(d)** Bilateral modified Schobinger incision.

a

b

c

d

undergo postoperative radiation. Subplatysmal flaps are raised. The external jugular vein and the greater auricular nerve should be preserved. Superior flap dissection should be performed exactly at the level of the platysma so as to not disrupt the marginal mandibular nerve. The marginal mandibular nerve is identified, traced, and preserved (▶ Fig. 9.2). The dissection begins inferior to the submandibular gland, where the posterior belly of the digastric muscle is identified and traced anteriorly to skeletonize the anterior belly of the muscle. The fibrofatty contents of the area between the two anterior bellies of the digastric and superficial to the mylohyoid should be removed as midline level IA neck dissection. Level IA can be transected and sent as a separate specimen. Attention is then brought back toward the submandibular gland, which is retracted inferiorly and anteriorly. The hypoglossal nerve should be identified just superior to the posterior belly of the digastric, and deep to the submandibular gland. The lateral edge of the mylohyoid muscle is skeletonized and retracted; part of the gland will wrap around the lateral edge of this muscle. The nerve to the mylohyoid is a branch of the inferior alveolar nerve and needs to be transected. As you free the submandibular

gland up on its posterior surface, you will identify the lingual nerve. The lingual nerve is always superior to the hypoglossal nerve, and both nerves should be clearly identified prior to proceeding with the next steps. The submandibular ganglion of the lingual nerve is then transected. The submandibular duct will be visible and should be ligated. The facial artery and vein will be noted at the posterior aspect of the submandibular gland. The artery may be entering the submandibular gland itself, or often just sends off a large branch into the gland. The facial artery can be dissected distally to preserve as much length as possible if free flap reconstruction is anticipated. The facial nodes around the facial vein and facial artery should also be removed with the specimen. It is wise to always go back and palpate this area to ensure no lymph nodes have been left behind. This completes the level Ib dissection.

The upper jugular nodes are then addressed. The posterior belly of the digastric muscle is exposed, and the tail of the parotid is identified at its posterior aspect. The dissection proceeds just inferior to the posterior belly of the digastric, where the tissue is divided in plane parallel to muscle to identify the jugular vein. Be cautious as there may be a large retromandibular vein

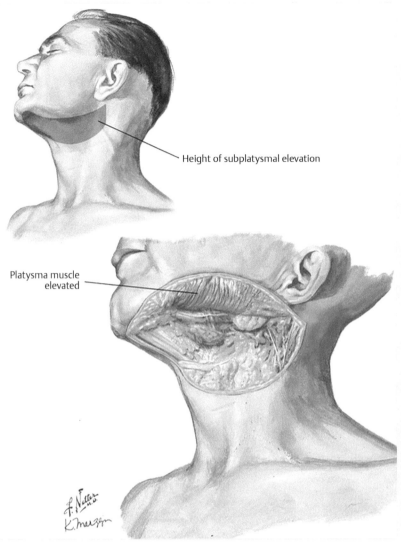

Height of subplatysmal elevation

Platysma muscle
elevated

joining the internal jugular vein in a "Y" configuration. The hypoglossal nerve and its associated *ranine veins* can also be identified in this area, as well as the *ansa cervicalis* descending from the hypoglossal nerve (▶ Fig. 9.3). The dissection then proceeds laterally, toward the sternocleidomastoid muscle. The fascia of the sternocleidomastoid muscle should be incised along its anterior border. It is not necessary to resect external jugular nodes for aerodigestive tract cancers, but external jugular node dissection is indicated for cutaneous malignancies. Keeping the fascia along the anterior aspect of the sternocleidomastoid muscle intact may help prevent fibrosis, stressing the importance of incising the fascia along the anterior/medial border of the muscle. The fascia along the posteromedial aspect of the sternocleidomastoid muscle—part of the superficial layer of the deep cervical fascia—is dissected off the muscle. As we approach the posterior border of the muscle, the angle of the dissection is changed from posterior to medial, and the superficial layer of the deep cervical fascia is incised to expose the fibrofatty contents lying deep to it. These are then grasped with Allis clamps and reflected anteromedially. The upper cervical rootlets are preserved, and dissected medially, thus releasing the posterior attachments of the specimen. The spinal accessory nerve is exposed and traced toward the posterior belly of the digastric.

Most commonly, the spinal accessory nerve will course lateral to the internal jugular vein, but rarely it may "split" the vein or course medial to it. The prominence of the transverse process of C2 can routinely be palpated at this point. When searching for the spinal accessory nerve, it is important to know that a branch of the occipital artery is often within a few millimeters of the nerve, lying in a plane immediately superficial to it. This vessel can be used as a landmark to help identify the nerve, and it may be safely ligated. If level IIB are to be resected, limit the retraction and manipulation of the spinal accessory nerve as traction injury is common. The omohyoid muscle is exposed lower in the neck, and used as the inferior boundary for the dissection. The internal jugular vein can be consistently identified under the tendon of this muscle, and its lateral aspect should be exposed. There should not be any lateral branches off the internal jugular vein. The fibrofatty contents of levels II and III are reflected medially and dissected off the deep muscles of the neck, internal carotid artery, and internal jugular vein. Caution should be used to not injure the vagus nerve with the Bovie during this maneuver. This completes the level II and III neck dissection. The specimen should be divided into levels and sent separately ex vivo, to allow each lymphatic level to be examined and recorded in the pathological report.

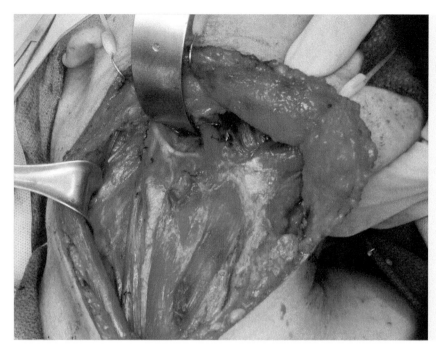

Fig. 9.3 Intraoperative photograph of a completed supraomohyoid neck dissection. The posterior belly of the digastric muscle is retracted to show the hypoglossal nerve. Posteriorly, the spinal accessory nerve can be visualized as it enters the sternocleidomastoid muscle.

9.5 Controversies

A few technical aspects of the supraomohyoid neck dissection are controversial. These include preservation of the submandibular gland, nodal yield, and the need for resection of level IIB in patients with occult oral cavity disease.

Is it absolutely necessary to remove the submandibular gland during a supraomohyoid neck dissection? The submandibular gland should of course be removed if tumor is invading directly into it. Advocates of standard removal also suggest that it is easier to address the adjacent facial nodes when the submandibular gland has been removed. Opponents to routine removal argue that—as opposed to the parotid—there are no lymph nodes within the substance of the submandibular gland. In Bocca's landmark 1967 paper "A Conservation Technique in Radical Neck Dissection," he proposed preserving the submandibular gland, as there is no lymphatic drainage within the gland.[4] He argued that the fascial layers of the neck convolve around the gland, and hence the lymph nodes would be outside that fascia, therefore making it oncologically safe to spare the gland. The goal of submandibular gland preservation would be to maintain its salivary function in order to prevent xerostomia. Radiation therapy to any salivary gland results in loss of salivary function above 39 Gy.[15] Therefore, if the primary tumor already has indications for postoperative radiation (bone or perineural invasion), and the submandibular area is going to be radiated postoperatively, it is best to resect the submandibular gland. The salivary function of the gland will be negligible after radiation therapy, and its removal will ensure that all the facial nodes are properly addressed. In addition to prevention of xerostomia, advocates of preservation also cite the incidence of marginal mandibular, hypoglossal, and lingual nerve injuries as justifications to spare the gland.[16,17]

The dissection of level IIB—lateral to the spinal accessory nerve—can result in symptomatic shoulder dysfunction, even if the nerve is anatomically intact. This is likely due to traction injury during dissection. In continued efforts to reduce morbidity associated with neck dissection, the need for dissection of level IIb in cN0 or low-volume nodal disease has been questioned. As it relates to oral cavity disease, the consensus seems to be that level IIB need not be dissected if level IIA is negative, with consideration for elective dissection in lateral tongue disease.[18,19] Elsheikh et al examined 48 patients with oral cancer and cN0 necks, and studied the level IIb nodes, specifically looking for micrometastasis.[20] They found a 10% rate of micrometastasis to the IIB nodal basin, including all oral tongue primary subsites. As such, they recommended elective dissection of level IIB for all oral tongue cancers, but not for other oral cavity sites. In terms of the oncological benefits of elective neck dissection, the best evidence comes from a landmark study by Vaish et al.[21] They prospectively studied patients with early oral cavity cancer with cN0 necks. Patients were randomized to elective neck dissection versus observation with a therapeutic (or salvage) neck dissection if regional metastasis developed. Patients with upfront elective neck dissection had improved survival compared to those who underwent a therapeutic (salvage) neck dissection.

The yield of lymph nodes has been studied as a guide to help define an oncologically complete supraomohyoid neck dissection. Pou et al found a significantly higher rate of positive nodes in specimens that contained more than 18 nodes (36 vs. 15%) and suggested further study.[22] It is always best practice to review the pathological report to determine the number of nodes removed; any specimen containing less than 10 lymph nodes is suggestive of an incomplete dissection. In this regard, the practice of "berry picking" lymph nodes is strongly discouraged, and every effort should be made to perform a standardized, compartment-oriented dissection of the neck levels to be addressed.

In conclusion, the supraomohyoid neck dissection is considered by many as the standard of care for cN0 or low-volume oral cavity cancer. When compared to the radical neck dissection, or MRND, this procedure yields similar oncologic outcomes but improved functional status.

References

[1] Patel KN, Shah JP. Neck dissection: past, present, future. Surg Oncol Clin N Am. 2005; 14(3):461–477, vi

[2] Crile G. Landmark article Dec 1, 1906: excision of cancer of the head and neck. With special reference to the plan of dissection based on one hundred and thirty-two operations. By George Crile. JAMA. 1987; 258(22):3286–3293

[3] Ward GE, Robben JO. A composite operation for radical neck dissection and removal of cancer of the mouth. Cancer. 1951; 4(1):98–109

[4] Bocca E, Pignataro O. A conservation technique in radical neck dissection. Ann Otol Rhinol Laryngol. 1967; 76(5):975–987

[5] Suarez O. El problema de las metástasis linfáticas y alejadas del cáncer de laringe e hipofaringe. Rev Otorrinolaringol. 1963; 23:83–99

[6] Ferlito A, Rinaldo A. Osvaldo Suárez: often-forgotten father of functional neck dissection (in the non-Spanish-speaking literature). Laryngoscope. 2004; 114 (7):1177–1178

[7] Lindberg R. Distribution of cervical lymph node metastases from squamous cell carcinoma of the upper respiratory and digestive tracts. Cancer. 1972; 29 (6):1446–1449

[8] Byers RM, Wolf PF, Ballantyne AJ. Rationale for elective modified neck dissection. Head Neck Surg. 1988; 10(3):160–167

[9] Medina JE, Byers RM. Supraomohyoid neck dissection: rationale, indications, and surgical technique. Head Neck. 1989; 11(2):111–122

[10] Spiro JD, Spiro RH, Shah JP, Sessions RB, Strong EW. Critical assessment of supraomohyoid neck dissection. Am J Surg. 1988; 156(4):286–289

[11] Brazilian Head and Neck Cancer Study Group. Results of a prospective trial on elective modified radical classical versus supraomohyoid neck dissection in the management of oral squamous carcinoma. Am J Surg. 1998; 176(5):422–427

[12] Goldstein DP, Ringash J, Bissada E, et al. Scoping review of the literature on shoulder impairments and disability after neck dissection. Head Neck. 2014; 36(2):299–308

[13] Spalthoff S, Zimmerer R, Jehn P, Gellrich NC, Handschel J, Krüskemper G. Neck dissection's burden on the patient: functional and psychosocial aspects in 1,652 patients with oral squamous cell carcinomas. J Oral Maxillofac Surg. 2017; 75(4):839–849

[14] Abu-Ghanem S, Yehuda M, Carmel NN, et al. Elective neck dissection vs observation in early-stage squamous cell carcinoma of the oral tongue with no clinically apparent lymph node metastasis in the neck: a systematic review and meta-analysis. JAMA Otolaryngol Head Neck Surg. 2016; 142(9):857–865

[15] Murdoch-Kinch CA, Kim HM, Vineberg KA, Ship JA, Eisbruch A. Dose-effect relationships for the submandibular salivary glands and implications for their sparing by intensity modulated radiotherapy. Int J Radiat Oncol Biol Phys. 2008; 72(2):373–382

[16] Razfar A, Walvekar RR, Melkane A, Johnson JT, Myers EN. Incidence and patterns of regional metastasis in early oral squamous cell cancers: feasibility of submandibular gland preservation. Head Neck. 2009; 31(12):1619–1623

[17] Malgonde MS, Kumar M. Practicability of submandibular gland in squamous cell carcinomas of oral cavity. Indian J Otolaryngol Head Neck Surg. 2015; 67 s uppl 1:138–140

[18] Lim YC, Song MH, Kim SC, Kim KM, Choi EC. Preserving level IIb lymph nodes in elective supraomohyoid neck dissection for oral cavity squamous cell carcinoma. Arch Otolaryngol Head Neck Surg. 2004; 130(9):1088–1091

[19] Bhattacharya A, Adwani D, Adwani N, Sharma V. Is it worthy? Removal of level IIB nodes during selective neck dissection (I-III) for oral carcinomas. Ann Maxillofac Surg. 2015; 5(1):20–25

[20] Elsheikh MN, Mahfouz ME, Elsheikh E. Level IIb lymph nodes metastasis in elective supraomohyoid neck dissection for oral cavity squamous cell carcinoma: a molecular-based study. Laryngoscope. 2005; 115(9):1636–1640

[21] Vaish R, Gupta S, D'Cruz AK. Elective versus therapeutic neck dissection in oral cancer. N Engl J Med. 2015; 373(25):2477

[22] Pou JD, Barton BM, Lawlor CM, Frederick CH, Moore BA, Hasney CP. Minimum lymph node yield in elective level I-III neck dissection. Laryngoscope. 2017; 127(9):2070–2073

10 Salvage Neck Dissection: Indications, Workup, and Technical Considerations

Mingyann Lim and Mark Zafereo

Abstract

A salvage neck dissection is defined as a neck dissection in a neck that has been previously treated with radiation, chemotherapy, surgery, or a combination of these three modalities. This procedure can be planned or unplanned, and there is mounting evidence to suggest that planned salvage neck dissection is unnecessary in most circumstances. Salvage neck dissection should be performed for nodal disease that is in partial remission following radiation or chemoradiation, as well as cases of recurrent disease. Preoperative workup may include cross-sectional imaging (CT or MRI), PET scan, and/or ultrasound-guided fine-needle aspiration (FNA). Following definitive chemoradiation of neck disease, PET scan has a very high negative predictive value, such that patients with a negative PET at 12 weeks posttreatment have an exceedingly low risk of residual nodal disease. Selective or superselective salvage neck dissections are generally favored over a comprehensive neck dissection in the salvage setting. Important intra- and postoperative considerations with salvage neck surgery include awareness of the importance of en bloc disease resection, achieving negative margin status, possible need for vascularized tissue, and potential indication for adjuvant external beam radiation or brachytherapy.

Keywords: salvage neck dissection, radiation therapy, brachytherapy, head and neck squamous cell carcinoma, recurrence

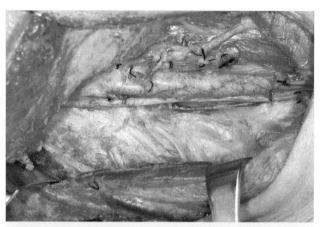

Fig. 10.1 Salvage modified radical neck dissection after chemoradiation therapy for squamous cell carcinoma of the oropharynx, with sacrifice of the internal jugular vein, and preservation of the sternocleidomastoid muscle and spinal accessory nerve. Vagus and hypoglossal nerves are preserved and visible. Dense fibrotic tissue in the neck encasing the cervical rootlets demonstrates the extent of treatment-related soft-tissue fibrosis and scarring.

10.1 Introduction

Salvage neck dissection is defined as a neck dissection for a neck that has been previously treated with radiation, chemotherapy, surgery, or a combination of these three modalities. Salvage neck dissection can be either a planned or unplanned dissection. A planned neck dissection occurs following radiotherapy or chemoradiotherapy (CRT), where, in anticipation of possible residual disease, the neck dissection is sequentially performed as part of the overall initial treatment plan. Unplanned neck dissection refers to the scenario where there is initially no plan to perform neck dissection after therapy, but the decision for the neck dissection follows later due to residual disease or disease recurrence. In the literature, the terminology can be confusing as some authors refer to only unplanned neck dissections as salvage neck dissections, whereas others refer to both planned and unplanned posttreatment neck dissections as salvage dissections.

Salvage neck dissections are characterized by a technically more challenging surgery, due to the presence of scarring and fibrosis from previous treatments (▶ Fig. 10.1). In general, the potential acute and long-term morbidity of a salvage neck dissection is higher than in primary procedures. It is also well documented that after radiation, neck dissection has an increased rate of postsurgical complications, in addition to increased subdermal fibrosis, neck and shoulder stiffness, pain, and dysphagia.[1] Additionally,

disease control with salvage neck dissection is poorer than with primary neck dissection, as the disease tends to be biologically more aggressive and may be resistant to adjuvant treatment. Furthermore, fewer adjuvant treatment options may be available due to toxicity from previous therapies.[2] Finally, it is critically important to place salvage neck surgery in the overall context of the patient, and the overall disease burden. Patients with local disease recurrence in addition to regional disease recurrence often have poorer prognosis and are faced with more significant morbidity and radical changes to their quality of life in the setting of salvage surgery. In these patients, the prognosis and morbidity tend to be highly correlated with the site of recurrence. Generally, among patients presenting with synchronic local and regional recurrence, those with laryngeal or oral cavity primaries tend to fare better than those with oropharyngeal disease.[3] Given these inherent challenges, it is crucial for clinicians to be familiar with the workup, decision-making process, and technical considerations associated with nodal disease that may necessitate a salvage neck dissection.

10.2 Indications

There are several clinical scenarios in which a salvage neck dissection may be considered: (1) partial nodal remission following (chemo)radiation therapy; (2) complete nodal remission in a post(chemo)radiotherapy neck as part of a planned neck dissection; (3) disease recurrence in the neck following previous surgery (with or without radiation); (4) local disease recurrence in a previously treated N0 neck. These four potential indications for salvage surgery will be sequentially reviewed in subsequent subsections.

10.2.1 Partial Nodal Remission Following (Chemo)radiation Therapy or Complete Remission in a Post(chemo) radiotherapy Neck as Part of a Planned Neck Dissection

The most common scenario in which a salvage neck dissection is performed is in the context of a patient who has had (chemo) radiotherapy as initial treatment for a head and neck cancer. Chemoradiation—as a combined modality for advanced head and neck cancer—has allowed for improved organ preservation, with generally equivalent rates of locoregional control compared to surgery and adjuvant treatment. A patient who has been treated with (chemo)radiotherapy can have either a complete or an incomplete response to treatment.

There is an inverse relationship between the likelihood of complete response to treatment in relation to the size and overall burden of nodal disease,[4] with N1 nodal disease showing the best complete response to (chemo)radiotherapy, with relatively less complete response among patients with N2 and N3 disease.[5] For patients with less than complete response in neck lymph nodes, salvage neck dissection should be performed assuming the disease is surgically resectable.[6,7] For patients who have had complete remission of disease in response to therapy, those with original N1 disease do not require a salvage neck dissection.[8,9] It is among the N2 and N3 group patients wherein controversy has existed over whether a salvage neck dissection should be performed, even with complete response in the neck to (chemo)radiotherapy. The evidence for and against planned neck dissection for patients with N2/N3 disease will be explored in the following three subsections.

10.2.2 Evidence Supporting Planned Neck Dissection for N2/N3 Disease Following (Chemo)radiotherapy

Several studies lend support to planned neck dissection following irradiation only for head and neck squamous cell carcinoma (SCC) patients with N2/N3 disease. Mendenhall et al looked at 161 patients (oral cavity, oropharynx, nasopharynx, hypopharynx, supraglottic larynx, unknown head and neck primary) and found that after radiotherapy, initial control of neck disease dropped from 92% for N1 disease to 65% for N2a disease.[10] Dubray et al found similar poor results for N2/N3 necks after radiotherapy. In a series of 1,251 consecutive patients with node-positive oropharyngeal or pharyngolaryngeal SCC, the overall 3-year actuarial neck failure rates were 33% for N2 ($n = 103$) and 45% for N3 disease ($n = 699$).[11]

Studies incorporating both, radiotherapy arms and concurrent CRT arms, show similar results. In Lavertu et al's[9] retrospective review of a 100-patient, phase III randomized clinical trial comparing definitive concurrent CRT with radiotherapy alone, 35 of 53 patients with N2/N3 disease had a neck dissection. None of the patients in this cohort who had a complete response in the neck, and who also underwent a posttreatment neck dissection, experienced regional recurrence. In contrast, 25% of the patients who had a clinically complete response but did not undergo posttreatment neck dissection had regional neck recurrence.

From a histopathologic perspective, several studies have shown that a significant proportion of patients with N2/N3 disease continue to have pathologic disease, despite achieving a clinically complete response post-CRT.[12,13] McHam et al,[12] for example, looked at a series of 109 patients with head and neck SCC (excluding nasopharynx, paranasal sinus, and salivary gland tumors) who had N2 and N3 disease. All patients underwent CRT and a subsequent planned neck dissection at least 6 weeks after treatment. The authors found that 28% of N2 disease patients, and 42% of N3 disease patients had pathologic evidence of disease in the neck dissection specimens.

Additionally, it is also argued that salvage surgery in an unplanned fashion, when disease recurs, is often not successful, with local control rates ranging from 22 to 35%.[14] This is due to difficulty in achieving microscopically clear margins in a treated/fibrotic neck, coupled with limited adjuvant treatment options for microscopic disease. Finally, despite increased technical challenge, the immediate reported postoperative complication rates of planned neck dissection remain relatively low. Lavertu et al looked at a series of 100 patients treated in a phase 3 trial comparing radiotherapy alone with concurrent CRT for stage III and IV head and neck SCC. Twenty-nine planned neck dissections were performed for persistent neck disease or initial-stage N2 or greater. They found a major complication rate of 7% after neck dissection for radiation only, and 0% after neck dissection for chemoradiation.[15]

10.2.3 Evidence Refuting Planned Neck Dissection for N2/N3 Disease Following (Chemo)radiotherapy

Other studies have shown relatively low rates of neck failure after treatment with radiotherapy and CRT. Greven et al retrospectively reviewed 103 patients with stage III/IV, node-positive SCC (larynx, oropharynx, oral cavity, and hypopharynx) who had been treated with definitive radiotherapy or chemoradiation at a single institution with median follow-up of 42 months. CT scans were performed at a median of 4 weeks after treatment. The authors found that patients who had a radiographic complete response on posttreatment CT, and who underwent a neck dissection, had a nodal control rate of 94%, compared with 97% among those without neck dissection. On the other hand, patients with partial radiographic response who were treated with neck dissection had a nodal control rate of 94% compared with 73% among those without neck dissection. The authors concluded that patients who had a complete radiographic response on posttreatment imaging 4 to 6 weeks after radiation did not need a neck dissection.[16]

A series of 62 node-positive patients with oropharyngeal cancer from MD Anderson Cancer Center were treated with concomitant boost radiation and observed following complete response. The isolated neck failure rate was less than 5%, suggesting that observation is a reasonable approach in patients with nodal complete remission.[17] Subsequently, the same group looked at 880 patients with T1–T4, N1–N3 M0 SCC of the oropharynx, larynx, or hypopharynx who received CRT or radiotherapy alone. Nodal complete response occurred in 377 (43%) patients, of whom 365 patients did not undergo nodal dissection. The 5-year actuarial regional control rate of patients with complete response was 92%. Two hundred sixty-eight (53%) of the remaining 503 patients without complete response underwent salvage neck dissections, and the 5-year actuarial regional control rate for patients without a complete response was 84%. Those who had a neck dissection fared better, with 5-year actuarial regional control rates of 90% for those operated, versus 76% for those not operated ($p < 0.001$). Following initial (chemo) radiotherapy, this large study thus supports observation for patients with complete nodal response, but salvage surgery for patients with partial nodal response.[18]

10.2.4 Planned Neck Dissection for N2/N3 Disease: Current Evidence-Based Recommendations

Drawing conclusions from studies that support and refute the decision for planned salvage neck dissection for N2/N3 disease can be challenging, due to significant heterogeneous and confounding factors inherent in individual studies. Many factors influence neck disease remission following CRT, including location of the primary tumor (e.g., the high response rate observed in nasopharyngeal and human papillomavirus–associated oropharyngeal cancer) and nodal disease burden.

In particular, for posttreatment neck dissections that demonstrate positive pathologic disease, the timing of the neck dissection may be crucial in interpreting results. Even among patients with complete radiologic response to therapy, as many as 30 to 40% of neck dissection pathologic specimens may contain cancer.[19,20] However, neck dissections in such studies were performed relatively early posttreatment (4–6 weeks). Surgical pathology from an early (4–6 week) posttreatment neck dissection may produce falsely positive results related to tumor cells that are in the process of dying, but yet appear histopathologically positive in the initial posttreatment period. The use of proliferation markers such as Ki-67 may be useful in differentiating active proliferating tumor cells versus nonviable tumor cells.[21] When long-term clinical outcomes are analyzed, rather than analysis of early neck dissection pathology results, patients who obtain a complete clinical and radiological response to chemoradiation have a low (< 5%) risk of isolated neck recurrence.[22]

It has been difficult to prove significant benefit of salvage planned neck surgery for post(chemo)radiotherapy patients with complete radiographic response in the neck, regardless of the initial N staging.[9,23,24] It is now generally agreed that it is reasonable to observe an N2/N3 neck after (chemo)radiotherapy if there is no evidence of disease on cross-sectional imaging at 6 weeks after treatment. A negative PET scan at 12 weeks (to be discussed in subsequent sections) makes this approach even more attractive. A routine neck observation approach following CRT is especially favored if patients are reliable to undergo appropriate follow-up imaging at regular intervals. Hence, patient factors and relevant resources of the health care system may also be taken into account. Surveillance post-CRT, rather than planned neck dissection, is now widely accepted as a recommended practice.[25,26] However, in select cases, a planned neck dissection may be appropriate in the setting of adverse risk factors, which predispose to poorer ultimate regional control. For example, one may consider a planned salvage neck dissection in the context of large nodal disease burden (especially N3 disease) in non-nasopharyngeal, nonoropharyngeal SCC.

10.2.5 Disease Recurrence in the Neck Following Previous Surgery (with or without Radiation)

Salvage neck dissection may also be performed after a patient has been treated with previous neck dissection (with or without adjuvant postoperative therapy after the neck dissection). Disease recurrence may result from missed lymph nodes in dissected neck levels, extracapsular nodal disease extension that recurs in the soft tissues of the neck, or recurrence in lymph nodes in areas not previously dissected. Aggressive tumor histology has been found to be associated with recurrent neck disease.[27] In general, patients with recurrent nodal disease following a neck dissection should be offered a salvage neck dissection provided the disease is grossly resectable.

In a retrospective review of 699 radical neck dissections, Jones et al found that 119 patients who had undergone a radical neck dissection developed a nodal recurrence; of these, 69 were considered candidates for salvage surgery. Factors that increased the risk of neck recurrence were neck node (N) status and absence of adjuvant radiotherapy. The 5-year survival for salvage neck dissection was 31%, with younger patients and low T and N classification having improved survival.[28]

10.2.6 Local Disease Recurrence in an N0 Neck Previously Treated with (Chemo)radiation Therapy

Salvage neck dissection may be considered in the context of a patient with local disease recurrence, and an N0 neck after previous (chemo)radiotherapy. Salvage neck dissections in this scenario typically yield relatively low rates of neck nodal involvement (< 10%).[29] Radiation causes hyalinization and fibrosis of lymphatic structures, resulting in eventual narrowing of these structures,[30] which may explain the relative lower rates of subsequent nodal involvement when the primary tumor recurs.

Additionally, neck dissection performed in this setting seems to increase late adverse effects of radiation therapy (RT). In an analysis of three separate Radiation Therapy Oncology Group (RTOG) trials, severe late toxicity after CRT was quite common at 43%, and neck dissection after CRT was an independent risk factor for severe late toxicity with an odds ratio of 2.4.[31]

Dagan et al performed a retrospective review of patients treated with elective nodal radiation for T1–T4 N0 M0 SCC of the oropharynx, hypopharynx, or larynx who later developed an isolated local recurrence and remained N0. Fifty-seven patients were salvaged, 40 with neck dissection and 17 with neck observation. Four of 46 (9%) heminecks were found to have occult metastases in the surgical specimen. The 5-year local–regional control rate was 75% for all patients. Neck dissection resulted in poorer outcomes compared with observation. In the dissected group, the 5-year local control, regional control, cause-specific survival, and overall survival rates were 71, 87, 60, and 45%, respectively, compared to 82, 94, 92, and 56%, respectively, for the observation group. Toxicity was more likely with neck dissection. The authors concluded that in the setting of previous elective nodal irradiation, routine elective neck dissection should not be included during salvage surgery for locally recurrent head and neck SCC. The risk of occult neck disease is low, outcomes do not improve, and the likelihood of adverse effects increases.[29] For the case of elective salvage neck dissection associated with larynx cancer, the rate of occult nodal metastases has been shown to be about 5%, and there has not been demonstrated a regional control benefit to elective salvage neck dissection in this setting.[32]

In summary, elective salvage neck dissection in the locally recurrent primary with an already treated neck is not typically recommended. However, it should be recognized that many patients with local recurrence for head and neck SCC require free flap reconstruction of the primary site. Since in these cases the neck must be explored for flap recipient blood vessels, it is reasonable to resect any nodal basin(s) in the area of the respective exploration.

10.3 Workup

10.3.1 Confirmation of Disease

Some authors make an arbitrary distinction between residual and recurrent diseases, wherein residual disease is disease that remains after treatment (i.e., no disease-free interval) and recurrent disease is disease that becomes apparent after at least 6 months of complete regression. Regional, residual, or recurrent disease can be detected on clinical or radiologic follow-up. Depending on the philosophy and resources of the treating institution, follow-up imaging may be performed at various intervals in the first 5 years after treatment, and may take the form of ultrasound, CT, MRI, or PET scan.

CT scan with contrast is a quick and efficient means of obtaining a radiologic evaluation of the neck nodal status. The performance of CT scan in the post-CRT setting has been reported as 57 to 85% sensitivity, 24 to 79% specificity, 22 to 59% positive predictive value, and 73 to 94% negative predictive value.[20,33,34] In some institutions, MRI is the preferred modality of imaging for surveillance. MRI, with the use of diffusion weighted imaging (DWI) protocols based on tissue cellularity, may aid in discriminating between metastatic and benign neck adenopathy, with metastatic adenopathy demonstrating significantly higher apparent diffusion coefficient.[35]

Additionally, some have suggested that MRI may be better in distinguishing posttreatment changes versus recurrence in the primary tumor bed, based on T2 signal characteristics.[36] Hence, the neck is followed with the same imaging modality as the primary in this setting. However, other studies suggest that the superiority of MRI over CT scan in the follow-up of the primary bed is exclusively for nasopharyngeal cancers, rather than laryngeal and pharyngeal neoplasms.[37] A large meta-analysis by de Bondt et al comparing CT and MRI in the detection of lymph node metastases pretreatment in head and neck cancer showed

that MRI and CT scan had similar accuracy.[38] In many centers, CT is employed as a relatively cheap, quick, and readily available means of imaging surveillance.

While ultrasound-guided FNA biopsy is not first line in the routine surveillance of neck disease, it can be useful to confirm the presence of disease suspected on imaging on CT/MRI before committing to salvage surgery. In the de Bondt et al meta-analysis, the authors concluded that ultrasound-guided FNA biopsy was the most accurate imaging modality to detect cervical lymph node metastases. Ultrasound-guided FNA biopsy showed the highest diagnostic odds ratio (DOR) of 260, compared to ultrasound without FNA (DOR = 40), CT (DOR = 14), and MRI (DOR = 7).[38] Nonetheless, it must be stated that ultrasound-guided FNA biopsy is only useful with a positive result. In situations where cytological proof cannot be obtained from an ultrasound-guided FNA biopsy, intraoperative frozen section can be performed to confirm presence of disease before proceeding with surgical resection. In most cases, however, intraoperative frozen section is not feasible due to potential oncologic compromise in obtaining the samples (vs. favored en bloc specimen removal). As such, preoperative counseling and disclosure regarding the possibility of a pathologically negative specimen is a recommended practice.

PET-CT scan has a very high negative predictive value in the posttreatment neck. If the PET-CT is negative, it is very unlike that there is viable tumor present in the lymph nodes, even if there are persistent lymphadenopathies on other imaging modalities (CT, MRI, ultrasound). Its negative predictive value of 93 to 95% for the primary site, and of 94 to 100% for the neck, makes this imaging modality an attractive choice for the initial posttreatment follow-up regimen.[39] PET scans have the additional advantage of simultaneous assessment of distant disease; although these tests are resource intensive, patients with negative PET scan at 12 weeks posttreatment have a very low risk of subsequent failure.[40,41]

A large, multicentric randomized phase 3 trial involving 37 head and neck cancer centers in the United Kingdom recruited 564 patients to study the utility of PET in the evaluation of planned neck dissection post-CRT. The patients were randomized to planned neck dissection before or after CRT (control), or CRT followed by fludeoxyglucose PET-CT 10 to 12 weeks post-CRT with neck dissection only if PET-CT showed incomplete or equivocal response of nodal disease (intervention). There were 54 neck dissections performed in the surveillance arm, with 22 surgical complications, and 221 neck dissections in the neck dissection arm, with 85 complications. Quality-of-life scores were slightly better in the surveillance arm. The authors concluded that PET-CT-guided active surveillance after CRT showed similar survival outcomes compared to planned neck dissection but resulted in considerably fewer neck dissections, fewer complications, and lower cost, supporting the routine use of PET imaging in the posttreatment setting.[42] Although PET is useful in surveillance of the primary and neck after CRT, the resources of the treating institution and country must be taken into account when considering this as a standard practice. A resource-balanced approach that is employed in many centers in the United States is a single PET scan at 12 weeks posttreatment to rule out residual active tumor in nodal remnants, with further follow-up imaging (if necessary) limited to more cost-efficient modalities such as CT.

10.3.2 Extent of Disease and Operative Planning

Imaging is not only important in oncologic surveillance, but also in determining the extent of recurrent disease in order to assess resectability, develop an appropriate surgical plan, and counsel the patient on the potential morbidity of the procedure. Cross-sectional imaging (CT or MRI) can delineate disease extending beyond the confines of a lymph node to include involvement of the sternocleidomastoid muscle or internal jugular vein, either of which may require sacrifice with a salvage surgery. Sacrifice of a unilateral internal jugular vein has little functional consequence other than increased preponderance for postoperative lymphedema, while sacrifice of the entire sternocleidomastoid muscle will generally require vascularized tissue transfer (often a pectoralis muscle rotational flap into the neck) to cover the carotid artery. Most importantly, extranodal disease near the carotid sheath or in levels I and II of the neck may involve the vagus, hypoglossal, and/or spinal accessory nerves, all of which have important functional consequences in the event of sacrifice. Extranodal disease extending above the mandible or below the clavicle has implications on surgical access, which generally render disease not meaningfully resectable in a salvage setting for SCC. Carotid artery encasement (> 270 degrees) and involvement of the prevertebral fascia or brachial plexus are general contraindications to salvage surgery for SCC due to the combination of high morbidity and low prospects of long-term regional control.

10.3.3 Timing of Posttreatment Imaging

The timing of posttreatment imaging is critically important. False-positive results commonly occur if imaging is performed too early, as nodal remnants and hypermetabolic activity often continue to resolve over time.[43] However, delaying posttreatment imaging too long may result in loss of opportunity to intervene in the optimal surgical window following (chemo) radiation therapy. This window represents a short time frame, when fibrosis is less marked and surgery is technically easier to perform, or between resolution of the acute CRT injury and the onset of chronic CRT injury. Another obvious risk in delaying too long is the risk for disease progression. It is, therefore, recommended that CT or MRI be performed approximately 8 to 12 weeks after completion of CRT.[22]

For PET and PET-CT, the timing posttreatment is equally important. As treatment-related inflammation abates, false-positive results on posttreatment PET scan decrease proportionally (increased specificity and negative predictive as time from treatment completion increases).[40] The current recommendation for optimal timing of PET is approximately 12 weeks posttreatment.[22,40]

10.4 Technical Considerations

10.4.1 Which Neck Levels Should Be Included in Salvage Dissection?

The appropriate neck level to address in salvage dissection depends on the primary site, extent of original nodal disease, and current nodal status post(chemo)radiotherapy. Historically, neck dissection performed for presumed residual disease after (chemo)radiotherapy was performed as a comprehensive radical neck dissection to encompass all levels of disease (▶ Fig. 10.2a). However, in recent decades, modified radical and selective neck dissections have been demonstrated to offer equivalent disease control and decreased morbidity, unless there is invasion of the sternocleidomastoid muscle, internal jugular vein, and/or spinal accessory nerve.

Neck dissection after chemoradiation for advanced head and neck cancer is not without risks, especially related to wound healing. Davidson et al showed that a preoperative radiotherapy dose greater than 70 Gy was associated with complications in 58% of the patients, versus 29% if the dose was less than 70 Gy ($p = 0.09$). This trend was reflected primarily in wound complications, and reached significance for skin flap necrosis.[44] Others have shown initial increased incidence of spinal accessory nerve dysfunction, and a negative impact on quality of life, when all five neck levels were dissected.[45] In general, more extensive neck dissections with associated removal of fibrofatty tissue result in greater long-term fibrosis with subsequent deleterious effects on swallowing and neck mobility.[46]

Selective neck dissection is generally preferred to comprehensive neck dissection in the salvage setting. A selective neck dissection is one that involves the removal of at least three contiguous neck levels (▶ Fig. 10.3), whereas a superselective neck dissection is a neck dissection where only two contiguous levels are addressed (▶ Fig. 10.4). The concept of selective neck dissection is based on predictable patterns of lymphatic drainage, and lymphatic tumor spread in association with upper aerodigestive tract cancers.[47,48] However, this philosophy is based on the understanding of lymphatic drainage and lymphatic tumor spread in the untreated neck. In the situation of previous CRT, drainage patterns may potentially change. Nonetheless, several studies have shown that a selective or even superselective neck dissection is generally the preferred salvage option to both limit morbidity and ensure appropriate oncologic disease control.[49,50]

A study examining 28 postradiotherapy neck dissections for SCC found that only 1 of 28 neck dissections (23 of which were comprehensive) revealed cancer outside nodal levels II, III, and IV. Primary sites in this study were oropharynx ($n = 19$), nasopharynx ($n = 3$), and larynx/hypopharynx ($n = 3$). The one case with nodal disease outside levels II to IV was a patient with a 10-cm neck mass.[51] Another study by Stenson et al[13] suggests that level V need not be addressed unless there is gross disease in this level prior to RT.

Robbins et al examined a series of 106 neck dissections performed after concurrent intra-arterial chemoradiation. The extent of neck dissection was determined by extent of disease, as elucidated by posttreatment imaging. Three subgroups of patients were delineated by the extent of neck dissection: radical or modified radical neck dissection, selective neck dissection, and superselective neck dissection. With a median follow-up of 58 months, regional failure occurred in 11 (5%) of 240 patients: 2/12 (17%) in the modified radical neck dissection group, 3/65 (5%) in the selective neck dissection group, 0/7 in the superselective neck dissection group, and 6/156 (4%) in the no neck dissection group. The rates of overall survival and distant metastases were not significantly different among the three neck dissection subsets. Notwithstanding the selection bias

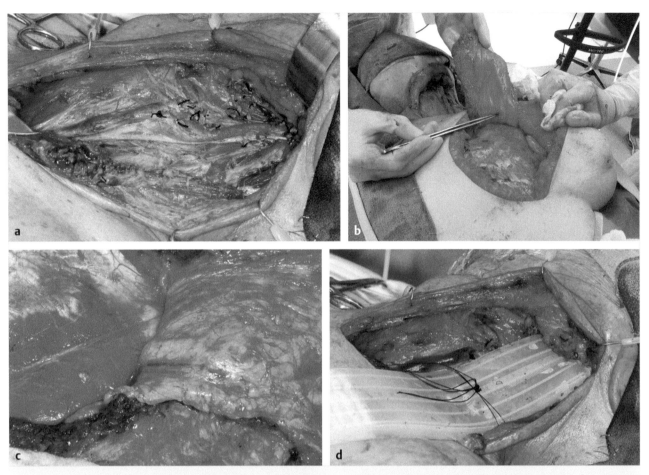

Fig. 10.2 (a) Radical neck dissection (with sacrifice of the spinal accessory nerve, internal jugular vein, and sternocleidomastoid muscle for recurrent neck squamous cell carcinoma, 2.5 years after definitive chemoradiation therapy an oropharyngeal primary. Dense, fibrotic scar tissue can be seen along the floor of the neck. (b) Harvesting of a pectoralis muscle flap for coverage of the carotid artery. (c) Closer view of the pectoralis muscle flap with several vascular pedicles. Note the thinning of the flap around the pedicle to allow for maximum length, so as to reach to the mastoid area. (d) Intraoperative insertion of brachycatheters. Catheters are typically placed at about 1-cm intervals along the tumor bed. The pectoralis muscle flap is then rotated into the neck to cover the brachycatheters.

among treatment groups, the authors concluded that selective and superselective neck dissections are viable therapeutic alternatives for patients with residual disease confined to one neck level after intra-arterial chemoradiation, and possibly other chemoradiation protocols.[52]

In another study by Robbins et al involving intra-arterial chemotherapy with concurrent radiation, 57 salvage neck dissections (the majority of which were selective neck dissections rather than modified radical neck dissections) were performed in 54 patients. A comparison was made between clinical and radiological findings, prior to neck dissection and review of final pathology. Only 2 of the 54 patients had evidence of pathologic disease extending beyond a single neck level: one had disease in a contiguous neck level, and the other had disease in a non-contiguous level. The use of superselective neck dissection with removal of only two contiguous neck levels would have encompassed known disease in all but one patient. The authors concluded that superselective neck dissection is a reasonable option for persistent nodal disease confined to one neck level.[49]

In summary, with the exception of oral cavity and nasopharyngeal cancers, levels I and V have a low incidence of nodal involvement,[13,50] implying that a comprehensive neck dissection

is not generally necessary for a curative resection post-CRT/RT. Selective and superselective neck dissections are favored in the salvage setting, and levels of dissection should be based on the presence of residual disease, and the site of origin of the primary tumor.

10.4.2 Timing of Neck Dissection

For cases where there is residual disease posttreatment (or in the setting of a planned salvage neck dissection), the timing of a salvage neck dissection is in many cases associated with the timing of posttreatment imaging (See section 3.1.3). Several studies have suggested that performing a salvage neck dissection between 8 and 12 weeks following completion of RT may be an optimal time frame as indicated by a low surgical complication rate for neck dissections performed in this interval.[13,15] This has been described as a surgical window between resolution of the acute (chemo)radiation injury and the onset of chronic chemo(radiation) injury. Lavertu et al observed a statistically significant higher rate of major surgical complications (20 vs. 3%), and overall complications (60 vs. 31%) after salvage neck dissection as compared to earlier planned neck dissection.[15]

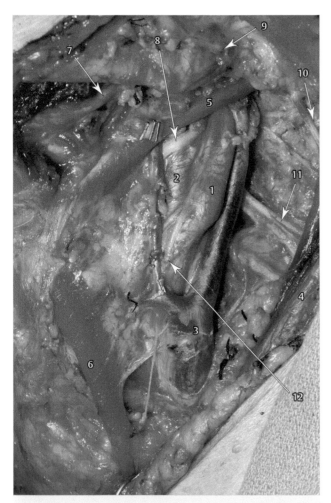

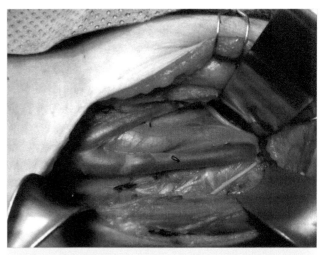

Fig. 10.4 Superselective neck dissection of levels II and III for residual squamous cell carcinoma of the neck at 14 weeks following chemo-radiation therapy. Visible preserved structures include the internal jugular vein, sternocleidomastoid muscle, spinal accessory nerve, and hypoglossal nerve. Dense fibrotic scar tissue can be noted along the floor of the neck with accompanying cervical rootlets.

Fig. 10.3 Selective neck dissection of levels I, II, and III following chemoradiation for oral cavity squamous cell carcinoma. Important neurovascular and muscular structures are labeled as follows: 1 = external carotid artery; 2 = internal carotid artery; 3 = internal jugular vein; 4 = sternocleidomastoid muscle; 5 = posterior belly of digastric; 6 = omohyoid muscle; 7 = lingual nerve; 8 = hypoglossal nerve; 9 = marginal mandibular nerve; 10 = accessory nerve; 11 = cervical rootlets; and 12 = ansa cervicalis.

However, a retrospective study by Goguen et al did not concur. This study compared the complication rate, and relapse rate, between neck dissections performed before 12 weeks and those performed after 12 weeks of completion of treatment. Sixty-seven neck dissections were performed less than 12 weeks posttreatment, while 38 were performed 12 weeks or more after completion of radiation. There was no statistically significant difference in the rate of major or minor complications between the two groups. There was also no difference in the regional relapse rate, progression-free survival, and overall survival between the two groups, with a median follow-up time for surviving patients of 56 (range 3–136) months. This author concluded that the timing of neck dissection may not influence oncologic outcomes or risk of complications.[53]

Notwithstanding the above study, delaying a salvage neck dissection in the presence of suspected disease (especially if the residual disease is sizeable) may lead to regional disease progression with the development of resistant clones.[1] Hence, all things considered, a common approach to imaging and potential neck dissection following (chemo)radiation therapy is to obtain cross-sectional imaging of the neck 6 to 8 weeks after treatment. Patients who have neck nodal remnants deemed as suspicious in axial imaging may undergo PET imaging no sooner than 12 weeks after completion of treatment. If the residual nodal disease is PET positive, a neck dissection is indicated, while patients with equivocal PET activity (low residual fluorodeoxyglucose activity) may either undergo ultrasound FNA, short-term observation with follow-up imaging, or proceed to salvage neck dissection.

10.4.3 Intraoperative and Postoperative Salvage Surgery Considerations

Typically, neck dissection following RT/CRT is technically more challenging due to fibrotic tissue planes. This fibrosis may be more pronounced in patients treated with chemoradiation as opposed to radiation alone. Blunt-tipped instruments, such as the Cooley Mayo-tipped scissors, may be particularly useful in this setting, especially when dissecting around the carotid artery. A significant challenge in the realm of salvage surgery is delineation of disease boundaries, which can be significantly obscured by fibrosis. It is critically important to excise circumferential margins around areas of residual disease, balancing this primary goal with a very close secondary goal of preservation of critical neurovascular structures.

In a salvage setting, if disease is adherent to surrounding muscle (e.g., sternocleidomastoid, digastric), then at least a cuff of muscle should be resected en bloc with the disease. In some cases where the disease is significantly invading the muscle, a complete resection of the muscle may be required. In these cases, mobilization of nonradiated, well-vascularized tissue is usually necessary to cover the exposed carotid artery. The most commonly used alternative for this purpose is reconstruction with a pectoralis muscle pedicled flap (▶ Fig. 10.2b,c). This flap is relatively easy to harvest, and has a robust pedicle and blood supply, making it extremely reliable

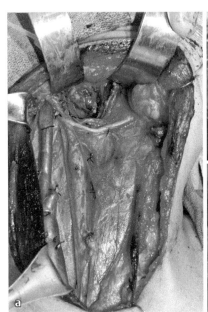
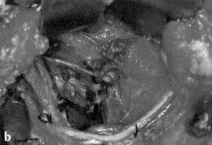
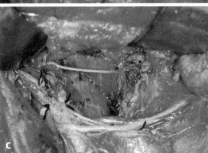

Fig. 10.5 (a) A 3.5-cm right retropharyngeal nodal metastasis. The right lateral neck levels II, III, and IV have been dissected, and the posterior belly of the digastric and stylohyoid muscles has been divided to expose the retropharyngeal space. The submandibular gland is preserved and retracted anteriorly. **(b)** Closer view of the 3.5-cm right retropharyngeal nodal metastasis. The disease underlies the glossopharyngeal nerve and internal carotid artery. The hypoglossal nerve is preserved inferiorly. **(c)** View of the retropharyngeal space following removal of the nodal metastasis, with preservation of glossopharyngeal nerve. The internal carotid artery is retracted laterally.

with the appropriate technique. Another reconstructive option is free tissue transfer (e.g., anterolateral thigh, radial forearm free flap), although this is technically more challenging and requires appropriate recipient vessels in the neck. In lieu of other recipient vessel options, which may be compromised by disease and/or fibrosis, the transverse cervical vessels should be remembered as a potential alternative.

In general, major cranial nerves (e.g., hypoglossal nerve, spinal accessory nerve, vagus nerve) should be resected only if grossly involved or completely encased by disease, but should not otherwise be resected to achieve a surgical margin. Sacrificing the internal jugular vein, on the other hand, is significantly less morbid, and this structure should be resected en bloc with the nodal specimen if there are any concerns for tumoral invasion.

An area of particular difficulty with dissection in a salvage setting, after previous surgery and/or (chemo)radiation, is the retropharyngeal area. Retropharyngeal nodal metastases are most common with pharyngeal and thyroid cancers, and surgical excision of retropharyngeal lymph nodes can be performed transcervically or transorally, although transcervical resection is generally favored in a salvage setting (► Fig. 10.5a–d). Treatment options for recurrent retropharyngeal nodal metastases include stereotactic re-irradiation, versus surgery, with or without postoperative adjuvant stereotactic reirradiation.[54] Since the hypoglossal and glossopharyngeal nerves often must be skeletonized and mobilized for access to the retropharyngeal area, these nerves are at particular risk for paresis in the setting of salvage surgery following radiation. Additionally, many small nerve branches innervating the upper pharyngeal constrictor must be divided when surgically removing retropharyngeal disease. In the setting of previous radiation, patients very often have temporary dysphagia, and a minority may even require temporary (or permanent) gastrostomy tube.

For patients who have recurrent neck disease beyond the initial postradiation period (i.e., after an initial negative postradiation scan), postoperative therapeutic options must be considered. Interstitial brachytherapy,[55] re-irradiation with intensity-modulated RT,[56] and proton therapy[57] have been demonstrated to improve locoregional control with reasonable

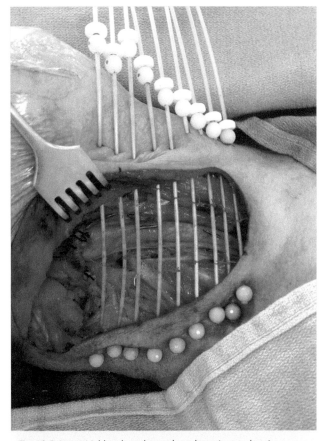

Fig. 10.6 Interstitial brachycatheters have been inserted at 1-cm intervals following salvage neck dissection for recurrent squamous cell carcinoma. Metallic clips mark the tumor boundary to facilitate postoperative dosimetry planning. A pectoralis muscle flap will be rotated into the neck to cover the brachycatheters.

tolerance and treatment-related morbidity (► Fig. 10.6). It should be emphasized that the decision for brachytherapy must be determined prior to surgery (since the catheters are inserted intraoperatively) and that vascularized tissue (e.g., pectoralis flap, free tissue flap) is generally necessary to improve tolerance and reduce morbidity and postoperative complications associated with postoperative adjuvant brachytherapy or re-irradiation. Finally, the importance of multidisciplinary discussion in the evaluation of patients for salvage neck surgery cannot be overemphasized, as intraoperative strategy and decision-making will be greatly influenced by preoperative multidisciplinary discussion and planning.

References

[1] Lango MN, Myers JN, Garden AS. Controversies in surgical management of the node-positive neck after chemoradiation. Semin Radiat Oncol. 2009; 19 (1):24–28

[2] Zafereo M. Surgical salvage of recurrent cancer of the head and neck. Curr Oncol Rep. 2014; 16(5):386

[3] Zafereo ME, Hanasono MM, Rosenthal DI, et al. The role of salvage surgery in patients with recurrent squamous cell carcinoma of the oropharynx. Cancer. 2009; 115(24):5723–5733

[4] Barkley HT, Jr, Fletcher GH, Jesse RH, Lindberg RD. Management of cervical lymph node metastases in squamous cell carcinoma of the tonsillar fossa, base of tongue, supraglottic larynx, and hypopharynx. Am J Surg. 1972; 124(4):462–467

[5] Armstrong J, Pfister D, Strong E, et al. The management of the clinically positive neck as part of a larynx preservation approach. Int J Radiat Oncol Biol Phys. 1993; 26(5):759–765

[6] Wolf GT, Fisher SG. Effectiveness of salvage neck dissection for advanced regional metastases when induction chemotherapy and radiation are used for organ preservation. Laryngoscope. 1992; 102(8):934–939

[7] Simon C, Goepfert H, Rosenthal DI, et al. Presence of malignant tumor cells in persistent neck disease after radiotherapy for advanced squamous cell carcinoma of the oropharynx is associated with poor survival. Eur Arch Otorhinolaryngol. 2006; 263(4):313–318

[8] Brizel DM, Prosnitz RG, Hunter S, et al. Necessity for adjuvant neck dissection in setting of concurrent chemoradiation for advanced head-and-neck cancer. Int J Radiat Oncol Biol Phys. 2004; 58(5):1418–1423

[9] Lavertu P, Adelstein DJ, Saxton JP, et al. Management of the neck in a randomized trial comparing concurrent chemotherapy and radiotherapy with radiotherapy alone in resectable stage III and IV squamous cell head and neck cancer. Head Neck. 1997; 19(7):559–566

[10] Mendenhall WM, Million RR, Cassisi NJ. Squamous cell carcinoma of the head and neck treated with radiation therapy: the role of neck dissection for clinically positive neck nodes. Int J Radiat Oncol Biol Phys. 1986; 12(5):733–740

[11] Dubray BM, Bataini JP, Bernier J, et al. Is reseeding from the primary a plausible cause of node failure? Int J Radiat Oncol Biol Phys. 1993; 25(1):9–15

[12] McHam SA, Adelstein DJ, Rybicki LA, et al. Who merits a neck dissection after definitive chemoradiotherapy for N2-N3 squamous cell head and neck cancer? Head Neck. 2003; 25(10):791–798

[13] Stenson KM, Haraf DJ, Pelzer H, et al. The role of cervical lymphadenectomy after aggressive concomitant chemoradiotherapy: the feasibility of selective neck dissection. Arch Otolaryngol Head Neck Surg. 2000; 126(8):950–956

[14] Kutler DI, Patel SG, Shah JP. The role of neck dissection following definitive chemoradiation. Oncology (Williston Park). 2004; 18(8):993–998, discussion 999, 1003–1004, 1007

[15] Lavertu P, Bonafede JP, Adelstein DJ, et al. Comparison of surgical complications after organ-preservation therapy in patients with stage III or IV squamous cell head and neck cancer. Arch Otolaryngol Head Neck Surg. 1998; 124(4):401–406

[16] Greven KM, Williams DW, III, Browne JD, McGuirt WF, Sr, White DR, D'Agostino RB, Jr. Radiographic complete response on post treatment CT imaging eliminates the need for adjuvant neck dissection after treatment for node positive head and neck cancer. Am J Clin Oncol. 2008; 31(2):169–172

[17] Peters LJ, Weber RS, Morrison WH, Byers RM, Garden AS, Goepfert H. Neck surgery in patients with primary oropharyngeal cancer treated by radiotherapy. Head Neck. 1996; 18(6):552–559

[18] Thariat J, Ang KK, Allen PK, et al. Prediction of neck dissection requirement after definitive radiotherapy for head-and-neck squamous cell carcinoma. Int J Radiat Oncol Biol Phys. 2012; 82(3):e367–e374

[19] Boyd TS, Harari PM, Tannehill SP, et al. Planned postradiotherapy neck dissection in patients with advanced head and neck cancer. Head Neck. 1998; 20 (2):132–137

[20] Velázquez RA, McGuff HS, Sycamore D, Miller FR. The role of computed tomographic scans in the management of the N-positive neck in head and neck squamous cell carcinoma after chemoradiotherapy. Arch Otolaryngol Head Neck Surg. 2004; 130(1):74–77

[21] Strasser MD, Gleich LL, Miller MA, Saavedra HI, Gluckman JL. Management implications of evaluating the N2 and N3 neck after organ preservation therapy. Laryngoscope. 1999; 109(11):1776–1780

[22] Wee JT, Anderson BO, Corry J, et al. Asian Oncology Summit. Management of the neck after chemoradiotherapy for head and neck cancers in Asia: consensus statement from the Asian Oncology Summit 2009. Lancet Oncol. 2009; 10 (11):1086–1092

[23] Goguen LA, Posner MR, Tishler RB, et al. Examining the need for neck dissection in the era of chemoradiation therapy for advanced head and neck cancer. Arch Otolaryngol Head Neck Surg. 2006; 132(5):526–531

[24] Clayman GL, Johnson CJ, II, Morrison W, Ginsberg L, Lippman SM. The role of neck dissection after chemoradiotherapy for oropharyngeal cancer with advanced nodal disease. Arch Otolaryngol Head Neck Surg. 2001; 127 (2):135–139

[25] Paleri V, Urbano TG, Mehanna H, et al. Management of neck metastases in head and neck cancer: United Kingdom National Multidisciplinary Guidelines. J Laryngol Otol. 2016; 130 S2:S161–S169

[26] Hermann RM, Christiansen H, Rödel RM. Lymph node positive head and neck carcinoma after curative radiochemotherapy: a long lasting debate on elective post-therapeutic neck dissections comes to a conclusion. Cancer Radiother. 2013; 17(4):323–331

[27] Petruzzelli GJ, Benefield J, Yong S. Mechanism of lymph node metastases: current concepts. Otolaryngol Clin North Am. 1998; 31(4):585–599

[28] Jones AS, Tandon S, Helliwell TR, Husband DJ, Jones TM. Survival of patients with neck recurrence following radical neck dissection: utility of a second neck dissection? Head Neck. 2008; 30(11):1514–1522

[29] Dagan R, Morris CG, Kirwan JM, et al. Elective neck dissection during salvage surgery for locally recurrent head and neck squamous cell carcinoma after radiotherapy with elective nodal irradiation. Laryngoscope. 2010; 120(5):945–952

[30] Burge JS. Histological changes in cervical lymph nodes following clinical irradiation. Proc R Soc Med. 1975; 68(2):77–79

[31] Machtay M, Moughan J, Trotti A, et al. Factors associated with severe late toxicity after concurrent chemoradiation for locally advanced head and neck cancer: an RTOG analysis. J Clin Oncol. 2008; 26(21):3582–3589

[32] Sandulache VC, Vandelaar LJ, Skinner HD, et al. Salvage total laryngectomy after external-beam radiotherapy: a 20-year experience. Head Neck. 2016; 38 Suppl 1:E1962–E1968

[33] Inohara H, Enomoto K, Tomiyama Y, et al. The role of CT and (18)F-FDG PET in managing the neck in node-positive head and neck cancer after chemoradiotherapy. Acta Otolaryngol. 2008; 7:1–7

[34] Tan A, Adelstein DJ, Rybicki LA, et al. Ability of positron emission tomography to detect residual neck node disease in patients with head and neck squamous cell carcinoma after definitive chemoradiotherapy. Arch Otolaryngol Head Neck Surg. 2007; 133(5):435–440

[35] Sumi M, Sakihama N, Sumi T, et al. Discrimination of metastatic cervical lymph nodes with diffusion-weighted MR imaging in patients with head and neck cancer. AJNR Am J Neuroradiol. 2003; 24(8):1627–1634

[36] King AD, Keung CK, Yu KH, et al. T2-weighted MR imaging early after chemoradiotherapy to evaluate treatment response in head and neck squamous cell carcinoma. AJNR Am J Neuroradiol. 2013; 34(6):1237–1241

[37] Hermans R. Head and neck cancer: how imaging predicts treatment outcome. Cancer Imaging. 2006; 6:S145–S153

[38] de Bondt RB, Nelemans PJ, Hofman PA, et al. Detection of lymph node metastases in head and neck cancer: a meta-analysis comparing US, USgFNAC, CT and MR imaging. Eur J Radiol. 2007; 64(2):266–272

[39] Gupta T, Master Z, Kannan S, et al. Diagnostic performance of post-treatment FDG PET or FDG PET/CT imaging in head and neck cancer: a systematic review and meta-analysis. Eur J Nucl Med Mol Imaging. 2011; 38 (11):2083–2095

[40] Porceddu SV, Jarmolowski E, Hicks RJ, et al. Utility of positron emission tomography for the detection of disease in residual neck nodes after (chemo)radiotherapy in head and neck cancer. Head Neck. 2005; 27 (3):175–181

[41] Yao M, Graham MM, Hoffman HT, et al. The role of post-radiation therapy FDG PET in prediction of necessity for post-radiation therapy neck dissection in locally advanced head-and-neck squamous cell carcinoma. Int J Radiat Oncol Biol Phys. 2004; 59(4):1001–1010

[42] Mehanna H, McConkey CC, Rahman JK, et al. PET-NECK: a multicentre randomised Phase III non-inferiority trial comparing a positron emission tomography-computerised tomography-guided watch-and-wait policy with planned neck dissection in the management of locally advanced (N2/N3) nodal metastases in patients with squamous cell head and neck cancer. Health Technol Assess. 2017; 21(17):1–122

[43] Liauw SL, Mancuso AA, Morris CG, Amdur RJ, Mendenhall WM. Definitive radiotherapy for head-and-neck cancer with radiographically positive retropharyngeal nodes: incomplete radiographic response does not necessarily indicate failure. Int J Radiat Oncol Biol Phys. 2006; 66(4):1017–1021

[44] Davidson BJ, Newkirk KA, Harter KW, Picken CA, Cullen KJ, Sessions RB. Complications from planned, posttreatment neck dissections. Arch Otolaryngol Head Neck Surg. 1999; 125(4):401–405

[45] Kuntz AL, Weymuller EA, Jr. Impact of neck dissection on quality of life. Laryngoscope. 1999; 109(8):1334–1338

[46] Agarwal J, Kundu S. Salvage neck dissection after chemoradiation in head and neck cancer: practice and pitfalls. Int J Head Neck Surg. 2012; 3(1):15–21

[47] Lindberg R. Distribution of cervical lymph node metastases from squamous cell carcinoma of the upper respiratory and digestive tracts. Cancer. 1972; 29 (6):1446–1449

[48] Shah JP. Patterns of cervical lymph node metastasis from squamous carcinomas of the upper aerodigestive tract. Am J Surg. 1990; 160(4):405–409

[49] Robbins KT, Shannon K, Vieira F. Superselective neck dissection after chemoradiation: feasibility based on clinical and pathologic comparisons. Arch Otolaryngol Head Neck Surg. 2007; 133(5):486–489

[50] Doweck I, Robbins KT, Mendenhall WM, Hinerman RW, Morris C, Amdur R. Neck level-specific nodal metastases in oropharyngeal cancer: is there a role for selective neck dissection after definitive radiation therapy? Head Neck. 2003; 25(11):960–967

[51] Yao M, Roebuck JC, Holsinger FC, Myers JN. Elective neck dissection during salvage laryngectomy. Am J Otolaryngol. 2005; 26(6):388–392

[52] Robbins KT, Doweck I, Samant S, Vieira F. Effectiveness of superselective and selective neck dissection for advanced nodal metastases after chemoradiation. Arch Otolaryngol Head Neck Surg. 2005; 131(11):965–969

[53] Goguen LA, Chapuy CI, Li Y, Zhao SD, Annino DJ. Neck dissection after chemoradiotherapy: timing and complications. Arch Otolaryngol Head Neck Surg. 2010; 136(11):1071–1077

[54] Pollard C, III, Nguyen TP, Ng SP, et al. Clinical outcomes after local field conformal reirradiation of patients with retropharyngeal nodal metastasis. Head Neck. 2017; 39(10):2079–2087

[55] Kupferman ME, Morrison WH, Santillan AA, et al. The role of interstitial brachytherapy with salvage surgery for the management of recurrent head and neck cancers. Cancer. 2007; 109(10):2052–2057

[56] Takiar V, Garden AS, Ma D, et al. Reirradiation of head and neck cancers with intensity modulated radiation therapy: outcomes and analyses. Int J Radiat Oncol Biol Phys. 2016; 95(4):1117–1131

[57] Phan J, Sio TT, Nguyen TP, et al. Reirradiation of head and neck cancers with proton therapy: outcomes and analyses. Int J Radiat Oncol Biol Phys. 2016; 96 (1):30–41

11 Complications of Neck Dissection

David J. Hernandez and Chad E. Galer

Abstract

The boundaries of the neck dissection bring the surgeon in close proximity to a number of nerves that are important for facial symmetry, voice production, swallowing, tongue sensation and movement, and diaphragm contraction. Under most circumstances, injury to any of these nerves should be considered an unanticipated complication during a neck dissection and often results in reduced patient quality of life. Mastery of the anatomy and a keen awareness of the potential pitfalls are required to minimize complications during a neck dissection. Early recognition of complications allows the surgeon to manage them expediently, which often spares the patient further morbidity and potentially mortality. The surgeon must have a clear understanding of the cranial nerves, arteries, veins, and lymphatics of the neck and be able to utilize landmarks and maneuvers to removal nodal packet contents safely. Nevertheless, the only effective way to completely avoid complication is to not operate at all. Thus, surgeons must also be versed in the recognition and management of complications as well as appreciate when to seek consultation with other physicians or surgeons.

Keywords: complication, neck dissection, anatomy, infection, blowout, stroke, nerve injury, chyle leak, air embolism, pneumothorax, hypoparathyroidism, blindness

11.1 Introduction

This chapter explores the various pitfalls encountered during neck dissections. A strong emphasis on mastering the anatomy will help avoid unnecessary morbidity. Every surgeon who performs neck dissections should be keenly aware of the potential complications he or she might face, be able to quickly diagnose them (especially if they are life threatening), and be capable of managing them to minimize further morbidity and potential mortality.

This chapter will focus on surgical complications specific to the neck dissection, and will not cover morbidity associated with primary tumor ablation (pharyngocutaneous fistula, thyroidectomy, etc.), reconstruction, and nonsurgical complications.

11.2 Wound Infection/Dehiscence

The excellent blood supply of the neck limits the rate of wound infection and dehiscence. In the absence of communication with the aerodigestive tract, neck dissection is a clean procedure and carries a wound infection rate of approximately 1%. This increases considerably when the aerodigestive tract is entered, with studies showing surgical site infection (SSI) rates (as strictly defined by the Centers for Disease Control and Prevention [CDC]) of between 3 and 41%.[1,2] Antibiotic prophylaxis can decrease this risk to about 13%.[1] Multiple antibiotic combinations have been tested, with the most common being cefazolin for clean procedures, and ampicillin-sulbactam for clean-contaminated. Clindamycin alone has been shown to be inferior to ampicillin-sulbactam, and it is recommended to add gram-negative coverage for patients who are allergic to penicillins.[3,4] Duration of antibiotic prophylaxis longer than 24 hours does not correlate with improvement in SSI rate.[5,6,7] Multiple factors have been shown to increase risk of SSI including medical (hypothyroidism, diabetes, smoking, methicillin-resistant *Staphylococcus aureus* colonization, hypoalbuminemia, history of previous radiation therapy) and surgical (operative time, operative blood loss, flap failure, operative takebacks, concomitant tracheostomy, osteocutaneous free flaps).[8,9,10] When possible, these should be addressed to reduce the risk of infection.

Wound dehiscence is often closely related to wound infection; however, it can occur primarily. Careful attention to incision planning, particularly in the case of previous surgery or radiation, is critical to avoid flap loss and subsequent dehiscence. Avoiding trifurcated incisions when possible, gentle tissue handling, subplatysmal dissection, meticulous closure, and elimination of dead spaces are all technical considerations that reduce the risk of wound complications. Similarly, avoidance of excess tension on the skin—particularly if skin is resected with the specimen—is mandatory to avoid diminished vascularity and secondary tissue loss.

11.3 Vascular Complications

11.3.1 Hemorrhage

Bleeding complications after a neck dissection typically cause issues related to local compression, rather than loss of blood volume and resultant hemodynamic instability. Hematomas typically develop in the immediate postoperative time frame, but there are reports of patients presenting 1 week postoperatively with acute hematomas requiring surgical treatment. Most hematomas should be managed with exploration in the operating room with control of any offending vessels. The overall incidence of postoperative hematoma after neck surgery is estimated to be 1 to 1.7%.[11]

Patients may develop difficulty breathing when a hematoma expands, and causes venolymphatic obstruction that leads to supraglottic edema (▶ Fig. 11.1). For this reason, once a hematoma is identified, it should be managed expediently, and, occasionally, bedside drainage is necessary to prevent upper airway obstruction if patients show signs of respiratory distress. The airway should be secured as soon as an expansile hematoma is identified.

Hematomas are best avoided by ensuring meticulous hemostasis during the dissection and prior to closing the wound. Many surgeons evaluate for bleeding using intraoperative Valsalva maneuver or Trendelenburg tilt. Several studies have shown that these maneuvers identify small bleeding points, but their use does not correlate with a reduction in hematoma formation.[12,13]

Numerous attempts have been made using specialized instruments (e.g., Harmonic scalpel) or hemostatic products to decrease intraoperative bleeding, and reduce rate of hematoma. Studies have shown some nonclinically significant improvement in intraoperative bleeding and postoperative drainage, but unfortunately are underpowered to detect differences in hematoma rates.[14,15,16,17,18] Proper patient selection, meticulous surgical technique, and thorough hemostasis are still the best practices for preventing postoperative hematoma.

Arterial spasm may also deceive the surgeon intraoperatively. Thus, it is advisable to routinely examine the superior thyroid, occipital, transverse cervical, and facial arteries at the end of a case if the nodal packets near these vessels were dissected.

Another rare but potentially serious bleeding complication can arise during a neck dissection if the patient has a tortuous

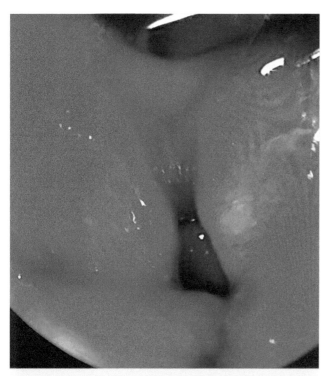

Fig. 11.1 Edematous false vocal folds and partially obstructed airway in a patient being intubated due to airway compromise caused by a neck hematoma.

carotid artery that results in a laterally displaced segment of carotid artery.[19] This can be particularly prominent in elderly patients (▶ Fig. 11.2). Such a segment of distorted carotid artery is prone to injury when dissecting the lateral nodal contents off the transition point between the floor of the neck and the carotid sheath. Vascular injury in these cases may be avoided by routinely reviewing the preoperative CT scan. Injury to the carotid artery during a neck dissection may result in life-threatening blood loss and stroke.

11.3.2 Internal Jugular Vein Blowout

Internal jugular vein (IJV) blowout has been reported and is usually associated with circumferential dissection of the vessel, desiccation of the vessel adventitia, and/or a concomitant salivary fistula.[20] This is a low-pressure system; therefore, bleeding is typically not florid, but it may be intermittent and associated with increased venous pressure as it occurs with coughing. At the time of surgical intervention, the carotid sheath should be carefully inspected, and consideration given to flap coverage in the context of a salivary fistula, as this situation also puts the carotid at risk of blowout.

11.3.3 Carotid Blowout Syndrome

This is defined as rupture of the carotid artery or branches caused by tumor involvement of the vessel, or as a result of late radiation toxicity. The level of severity is further subdivided into three clinical syndromes: *threatened blowout*, which refers to a clinically exposed vessel or radiologic evidence of tumor invasion to the vascular structure; *impending blowout*, when a herald bleed has settled spontaneously; and *acute carotid blowout syndrome*, with profuse, uncontrollable bleeding. When a carotid artery blowout is suspected, the surgeon typically has little time to act and mobilize resources. Radiation treatment and, particularly, re-irradiation place patients at increased risk of carotid blowout. Other contributing factors include a history of a neck dissection (particularly a radical neck dissection), fistula,

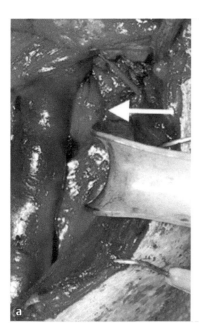
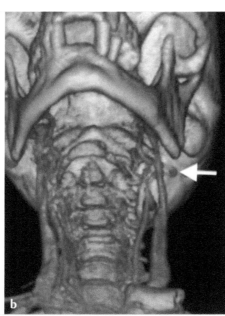

Fig. 11.2 **(a)** A tortuous segment of internal carotid artery (*white arrow*) is noted after a left neck dissection. This knuckle of artery may be mistaken for a prominent lymph node if care is not taken. **(b)** CT angiogram of a different patient with a more extreme example of an ectatic internal carotid artery (*white arrow*) on the left. (Image b reproduced with permission of Agarwal G, Gupta A, Chaudhary V, Mazhar H, Tiwari S. Rare anatomical variant of the cervical internal carotid artery. Br J Oral Maxillofac Surg 2017;55:530–532.)

devitalized soft tissue overlying the carotid, and cancer overlying or encasing the carotid.

Since survival is not guaranteed after developing this severe complication, extreme measures must be employed in managing it. This typically involves placing constant digital pressure over the area of hemorrhage, mobilizing a code team to actively start resuscitation while transporting the patient to the operating room, or to the interventional radiology suite, to ligate, bypass, stent, or embolize the carotid artery. In the case of operative intervention, the finger is prepped into the field and continuous pressure is maintained while wide exposure is obtained. If available, vascular surgeons may be of great assistance in managing this complex surgical scenario. More recently, excellent results have been obtained using endovascular stenting of the carotid artery.[21,22]

In patients with a known substantial risk of carotid blowout (e.g., patient with unresectable carcinoma encasing the carotid, with contiguous disease involving the skin or pharynx), a frank discussion should be undertaken with the patient regarding this often-fatal complication and the potential role of prophylactic endovascular intervention. Advanced directives should be strongly encouraged for these patients.

11.4 Neurologic Complications

11.4.1 Stroke

Stroke is a rare, but functionally devastating complication of neck dissection. The risk of stroke in older series ranged as high as 4.8%. These studies, however, were retrospective and did not account for variables such as smoking, which is also correlated with the risk of stroke.

In a systematic review of NSQIP (National Surgical Quality Improvement Program) data, Cramer et al reported an increased risk of stroke following a neck dissection in patients with at least two carotid artery stenosis (CAS) risk factors (age older than 65 years, smoking, diabetes mellitus, hypertension, congestive heart failure, renal failure, history of stroke or transient ischemic attack).[23] The risk for such patients was measured at 2.86% for bilateral neck dissections, 0.41% for unilateral neck dissection, and 0.24% for no neck dissection. Additionally, stroke was significantly associated with 30-day mortality (7.4%). Another large database study from Canada showed a similar stroke rate in 30 days following surgery (0.7%) as compared to non–head and neck major surgery. Similar risk factors were identified, but the data were not reported separately for the high-risk group.[24] Additionally, the authors found a significant decrease in incidence from 1995 to 2012 (1.1–0.3%).

In patients with carotid artery disease, or risk factors for CAS, extra care should be taken to avoid retraction of the carotid sheath, and unnecessary manipulation of the carotid. If a very high-grade stenosis is identified on imaging, consideration can be made for preoperative endarterectomy, with careful consideration of the risk in the oncologic context.

11.4.2 Spinal Accessory Injury

Spinal accessory nerve injuries are best avoided by understanding not only the anatomic relationships of the nerve within the neck, but also that many patients with shoulder dysfunction after a neck dissection have an anatomically intact nerve. While the

rate of unintended transection of the spinal accessory nerve is exceedingly low in experienced hands, the rate of shoulder syndrome after radical neck dissection is estimated to be 47 to 100%.[25] In addition, careful evaluation of shoulder function after neck dissection shows an approximately 20% reduction in function following a selective neck dissection, and up to 50% reduction following a modified radical neck dissection (with dissection of spinal accessory in level V as well). A program of physical therapy in the postoperative period is helpful in reversing weakness and postoperative pain, and it is routinely offered to patients after neck dissection at many institutions.[26,27]

Injury to the spinal accessory nerve during a neck dissection may result from excessive traction and/or devascularization of the nerve. Direct traction on the nerve with a retractor should be avoided at all times during the procedure. If needed, a retractor may be placed on the sternocleidomastoid muscle (SCM) immediately cranial or caudal to the insertion of the spinal accessory nerve. Devascularization of a segment of the nerve is often difficult to avoid during dissection of level IIB (in addition to level IIA).[28] Bipolar electrocautery or cold techniques are best used near the nerve to avoid thermal injury as well. An additional area of concern for spinal accessory injury is in the posterior triangle of the neck, where the nerve is very superficial and can be injured while raising the skin flaps. Furthermore, in this area the nerve tends to be tortuous and may have a branching pattern, so meticulous attention to its meandering is critical to avoid injury.

Technically, the nerve is easily identified in the carotid triangle by slowly unwrapping the fascia of the SCM. The tendinous portion of the SCM is superficial to the nerve. The occipital perforating vessels supplying the upper portion of the SCM are found immediately superficial to the nerve (▶ Fig. 11.3). The bony landmark for the point where the nerve intersects with the IJV is the transverse process of the atlas, or C1.[29] Typically, the nerve traverses the IJV superficial—or lateral—to the vein (40–96%).[30] Occasionally, the nerve crosses deep—or medial—to the nerve (3–57%), and, rarely, the nerve courses through a fenestrated or bifurcating vein (▶ Fig. 11.3). There is even a report of the nerve splitting around the vein.[27] Given the variable relationship between the spinal accessory nerve and the IJV, it is prudent that surgeons be aware of this variability to avoid unnecessary injury to the IJV or spinal accessory nerve.

Dissection of level V places the nerve at increased risk due to its superficial course in this location. A firm grasp of the surgical planes and the course of the nerve in the posterior triangle is key to avoid injury. Identifying the anterior border of the trapezius is most helpful, since the nerve typically courses 1 to 2 cm inferior and parallel to this landmark. The nerve typically enters the anterior surface of the trapezius 2 to 5 cm superior to the clavicle. Along the posterior border of the SCM, the spinal accessory nerve is located typically within 1 cm superior to Erb's point.[29]

11.4.3 Marginal Mandibular Nerve Injury

The marginal mandibular nerve (MMN) is most relevant during a level I neck dissection, and to a lesser extent during access to the superior limit of level II. This branch of the facial nerve is responsible for innervating the depressors of the lower lip: the depressor anguli oris and depressor labii inferioris muscles. The

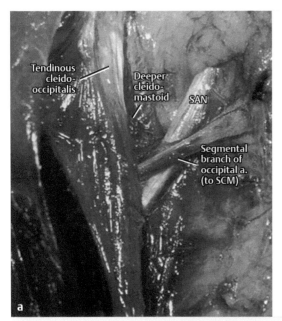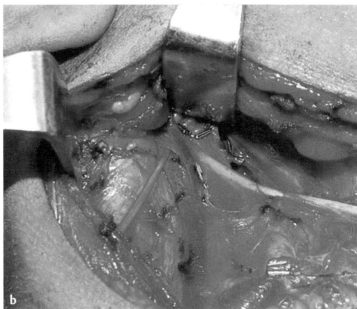

Fig. 11.3 **(a)** Right spinal accessory nerve identified immediately deep to the perforating occipital vessels supplying the superior sternocleidomastoid muscle. **(b)** Rare example of a spinal accessory nerve traversing between a fenestrated internal jugular vein. (Reproduced with permission of Tatla T, Kanagalingam J, Majithia A, Clarke PM. Upper neck spinal accessory nerve identification during neck dissection. J Laryngol Otol 2005;119:906–908.)

consequence of the injury is an asymmetric smile, as well as some perceived difficulty with drinking and eating.[31]

Using the traditional House–Brackmann scale to assess lower domain facial nerve function, Møller et al reported a 14% rate of weakness at 2 weeks post-op, which had decreased to about 4% on long-term follow-up.[32] In another study by Batstone et al, up to a 23% incidence of weakness, 31% initially and decreasing to 13% between 1 and 2 years, was identified.[31] A subgroup of patients experience significant distress over this.

Transient lower lip weakness often develops after a neck dissection due to the disruption of the cervical branch of the facial nerve, which innervates the platysma. The weakness of the lower lip due to loss of platysmal function is self-limiting when the MMN is left intact.[33] The key to avoiding injury to the MMN —as is the case with avoiding injury to any other nerve—is having a firm grasp of the anatomy.

The MMN may actually consist of more than one nerve branch. It typically crosses the facial artery 1.73 mm inferior to the lower border of the mandible.[34] Thus, the facial notch is a very reliable landmark when identifying the MMN. Subplatysmal flap elevation will avoid injury to the MMN since the nerve lies in a fascial layer deep to the platysma. The nerve is found superficial to the facial artery and vein. The Hayes Martin maneuver consists in ligating the facial vein inferior to the mandible (approximately at the level of the inferior border of the submandibular gland) retracting the superior vein stump superiorly. This protects the nerve in the fascial plane, superficial to the facial vein, without definitively identifying it. However, whenever perifacial node dissection is necessary, the MMN must be skeletonized and retracted above the level of the mandible. It is recommended that careful dissection of the nerve begin at the level of the facial notch, as this is a consistent landmark as noted earlier. Once the nerve is identified at the facial notch, it should be dissected anteriorly and posteriorly until it may be retracted above the level of the mandible.

Unilateral MMN paralysis may result in an asymmetric smile, asymmetry during expression of certain facial emotions, oral incompetence, drooling, and lip biting.[35] Treatment of a unilateral MMN injury, should it prove to be a permanent paralysis, is centered on restoring symmetry to the lower lip. This may be accomplished in a number of methods aimed at either restoring mobility to the lip on the unilateral side or paralyzing the contralateral lower lip. The contralateral lower lip depressors may be paralyzed temporarily with injection of botulinum toxin[33] or by resecting the contralateral depressor labii inferioris muscle.[35] Alternatively, procedures aimed at restoring movement of the paralyzed lower lip include the anterior belly digastric muscle flap[33,36] and the extensor digitorum brevis free flap.[33]

11.4.4 Vagus Nerve Injury

The vagus nerve is at greatest risk for injury when a radical neck dissection is performed. On occasion, the neck disease may directly involve the vagal nerve as it may involve the IJV and the carotid artery. During sacrifice of the IJV, it is prudent to ensure that the vagus nerve is not inadvertently ligated. This is best avoided by carefully dissecting the IJV circumferentially in order to exclude the vagal nerve. If possible, visually confirming the location of the vagal nerve within the carotid sheath should also reassure the surgeon that it is not injured during dissection within the carotid sheath.

The vagal nerve is situated posteriorly within the carotid sheath, between the IJV and the carotid artery, and the most common clinical manifestation in case of an injury is ipsilateral vocal cord paralysis. Depending on the location of injury, vagal nerve fibers that supply the superior vagal nerve may also be affected, which may affect laryngeal sensation and contribute to aspiration. Dysphagia may also result from a high vagal nerve injury, due to the vagal nerve branches that innervate the pharyngeal constrictors and other muscles involved with deglutition.

Immediate neurography should be performed after a vagal nerve injury is identified, while an interposition nerve graft should be attempted if there is anatomical discontinuity of the nerve. When the nerve is injured, patients will acutely present with a hoarse, breathy voice in the immediate postoperative period. Since aspiration is a common associated feature, a formal evaluation of swallowing is recommended prior to resuming oral diet. The management of the vocal cord paralysis will depend on the nature of the injury, and the prognosis for full recovery. A temporary vocal cord medialization can provide significant symptomatic relief while allowing time to observe for nerve regeneration. If the functional prognosis is estimated to be poor—or if the patient has failed to improve—more definitive approaches such as a type I thyroplasty are indicated. Involving a laryngologist early after the injury can be very helpful to inform these decisions.

11.4.5 Phrenic Nerve Injury

The phrenic nerve is derived from the third, fourth, and fifth cervical nerves. It takes a slightly lateral-to-medial course in the neck, along the anterior surface of the anterior scalene muscle (▶ Fig. 11.4). It is at greatest risk to injury during dissection of levels III and IV. The phrenic nerve lies immediately deep to the fascia overlying the anterior scalene muscle (prevertebral fascia),

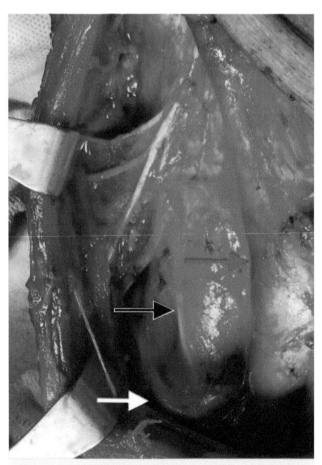

Fig. 11.4 Following a right neck dissection, the phrenic nerve (*black arrow*) is seen coursing from lateral to medial overlying the anterior scalene muscle. The transverse cervical artery (*white arrow*), the internal jugular vein (*blue arrow*), and cervical rootlets are pictured as well. The sternocleidomastoid muscle is retracted laterally.

which comprises part of the floor of the neck. During a neck dissection, phrenic nerve injury is avoided by carefully preserving this fascial layer while detaching the contents of levels III and IV from the floor of the neck. It is also necessary to be prudent with the use of electrocautery in this area, particularly in the event of an injury to the transverse cervical vessels.

Injury to the phrenic nerve results in hemidiaphragm paralysis. Hemidiaphragm paralysis can also occur with an intact phrenic nerve if the branches from the third to fifth cervical nerves are damaged near the cervical plexus. This diagnosis may be suspected on chest X-ray, but the more confirmatory diagnostic would be chest fluoroscopic radiography in which a patient is asked to sniff or inspire forcefully. The affected diaphragm fails to depress during this maneuver when it is paralyzed. This complication is typically not accompanied by long-term respiratory insufficiency as long as the other phrenic nerve is intact, provided that the patient's respiratory function is not marginal at baseline. It can lead to exertional dyspnea, however. Bilateral phrenic nerve paralysis is more likely to require artificial respiratory support. Plication of the paralyzed diaphragm is a potential treatment option for a paralyzed diaphragm.

11.4.6 Hypoglossal Nerve

The hypoglossal nerve is typically not in great danger of injury during a neck dissection, except during a radical or extended neck dissection with disease involving the nerve. The hypoglossal nerve is deep to the ranine veins, which are encountered just deep and inferior to the posterior belly of the digastric muscle. The proximal nerve is located posterior to the carotid artery and distally it is found on the lateral surface of the hyoglossus muscle. Dissecting superficial to the ranine veins and keeping these vessels intact will ensure the hypoglossal nerve is not injured and prevent the nuisance bleeding that may be encountered from these veins. Anecdotally, it is during attempts to control bleeding from ranine veins that accidental injury to the hypoglossal nerve may result. Thus, the ranine veins are not necessarily ligated during a neck dissection. The hypoglossal nerve should also be routinely identified prior to ligating the facial artery in level IB, as the proximal segment of the hypoglossal nerve often runs parallel to and has a similar caliber to the facial artery.

11.4.7 Lingual Nerve

The lingual nerve is encountered during dissection of the submandibular triangle, in the context of either level IB neck dissection or submandibular gland excision. While there is a paucity of data regarding lingual nerve injury in neck dissection, the incidence has been reported between 0 and 4.4% in submandibular gland excision. Generally, unless involved by tumor, the lingual nerve is robust and easily identified during the procedure. However, care must be taken while dividing the submandibular ganglion to place clamps far enough from the "elbow" of the lingual nerve to avoid crush injury.

11.4.8 Brachial Plexus

The brachial plexus is located between the anterior and middle scalene muscles. It is identified in level IV and V dissections. As with the phrenic nerve, it is deep to the prevertebral fascia, so careful dissection superficial to this plane will prevent injury. Fortunately, this nerve complex is rarely injured during neck dissection although it has been reported in the literature.

11.4.9 Sympathetic Chain

The sympathetic chain and ganglion lie posterior to the carotid artery. Injury will result in ipsilateral Horner's syndrome (miosis, ipsilateral ptosis, and anhidrosis). To avoid encountering the sympathetic chain, the surgeon must remember to "climb the mountain" and transition from dissecting along the prevertebral fascia laterally to coming over the great vessels medially.

11.4.10 Cervical Rootlets

Another consideration to be made during a neck dissection is to the preservation of the cervical root branches. Garzaro et al reported significantly improved shoulder mobility and quality of life in patients who preserved cervical root branches compared to patients who had these nerves transected during their neck dissection.[37] There was also significantly less loss of cutaneous sensation in the preservation group. Another study also noted lower pain scores and less head and neck pain when the spinal accessory nerve was spared during a neck dissection.[38] This study also found that dissection of level V, which typically involves sacrifice of the cervical rootlets, is associated with worse pain and quality of life, even when the spinal accessory nerve is spared. Thus, cervical root branches should be spared during a selective neck dissection, especially when performed in the context of an N0 neck, to minimize perioperative morbidity.

11.5 Chyle Leak

Dissection of the left level IV nodal packet should always be done cautiously and with attention to the area of the thoracic duct. While encountering and injuring the thoracic duct itself is not a serious complication, an unidentified thoracic duct injury that is not addressed intraoperatively may result in a postoperative chylous fluid leak, or chyle leak. This complication often presents as turbid, opaque, and often milky fluid drainage that shows up in the bulb of a closed suction drain, particularly after the patient begins to eat (▶ Fig. 11.5). Thus, it may present somewhat delayed if the patient's enteral nutrition is restricted in the immediate postoperative period. The thoracic duct transports chyle, which consists of lymph and free fatty acids (emulsified fats), from the abdomen to the left neck. It empties into the systemic circulation at the junction between the left IJV and the left subclavian vein (▶ Fig. 11.5). It is the largest lymphatic duct in the body. The right lymphatic duct empties in a similar location in the right neck. While we often think of chyle leaks occurring in the left level IV neck, approximately 25% of the time chyle leaks occur on the right,[39] but these tend to be self-limited and can be managed conservatively. The overall incidence of chyle leaks is around 3%, although estimates range up to 5.7%.

Intraoperatively, it is prudent to always inspect level IV after a lateral neck dissection, to look for any frank chyle fluid. Most clinically significant chyle leaks are first identified intraoperatively. A Valsalva maneuver may help identify and localize a

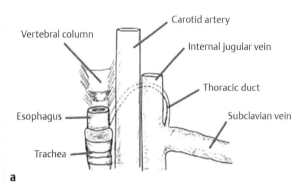

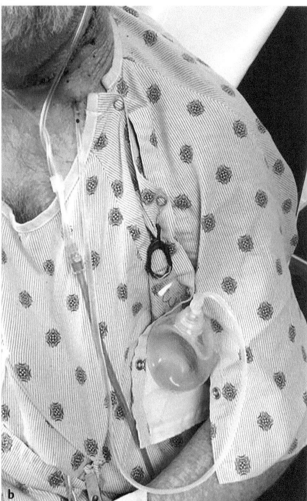

Fig. 11.5 (a) Illustration of the thoracic duct as it empties into the junction of the left internal jugular vein and subclavian vein. (Adapted from Delaney et al.[41]) (b) Post-op day 1 picture of a patient with a bulb suction drain collecting fluid consistent with a chylous leak.

lymphatic leak, as the increased intrathoracic pressure acts to advance chyle within the thoracic duct. If a chyle leak is identified intraoperatively, it should be clipped, tied, or suture ligated. If possible, the duct should be ligated with some associated soft tissue, as the thin wall is easily torn. A Valsalva maneuver should be repeated after the repair to ensure the leak has been addressed. In these cases, the suction drain output should be watched closely postoperatively.

If a chyle leak is suspected in the postoperative setting, conservative measures should be taken initially. The patient should be started on a medium chain fatty acid diet or enteral feeding depending on the circumstances. Fluids and electrolytes should be monitored and repleted as needed. The head of bed should be elevated, activity should be restricted, and stool softeners should be given. These measures reduce the flow of chyle fluid in the thoracic duct by limiting increases in intrathoracic pressure. At times, pressure dressings are utilized, but many surgeons find them ineffective and risk pressure necrosis of the skin flaps. Close monitoring of the drain output can be used to assess the patient's progress.

Octreotide is a synthetic formulation of somatostatin, which is a neuroendocrine hormone that inhibits the release of a variety of gastrointestinal hormones that regulate digestion and absorption. It reduces the production of chyle, and decreases the flow of lymphatic and chylous fluid. This medication has proven to be an important adjunct in the armamentarium against chyle leaks.[40,41]

Historically, chyle leaks have been divided into low- and high-output leaks depending on the amount of chyle collected from the drain, with the arbitrary cutoff value of typically 500 mL/d. More important than focusing on a value of drain output is assessing the response to conservative treatment. Persistent chyle leaks should be managed more aggressively. This may entail transcervical exploration with ligation of any identifiable offensive lymphatic channels. Additionally, consideration should be made to rotating some muscle into the area of the leak and/or applying a topical agent such as a cyanoacrylate adhesive, fibrin glue, or polyglactin mesh.[42,43] Other interventions reserved for the most recalcitrant chyle leaks include embolization and thoracoscopic thoracic duct ligation.[41,44] Total parenteral nutrition (TPN) may also be utilized in cases refractory to conservative measures; however, the risks of TPN—such as infection—must be weighed heavily prior to pursuing this approach.

11.6 Venous Air Embolus

This is a rare but potentially fatal complication that merits attention. A venous air embolism may occur when atmospheric air is exposed to a large vein, such as the IJV, and there exists a gradient for air to enter the systemic venous circulation, which may occur if the neck is slightly elevated above the heart. This complication may present with a sudden drop in end-tidal CO_2 and arterial blood pressure. A "mill-wheel" murmur may be heard over the precordial area. If this complication is suspected, local pressure with a moist lap should be applied to the neck or the bleeding should be controlled quickly. The patient should then be placed in the left lateral decubitus (Durant's maneuver) and simultaneously in the Trendelenburg position. This maneuver lodges the air bubble in the apex of the right ventricle and prevents its propagation into the pulmonary arteries, which may result in right ventricular outflow obstruction. In severe or extreme cases, a central venous catheter should be used to aspirate the air from the right atrium. Advanced cardiac life support (ACLS) protocol should be followed as necessary. The definitive treatment of venous air emboli, as is the treatment of decompression syndrome, is hyperbaric oxygen.[45]

11.7 Pneumothorax

Dissection that involved levels IV and V, particularly level VB or the supraclavicular nodes, potentially places the lung apices at risk for pleural violation. This rare complication is avoided by properly demarcating the dissection inferiorly. The clavicle and transverse cervical vessels are useful landmarks to avoid dissection beyond the inferior limits of a level IV and V neck dissection. In certain patients, superiorly displaced lung apices may redispose to this injury. Patients with bulky level IV and V nodal disease are also at increased risk of pneumothorax.

If the pleural space is violated during a neck dissection, the pleura should be repaired primarily with suture whenever possible, and rarely requires any further intervention if identified and repaired promptly. When this complication is not identified immediately, the patient may develop tachycardia, hypotension, hypercapnia, and hypoxia. This may occur intraoperatively or in the postanesthetic care unit. If the patient is awake and conscious, they may complain of chest pain. If these symptoms and/or signs develop, a tension pneumothorax should be suspected and requires immediate treatment. This can be confirmed by auscultation of breath sounds and confirmed with a chest X-ray. However, when emergent intervention is required, the patient should be intubated (if not already) and a chest tube should be placed immediately. Conversely, if a small pneumothorax is identified on chest X-ray in a stable, asymptomatic patient who is spontaneously breathing via his or her native airway, it can likely be followed clinically and radiographically with serial chest X-rays. These pneumothoraxes normally resorb spontaneously. If this same patient were receiving positive pressure ventilation, a chest tube would likely be required. Typically, consultation with a thoracic surgeon is prudent to ensure proper management of this rare complication.

11.8 Hypoparathyroidism/ Hypocalcemia

The risk of hypocalcemia as a result of surgical hypoparathyroidism is not only associated with endocrine surgery, but may also develop following procedures involving central neck compartments such as total laryngectomy. In the literature, the rate of transient hypoparathyroidism and hypocalcemia has been reported at greater than 50% when a bilateral central neck dissection is performed in addition to the thyroidectomy.[46,47] The rate of permanent hypoparathyroidism and hypocalcemia after this procedure has been reported at 12 to 16%.[48,49]

The keys to avoid this complication are proper patient selection and judicious indication of bilateral central neck dissections. Updated ATA (American Thyroid Association) guidelines[50] recommend against prophylactic central neck dissection for T1–T2, noninvasive, clinically node-negative papillary thyroid carcinoma, and most follicular cancers. In fact, according to these guidelines, only a weak recommendation could be made for *considering* a prophylactic central neck dissection: (1) node-negative T3–T4 papillary thyroid cancer, (2) presence of metastatic lateral neck nodes, or (3) gather information that will aid for further treatment planning.

When deciding on the need for an elective dissection of the central compartment in the context of squamous cell carcinoma of the hypopharynx, it is relevant to know the risk of central nodal disease based on the subsite of the primary. Joo et al reports the rate of paratracheal—or central neck nodal disease—for postcricoid, piriform sinus, and posterior pharyngeal wall cancers at 58, 20, and 8%, respectively.[51]

In terms of surgical technique, prevention of hypoparathyroidism depends on properly identifying parathyroids and preserving their blood supply during a central neck dissection. Any overtly devascularized parathyroid glands should be reimplanted in a well-vascularized muscle, after previous confirmation of histology on frozen section analysis. While the superior parathyroid glands are typically located dorsal to the recurrent laryngeal nerve, and the inferior parathyroids are generally ventral to the nerves, the location of parathyroid glands is highly variable, and the glands may be intrathyroidal, in nonstandard locations in the neck, or within the mediastinum.

11.9 Cerebral Edema/Blindness

Ligation of bilateral IJVs may result in severe facial edema and increased intracranial pressure (ICP). The elevated ICP is typically accompanied by systemic hypertension as a result of Cushing's reflex. This may manifest in altered mental status in addition to the obvious facial edema. Even when only unilateral ligation of the IJV is performed, thrombosis of the contralateral IJV may result in this complication. In general, performing bilateral IJV ligation should be avoided whenever possible. It is worthwhile being aware that even when an IJV is preserved, postoperative thrombosis may occur, but this risk is minimized by preventing desiccation of the vessel and minimizing surgical trauma. It should also be noted that performing unilateral neck dissection may result in elevated ICP if the contralateral neck has been previously dissected or treated with radiation. Thus, whenever possible, preservation of the superficial venous drainage such as external jugular veins should be attempted. The management of this complication includes head of bed elevation, fluid restriction, corticosteroids, mannitol, and hyperventilation. The ICP normalizes within 24 hours usually.

Another rare but devastating complication to consider is blindness. Typically, blindness is associated with bilateral radical neck dissections, but reports have been made of this occurring following less radical surgery. The blindness is described as nonarteritic anterior (or posterior) ischemic optic neuropathy. The etiology of this complication is likely multifactorial and is associated with hypotension, anemia, and increased intracranial venous pressure, which is likely to occur after bilateral IJV sacrifice. The blindness presents postoperatively and is typically bilateral. If the IJVs were resected or ligated, the prognosis is poorer and typically permanent. If vision loss or blindness occurs in the setting of at least one preserved IJV, the prognosis is improved for recovery of vision. In addition to ophthalmologic consultation, steroids and diuretics may be given empirically, but this has not been proven to be very effective.[52]

11.10 Conclusion

Neck dissection is an essential part of the treatment of many head and neck cancers. In experienced and vigilant hands,

nodal clearance can be successfully performed with acceptable morbidity. Many pitfalls await the unwary.

References

[1] Jain U, Somerville J, Saha S, et al. Oropharyngeal contamination predisposes to complications after neck dissection: an analysis of 9462 patients. Otolaryngol Head Neck Surg. 2015; 153(1):71–78

[2] Cannon RB, Houlton JJ, Mendez E, Futran ND. Methods to reduce postoperative surgical site infections after head and neck oncology surgery. Lancet Oncol. 2017; 18(7):e405–e413

[3] Weber RS, Raad I, Frankenthaler R, et al. Ampicillin-sulbactam vs clindamycin in head and neck oncologic surgery. The need for gram-negative coverage. Arch Otolaryngol Head Neck Surg. 1992; 118(11):1159–1163

[4] Pool C, Kass J, Spivack J, et al. Increased surgical site infection rates following clindamycin use in head and neck free tissue transfer. Otolaryngol Head Neck Surg. 2016; 154(2):272–278

[5] Mitchell RM, Mendez E, Schmitt NC, Bhrany AD, Futran ND. Antibiotic prophylaxis in patients undergoing head and neck free flap reconstruction. JAMA Otolaryngol Head Neck Surg. 2015; 141(12):1096–1103

[6] Cohen LE, Finnerty BM, Golas AR, et al. Perioperative antibiotics in the setting of oropharyngeal reconstruction: less is more. Ann Plast Surg. 2016; 76 (6):663–667

[7] Khariwala SS, Le B, Pierce BH, Vogel RI, Chipman JG. Antibiotic use after free tissue reconstruction of head and neck defects: short course vs long course. Surg Infect (Larchmt). 2016; 17(1):100–105

[8] Benatar MJ, Dassonville O, Chamorey E, et al. Impact of preoperative radiotherapy on head and neck free flap reconstruction: a report on 429 cases. J Plast Reconstr Aesthet Surg. 2013; 66(4):478–482

[9] Cannady SB, Hatten KM, Bur AM, et al. Use of free tissue transfer in head and neck cancer surgery and risk of overall and serious complication(s): an American College of Surgeons-National Surgical Quality Improvement Project analysis of free tissue transfer to the head and neck. Head Neck. 2017; 39(4):702–707

[10] Penel N, Lefebvre D, Fournier C, Sarini J, Kara A, Lefebvre JL. Risk factors for wound infection in head and neck cancer surgery: a prospective study. Head Neck. 2001; 23(6):447–455

[11] Matory YL, Spiro RH. Wound bleeding after head and neck surgery. J Surg Oncol. 1993; 53(1):17–19

[12] Tokaç M, Dumlu EG, Bozkurt B, et al. Effect of intraoperative valsalva maneuver application on bleeding point detection and postoperative drainage after thyroidectomy surgeries. Int Surg. 2015; 100(6):994–998

[13] Moumoulidis I, Martinez Del Pero M, Brennan L, Jani P. Haemostasis in head and neck surgical procedures: Valsalva manoeuvre versus Trendelenburg tilt. Ann R Coll Surg Engl. 2010; 92(4):292–294

[14] Bajwa MS, Tudur-Smith C, Shaw RJ, Schache AG. Fibrin sealants in soft tissue surgery of the head and neck: a systematic review and meta-analysis of randomised controlled trials. Clin Otolaryngol. 2017; 42(6):1141–1152

[15] Ren ZH, Xu JL, Fan TF, Ji T, Wu HJ, Zhang CP. The harmonic scalpel versus conventional hemostasis for neck dissection: a meta-analysis of the randomized controlled trials. PLoS One. 2015; 10(7):e0132476

[16] Lin WJ, Wang CC, Jiang RS, Huang YC, Ho HC, Liu SA. A prospective randomised trial of LigaSure Small Jaw® versus conventional neck dissection in head and neck cancer patients. Clin Otolaryngol. 2017; 42(2):245–251

[17] Fritz DK, Matthews TW, Chandarana SP, Nakoneshny SC, Dort JC. Harmonic scalpel impact on blood loss and operating time in major head and neck surgery: a randomized clinical trial. J Otolaryngol Head Neck Surg. 2016; 45(1):58

[18] Shin YS, Koh YW, Kim S-H, Choi EC. The efficacy of the harmonic scalpel in neck dissection: a prospective randomized study. Laryngoscope. 2013; 123 (4):904–909

[19] Pfeiffer J, Becker C, Ridder GJ. Aberrant extracranial internal carotid arteries: new insights, implications, and demand for a clinical grading system. Head Neck. 2016; 38 Suppl 1:E687–E693

[20] Cleland-Zamudio SS, Wax MK, Smith JD, Cohen JI. Ruptured internal jugular vein: a postoperative complication of modified/selected neck dissection. Head Neck. 2003; 25(5):357–360

[21] Manzoor NF, Rezaee RP, Ray A, et al. Contemporary management of carotid blowout syndrome utilizing endovascular techniques. Laryngoscope. 2017; 127(2):383–390

[22] Bond KM, Brinjikji W, Murad MH, Cloft HJ, Lanzino G. Endovascular treatment of carotid blowout syndrome. J Vasc Surg. 2017; 65(3):883–888

[23] Cramer JD, Patel UA, Maas MB, Samant S, Smith SS. Is Neck Dissection Associated with an Increased Risk of Postoperative Stroke? Otolaryngol Head Neck Surg. 2017; 157(2):226–232

[24] Thompson SK, Southern DA, McKinnon JG, Dort JC, Ghali WA. Incidence of perioperative stroke after neck dissection for head and neck cancer: a regional outcome analysis. Ann Surg. 2004; 239(3):428–431

[25] van Wilgen CP, Dijkstra PU, van der Laan BF, Plukker JT, Roodenburg JL. Shoulder complaints after neck dissection; is the spinal accessory nerve involved? Br J Oral Maxillofac Surg. 2003; 41(1):7–11

[26] Eickmeyer SM, Walczak CK, Myers KB, Lindstrom DR, Layde P, Campbell BH. Quality of life, shoulder range of motion, and spinal accessory nerve status in 5-year survivors of head and neck cancer. PM R. 2014; 6(12):1073–1080

[27] McNeely ML, Parliament MB, Seikaly H, et al. Effect of exercise on upper extremity pain and dysfunction in head and neck cancer survivors: a randomized controlled trial. Cancer. 2008; 113(1):214–222

[28] Cappiello J, Piazza C, Nicolai P. The spinal accessory nerve in head and neck surgery. Curr Opin Otolaryngol Head Neck Surg. 2007; 15(2):107–111

[29] Durazzo MD, Furlan JC, Teixeira GV, et al. Anatomic landmarks for localization of the spinal accessory nerve. Clin Anat. 2009; 22(4):471–475

[30] Taylor CB, Boone JL, Schmalbach CE, Miller FR. Intraoperative relationship of the spinal accessory nerve to the internal jugular vein: variation from cadaver studies. Am J Otolaryngol. 2013; 34(5):527–529

[31] Batstone MD, Scott B, Lowe D, Rogers SN. Marginal mandibular nerve injury during neck dissection and its impact on patient perception of appearance. Head Neck. 2009; 31(5):673–678

[32] Møller MN, Sørensen CH. Risk of marginal mandibular nerve injury in neck dissection. Eur Arch Otorhinolaryngol. 2012; 269(2):601–605

[33] Tulley P, Webb A, Chana JS, et al. Paralysis of the marginal mandibular branch of the facial nerve: treatment options. Br J Plast Surg. 2000; 53(5):378–385

[34] Balagopal PG, George NA, Sebastian P. Anatomic variations of the marginal mandibular nerve. Indian J Surg Oncol. 2012; 3(1):8–11

[35] Hussain G, Manktelow RT, Tomat LR. Depressor labii inferioris resection: an effective treatment for marginal mandibular nerve paralysis. Br J Plast Surg. 2004; 57(6):502–510

[36] Tan ST. Anterior belly of digastric muscle transfer: a useful technique in head and neck surgery. Head Neck. 2002; 24(10):947–954

[37] Garzaro M, Riva G, Raimondo L, Aghemo L, Giordano C, Pecorari G. A study of neck and shoulder morbidity following neck dissection: the benefits of cervical plexus preservation. Ear Nose Throat J. 2015; 94(8):330–344

[38] Terrell JE, Welsh DE, Bradford CR, et al. Pain, quality of life, and spinal accessory nerve status after neck dissection. Laryngoscope. 2000; 110(4):620–626

[39] Smith ME, Riffat F, Jani P. The surgical anatomy and clinical relevance of the neglected right lymphatic duct: review. J Laryngol Otol. 2013; 127(2):128–133

[40] Jain A, Singh SN, Singhal P, Sharma MP, Grover M. A prospective study on the role of octreotide in management of chyle fistula neck. Laryngoscope. 2015; 125(7):1624–1627

[41] Delaney SW, Shi H, Shokrani A, Sinha UK. Management of chyle leak after head and neck surgery: review of current treatment strategies. Int J Otolaryngol. 2017; 2017:8362874

[42] Kim HK, Kim SM, Chang H, et al. Clinical experience with n-butyl-2-cyanoacrylate in performing lateral neck dissection for metastatic thyroid cancer. Surg Innov. 2016; 23(5):481–485

[43] Cheng L, Lau CK, Parker G. Use of TissuePatch™ sealant film in the management of chyle leak in major neck surgery. Br J Oral Maxillofac Surg. 2014; 52 (1):87–89

[44] Wilkerson PM, Haque A, Pitkin L, Soon Y. Thoracoscopic ligation of the thoracic duct complex in the treatment for high-volume chyle leak following modified radical neck dissection: safe, feasible, but underutilised. Clin Otolaryngol. 2014; 39(1):73–74

[45] Moon RE. Hyperbaric oxygen treatment for air or gas embolism. Undersea Hyperb Med. 2014; 41(2):159–166

[46] McMullen C, Rocke D, Freeman J. Complications of bilateral neck dissection in thyroid cancer from a single high-volume center. JAMA Otolaryngol Head Neck Surg. 2017; 143(4):376–381

[47] Cavicchi O, Piccin O, Caliceti U, De Cataldis A, Pasquali R, Ceroni AR. Transient hypoparathyroidism following thyroidectomy: a prospective study and multivariate analysis of 604 consecutive patients. Otolaryngol Head Neck Surg. 2007; 137(4):654–658

[48] Giordano D, Valcavi R, Thompson GB, et al. Complications of central neck dissection in patients with papillary thyroid carcinoma: results of a study on 1087 patients and review of the literature. Thyroid. 2012; 22(9):911–917

[49] Roh JL, Kim JM, Park CI. Lateral cervical lymph node metastases from papillary thyroid carcinoma: pattern of nodal metastases and optimal strategy for neck dissection. Ann Surg Oncol. 2008; 15(4):1177–1182

[50] Haugen BR, Alexander EK, Bible KC, et al. 2015 American Thyroid Association Management Guidelines for Adult Patients with Thyroid Nodules and Differentiated Thyroid Cancer: The American Thyroid Association Guidelines Task Force on Thyroid Nodules and Differentiated Thyroid Cancer. Thyroid. 2016; 26(1):1–133

[51] Joo YH, Sun DI, Cho KJ, Cho JH, Kim MS. The impact of paratracheal lymph node metastasis in squamous cell carcinoma of the hypopharynx. Eur Arch Otorhinolaryngol. 2010; 267(6):945–950

[52] Pazos GA, Leonard DW, Blice J, Thompson DH. Blindness after bilateral neck dissection: case report and review. Am J Otolaryngol. 1999; 20(5):340–345

12 Rehabilitation After Neck Dissection

Peter S. Vosler and Douglas B. Chepeha

Abstract

Rehabilitation after neck dissection is perceived as important, but there has been little research on specific regimens or protocols to help patients recover after neck dissection. This chapter evaluates the types of impairment following neck dissection, treatment factors that influence impairment, the assessment tools used to evaluate function, and optimal rehabilitation following neck dissection. Emphasis is placed on evidence regarding the impact of the extent and type of treatment on shoulder impairment. The literature is reviewed to determine the evidence supporting different rehabilitation modalities for both shoulder impairment and lymphedema. Best practice suggestions are provided based on synthesis of the content of the chapter in the conclusion section.

Keywords: neck dissection, rehabilitation, shoulder impairment, lymphedema, pain, dysphagia, head and neck cancer

12.1 Introduction

Neck dissection is a surgical procedure commonly performed to improve regional control of head and neck malignancy of the upper aerodigestive tract, thyroid, parotid, or skin. The extent of neck dissection is determined by the primary tumor and the presence and location of regional metastasis.

Most patients undergoing selective neck dissection (SND) experience relatively little disability. When neck dissection is more extensive, and when there is injury to the accessory nerve or when multiple treatment modalities are employed, there is an increased likelihood of impairment. The impairments include loss of skin sensation, paresthesia, loss of depressor anguli oris function, decreased range of motion of the neck and shoulder, neck pain, neck stiffness, and loss of strength for lifting of objects. Recent research has evaluated psychosocial and psychological sequelae in addition to functional impairments of neck dissection that warrant consideration in proper rehabilitation. This chapter describes the impairment following neck dissection, the treatment factors that influence impairment, the assessment tools used to evaluate function, and optimal rehabilitation following neck dissection.

12.1.1 Prevalence of Impairment Following Neck Dissection

Shoulder impairment following radical neck dissection (RND) was first described by Ewing and Martin in 1952.[1] The prevalence of impairment following neck dissection, predominantly manifested by shoulder and upper limb impairment, ranges between 18 and 77%.[2] Prevalence is difficult to report on because of the different types of neck dissection, the different primary site treatments associated with neck dissection, and the number of different measures that are used to assess neck dissection–related impairment.

12.1.2 General Factors That Affect Functional Outcome after Neck Dissection

There are a number of patient factors that can contribute to the difficulty of neck dissection and potential complications postoperatively. Factors that limit surgical exposure such as morbid obesity and decreased range of motion of the neck increase likelihood of damage to the neural and vascular structures in the neck. Patient comorbidities such as smoking, alcohol consumption, diabetes, and coagulopathy can increase the likelihood of a wound complication that in turn can increase postoperative scarring and mobility. Patients with a history of atherosclerosis have an increased likelihood of stroke.

12.1.3 Late Effects of Neck Dissection

The late effects of neck dissection include impaired neck and shoulder mobility and strength, cervical paresthesia, pain, lymphedema, dysphagia, psychosocial issues,[3] and impaired quality of life.[4] Evaluation of patients who underwent neck dissection and comparing to patients without neck dissection revealed impairments in intelligibility of speech, health-related quality of life, and decreased employment.[3] Similar results were obtained using the University of Washington-QOL and Functional Assessment of Cancer Therapy Head and Neck questionnaires in patients who did and did not undergo neck dissection. Five years after treatment, patients who underwent neck dissection had worse scores with regard to aesthetics, willingness to eat in public, decreased levels of activity, and decreased involvement with recreation or entertainment than patients who did not undergo neck dissection.[4]

12.2 Components of Impairment after Neck Dissection

There are critical structures in each level of the neck that, when dissected, can contribute to impairment following neck dissection (▶ Table 12.1).

12.2.1 Level I

Component of level I include the following: level Ia, the submental nodes, extending from the mandible anteriorly, bordered by the anterior belly of the digastric bilaterally, and the hyoid inferiorly. Removal of fibrofatty tissue from this area can lead to a cosmetic contour deformity. The area can be not only depressed, but also excessively full due to lymphedema. It is generally thought that there is no treatment for these sequelae.

Table 12.1 Contributors to neck and shoulder disability based on level of neck dissection

Anatomical level	Structure affected	Impairment/disability
Level Ia	Fibrofatty tissue	Mild cosmetic deformity
Level Ib	Hypoglossal N	Ipsilateral tongue hemiplegia, dysphagia, dysarthria
	Lingual N	Ipsilateral tongue paresthesia, dysphagia, dysgeusia, dysarthria
	Marginal mandibular N	Paralysis of lower lip depressor, cosmetic deformity, lower lip trauma
Level IIa	Spinal accessory N	Shoulder and neck ROM and strength
	Hypoglossal N	Ipsilateral tongue hemiplegia, dysphagia, dysarthria
	Great auricular N	Ipsilateral pinna paresthesia
Level IIb	Spinal accessory N	Shoulder and neck ROM and strength
Level III	Phrenic N	Hemi diaphragm paralysis/DOE, pneumonia
	Ansa cervicalis N	Hyolaryngeal elevation
Level IV	Phrenic N	Hemidiaphragm paralysis/DOE, pneumonia
	Thoracic duct	Chyle leak
Levels II–IV	Jugular vein	Lymphedema
	Vagus N	Ipsilateral vocal cord paralysis, dysphonia, aspiration
	Cervical rootlets	Cervical paresthesia
	Sympathetic trunk	Horner's syndrome[a]
	Carotid artery	TIA, stroke
Level V	Spinal accessory N[b]	Shoulder and neck ROM and strength
	Brachial plexus	Hand and arm paresthesias and weakness, hand or arm paralysis, severe pain
	Cervical rootlets	Cervical paresthesia

Abbreviations: DOE, dyspnea on exertion; N, nerve; ROM, range of motion; TIA, transient ischemic attack.
[a]Horner's syndrome: triad of ptosis, meiosis, and anhydrosis resulting from injury to the cervical sympathetic trunk.
[b]Increased shoulder impairment with dissection of this level.

Level Ib, which is bordered by the mandible superiorly, and the digastric muscle inferiorly, contains multiple neurovascular structures. The most notable structures include the hypoglossal and lingual nerves. Injury to the hypoglossal nerve, which supplies ipsilateral motor innervation to the tongue, can lead to dysphagia and dysarthria. The ansa hypoglossi is a branch of C1 and travels with the hypoglossal nerve to innervate the thyrohyoid and the geniohyoid. The nerve branch to the thyrohyoid (which passes to level III) is frequently cut during neck dissection, but the impact of this transection is not well understood. The lingual nerve supplies sensory innervation to the ipsilateral tongue. Dysgeusia is very uncommon after neck dissection.

The marginal mandibular nerve is a branch of the facial nerve and it innervates the depressor anguli oris muscle, which depresses the ipsilateral corner of the mouth. The nerve courses inferior to the mandible within the fascia overlying the submandibular gland and can be injured during dissection of this level. Rates of injury are reported to be up to 23% in one observational study of 66 patients.[5] The main complaint of patients following injury to the nerve is cosmetic deformity manifested by smile asymmetry. Patients may also complain of biting their lower lip when eating and some difficulties with oral competence.

12.2.2 Level II

Level II extends from the skull base superiorly to the hyoid inferiorly. The medial border is the deep cervical fascia overlying the paravertebral muscles and the levator scapulae. Level II is divided into level IIa that is superior to the spinal accessory nerve (SAN; cranial nerve [CN] XI) and with level IIb that is below CN XI.

CN XI supplies motor innervation to the sternocleidomastoid muscle (SCM). The motor innervation of the upper trapezius is supplied by variable contributions of CN XI and the cervical plexus. The sacrifice of CN XI results in shoulder impairment in 60 to 80% of patients.[6] Even when intact, the extent of CN XI dissection is correlated with the degree of shoulder impairment.[7,8] Deficits in shoulder function from dissection or sacrifice include reduced abduction and decreased range of motion, scapular winging, scapular droop, neck stiffness, and neck pain.

12.2.3 Level III

The boundaries of level III include the hyoid superiorly to the inferior border of the cricoid inferiorly, and the sternohyoid and deep cervical fascia over the paravertebral muscles medially. The largest segment of the ansa cervicalis provides motor innervation to the infrahyoid strap muscles to induce hyolaryngeal stabilization and depression. The contribution of these muscles is not well understood. The infrahyoid strap muscles are a counterbalance to the suprahyoid muscles. Contraction of the suprahyoid musculature produces hyoid and laryngeal elevation and causes the base of tongue to cover the laryngeal inlet and fold over the epiglottis (epiglottic inversion). The infrahyoid strap muscles provide a counterbalance to this swallowing action. Transection or resection of the ansa branches or the infrahyoid strap muscles do not seem to result in swallowing or airway impairment. If the patient undergoes multimodality (radiation) treatment that includes extensive resection including the SCM and the infrahyoid musculature, decreased hyoid elevation is observed during swallowing that can lead to increased incidence of aspiration.

The phrenic nerve arises in level III from contributions of C3–C5, traverses superficial to the anterior scalene muscle, and runs in a lateral-to-medial direction. Damage to the phrenic nerve during a neck dissection usually results in elevation of the hemidiaphragm, and this can impair respiration.

12.2.4 Level IV

Level IV is bounded by the cricoid superiorly and the clavicle inferiorly. The medial border is the deep cervical fascia over the paravertebral muscles. The posterior border is aligned with the posterior border of the SCM. The structure most commonly injured in level IV is the thoracic duct, which is on the left, although there are large lymphatics found on the right. Injury to the lymphatics in level IV can lead to a chylocele that, in some cases, does not spontaneously resolve and may need treatment to resolve electrolyte loss that can lead to electrolyte abnormalities.

12.2.5 Common Structures in Levels II to IV

Structures common to levels II to IV include the internal jugular vein (IJV), carotid artery, vagus nerve, sympathetic trunk, and the SCM. Sacrifice of a single IJV contributes to lymphedema of the neck that can result in increased neck stiffness and an impaired cosmetic appearance. If both IJVs are transected, life-threatening cerebral edema can result. If both are transected acutely, a bypass should be performed. Stroke can result from manipulation of the carotid vessels; however, there appears to be no long-term sequelae from ligation of the external carotid artery. The vagus nerve provides innervation important for swallowing and it innervates the ipsilateral vocal cord; therefore, injury to the vagus can result in dysphagia, dysphonia, and aspiration. Finally, the sympathetic trunk courses within the carotid sheath, and injury can result in Horner's syndrome of ptosis, meiosis, and anhydrosis.

12.2.6 Level V

The posterior triangle of the neck is bounded by the trapezius posteriorly, the clavicle inferiorly, and, for surgeons, the cervical rootlets anteriorly. It is divided into sublevels Va (superior) and Vb (inferior) by the plane of the inferior border of the cricoid. Level V contains CN XI. CN XI picks up branches of C2 as CN XI exits the SCM. The branches of C2 can variably provide motor innervation to the trapezius. Dissection of CN XI results in worse shoulder function in most patients.[7,8,9] Dissection or sacrifice, of cervical rootlets, can lead to neck, earlobe, or upper chest paresthesia.

12.2.7 Level VI

Level VI is bordered superiorly by the hyoid, inferiorly by the innominate artery, and laterally by the carotid arteries. The deep boundary is the visceral fascia around the thyroid and larynx. Critical structures include the recurrent laryngeal nerves and the parathyroid glands. Dissection of the recurrent laryngeal nerve or the external branch of the superior laryngeal nerve can lead to weakness and changes in voice production. Dissection of the inferior thyroid artery of the parathyroid glands can lead to hypocalcemia.

12.3 Treatment Factors

If a neck dissection includes more levels, there will be more impairment—particularly if level V is dissected. It is important to note the both radiation and radiation with chemotherapy also contribute to impairment after neck dissection.

12.3.1 Types of Neck Dissection

The underlying disease determines the extent of neck dissection, and it should be the foremost determinate as to the type of neck dissection performed. The classification of neck dissection includes RND, modified RND (MRND), and SND.

RND involves removal of the ipsilateral cervical lymph nodes from levels I to V with sacrifice of the SCM, CN XI, and the IJV. The other neck dissections are variations of the RND with regard to levels of dissection and preservation of nonlymphatic structures. MRND also involves removal of ipsilateral cervical lymph nodes in levels I to V, but with preservation of one or more of the aforementioned nonlymphatic structures (SCM, CN XI, IJV). Functional neck dissection is a term that is no longer used that describes preservation of the SCM, CN XI, IJV, part of the cervical plexus, or one or more levels of the neck. SND involves removal of one or more nodal levels with preservation of nonlymphatic structures.

12.3.2 Extent of Neck Dissection

RND is associated with the worst functional outcome by virtue of sacrifice of vital structures for shoulder and neck function as well as cosmetic deformity with removal of the SCM. A retrospective review that assessed 224 patients who underwent 308 neck dissections evaluated pain, impaired shoulder function by measuring shoulder drop, reach above and arm abduction, increased neck and shoulder stiffness, and increased neck constriction for patients undergoing radical, MRND or SND. Sacrifice of CN XI was associated with worse outcome across all measures. If level V was not dissected, then patients had better outcomes across all measures. Cosmetic outcome was associated with the preservation of the SCM.[10]

Multiple studies validate the association of dissection of CN XI and increased impairment with different outcome measures. A retrospective comparison of SND levels II to IV ($n = 20$) with SND levels II to V ($n = 20$) showed that level V dissection was associated with impaired shoulder muscle strength, shoulder range of motion limitation, shoulder droop, protraction, and flaring, and decreased electromyographic potentials.[7] Impairment in strength and function was predominately reported as mild. Similarly, retrospective review compared 15 patients who underwent MRND with preservation of the SCM, CN XI, and IJV with 17 patients who underwent SND levels II to IV. This study demonstrated a trend toward increased pain, increased disability as assessed by the Shoulder Pain Disability Index (SPDI), and decreased range of motion as measured by goniometry 6 months postoperatively in the MRND group despite sparing SCM, CN XI, and IJV.[11] This finding is further corroborated in a retrospective review of 121 SND and 46 SCM and CN XI–sparing MRND where impaired shoulder function was found using the Neck Dissection Impairment Index (NDII) in the patients who received MRND.[8]

12.3.3 Dissection of Sublevel IIb

There is controversy in the field regarding the utility of sublevel IIb dissection. Multiple papers have evaluated patients who have a clinical and radiological N0 classification neck and showed the incidence of positive level IIb nodes within a range of 0 to 10.4%.[12] Of note, there were only three episodes of isolated level IIb nodes out of 332 patients. None of the studies to date evaluate shoulder function when controlling for sublevel IIb dissection. In theory, dissection level IIb after level IIa dissection could lead to increased shoulder impairment postoperatively without improved oncologic control.

In summary, the literature supports the findings that sacrifice or dissection of key structures, particularly CN XI in level V, causes increased impairment.

12.3.4 Radiation and Chemotherapy

Adjuvant therapy for head and neck cancer also plays a role in head and neck cancer treatment-related morbidity. A multivariable analysis was performed using the NDII as the assessment tool to compare MRND sparing CN XI with SND, and adjuvant radiation or chemoradiation were independent predictors associated with shoulder impairment.[8]

Similarly, in a study of 25 who underwent SND levels I to III, and 86 who underwent extended SND (levels I–V) with sacrifice of SCM, the extended SND was associated with greater cervical range-of-motion deficit compared to SND levels I to III. In this study, 98 patients received radiation and the combination of extended SND and radiation produced additional impairments in cervical range of motion compared to extended SND alone. Radiation therapy as a single modality did not result in increased morbidity of cervical range of motion, mouth opening, swallowing, or lymphedema at 12 months posttreatment.[13] Postoperative radiation therapy after neck dissection was associated with impairment of upper limb function and increase shoulder pain as measured by the NDII and Quick Disabilities of the Arm, Shoulder, and Hand (DASH) survey in a retrospective study examining 89 patients treated with SCM and CN XI–sparing neck dissections.[14]

Primary radiation or chemoradiation for treatment of oropharyngeal and nasopharyngeal carcinomas allows for examination of posttreatment effects. Examination of patients presenting with dysphagia greater than 5 years postradiation or chemoradiation for head and neck cancer revealed dysarthria or dysphonia, cranial neuropathies, and pneumonia in 76, 46, and 86% of patients, respectively.[15] When looking at post–chemoradiation therapy (post-CRT) neck dissection for patients without complete response, nearly all patients had returned to a soft or regular diet by 2 years posttreatment with 10% of patients remaining gastrostomy tube dependent.[16] The rate of gastrostomy tube dependence did not appear to be associated with posttreatment neck dissection

Overall, chemoradiation does not seem to cause shoulder morbidity as a primary therapy within 2 years of treatment. Use of chemoradiation in the adjuvant setting exacerbates the morbidity caused by neck dissection.

12.3.5 Sentinel Lymph Node Biopsy

Sentinel lymph node biopsy (SNB) is the standard staging tool for the management of melanoma, and it has been studied for use in early classification (T1–T2) of oral cavity squamous cell carcinoma demonstrating a negative predictive value of 95%.[17] Few studies have been carried out examining the impairment of sentinel node biopsy versus elective neck dissection.

A retrospective comparison of 62 patients with early classification oral tongue lesions (T1–T2) who underwent either SNB ($n = 33$) or SNB followed by elective neck dissection ($n = 29$) demonstrated SNB was associated with less shoulder impairment than SNB followed by SND using the NDII and constant score as outcome measures.[18]

12.4 Assessment Tools for Neck Disability

There are many different tools available for the assessment of shoulder disability. ▶ Table 12.2 outlines the most commonly used questionnaires in the head and neck literature to assess shoulder function. Most of the assessment tools were designed to assess rotator cuff and/or glenohumeral joint disease.

The two patient-reported outcome (PRO) measures for assessment of shoulder function after neck dissection are the NDII and the DASH questionnaire. The NDII was specifically designed and validated in the head and neck cancer population.[19] The DASH has undergone the most rigorous psychometric analysis and validation of any of the questionnaires listed in ▶ Table 12.2, and it is the best tool for comprehensive assessment of upper extremity function. A comprehensive review of the outcome measures has been conducted and the NDII was found to be the most appropriate assessment tool at this time.[20]

The DASH questionnaire was validated in the head and neck cancer patient population in a cross-sectional study comparing RND, MRND, and SND. Evaluation of the DASH by both physicians and patients met sensibility criteria, which means the DASH questionnaire asked questions appropriate for patients who underwent neck dissection. The DASH was also able to discriminate between the different types of neck dissection, and it was also validated in this patient population with high correlation of the DASH with the head and neck cancer patient-validated NDII.[21] The Shoulder Disability Questionnaire (SDQ), NDII, and Shoulder Pain and Disability Index (SPADI) were also validated in a cohort of patients who underwent neck dissection; however, only the NDII was able to discriminate between types of neck dissection.[22]

In summary, there are two convenient questionnaires that are reliable constructs for evaluation of shoulder impairment following neck dissection—the NDII and DASH. Although the SPADI and SDQ are also validated in patients undergoing neck dissection, these measures do not appear to be as sensitive as the NDII and DASH.

Table 12.2 Patient-related outcome questionnaires for shoulder function

Instrument	# Questions	Recall period	Time to complete	Type of question	Scoring	Total score	Advantages	Disadvantages
Neck Dissection Impairment Index (NDII)	10	4 wk	<5 min	QOL, ADL, work- and activity-related questions	0–5: 0 worst, 5 best	100 (higher = less disability)	Designed and validated specifically to assess disability after neck dissection; simple, quick to complete; easy to score	No MDC or SEM
Disabilities of the Arm, Shoulder, and Hand Questionnaire (DASH)	30	1 wk	13 min	21 functional, 6 symptom items, and 3 social/role function items; 2 optional 4-question modules: assess shoulder function on work or sport/arts	0–5: 1 = no difficulty; 5 = extremely difficult	100 (higher = greater disability)[a]	Extensive development and psychometric property assessment Best tool for comprehensive assessment of upper extremity Can detect patients with nerve injury	Region specific, i.e., not specific to shoulder Longer time to complete
Constant's Shoulder Score (CSS)	10	1 wk	5–7 min	Combination of ROM and strength testing with pain and activity limitations	Pain 0–15 VAS; 0 = maximal; 15 = no pain Activity 0–5 Likert scale: 0 = worst; 5 = best Mobility 0–10: 0 = worst; 10 = best Strength 1 point/0.5 kg, max 25 points	100 (higher = less disability)	Clinically relevant content with high responsiveness, formal strength, and range of motion testing, very fast assessment for physical testing, used across many disease types	No psychometric assessment in H&N cancer patients
Shoulder Pain and Disability Index (SPADI)	13	1 wk	7 min	5 pain-related items; 8 disability/function-related items	0–10 VAS: 0 = none; 10 = worst	100 (higher = greater disability)	Content validity determined with expert review Most responsive shoulder instrument to detect impairment Validated in H&N cancer patients	Item reduction No direct patient input for development Main focus is on pain; less emphasis on other potential symptoms
Shoulder Disability Questionnaire (SDQ)	16	24 h	<5 min	13 pain-related questions; 3 questions–sleeping, need to rub, and irritability	Yes = 1, No = 0; no. of yes responses/ no. of completed items[a] 100 Higher score = more disability	Higher = greater disability	Able to differentiate clinically stable versus improvement (MDC 95%); Simple, quick to complete; Easy to score; Validated in H&N cancer patients	Poor content validity
American Shoulder and Elbow Surgeons standardized score (ASES)	11	1 wk	4 min	10 pain-related items; 1 function question	Score for both R & L shoulders Pain 0–10 VAS: 0 = none; 10 = worst Function 0–3: 0 = unable; 3 = no difficulty	Higher = less disability	Good construct validity, responsiveness, and reliability Quick to complete	No reliability or validity testing in H&N cancer patients Scoring complicated by VAS conversion Limited sensitivity

Continued

Table 12.2 continued

Instrument	# Questions	Recall period	Time to complete	Type of question	Scoring	Total score	Advantages	Disadvantages
Simple Shoulder Test (SST)	12	Time to completion	3 min	Questions regarding subjective component and activity-specific performance. Physical activity	1 = yes, 0 = no; max. score of 12 converted to percentage score out of 100	100% (higher = less disability)	Quick and easy to use. Can differentiate patients with various shoulder conditions	Limited functional items. Lack of construct validity in H&N cancer patients

Abbreviations: ADL, activities of daily living; H&N, head and neck; MDC, minimal detectable change; QOL, quality of life; R & L, right and left; ROM, range of motion; SEM, standard error of the mean; VAS, visual analogue scale.
[a]Work and sports/performing arts modules scored separately.

12.5 Shoulder Rehabilitation

Based on electromyographic studies, the type of injury that occurs during CN XI–persevering neck dissection is axonotmesis, and the expected recovery for nerve recovery is between 12 and 18 months.[23] During this time, the injury to the SAN results in trapezius muscle weakness causing malposition of scapula inferiorly, medially, and in abduction, resulting in decreased shoulder and arm range of motion and strength. If there is no physical therapy intervention, then patients acquire adhesive capsulitis, characterized by pain, decreased internal and external shoulder rotation, and limited shoulder abduction and flexion.[2] Treatment for adhesive capsulitis is unfortunately limited; therefore, prevention from physical therapy is the best practice following neck dissection. Overall, the goal of physical therapy is to maintain strength, length of muscles, range of motion, and prevent adhesive capsulitis.

12.5.1 Evidence Basis for Physiotherapy

Physiotherapy improves shoulder function following neck dissection; however, there is controversy regarding an optimal physiotherapy regimen. The pathophysiology underlying shoulder impairment following neck dissection is focused on CN XI injury that results in trapezius and scapular muscles that work synergistically with the trapezius. Exercises that target the glenohumeral joint or rotator cuff muscles are unlikely to improve the impairment caused by CN XI neuropraxia or axonotmesis.[23] Therefore, the type of physiotherapy should be modified based on type of nerve injury. If the nerve is transected, as in RND, then there is likely limited benefit to targeted strength training of the trapezius muscle. If the nerve is spared as in SND or MRND, then progressive resistance training has a higher theoretical benefit.

There is limited evidence regarding the benefit of physiotherapy following RND where the SCM and CN XI are sacrificed. In a Japanese study, rehabilitation with an undisclosed physiotherapy regimen improved arm abduction in patients who underwent SCM and CN XI sacrifice compared to patients with the same operation who did not receive rehabilitation.[10]

A Cochrane review of the only three randomized control trials conducted up to 2012 examining physical therapy exercises to treat shoulder impairment following neck dissection concluded that progressive resistance training reduced shoulder disability and pain, but it did not result in statistically significant reduction of neck dissection impairment and fatigue, or improved QOL.[24] Review of literature to evaluate the effectiveness of physiotherapy following neck dissection found poor scientific rigor in evaluation of efficacy and therefore little evidence-based literature for the type of physiotherapy modality employed. It was concluded that exercise-based physiotherapy has the greatest promise for improved function.[23]

A more recent prospective randomized control trial analyzed the efficacy of progressive scapular-strengthening exercises versus standard physiotherapy, consisting of generalized shoulder and neck exercises, in a cohort of 53 patients that underwent CN XI–preserving neck dissection. The prevalence of shoulder impairment across groups was 36.86%, and adherence to the therapy was 76.6 and 82.2% in the intervention and control groups, respectively. Overall, both the group receiving progressive scapular strengthening and the control group showed improvement in the SPADI and NDII. Shoulder abduction was increased with progressive scapular strengthening at 3 months, but there was no difference between the two groups at 6 and 12 months post–neck dissection.[25]

In summary, there is little evidence to support specific physiotherapy regimens following neck dissection, but sufficient evidence to support the recommendation that all patients who undergo either SAN-sacrificing or SAN-preserving neck dissection should undergo some shoulder physiotherapy regimen.

12.6 Rehabilitation of Pain

There are limited controlled trials evaluating pain management following neck dissection in the context of shoulder impairment. This is likely multifactorial as there is clinically significant cervical paresthesia from transection of cutaneous nerves and, in the case of level V dissection, cervical rootlet transection. Postoperative pain is most often due to shoulder impairment, and as many neck dissections occur in the context of a primary tumor site resection, it is difficult to distinguish if the cause of pain is from the neck dissection or primary tumor resection.

Inflammation is a significant component of postoperative pain. Nonsteroidal anti-inflammatory drugs (NSAIDs) inhibit inflammation and are safe to use postoperatively. Further, administration of NSAIDs decreases opioid requirements, thereby reducing opioid-related complications and improving patient satisfaction.[26] Patients with preoperative opioid requirements requiring long-acting opioids may benefit from consultation of acute pain or palliative care physicians.

12.7 Lymphedema

The surgical removal of lymphatics results in decreased lymphatic drainage of the head and neck; the addition of radiation causes lymphatic apoptosis, decreased dermal lymphatics, and reduction in lymph transport.

Both can result in lymphatic back flow, chronic inflammation, edema, and fibrosis, all of which can lead to functional deficits and aesthetic disfigurement.

Lymphedema affects from 50 to 75% of head and neck cancer survivors who undergo neck treatment.[27,28] Head and neck lymphedema (HNL) can occur internally within the mucosa of the upper aerodigestive tract or externally with visible swelling of the skin and soft tissues. The MD Anderson Cancer Center (MDACC) HNL scale is modified from Foldi's scale to allow for categorization of nuanced findings specific to HNL.[27] An evaluation protocol developed at the MDACC has been developed that combines seven facial measurements to calculate a composite facial score with three neck circumference measurements for a composite neck score to accurately assess lymphedema.[27] This protocol allows for pre- and posttreatment evaluation of HNL to assess for efficacy of therapy.

The gold standard for treatment of lymphedema of the head and neck or in the extremities is complete decompressive therapy (CDT). This includes manual decompressive therapy, application of compressive garments or bandages, exercises, and skin care.[29] A retrospective study out of MDACC examined 1,202 patients with posttreatment HNL and evaluated CDT response in 733 of those patients. CDT resulted in 60% of patients with improved HNL, and treatment response was significantly related to treatment adherence.[29]

A protocol for CDT developed at MDACC includes use of compression garments both before and after manual lymphatic drainage. Manual lymphatic drainage consists of massage of the supraclavicular region, followed by massage of the trunk, neck, and face. This is coupled with cervical range of motion exercises to facilitate drainage. These techniques are taught to patients in an outpatient setting and patients are given a decompressive regimen to perform at home daily.[27]

12.8 Rehabilitation of Swallowing

The incidence of dysphagia ranges from 37 to 82% of patients undergoing organ-preserving CRT for head and neck cancer.[16] However, there is a paucity of literature regarding dysphagia following primary neck dissection, which is likely related to limited swallowing impairment caused by neck dissection alone. Accordingly, examination of swallowing impairment in a QOL study comparing no neck dissection, nerve sparing neck dissection, and nerve-sacrificing neck dissections revealed no differences in dysphagia as measured by the University of Washington QOL questionnaire.[4]

Evaluation of patients that received post-CRT neck dissections for incomplete clinical response demonstrated dysphagia with trimodal therapy, with 10% of patients remaining gastrostomy tube dependent 24 months after completion of treatment. The incidence of post-CRT neck dissection is similar to published dysphagia and gastrostomy tube dependence in patients who underwent CRT alone, suggesting that addition of neck dissection did not exacerbate dysphagia.[16]

Therapy for dysphagia, regardless of treatment modality employed, necessitates involvement of speech-language pathologists for discussion of food consistency, swallowing exercises, and strategies.

12.9 Conclusion

In summary, neck dissection is essential for oncological staging and locoregional control in the management of head and neck cancer. While oncologic rationale is the primary objective, judicious selection of the levels of neck dissection should be based on known patterns of metastasis, and neck levels that are unlikely to harbor metastasis should be left untouched in order to mitigate complications. The evidence demonstrates that neuropraxia or axonotmesis occurs with all neck dissections involving the SAN as measured by strength, range of motion, pain, and electromyography. Accordingly, more extensive dissection of the SAN produces greater impairment, with the best evidence demonstrated for dissection of level V. There is limited evidence for greater impairment with dissection of level IIb, but there is are a small percentage of metastases to this sublevel; therefore, it is recommended that level IIb dissection be reserved for patients with known level IIa–positive nodes. Adjuvant chemotherapy and radiation contribute to shoulder impairment, but radiation and chemotherapy without surgical intervention show no immediate impairment. The potential late effects of chemotherapy, and especially, radiation therapy, particularly with regard to dysphagia, require further study, as the long-term complications from these treatments can be substantial.

Rehabilitation following neck dissection should focus on the two main complications—shoulder impairment and lymphedema. Progressive scapular resistance makes sense from a pathophysiology perspective for shoulder rehabilitation albeit the current evidence suggests that any shoulder physiotherapy is beneficial as long as it precedes formation of adhesive capsulitis. The current standard of care for HNL is CDT, and it should be utilized for all patients who have HNL. Finally, there are two complimentary and validated questionnaires in the head and neck cancer population that are recommended for evaluation of shoulder impairment—NDII and DASH. Standard use of these questionnaires in future research will improve interpretability of shoulder rehabilitation research involving neck dissection.

References

[1] Ewing MR, Martin H. Disability following radical neck dissection; an assessment based on the postoperative evaluation of 100 patients. Cancer. 1952; 5(5):873–883

[2] Bradley PJ, Ferlito A, Silver CE, et al. Neck treatment and shoulder morbidity: still a challenge. Head Neck. 2011; 33(7):1060–1067

[3] Spalthoff S, Zimmerer R, Jehn P, Gellrich N-C, Handschel J, Krüskemper G. Neck dissection's burden on the patient: functional and psychosocial aspects in 1,652 patients with oral squamous cell carcinomas. J Oral Maxillofac Surg. 2017; 75(4):839–849

[4] Eickmeyer SM, Walczak CK, Myers KB, Lindstrom DR, Layde P, Campbell BH. Quality of life, shoulder range of motion, and spinal accessory nerve status in 5-year survivors of head and neck cancer. PM R. 2014; 6(12):1073–1080

[5] Batstone MD, Scott B, Lowe D, Rogers SN. Marginal mandibular nerve injury during neck dissection and its impact on patient perception of appearance. Head Neck. 2009; 31(5):673–678

[6] Leipzig B, Suen JY, English JL, Barnes J, Hooper M. Functional evaluation of the spinal accessory nerve after neck dissection. Am J Surg. 1983; 146(4):526–530

[7] Cappiello J, Piazza C, Giudice M, De Maria G, Nicolai P. Shoulder disability after different selective neck dissections (levels II–IV versus levels II–V): a comparative study. Laryngoscope. 2005; 115(2):259–263

[8] Gallagher KK, Sacco AG, Lee JS-J, et al. Association between multimodality neck treatment and work and leisure impairment: a disease-specific measure to assess both impairment and rehabilitation after neck dissection. JAMA Otolaryngol Head Neck Surg. 2015; 141(10):888–893

[9] Terrell JE, Welsh DE, Bradford CR, et al. Pain, quality of life, and spinal accessory nerve status after neck dissection. Laryngoscope. 2000; 110(4):620–626

[10] Nibu K, Ebihara Y, Ebihara M, et al. Quality of life after neck dissection: a multicenter longitudinal study by the Japanese Clinical Study Group on Standardization of Treatment for Lymph Node Metastasis of Head and Neck Cancer. Int J Clin Oncol. 2010; 15(1):33–38

[11] Selcuk A, Selcuk B, Bahar S, Dere H. Shoulder function in various types of neck dissection. Role of spinal accessory nerve and cervical plexus preservation. Tumori. 2008; 94(1):36–39

[12] Lea J, Bachar G, Sawka AM, et al. Metastases to level IIb in squamous cell carcinoma of the oral cavity: a systematic review and meta-analysis. Head Neck. 2010; 32(2):184–190

[13] Ahlberg A, Nikolaidis P, Engström T, et al. Morbidity of supraomohyoidal and modified radical neck dissection combined with radiotherapy for head and neck cancer: a prospective longitudinal study. Head Neck. 2012; 34(1):66–72

[14] Gane EM, O'Leary SP, Hatton AL, Panizza BJ, McPhail SM. Neck and upper limb dysfunction in patients following neck dissection: looking beyond the shoulder. Otolaryngol Head Neck Surg. 2017; 157(4):631–640

[15] Hutcheson KA, Lewin JS, Barringer DA, et al. Late dysphagia after radiotherapy-based treatment of head and neck cancer. Cancer. 2012; 118 (23):5793–5799

[16] Chapuy CI, Annino DJ, Snavely A, et al. Swallowing function following postchemoradiotherapy neck dissection: review of findings and analysis of contributing factors. Otolaryngol Head Neck Surg. 2011; 145(3):428–434

[17] Schilling C, Stoeckli SJ, Haerle SK, et al. Sentinel European Node Trial (SENT): 3-year results of sentinel node biopsy in oral cancer. Eur J Cancer. 2015; 51 (18):2777–2784

[18] Murer K, Huber GF, Haile SR, Stoeckli SJ. Comparison of morbidity between sentinel node biopsy and elective neck dissection for treatment of the n0 neck in patients with oral squamous cell carcinoma. Head Neck. 2011; 33 (9):1260–1264

[19] Taylor RJ, Chepeha JC, Teknos TN, et al. Development and validation of the neck dissection impairment index: a quality of life measure. Arch Otolaryngol Head Neck Surg. 2002; 128(1):44–49

[20] Goldstein DP, Ringash J, Bissada E, et al. Evaluation of shoulder disability questionnaires used for the assessment of shoulder disability after neck dissection for head and neck cancer. Head Neck. 2014; 36(10):1453–1458

[21] Goldstein DP, Ringash J, Irish JC, et al. Assessment of the Disabilities of the Arm, Shoulder, and Hand (DASH) questionnaire for use in patients after neck dissection for head and neck cancer. Head Neck. 2015; 37(2):234–242

[22] Stuiver MM, ten Tusscher MR, van Opzeeland A, et al. Psychometric properties of 3 patient-reported outcome measures for the assessment of shoulder disability after neck dissection. Head Neck. 2016; 38(1):102–110

[23] McGarvey AC, Chiarelli PE, Osmotherly PG, Hoffman GR. Physiotherapy for accessory nerve shoulder dysfunction following neck dissection surgery: a literature review. Head Neck. 2011; 33(2):274–280

[24] Carvalho AP, Vital FM, Soares BG. Exercise interventions for shoulder dysfunction in patients treated for head and neck cancer. Cochrane Database Syst Rev. 2012; 18(4):CD008693

[25] McGarvey AC, Hoffman GR, Osmotherly PG, Chiarelli PE. Maximizing shoulder function after accessory nerve injury and neck dissection surgery: a multicenter randomized controlled trial. Head Neck. 2015; 37(7):1022–1031

[26] Gupta A, Bah M. NSAIDs in the treatment of postoperative pain. Curr Pain Headache Rep. 2016; 20(11):62

[27] Smith BG, Lewin JS. Lymphedema management in head and neck cancer. Curr Opin Otolaryngol Head Neck Surg. 2010; 18(3):153–158

[28] Shaitelman SF, Cromwell KD, Rasmussen JC, et al. Recent progress in the treatment and prevention of cancer-related lymphedema. CA Cancer J Clin. 2015; 65(1):55–81

[29] Smith BG, Hutcheson KA, Little LG, et al. Lymphedema outcomes in patients with head and neck cancer. Otolaryngol Head Neck Surg. 2015; 152 (2):284–291

13 Cross-sectional Imaging

Ryan T. Fitzgerald

Abstract

Cross-sectional imaging has become an integral part of the workup, treatment planning, and surveillance for patients with neoplasms arising within or otherwise involving the head and neck and directly impacts decision-making regarding neck dissections. This chapter is organized around imaging anatomy as it applies to neck dissection, imaging approaches to staging, and surveillance imaging. Much of the discussion revolves around in computed tomography (CT), but MRI and combined CT/PET strategies are also briefly touched upon.

Keywords: CT, MRI, neck dissection, lymphadenopathy, head and neck cancer, squamous cell carcinoma

13.1 Introduction

Imaging plays an integral role in the staging, treatment planning, and surveillance for squamous cell carcinoma (SCC) and other malignancies occurring in the head and neck. Advances in CT and MRI in recent years have led to improvement in each of these imaging modalities as they apply to the management of head and neck cancer including their role in determination of the necessity of neck dissection.

Modern imaging and its interpretation are challenging endeavors due to the complexity of the hardware and software technologies that form the basis of image generation. Although this chapter will cover some important technical considerations that impact image acquisition and interpretation, the bulk of the material will focus on how imaging can be applied to maximize diagnostic certainty while at the same time maintaining efficiency and cost-effectiveness. Discussion of neck anatomy as it applies to the search for, and description of, cervical lymph node disease is covered briefly herein and more extensively in other chapters. Rather than organizing this chapter around imaging modalities, an outline based on imaging features of nodal metastases across multiple imaging modalities will instead be followed. Given its high prevalence relative to other malignancies, the bulk of the text is based on data from studies of nodal disease attributable to SCC. Nevertheless, many of the concepts such as imaging features indicative of lymph node metastases are broadly applicable across a wide spectrum of neoplasms. In the face of ever-evolving imaging techniques applied to head and neck malignancy, the goal has been to collate peer-reviewed evidence from the past decade. That said, in some cases it has been necessary to cite earlier work upon which more recent investigations have built. After a short synopsis of imaging-based neck anatomy, the bulk of this chapter will focus on the imaging approach to neck staging and thereafter conclude with a discussion of the imaging approach to surveillance of the neck.

13.2 Imaging Anatomy

Image-based classification of cervical lymph nodes in the context of head and neck malignancy has been widely adopted due to the ubiquity of imaging as part of cancer staging for most patients, the ability of imaging to detect clinically occult nodal metastases, and the high level of reproducibility with which modern cross-sectional imaging can localize metastatic nodes in relation to anatomic landmarks.[1] In 2000, Som et al proposed the most widely utilized radiologic classification system for cross-sectional imaging assessment of cervical lymph nodes, which complements the clinically based classification espoused by the American Joint Committee on Cancer and the American Academy of Otolaryngology–Head and Neck Surgery.[1] In this system, landmarks forming the borders of each nodal level are based on axial image sections. Level I includes lymph nodes superior to the hyoid bone, below the mylohyoid muscle, and anterior to the posterior borders of the submandibular glands. Levels II and III refer to lymph nodes that reside anterior to a transverse line along the posterior borders of the sternocleidomastoid muscles. Level II nodes are posterior to the posterior margin of the submandibular gland, lie between the skull base and inferior margin of the hyoid bone, and are positioned lateral to the medial border of the internal carotid artery. Below level II, level III describes a contiguous compartment that extends inferiorly to the lower border of the cricoid cartilage. Further inferiorly, level IV extends to the level of the clavicle. In contrast to levels II and III, level IV nodes lie anterior and medial to an oblique line drawn through the posterior edge of the sternocleidomastoid muscle and the posterior lateral edge of the anterior scalene muscle. Level V describes nodes that are dorsal to the posterior border of levels II to IV and lie anterior to a transverse line through the anterior edge of the trapezius muscles. Level VI refers to lymph nodes that lie inferior to the lower body of the hyoid bone, superior to the upper border of the manubrium, and medial to the medial borders of the common/internal carotid arteries. Level VII lymph nodes lie between the upper border of the manubrium and brachiocephalic veins and are also medial to the medial borders of the common carotid arteries. CT-based examples of the Som classification scheme are available in their original publication.[1]

Anatomic localization of suspected nodal metastases is important not only for staging and treatment planning, but can also provide guidance for further investigation if the site of primary neoplasm is not readily apparent. For example, nodal metastases isolated to level II would draw attention to the oral cavity or oropharyngeal mucosal space rather than the thyroid gland, whereas the finding of abnormal nodes confined to levels VI and VII would be much more likely to emanate from a thyroid primary. In cases in which the primary neoplasm is known, such knowledge can direct scrutiny to first-level nodal drainage areas and thus maximize the detection of early or subtle signs of metastatic involvement of cervical lymph nodes.

13.3 Imaging Approach to Neck Staging

In cases of SCC arising in the head and neck as well as other neck neoplasms, the presence or absence of metastatic lymph nodes substantially impacts treatment options and prognosis. Given the accuracy of modern cross-sectional imaging to identify and localize nodal metastases, imaging has become a necessary adjunct to the clinical examination for treatment planning. CT is currently the most widely utilized imaging modality for neck staging owing to its wide availability and technical capabilities. Much of the following section will thus focus on the application of CT in the neck staging, largely due to the fact that the preponderance of literature on the subject is CT based. MRI may also play a role in select cases such as patient for whom iodinated CT contrast agents are contraindicated (e.g., prior anaphylactic reaction after iodinated contrast) or for problem solving in the setting of suspected skull base invasion or perineural tumor spread owing to the superior sensitivity of MR for these applications. Among the barriers to expanded use of MRI are longer scan times relative to CT, increased cost, issues of claustrophobia, and the direct relationship between scan time and image degradation secondary to patient motion.

13.4 Lymph Node Characteristics Related to Metastatic Involvement

13.4.1 Size

Although size is frequently invoked in the discussion of lymph node metastases, it is a poor marker of metastatic involvement relative to other factors discussed later. At many centers, lymph node size is reported as long-axis diameter on an axial image section and may also include a long-axis measurement in another plane if such a measurement would impact staging. Long-axis measurements, in contrast to short-axis measurements that are employed at other locations such as the mediastinum, best replicate the clinical determination of palpable lymph node enlargement. Measurement in the long axis is the most frequently employed methodology across the literature and is the metric utilized in the TNM classification of the American Academy of Otolaryngology–Head and Neck Surgery.

Underlying the limitations of lymph node size as a primary determinant of metastatic involvement is the frequency of pathologic confirmation of metastases in lymph nodes of normal size (▶ Fig. 13.1). As an example, in a study of subjects with head and neck SCC, Don et al found that 67% of metastatic nodes had a longitudinal diameter smaller than 1 cm.[2] Lymph node enlargement may be a late manifestation of metastatic involvement that is proceeded by heterogeneous enhancement or other more sensitive imaging biomarkers.[3] The specificity of lymph node size as an indicator of metastatic involvement is lacking due to the propensity of lymph nodes to become enlarged as a response to infection and inflammation. The existence of multiple disagreeing size criteria and differences in accepted size thresholds based on location and patient age further confounds the application of size to the staging assessment.[3] For instance, the application of a 1-cm threshold within levels II and VI would yield a substantial difference in the specificity of nodal metastases, as nodes measuring above 1 cm are frequently encountered in level II of normal subjects. As such, many practitioners use a tiered threshold in which the size threshold for levels I and II is higher than that for more caudal levels. Asymmetry can serve as

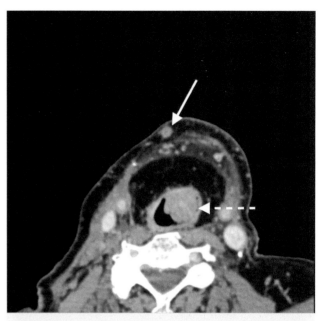

Fig. 13.1 Axial image from a contrast-enhanced CT scan in a patient with a history of laryngeal carcinoma reveals tumor recurrence (*dashed arrow*) along the ventral wall of the neopharynx reconstruction. A 4-mm lymph node within the nearby subcutaneous compartment was positive for metastases at resection despite its small size (*solid arrow*). Poorly defined margins and central low attenuation indicative of necrosis were prospectively suggestive of metastatic involvement.

another useful discriminator regarding the significance of lymph node enlargement, whereby enlarged lymph nodes that are unilateral and/or confined to a single anatomic level are more likely to be true positives than cases in which nodal enlargement is more widespread (▶ Fig. 13.2). Despite the suboptimal sensitivity and specificity of size as a marker of nodal metastases, lymph node enlargement can be a useful tool toward identification of nodes requiring further scrutiny, but as an isolated feature it is not necessarily sufficient for the determination of metastatic involvement in the absence of additional markers of nodal metastases such as irregular margins or internal necrosis.

13.4.2 Morphology and Architecture

Physiologic lymph nodes are reniform (kidney) in shape and are composed of intermediate-density tissues surrounding an eccentric fatty hilum. As metastatic cells proliferate within a lymph node, concentric centrifugal expansion tends to alter the morphology of the node toward a more rounded shape. Thus, round lymph nodes, regardless of size, appropriately raise suspicion for metastatic involvement. In nonmetastatic reactive lymph nodes, the ratio of the long axis diameter to the short axis diameter exceeds 2:1 in 86% of cases.[4]

Lymph node enhancement is another feature that can be applied toward the determination of metastatic involvement. The parenchyma of physiologic lymph nodes enhances homogeneously, whereas nodes harboring metastases may show areas of heterogeneity, typically hypoenhancement, that is of moderate specificity for metastatic involvement. The finding of hyperphysiologic enhancement is both a poorly sensitive

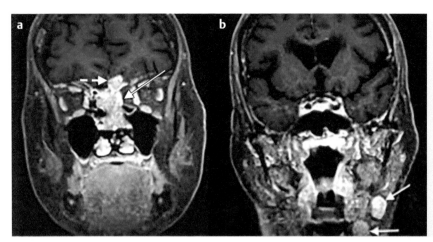

Fig. 13.2 Coronal **(a)** contrast-enhanced T1-weighted MR image shows an enhancing mass (esthesioneuroblastoma) arising in the left sinonasal cavity (*solid arrow*) and extending across the anterior skull base into the anterior cranial fossa (*dashed arrow*). **(b)** A coronal contrast-enhanced T1-weighted MR image more anteriorly in the same patient revealed enlarged, enhancing lymph nodes (*arrows*) in left level II that were positive for metastatic involvement at resection.

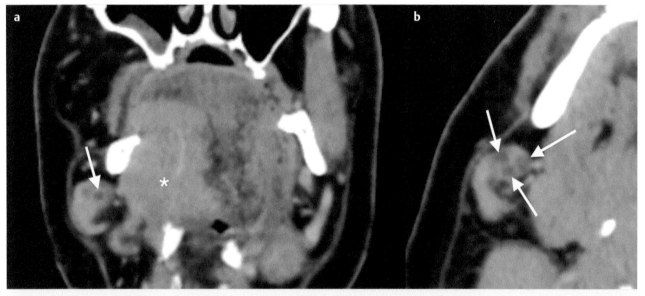

Fig. 13.3 Coronal **(a)** and axial **(b)** images from a contrast-enhanced neck CT show an enlarged lymph node lateral to the right submandibular gland that contains internal areas of hypoenhancement (*arrows*) indicative of necrosis. Although the node maintained a normal fatty hilum, on resection it was positive for metastatic involvement. On the axial image **(a)**, the primary neoplasm (squamous cell carcinoma) involving the right oral tongue and floor of mouth is indicated by an asterisk.

and poorly specific marker of metastatic involvement as it is commonly encountered in reactive lymph nodes (in the setting of infection/inflammation) and often persists in nodes previously treated by chemotherapy and radiation. Among the most specific markers of metastasis is the presence of intranodal necrosis (▶ Fig. 13.3, ▶ Fig. 13.4). Careful attention may be required to distinguish between the physiologic fatty hilum and necrotic tissue, particularly in lymph nodes that are not significantly enlarged. CT has been shown to be superior to MR for the detection of nodal necrosis.[5]

Cystic nodal metastases can be encountered in metastatic SCC from any primary site; however, there is an established predilection for the development of cystic nodes in association within primary cancers arising within Waldeyer's ring.[6] Thus, the discovery of cystic lymph nodes, particularly across levels II and III, should prompt scrutiny of pharyngeal lymphoid tissue. More recently, an association has been described between cystic nodal morphology and human papillomavirus (HPV) positive SCC.[7,8] In a study of 136 oropharyngeal SCC (OPSCC), metastases associated with HPV-positive tumors

demonstrated cystic features in 36% of cases versus in 9% of cases for nodal metastases attributed to HPV-negative primaries.[8] Papillary carcinoma of the thyroid is another primary tumor that is frequently implicated in the development of cystic nodal metastases. Thus, cystic nodal metastases within levels IV, VI, and VII and sparing of level II/III would appropriately focus attention to the thyroid gland (▶ Fig. 13.5).

13.4.3 Margins

Physiologic lymph nodes display clear, sharp margins bordered by homogeneous fat. Relative to size, the development of marginal irregularity is a specific marker of metastasis, as lymph nodes reacting to local of systemic infections may become enlarged but in most cases maintain normal margins. Extension of metastatic growth across and beyond the nodal capsule can also elicit stranding within adjacent fat. Loss of nodal margins should also prompt assessment for potential invasion of adjacent structures such as the carotid sheath vasculature, musculature, or glandular tissue, as such findings impact staging

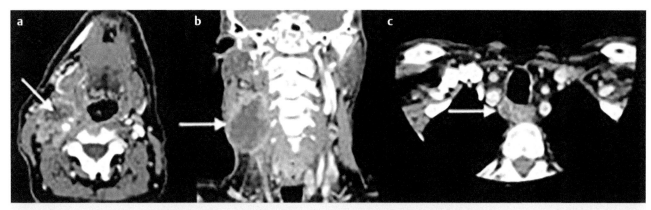

Fig. 13.4 (a) Axial contrast-enhanced CT image at across level II shows a metastatic nodal mass with peripherally enhancing margins and an irregular necrotic core (*arrow*). Tumor encases the right carotid sheath. (b) Coronal contrast-enhanced CT image provides an additional view of the necrotic lymph node conglomerate displays in panel A. (c) In a more caudal image from the same contrast-enhanced neck CT, necrosis with a 1.1-cm right tracheoesophageal lymph node (*arrow*) denotes mediastinal metastatic involvement.

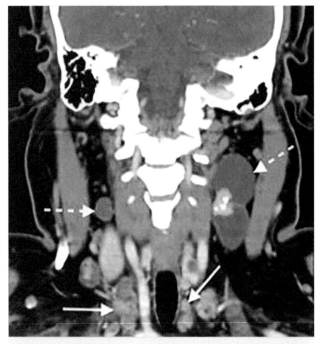

Fig. 13.5 Coronal contrast-enhanced image through the neck reveals numerous predominantly solid (*dashed arrows*) lymph nodes within levels IV and VI and several predominantly cystic lymph nodes (*solid arrows*) more superiorly centered within level III. Cystic nodes in the lower neck prompted investigation of the thyroid gland that yielded a diagnosis of papillary thyroid carcinoma.

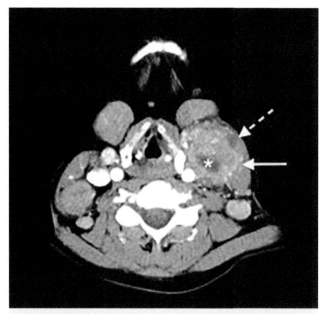

Fig. 13.6 Axial contrast-enhanced CT shows a centrally necrotic (*asterisk*) metastatic lymph node spanning left levels II and III. Margins of the node are irregular (*solid arrow*) and there is no clear fat plane between the node and the sternocleidomastoid muscle (SCM). Asymmetric enlargement of the left SCM and intramuscular edema (*dashed arrow*) are evidence of extracapsular spread and neoplastic infiltration of the muscle.

(▶ Fig. 13.6). A discussion of lymph node margin status as it applies to extracapsular disease spread can be found in the following section.

13.4.4 Extracapsular Spread

Extracapsular spread (ECS) of nodal metastases from head and neck SCC has been established as a poor prognostic indicator in terms of 5-year overall survival and also confers an increased probability of locoregional recurrence and distant metastases.[9,10] Although histologic determination of ECS is the gold standard, radiographically determined ECS also confers poor distant control of disease and attenuated survival.[11] Pretherapy, radiologic determination of ECS status may hold particular importance for patients with oropharyngeal cancers (OPSCC), which are often HPV related and amenable to treatment with radiation alone for early-stage disease and combined radiation and chemotherapy in more advanced disease.[12] Based on studies showing the survival benefit of chemotherapy in addition to routine postoperative radiation in OPSCC patients with positive margins or ECS, surgery could be reasonably deferred for OPSCC patients with radiologically determined ECS and reserved for cases that eventually require salvage therapy.[13]

While the potential for noninvasive determination of ECS status is promising, studies examining the test characteristics of CT and MRI for the detection of ECS have failed to show high degrees of reliability. A summary of reported sensitivities across studies using both CT and MR yielded suboptimal sensitivities ranging from 62.5 to 80.9% and specificities from 60 to 93%.[13] A large study of 432 patients with head and neck SCC undergoing neck dissection found a CT-derived specificity of 97.7% although the sensitivity in the study was only 43%.[14] Positive predictive values for CT-based ECS determination have been reported from 71 to 84% and negative predictive values from 48 to 49%.[15] Given the impact of ECS determination on recent management trends, examination of techniques that could potentially boost the sensitivity of ECS detection will be important going forward.

Inclusion of both macroscopic and microscopic extracapsular spread of disease on histopathology as ECS positive is almost certainly responsible in part for the suboptimal sensitivity of imaging-based determination of ECS status based on the constraints of spatial resolution inherent in current techniques. The predilection of some head and neck cancer metastases, particularly those from HPV-positive OPSCC, to exhibit cystic features may also complicate the assessment for ECS. In their study of 111 patients with OPSCC, Aiken et al found that intranodal necrosis was the most robust radiologic predictor of pathologically proven ECS, whereas irregular borders and gross invasion approached, but did not meet, statistical significance.[13] The overlap between the imaging appearance of internal necrosis and cyst formation may partially explain the lack of robust sensitivity of radiologic ECS determination across prior conventional cross-sectional imaging studies.

13.5 Imaging Approach to Surveillance

Imaging not only is applicable for staging and treatment planning but also plays an important role in the posttreatment setting for patients with head and neck malignancies in order to assess the response to treatment, guide further treatment, and also to establish a new baseline examination to which future radiologic surveillance studies can be compared. The timing and methods employed for surveillance vary across institutions, but in general patients who have received definitive radiation therapy and/or chemoradiotherapy undergo imaging 12 weeks after the conclusion of treatment. The typical 3-month gap between completion of therapy and imaging facilitates the evolution of treatment effects including tumor involution and thus reduces the possibility of false-positive results that can occur if imaging is obtained during or soon after treatment. For patients amenable to surgical treatment with curative intent, surveillance imaging is typically performed within the first 6 months after treatment.

CT continues to serve as the most widely utilized modality for imaging surveillance in patients with SCC of the head and neck for both the initial posttreatment examination and subsequent surveillance studies. The frequency and duration of surveillance radiographic assessment is patient specific and may vary according to pretreatment disease severity and treatment response. In general, surveillance imaging is performed every 3 to 12 months

for up to 3 years. Any clinical suspicion of neoplastic recurrence during this time frame and beyond would appropriately prompt imaging for confirmation (ultrasound- or CT-directed biopsy) and restaging.

Surveillance imaging can place a burden on patients with head and neck cancer in terms of both cost and frequency. Rather than following a traditional CT-based algorithm, some groups have explored the application of PET/CT-based strategy. McDermott et al reported in 2013 that two consecutive negative PET/CT examinations within a 6-month period after the conclusion of treatment resulted in a negative predictive value for neoplastic recurrence of 98%, which could obviate the necessity of further radiologic imaging in the absence of clinical signs of recurrence.[16] The potential of two PET/CT scans rather than a series of CT examinations over 3 years would likely result in an overall cost savings despite the higher relative cost of PET over CT. In a subset of head and neck cancer patients with advanced nodal disease (N2 or N3) receiving primary chemoradiotherapy, Mehanna et al showed that surveillance using combined CT/PET at 12 weeks, with neck dissection being performed only in cases showing an incomplete or equivocal response, was statistically equivalent to planned neck dissection in terms of survival.[17] Further, patients randomized to the imaging arm not only underwent fewer surgeries, but also incurred a substantially reduced cost of treatment.[17]

Imaging features of metastatic nodal involvement in the pretreatment neck such as altered nodal morphology/margins and lymph node enlargement continue to be applicable following surgery, radiation, chemotherapy, and combined treatments. That said, disturbance of anatomic relationships due to surgery and radiation-induced changes within superficial and deep soft-tissue compartments often complicate the typical anatomy-based search pattern in the posttreatment neck. Nodal contrast enhancement is of particularly poor specificity in the posttreatment setting and can be attributed to therapeutic irradiation or various chemotherapeutic and immunomodulatory agents[18] (▶ Fig. 13.7, ▶ Fig. 13.8).

13.6 Conclusion

Imaging plays an integral role in the determination of the necessity for and/or extent of neck dissection/radiation. This chapter has outlined relevant imaging anatomy and techniques, discussed criteria for the determination of metastatic lymph node involvement, and explored the implications of imaging features of nodal disease. Although modern techniques have greatly advanced the value of cross-sectional imaging for staging and surveillance of neoplastic disease in the head and neck, it is nonetheless important to recognize their limitations. The sensitivity of CT and MRI is constrained by the fact that up to 25% of clinical N0 necks harbor micrometastases that are beyond the spatial resolution of even the best current cross-sectional techniques.[19] Ultrasound and PET, covered in separate chapters, serve as complementary and/or adjunct modalities that further contribute to the workup, treatment planning, and surveillance for patients with head and neck cancers. Other burgeoning techniques such as molecular imaging are beyond the scope of the current text but may contribute to decision-making surrounding neck dissections in the future.

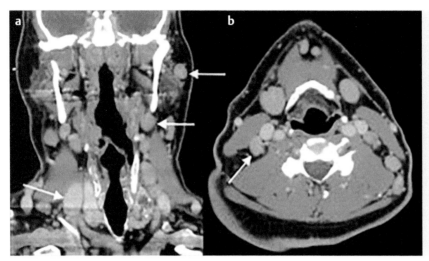

Fig. 13.7 Coronal **(a)** and axial **(b)** contrast-enhanced CT images show multiple enlarged, enhancing lymph nodes (*arrows*) bilaterally in this patient with a history of melanoma being treated with ipilimumab. See ▶ Fig. 13.8 for PET images and further discussion.

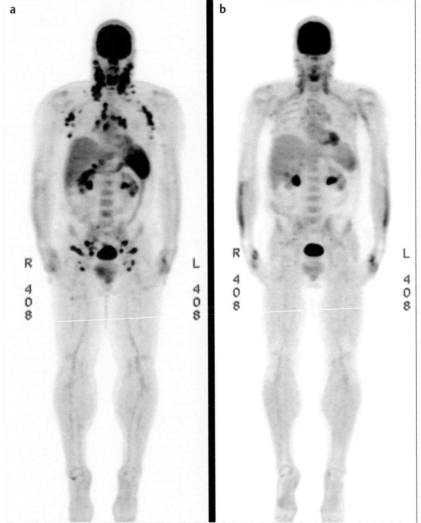

Fig. 13.8 Fluorodeoxyglucose (FDG) PET images from the same patient in ▶ Fig. 13.7 at baseline **(a)** and 2 months later **(b)** after the discontinuation of ipilimumab. The baseline examination **(a)** shows widespread FDG-avid lymphadenopathy that had fully resolved at 8 weeks **(b)**. Lymph node biopsy shortly after the baseline examination yielded reactive lymphadenitis and no malignant cells.

References

[1] Som PM, Curtin HD, Mancuso AA. Imaging-based nodal classification for evaluation of neck metastatic adenopathy. AJR Am J Roentgenol. 2000; 174(3):837–844

[2] Don DM, Anzai Y, Lufkin RB, Fu YS, Calcaterra TC. Evaluation of cervical lymph node metastases in squamous cell carcinoma of the head and neck. Laryngoscope. 1995; 105(7, pt 1):669–674

[3] Castelijns JA, van den Brekel MW. Imaging of lymphadenopathy in the neck. Eur Radiol. 2002; 12(4):727–738

[4] Bruneton JN, Balu-Maestro C, Marcy PY, Melia P, Mourou MY. Very high frequency (13 MHz) ultrasonographic examination of the normal neck: detection of normal lymph nodes and thyroid nodules. J Ultrasound Med. 1994; 13(2):87–90

[5] Curtin HD, Ishwaran H, Mancuso AA, Dalley RW, Caudry DJ, McNeil BJ. Comparison of CT and MR imaging in staging of neck metastases. Radiology. 1998; 207(1):123–130

[6] Goldenberg D, Sciubba J, Koch WM. Cystic metastasis from head and neck squamous cell cancer: a distinct disease variant? Head Neck. 2006; 28(7):633–638

[7] Goldenberg D, Begum S, Westra WH, et al. Cystic lymph node metastasis in patients with head and neck cancer: an HPV-associated phenomenon. Head Neck. 2008; 30(7):898–903

[8] Cantrell SC, Peck BW, Li G, Wei Q, Sturgis EM, Ginsberg LE. Differences in imaging characteristics of HPV-positive and HPV-negative oropharyngeal cancers: a blinded matched-pair analysis. AJNR Am J Neuroradiol. 2013; 34(10):2005–2009

[9] Kokemueller H, Rana M, Rublack J, et al. The Hannover experience: surgical treatment of tongue cancer: a clinical retrospective evaluation over a 30 years period. Head Neck Oncol. 2011; 3:27

[10] Jan JC, Hsu WH, Liu SA, et al. Prognostic factors in patients with buccal squamous cell carcinoma: 10-year experience. J Oral Maxillofac Surg. 2011; 69(2):396–404

[11] Kann BH, Buckstein M, Carpenter TJ, et al. Radiographic extracapsular extension and treatment outcomes in locally advanced oropharyngeal carcinoma. Head Neck. 2014; 36(12):1689–1694

[12] O'Sullivan B, Huang SH, Siu LL, et al. Deintensification candidate subgroups in human papillomavirus-related oropharyngeal cancer according to minimal risk of distant metastasis. J Clin Oncol. 2013; 31(5):543–550

[13] Aiken AH, Poliashenko S, Beitler JJ, et al. Accuracy of preoperative imaging in detecting nodal extracapsular spread in oral cavity squamous cell carcinoma. AJNR Am J Neuroradiol. 2015; 36(9):1776–1781

[14] Prabhu RS, Magliocca KR, Hanasoge S, et al. Accuracy of computed tomography for predicting pathologic nodal extracapsular extension in patients with head-and-neck cancer undergoing initial surgical resection. Int J Radiat Oncol Biol Phys. 2014; 88(1):122–129

[15] Chai RL, Rath TJ, Johnson JT, et al. Accuracy of computed tomography in the prediction of extracapsular spread of lymph node metastases in squamous cell carcinoma of the head and neck. JAMA Otolaryngol Head Neck Surg. 2013; 139(11):1187–1194

[16] McDermott M, Hughes M, Rath T, et al. Negative predictive value of surveillance PET/CT in head and neck squamous cell cancer. AJNR Am J Neuroradiol. 2013; 34(8):1632–1636

[17] Mehanna H, Wong W-L, McConkey CC, et al. PET-NECK Trial Management Group. PET-CT surveillance versus neck dissection in advanced head and neck cancer. N Engl J Med. 2016; 374(15):1444–1454

[18] Arellano K, Mosley JC, III. Case report of ipilimumab-induced diffuse, nonnecrotizing granulomatous lymphadenitis and granulomatous vasculitis. J Pharm Pract. 2017:897190017699762

[19] van den Brekel MW, van der Waal I, Meijer CJ, Freeman JL, Castelijns JA, Snow GB. The incidence of micrometastases in neck dissection specimens obtained from elective neck dissections. Laryngoscope. 1996; 106(8):987–991

14 Structures of the Neck Amenable to Ultrasound Evaluation

Donald Bodenner and Jamie Ferguson

Abstract

Ultrasound has become an important tool in the evaluation of the neck prior to a neck dissection. Ultrasound is safe, relatively inexpensive, available in the ambulatory setting, and, with the resolution of a few millimeters, is capable of characterizing even small structures in the neck. Ultrasound has proliferated in its use in the neck in the United States because of benign and malignant thyroid disease. This chapter will introduce the basic concepts of ultrasonography, largely from a thyroid perspective, and introduce common methods of evaluating the neck, and discuss normal and abnormal features of organs and structures in the neck that are important to appreciate prior to a neck dissection. There are multiple additional benefits to office-based neck ultrasound. The office utilization allows for direct communication from the physician to the patient in real time. Ultrasound is rapidly moving into outpatient clinical practice in endocrinology and surgery. Proficiency in thyroid ultrasound is now required for endocrine certification, and although not yet mandatory for otolaryngology and general surgery, certification is strongly encouraged.

Keywords: ultrasound, neck dissection, thyroid

14.1 Ultrasonography Basics

Ultrasound (US) is based on the reflection of generated sound waves. There have been tremendous advances in algorithms that transform the captured sound waves into a much more refined image. The depth that the sound waves reach is dependent upon frequency. Lower-frequency sound waves penetrate deeper but typically have poorer resolution. Higher-frequency sound waves do not penetrate as well but have superior resolution. Sound waves are reflected at the boundaries of tissues with different impedance, which is dependent on the density of the tissues and the velocity of the sound within a particular tissue.[1] Transducers both generate the sound waves and capture reflected sound. Transducers today commonly have variable frequency capabilities. A common frequency used to evaluate the thyroid lobes and superficial structures is 14 MHz. Slightly lower frequencies up to 12 MHz are often employed to localize parathyroid adenomas. Lower frequencies, from 7 to 10 MHz, are used to look at deep structures in the neck, up to 4 cm from the surface.[1]

To perform a US of the neck, the patient is typically positioned either supine or reclined up to an angle of 30 to 45 degrees. For some patients in a wheelchair or others who cannot lie supine, US can be performed in the near sitting position with the chin tilted back slightly. One common method to perform a US of the neck is to start in the thyroid gland with a frequency of 12 to 14 MHz. The transducer is placed transversely on the neck and the frequency is optimized for thyroid tissue. The transducer is slowly moved vertically to evaluate the thyroid lobe and nodules in transverse and anteroposterior dimensions. The transducer is then rotated 90 degrees to obtain the axial dimensions of structures of interest. Once the thyroid has been completely evaluated, the transducer is again placed in the

transverse orientation over the thyroid and moved caudally, paying particular attention to the area around the hyoid to pick up a possible thyroglossal duct cyst. With the transducer still in the transverse position, it is moved one-half to three-fourths of the width of the transducer laterally and then slowly moved inferior down to the clavicle. The transducer is tilted caudally for the sound beam to characterize lymph nodes or other structures beneath or inferior to the clavicle. This process is repeated moving into the contralateral neck to evaluate the presence of lymph nodes, the size and shape of the submandibular and parotid glands, and for the presence of any abnormal masses.

14.2 Thyroid/Parathyroid Gland

The thyroid gland is often a focus in the planning of a neck dissection. US of a normal thyroid gland is shown in ▶ Fig. 14.1. A normal thyroid gland is homogeneous with a density slightly brighter than that of the muscle. Thyroid tissue that arises from the isthmus and extends superiorly is known as a pyramidal lobe and may be present up to 30% of the time.

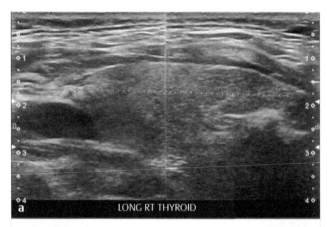

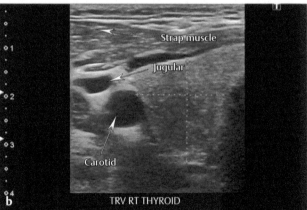

Fig. 14.1 (a) Normal thyroid lobe longitudinal view. (b) Normal thyroid lobe transverse view

There are many pathologic states that conceivably could influence the extent of neck dissection. Hashimoto's thyroiditis is a benign autoimmune disorder that can trigger an extensive inflammatory response potentially causing adhesions and difficulty during a dissection. The most common clinical presentation is a moderately enlarged gland, often one and a half times normal, that is very firm on physical examination. There are several US appearances of a Hashimoto gland.[2] The most common has been termed "giraffe skin" because of its mottled appearance with innumerable hypoechoic areas alternating with hyperechoic areas (▶ Fig. 14.2). These nodularities are typically small ranging from 3 to 5 mm. The hyperechoic areas are sometimes confluent, forming benign, well-defined nodules termed "white knights" (▶ Fig. 14.3). Hashimoto's thyroiditis can also manifest with large areas that are diffusely hypoechoic with some fibrous banding (▶ Fig. 14.4). Often, there is very little normal thyroid tissue present. The fibrous banding often forms pseudonodules, where in the transverse view the hypoechoic area appears exactly as a thyroid nodule; however, when the transducer is rotated to the longitudinal view, the nodule disappears. This form of Hashimoto's thyroiditis can appear almost identical to thyroid lymphoma (▶ Fig. 14.5) and any biopsy should always include a sample sent for flow cytometry in order to differentiate between the two possible diagnoses. A Hashimoto gland also may present as a hybrid of fibrous banding and hypoechogenicity, with hypoechoic areas often encompassing one-fourth or more of the thyroid gland with no normal tissue present and then the remainder of the thyroid lobe appearing relatively normal. Finally, the thyroid gland in early Hashimoto's thyroiditis may have a near-normal appearance. It is not unusual to see benign lymph nodes around the periphery of a Hashimoto gland. These can be mildly enlarged from 1 to 1.5 mm but are benign appearing with an elongated appearance and a good hilum.

There appears to be a correlation between the appearance of a Hashimoto gland and antithyroid peroxidase (thyroperoxidase [TPOAb]) and thyroglobulin antibody levels. Antibody levels are higher in homogeneously, hypoechoic glands and correlate with the degree of lymphocytic infiltration.[3] The prevalence of thyroid cancer in a Hashimoto gland is controversial. A large meta-analysis of over 10,000 papillary thyroid carcinoma (PTC) cases demonstrated that Hashimoto's gland was far more likely associated with PTC than normal thyroid tissue.[4] A second meta-analysis of over 64,000 patients showed a modest increase in PTC.[5] However, a recent, well-conducted meta-analysis compared studies categorized into a fine-needle aspiration biopsy (FNAB) group and an archival thyroidectomy group. The prevalence of PTC in the FNAB group was 1.2%, whereas in the archival thyroidectomy group it was 27%, strongly suggesting no real association.[6]

It is important to ascertain whether or not thyroid cancer is present. The characteristics of malignant or suspicious nodules that would trigger an FNAB will be discussed here, but the details of the workup of indeterminate nodules, etc., are beyond the scope of this publication. Four patterns of thyroid nodules are commonly associated with benign results[7]: (1) simple cysts with or without colloid clot that do not contain substantial solid element; (2) hyperechoic nodules or white knights (▶ Fig. 14.3) in a Hashimoto gland; (3) giraffe pattern (▶ Fig. 14.2) also in a Hashimoto gland; and (4) nodules resembling a wet sponge or "spongiform" nodules (▶ Fig. 14.6). However, the morphology of these benign lesions should be carefully standardized. As shown in ▶ Fig. 14.7, a nodule that closely resembled a spongiform nodule was found to be PTC on biopsy.

There are several US characteristics that suggest malignancy, with microcalcifications less than 1 mm having the highest specificity (▶ Fig. 14.8).[8] Intact eggshell calcifications are most

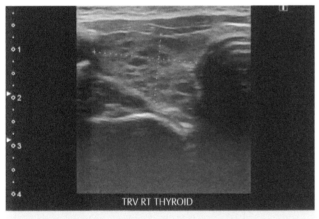

Fig. 14.2 Hashimoto's giraffe skin (moth-eaten) appearance.

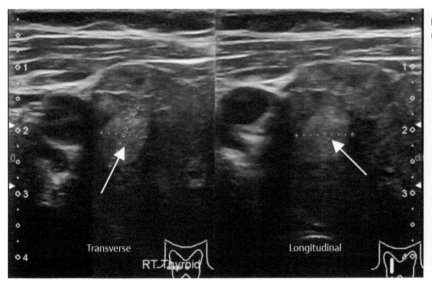

Fig. 14.3 Hashimoto's benign hyperechoic nodules (white knights).

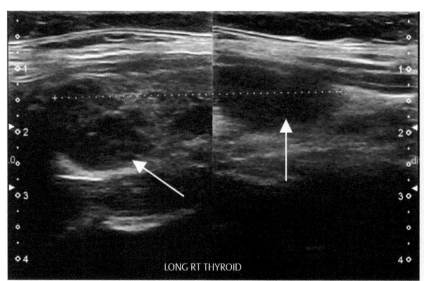

Fig. 14.4 Hashimoto's large hypoechoic areas.

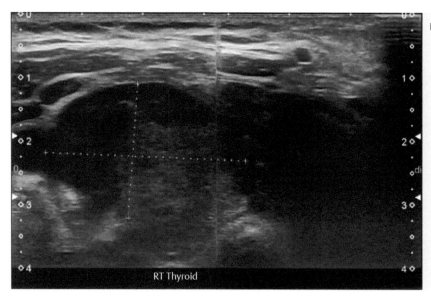

Fig. 14.5 Thyroid lymphoma.

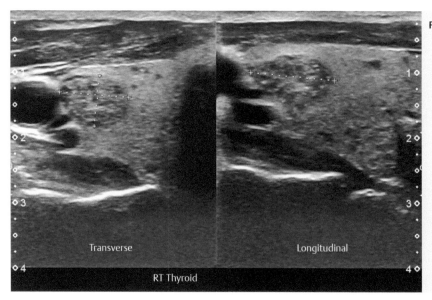

Fig. 14.6 Spongiform nodule.

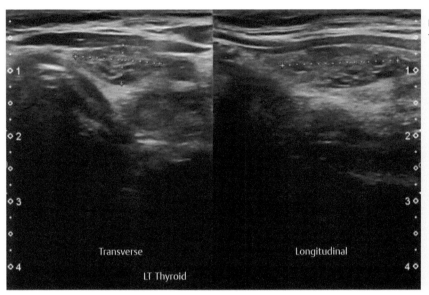

Fig. 14.7 Spongiform-appearing nodule positive for papillary thyroid carcinoma.

Transverse   Longitudinal

LT Thyroid

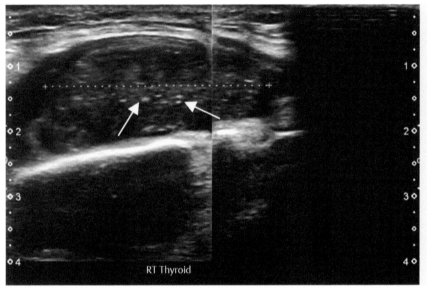

Fig. 14.8 Primary papillary thyroid carcinoma with microcalcifications.

RT Thyroid

often benign, but can be malignant depending upon the continuity of the calcifications. Incomplete eggshell calcifications and those with protruding elements are often malignant.[9] However, inspissated colloid can form bright objects that strongly resemble microcalcifications. The two can often be discriminated by shadowing often seen with microcalcifications that is rarely present with inspissated colloid.

It should be kept in mind that the presence of coarse calcification does not preclude the diagnosis of thyroid carcinoma, although usually, if malignant, they will be accompanied by microcalcifications (▶ Fig. 14.9). Hypoechogenicity is also a common finding in thyroid carcinoma.[10] The degree of hypoechogenicity is highly variable, ranging from an almost completely black appearance similar to the echogenicity of the carotid artery (▶ Fig. 14.8) to nodules that are just barely darker than the surrounding thyroid tissue (▶ Fig. 14.10). The sensitivity of hypoechogenicity is very high, but the specificity is rather low. For example, benign nodules can also be very hypoechoic. The continuity of the capsule is very important. If there is blebbing of the nodule out into

surrounding thyroid, or a very poorly defined capsule (▶ Fig. 14.9), this should be immediately concerning for the presence of malignancy.[11] A nodule that is taller than it is wide has been shown to have a higher propensity for malignancy.[11] The physiologic basis for this phenomenon is unclear, but it has been reported to have a specificity as high as 90%.[12] Size alone is a relatively poor indicator of malignancy. Generally, there is a positive correlation between the size of a nodule and its risk of malignancy. This is particularly true for nodules that are 2 cm or greater in size.[13] However, some studies have shown that nodules greater than 4 cm have a smaller chance of being malignant than nodules that are less than 4 cm.[14] In addition, there was no increased risk of malignancy in follicular neoplasms greater than 4 cm in size.[15] However, large nodules that are extremely hypoechoic, similar to that of the carotid artery, are highly suspicious and often are lymphoma (▶ Fig. 14.5) or poorly differentiated/anaplastic carcinoma (▶ Fig. 14.11).

Using the above criteria, there are some nodules that appear to be malignant immediately after the transducer is placed on

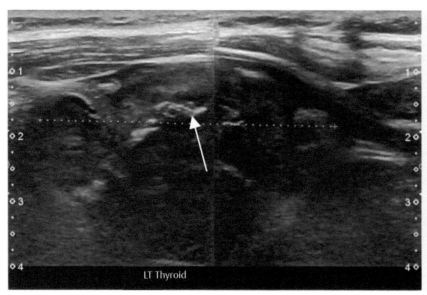

Fig. 14.9 Primary papillary thyroid carcinoma with coarse calcifications.

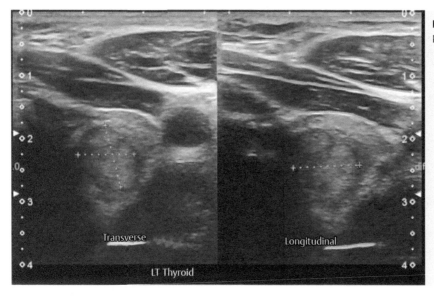

Fig. 14.10 Benign appearing thyroid nodule positive for papillary thyroid carcinoma.

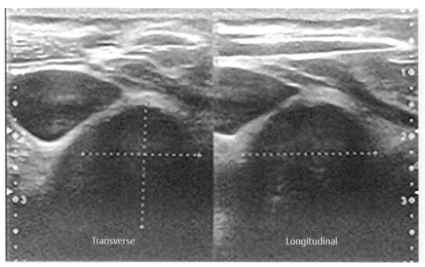

Fig. 14.11 Anaplastic thyroid carcinoma.

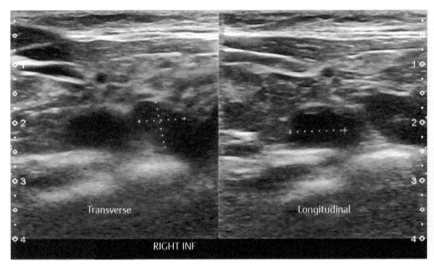

Fig. 14.12 Typical rounded, hypoechoic appearance of a parathyroid gland.

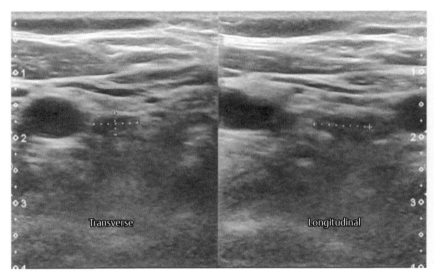

Fig. 14.13 Flattened, hyperechoic parathyroid gland.

the neck. However, this is not always the case. There are many instances where nodules are found to be malignant on FNAB with only mild hypoechogenicity on US (▶ Fig. 14.7).

Another structure that is amenable to evaluation by US is the parathyroid gland. There are typically four parathyroid glands, two off the inferior pole of the right and left lobe and two typically found posterior to the midportion of the thyroid lobes commonly referred to as superior parathyroid glands (▶ Fig. 14.12). The appearance of parathyroid glands on US imaging is typically rounded and hypoechoic. However, the gland is often irregularly shaped and may even be slightly hyperechoic (▶ Fig. 14.13). Parathyroid adenomas may show peripheral blood flow unlike central blood flow observed in lymph nodes. There may also be increased blood flow to the parathyroid capsule or adjacent thyroid tissue.[16,17] FNAB measuring parathyroid hormone in a saline washout is helpful in identifying an adenoma, particularly if an intrathyroidal parathyroid adenoma is suspected.[18] In a large meta-analysis of 20,000 patients, primary hyperparathyroidism (HPT) results from a single adenoma in approximately 88.9% of cases, double adenoma in 4.1%, and four-gland disease/hypertrophy in 5.8%.[19]

Ultrasound performs relatively poorly when multiple adenomas are present in renal failure or multiple endocrine neoplasia syndromes (MEN), and also in localizing an adenoma prior to

reoperation for persistent disease. In a study of 166 patients with HPT as a consequence of renal disease, sestamibi scan and US together failed to detect 61.5% of ectopic glands.[20] In 288 patients who required reoperation for persistent HPT, sestamibi provided the best results with 67% true-positive and no false-positive results. US only had a 48% true-positive and 21% false-positive results.[21] The ability to localize a parathyroid adenoma is reduced in the presence of thyroid nodules.[21]

14.3 Fine-Needle Aspiration Biopsy

FNAB is the gold standard in the evaluation of a thyroid nodule. FNAB can be performed with the needle either perpendicular or parallel to the transducer. The biopsy can be performed with a 25- or 23-gauge 1- to 1.5-inch needle. The choice of core needle biopsy versus fine-needle aspirate is still debated, but FNAB reveals more nuclear features, has fewer instances of bleeding, and overall is not inferior to core biopsy in terms of diagnostic yield in some[22] but not all[23] studies. Traditionally, lidocaine anesthesia was avoided because it could obscure nodule landmarks when the biopsy was performed without US guidance. We have found that 1 to 2 mL of lidocaine under the skin and along the probable needle track has markedly decreased patient anxiety and pain involved in the procedure. The only test that should precede an FNAB is a thyroid-stimulating hormone (TSH) determination. A suppressed TSH suggests a toxic adenoma and the diagnosis can be confirmed by thyroid scan and uptake. These lesions are rarely malignant and can be followed with serial US without FNAB. Thyroid scan in the absence of a suppressed TSH is typically not helpful, for benign nodules also are "cold."

FNAB should be reported according to the criteria established at the Bethesda conference in 2007,[24] which have recently been revised.[25] As shown in ▶ Table 14.1, moving from Bethesda III to Bethesda V dramatically increases the likelihood of malignancy. The most difficult Bethesda criteria to evaluate is Bethesda III and Bethesda IV. These nodules have approximately 30% chance of malignancy. In the past, at least a hemithyroidectomy was performed, with completion if the nodule was positive for malignancy. It is beyond the scope of this chapter to discuss gene classifier systems, but there are now several companies using this technology that are able to determine that a nodule is benign with a high degree of diagnostic accuracy. However, at the present time, these assays are quite poor in predicting malignancy, with a positive predictive value ranging from 15 to 20% to 60 to 70%. The American Thyroid Association (ATA) guidelines for the evaluation of thyroid nodules and well-differentiated thyroid carcinoma recommend a hemithyroidectomy for FNAB positive nodules that are less than 4 cm.[26] However, it must be kept in mind that these are just guidelines. Other considerations, such as appearance of the nodule on US or multiple nodules in the contralateral lobe, may result in a total thyroidectomy with a smaller lesion.

It is extremely important that the ipsilateral neck and at least levels II through V be evaluated by US. Metastatic disease as small as 3 mm within the lymph node can be identified and FNAB performed. Lateral neck ultrasonography can often prevent a second surgery. However, thyroid US performed in radiology departments will rarely examine the lateral neck unless this is requested. Reimbursement issues for performing both tests can be troublesome, because the CPT codes for thyroid US and neck US are identical and insurance companies will rarely pay for duplicate charges.

14.4 Lateral Neck Ultrasound

It is very important to perform a thorough and reproducible US of the lateral neck. One approach is to run the transducer in a transverse orientation and adjacent to the trachea from level I through the thyroid lobe down to lower level VI/VII. Then, move the transducer one-half to three-fourths of the width of the transducer laterally while maintaining a perpendicular orientation to the midline. This process should be repeated until the entire lateral neck has been examined to level V posterior to the sternocleidomastoid muscle. For each of these iterations, angle the transducer under the clavicle to look for far inferior lymph nodes. Benign lymph nodes are fairly easy to identify. They are almost always oblong or flattened with a ratio of any orthogonal axis less than 0.5. They also will contain a hilum most commonly represented as a thin hyperechoic band extending into the midportion of the lymph node (▶ Fig. 14.14). Malignant lymph nodes are typically rounded, with all ratios of orthogonal axis to another greater than 0.5 and often approaching 1.0, which represent the characteristics of a sphere (▶ Fig. 14.15). The hilum is effaced by tumor and absent (▶ Fig. 14.15). There is a wide range of echogenicity from completely hypoechoic (▶ Fig. 14.16) to hyperechoic similar to muscle (▶ Fig. 14.17). Calcifications are often present with metastatic PTC (▶ Fig. 14.17). Cystic lymph nodes are almost always malignant, most commonly with squamous cell or thyroid carcinoma (▶ Fig. 14.18). Metastatic squamous cell carcinoma involving lymph nodes in the neck is often more aggressive with obliteration of node architecture and erosion of the capsule (▶ Fig. 14.19).

14.5 Salivary Glands

The salivary glands include the parotid, submandibular, and sublingual gland. It is beyond the scope of this chapter to go into detail on all benign and malignant neoplasms of the salivary glands. In general, the echogenicity is similar between the three and a normal submandibular gland is shown in ▶ Fig. 14.20. They are typically hyperechoic and homogeneous, with the degree of hyperechogenicity dependent on the amount of fat present. Fatty glands are more hyperechoic.

The US evaluation of the salivary glands is similar to other structures in the neck. The transducer is initially transverse, fairly parallel to the mandible and canted slightly to visualize beneath. This is especially true when examining the parotid gland, which can extend considerably beneath the mandible. It is important to visualize the contralateral gland to compare size, echogenicity, and presence of lesions.

Table 14.1 The Bethesda System for Reporting Thyroid Cytopathology: risk of malignancy and usual clinical management

Diagnostic category		Risk of Malignancy (%)	Management
I.	Nondiagnostic or unsatisfactory	1-4	Repeat FNAB (ultrasound guidance)
II.	Benign	0-3	Clinical follow-up
III.	AUS or FLUS	5-15	Repeat FNAB (molecular testing)
IV.	Follicular neoplasm or suspicious for follicular neoplasm	15-30	Lobectomy (molecular testing)
V.	Suspicious for malignancy	60-75	Lobectomy or total thyroidectomy
VI.	Malignant	97-99	Lobectomy or total thyroidectomy

AUS, atypia of undetermined significance; FLUS, follicular lesion of undetermined significance; FNAB, fine-needle aspiration biopsy.

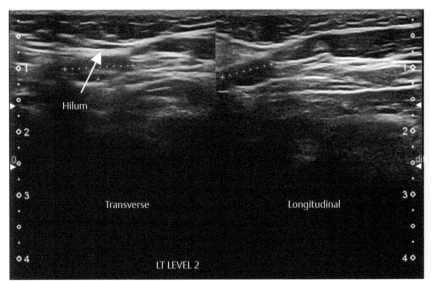

Fig. 14.14 Benign lymph node. Ovoid with defined hilum.

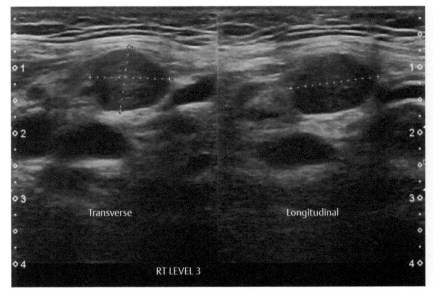

Fig. 14.15 Rounded hypoechoic lymph node positive for papillary thyroid carcinoma.

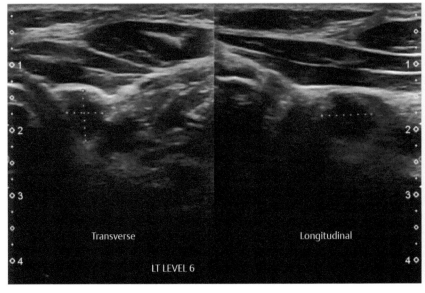

Fig. 14.16 Hypoechoic nodule in the thyroid bed positive for papillary thyroid carcinoma.

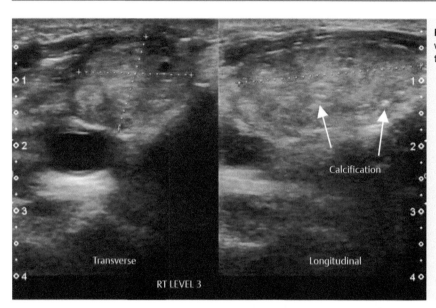

Fig. 14.17 Rounded hyperechoic lymph node with microcalcifications positive for papillary thyroid carcinoma.

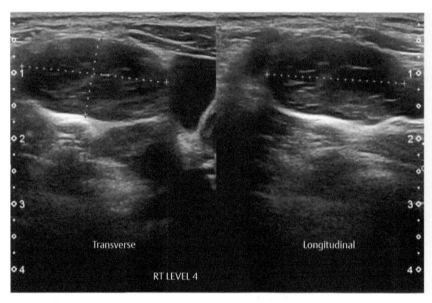

Fig. 14.18 Cystic lymph node positive for papillary thyroid carcinoma.

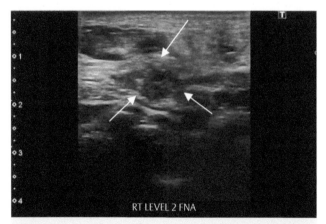

Fig. 14.19 Squamous cell node metastasis with obliteration of normal nodal architecture.

Both benign and malignant neoplasms arising from the salivary gland often have a similar appearance. They are typically hypoechoic and homogeneous with pleomorphic adenoma constituting the most common benign lesion. They are most commonly found in the parotid gland and are predominantly solitary.[27] Pleomorphic adenomas can be lobulated and contain calcifications but are poorly vascularized. Warthin's tumors have a very similar appearance to pleomorphic adenomas, hypoechoic, and oval shaped, but can be bilateral.

Malignant lesions of the salivary glands are predominantly represented by mucoepidermoid carcinoma and adenoid cystic carcinoma. They may present with lobulation and poor borders similar to other malignant neoplasms in the neck[28]; however, it is not uncommon to present as hypoechoic, well defined, and cystic.[29] Probably even more so than thyroid nodules, it is uncommon to be able to distinguish benign and malignant salivary gland tumors by US appearance; therefore, FNAB is mandatory.

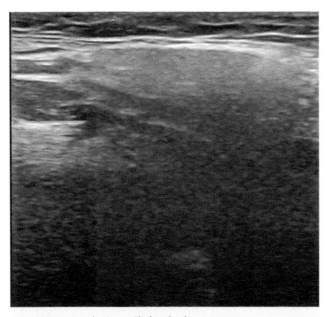

Fig. 14.20 Normal submandibular gland.

14.6 Conclusion

US of structures in the neck is safe and relatively inexpensive. Often US precludes more expensive and radiation-intensive imaging. Routine follow-up of thyroid nodules, neck surveillance in thyroid cancer survivors, and evaluation of neck nodes and salivary glands in high-risk individuals have become common in community-based surgical and endocrine practices. However, careful consideration should be given to the decision to pursue routine US-guided FNAB of these lesions. As with any procedure, practitioners need to be impartial in deciding their skill level and whether referral would be prudent.

References

[1] Kremkau F. Diagnostic Ultrasound: Principles and Instruments. St Louis, MO: Elsevier; 2006

[2] Anderson L, Middleton WD, Teefey SA, et al. Hashimoto thyroiditis: part 1, sonographic analysis of the nodular form of Hashimoto thyroiditis. AJR Am J Roentgenol. 2010; 195(1):208–215

[3] LiVolsi VA. Surgical Pathology of the Thyroid. Philadelphia, PA: Saunders; 1990

[4] Lee JH, Kim Y, Choi JW, Kim YS. The association between papillary thyroid carcinoma and histologically proven Hashimoto's thyroiditis: a meta-analysis. Eur J Endocrinol. 2013; 168(3):343–349

[5] Resende de Paiva C, Grønhøj C, Feldt-Rasmussen U, von Buchwald C. Association between Hashimoto's thyroiditis and thyroid cancer in 64,628 patients. Front Oncol. 2017; 7:53

[6] Jankovic B, Le KT, Hershman JM. Clinical review: Hashimoto's thyroiditis and papillary thyroid carcinoma: is there a correlation? J Clin Endocrinol Metab. 2013; 98(2):474–482

[7] Anderson L, Middleton WD, Teefey SA, et al. Hashimoto thyroiditis: part 2, sonographic analysis of benign and malignant nodules in patients with diffuse Hashimoto thyroiditis. AJR Am J Roentgenol. 2010; 195(1):216–222

[8] Solbiati L, Osti V, Cova L, Tonolini M. Ultrasound of thyroid, parathyroid glands and neck lymph nodes. Eur Radiol. 2001; 11(12):2411–2424

[9] Kim BM, Kim MJ, Kim EK, et al. Sonographic differentiation of thyroid nodules with eggshell calcifications. J Ultrasound Med. 2008; 27(10):1425–1430

[10] Kim EK, Park CS, Chung WY, et al. New sonographic criteria for recommending fine-needle aspiration biopsy of nonpalpable solid nodules of the thyroid. AJR Am J Roentgenol. 2002; 178(3):687–691

[11] Moon HJ, Sung JM, Kim EK, Yoon JH, Youk JH, Kwak JY. Diagnostic performance of gray-scale US and elastography in solid thyroid nodules. Radiology. 2012; 262(3):1002–1013

[12] Alexander EK, Marqusee E, Orcutt J, et al. Thyroid nodule shape and prediction of malignancy. Thyroid. 2004; 14(11):953–958

[13] Kamran SC, Marqusee E, Kim MI, et al. Thyroid nodule size and prediction of cancer. J Clin Endocrinol Metab. 2013; 98(2):564–570

[14] Shrestha M, Crothers BA, Burch HB. The impact of thyroid nodule size on the risk of malignancy and accuracy of fine-needle aspiration: a 10-year study from a single institution. Thyroid. 2012; 22(12):1251–1256

[15] Ibrahim Y, Mohamed SE, Deniwar A, et al. The impact of thyroid nodule size on the risk of malignancy in follicular neoplasms. Anticancer Res. 2015; 35(3):1635–1639

[16] Mohammadi A, Moloudi F, Ghasemi-Rad M. Preoperative localization of parathyroid lesion: diagnostic usefulness of color doppler ultrasonography. Int J Clin Exp Med. 2012; 5(1):80–86

[17] Mohammadi A, Moloudi F, Ghasemi-rad M. The role of colour Doppler ultrasonography in the preoperative localization of parathyroid adenomas. Endocr J. 2012; 59(5):375–382

[18] Devcic Z, Jeffrey RB, Kamaya A, Desser TS. The elusive parathyroid adenoma: techniques for detection. Ultrasound Q. 2013; 29(3):179–187

[19] Ruda JM, Hollenbeak CS, Stack BC, Jr. A systematic review of the diagnosis and treatment of primary hyperparathyroidism from 1995 to 2003. Otolaryngol Head Neck Surg. 2005; 132(3):359–372

[20] Andrade JS, Mangussi-Gomes JP, Rocha LA, et al. Localization of ectopic and supernumerary parathyroid glands in patients with secondary and tertiary hyperparathyroidism: surgical description and correlation with preoperative ultrasonography and Tc99m-Sestamibi scintigraphy. Rev Bras Otorrinolaringol (Engl Ed). 2014; 80(1):29–34

[21] Jaskowiak N, Norton JA, Alexander HR, et al. A prospective trial evaluating a standard approach to reoperation for missed parathyroid adenoma. Ann Surg. 1996; 224(3):308–320, discussion 320–321

[22] Kim SY, Lee HS, Moon J, et al. Fine-needle aspiration versus core needle biopsy for diagnosis of thyroid malignancy and neoplasm: a matched cohort study. Eur Radiol. 2017; 27(2):801–811

[23] Choi YJ, Baek JH, Suh CH, et al. Core-needle biopsy versus repeat fine-needle aspiration for thyroid nodules initially read as atypia/follicular lesion of undetermined significance. Head Neck. 2017; 39(2):361–369

[24] Baloch ZW, LiVolsi VA, Asa SL, et al. Diagnostic terminology and morphologic criteria for cytologic diagnosis of thyroid lesions: a synopsis of the National Cancer Institute Thyroid Fine-Needle Aspiration State of the Science Conference. Diagn Cytopathol. 2008; 36(6):425–437

[25] Cibas ES, Ali SZ. The 2017 Bethesda System for Reporting Thyroid Cytopathology. Thyroid. 2017; 27(11):1341–1346

[26] Haugen BR, Alexander EK, Bible KC, et al. 2015 American Thyroid Association Management Guidelines for Adult Patients with Thyroid Nodules and Differentiated Thyroid Cancer: The American Thyroid Association Guidelines Task Force on Thyroid Nodules and Differentiated Thyroid Cancer. Thyroid. 2016; 26(1):1–133

[27] Renehan A, Gleave EN, Hancock BD, Smith P, McGurk M. Long-term follow-up of over 1000 patients with salivary gland tumours treated in a single centre. Br J Surg. 1996; 83(12):1750–1754

[28] Howlett DC, Kesse KW, Hughes DV, Sallomi DF. The role of imaging in the evaluation of parotid disease. Clin Radiol. 2002; 57(8):692–701

[29] Howlett DC. High resolution ultrasound assessment of the parotid gland. Br J Radiol. 2003; 76(904):271–277

15 Integrated FDG-PET/CT for Head and Neck Malignancies

Twyla B. Bartel and Tracy L. Yarbrough

Abstract

Fluorine-18-fluorodeoxyglucose positron emission tomography/computed tomography (FDG-PET/CT) is now used routinely for the guidance of initial staging and for posttreatment monitoring as well as for the localization of an unknown primary in head and neck cancer patients. Along with qualitative image review, the semiquantitative parameter, standardized uptake value (SUV), allows not only assessment of a treatment response, but also provides prognostic information. In particular, one of the greatest utilities of FDG-PET/CT for head and neck malignancies is its high negative predictive value after treatment.

Keywords: head and neck, fluorodeoxyglucose, PET/CT

15.1 Introduction

Fluorine-18-fluorodeoxyglucose positron emission tomography (FDG-PET) provides in vivo functional information on the metabolic behavior of various tissues. It has proven to be very useful for head and neck (H&N) malignancies. When integrated with computed tomography (CT) as FDG-PET/CT, valuable combined functional and anatomical information is provided, which assists in the appropriate clinical management of patients. Also, by combining PET with CT, more accurate anatomic lesion localization and size measurements can be made than with PET alone. In most cases, PET/CT allows metabolically active malignancy to be differentiated from benign entities.

15.2 Technique

15.2.1 Fluorodeoxyglucose Dose and Administration

The patient should refrain from eating or drinking (water permitted) 6 to 8 hours prior to FDG injection. Typically, between 10 and 20 mCi (370–740 MBq) of FDG are administered intravenously (IV), and the patient is then placed in a quiet room with his or her eyes closed during what is termed the FDG "uptake period." During this time, the patient is discouraged from reading, chewing, or talking.

15.2.2 Image Acquisition

Approximately 1 hour after FDG administration, PET/CT imaging of the patient is acquired from the top of the head to the midthighs (occasionally extending to the soles of the feet in patients with tumors such as melanoma and myeloma). At some institutions, a second dedicated H&N PET/CT acquisition is acquired about 30 minutes later from the base of the skull through the aortic arch. This second set of images should be acquired with a higher matrix to improve visualization of H&N abnormalities and allow a longer uptake period for tumor accumulation of FDG. This second acquisition may also help differentiate between malignant and inflammatory or infectious

conditions (i.e., uptake in benign conditions may peak early on, while malignancies frequently have gradually increasing uptake over time).[1] Placing the head at a slightly greater tilt (increasing the degree of neck extension) during the second acquisition may also assist in visualization of oral cavity abnormalities when there is excessive dental artifact in the region.

15.2.3 Intravenous Contrast

Depending upon the institution, the CT portion of the examination will be performed with or without (more common) IV contrast enhancement. In the majority of cases, the CT portion of PET/CT is performed without IV contrast and used mainly for attenuation correction and localization purposes. The PET scan is attenuation corrected by utilizing coefficients obtained from scaling the CT numbers to the PET energy level of 511 keV.[2] It has been demonstrated that IV contrast does not interfere significantly with semiquantitative evaluation known as SUV.

15.3 Fluorodeoxyglucose Mechanism of Uptake

FDG is the most commonly utilized radiopharmaceutical for oncology imaging. It is a positron-emitting radionuclide with fluorine-18 (F-18) substituted for a hydroxyl group on the glucose molecule. FDG is essentially a "radioactive sugar," or glucose analog, which is taken up physiologically by various tissues in the body and, to a greater degree, by tumor cells. Once FDG enters a cell, it is trapped within that cell after initial phosphorylation by hexokinase without further metabolism. Essentially, FDG accumulates in the cells as FDG-6-phosphate and cannot enter glycolysis at this point. Given that tumor cells, in general, have a higher glucose utilization than nonmalignant tissues, there is an elevated amount of FDG trapped in these cells, and therefore greater radioactivity. Thus, the areas of increased radioactivity accumulation are visualized as "hot spots" when viewing FDG-PET images.

15.4 Standardized Uptake Value

If a region of interest (ROI) is drawn around any given "hot spot," an SUV can be calculated as an estimation of the metabolic activity within that specific tissue area or ROI. SUV is a semiquantitative measure of the metabolic activity of body tissues and corrects for the variability of FDG uptake related to differences in patient size and the dose of the injected FDG.[3] In general, the SUV is the ratio of the radioactivity concentration in the ROI (drawn on images on a computer monitor) divided by the whole-body concentration of the injected radioactivity:

$$SUV = (ROI\ radioactivity\ concentration)/(whole - body\ injected\ radioactivity\ concentration)$$

The SUV is especially useful in monitoring response to therapy, as the uptake at one time point can be compared to the uptake in that same tissue at a subsequent time point.

15.5 Lesion Size and Positron Emission Tomography Resolution

PET-reconstructed resolution is typically about 4 to 6 mm; therefore, evaluation of the metabolic activity of lesions below this size is not reliable. Newer time-of-flight (TOF) PET systems provide improved resolution, contrast, and signal-to-noise ratio.[4]

15.6 Indications for FDG-PET or FDG-PET/CT

15.6.1 TNM Staging

Accurate TNM (*t*umor size, *n*ode involvement, and *m*etastasis status) staging at the time of initial diagnosis is of utmost important in accurate treatment planning. An important benefit of FDG-PET and PET/CT in this aspect derives from the whole-body approach, thereby not only assessing the primary tumor, but also evaluating for nodal and/or distant metastases. FDG-PET has been reported to have higher sensitivity (87 compared to 62%) and specificity (89 compared to 73%) than CT for initial staging.[5] Integrated FDG-PET/CT has even higher sensitivity and specificity at greater than 90% each for this purpose.[6]

Primary Tumor

Tumor Extent

The literature suggests that FDG-PET/CT is at least as sensitive as anatomic imaging (i.e., CT or MRI) in detecting primary H&N malignancies (especially oral cancers), but may be somewhat lacking in providing assessment of the tumor extent and involvement of adjacent structures. Therefore, it is not routinely utilized clinically for this purpose. Contrast-enhanced MRI or CT typically provides greater anatomic soft-tissue details for this purpose. MRI is also superior to both FDG-PET/CT and CT alone for providing information on possible perineural

involvement of tumor. On the other hand, when IV contrast is given for the CT portion, FDG PET/CT, it may be the most practical single imaging study for management/surgical planning purposes by providing acceptable anatomic detail combined with functional information. This obviates the need to have the patient schedule two separate imaging sessions.

Unknown Primary

In the case of biopsy-proven cervical neck nodal metastases with an unknown primary H&N malignancy, FDG-PET/CT has been shown to successfully localize the primary malignancy in about 30 to 50% of cases when other imaging modalities do not.[7,8] A recent meta-analysis determined the overall sensitivity, specificity, and accuracy of FDG-PET/CT for detecting an unknown primary H&N malignancy as 82.5, 80.2, and 81.4%, respectively, without a significant difference between PET alone and combined PET/CT. The most common histological tumor type for unknown primary detection in these cases was squamous cell carcinoma (SCC; 68.6%), with the most common primary location being the tonsils at 21.6%[9,10] (▶ Fig. 15.1).

Nodal Metastases

FDG-PET/CT has been shown to play a role in both pretreatment evaluations of possible nodal metastases and posttreatment monitoring.

Pretherapy Evaluation

In the preoperative setting, FDG PET/CT yields a statistically significant improvement in detecting and predicting true pathologic cervical nodal metastasis in general (*p* = 0.005), and when occurring only in the contralateral neck (*p* = 0.013), as compared to CT or MRI, with sensitivity and specificity above 80%.[11,12] Regarding patients with clinically negative nodal disease, FDG-PET/CT is about twice as sensitive as conventional imaging (CT or MRI) in the detection of occult nodal metastases, thereby having a significant impact on treatment planning.[13,14]

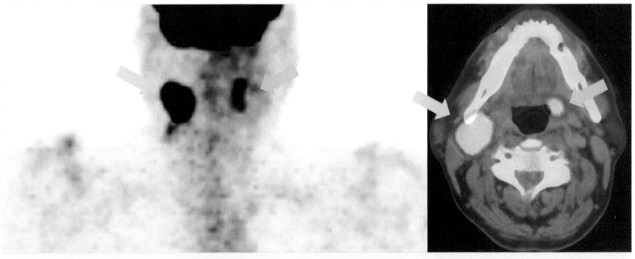

Fig. 15.1 This patient had biopsy-proven squamous cell carcinoma metastasis to a right neck node. The primary malignancy was unknown. A subsequent FDG-PET/CT scan showed uptake in the known right neck metastatic node (*green arrows*) and also localized the primary malignancy to the left tonsillar pillar (*blue arrows*).

Posttherapy Evaluation

It is recommended that FDG-PET/CT imaging be delayed for 10 to 12 weeks after completion of therapy, particularly after surgery or radiation treatment, in order to allow posttreatment inflammation to resolve and therefore to obtain higher diagnostic accuracy. This is true not only for nodal evaluation but also for the primary tumor. The high negative predictive value (NPV) of posttreatment FDG-PET/CT imaging is one of its greatest assets in directing management. If neck nodes are not metabolically active after treatment, they do not likely contain viable tumor. Therefore, if a postradiotherapy FDG-PET/CT scan is negative, neck dissection can be avoided with high confidence.

Distant Metastases

FDG-PET/CT offers a whole-body imaging approach, and therefore a single image acquisition to evaluate for possible distant metastatic disease; it has been shown to be very reliable for this purpose. Rohde et al[15] performed a recent prospective cohort study for head-to-head comparison of three imaging approaches for detection of distant metastases in patients with oral, pharyngeal, or laryngeal squamous cell cancer: (1) combined chest X-ray and H&N MRI (CXR/MRI), (2) combined chest CT and H&N MRI (CHCT/MRI), and (3) FDG-PET/CT. The study evaluated a total of 307 patients. FDG-PET/CT was shown to have a much higher detection rate for distant metastatic disease in this patient population as compared to the other two imaging approaches—CXR/MRI detected distant disease in 1% of patients, CHCT/MRI in 4%, and FDG-PET/CT in 8%. The most common site for distant metastasis was the lung (72% of cases). In addition, FDG-PET/CT was superior for the detection of synchronous carcinomas, with the most common site being a second H&N malignancy (20% of cases; ▶ Fig. 15.2).

15.6.2 Treatment Monitoring/Response

Anatomical response criteria applied to FDG PET/CT are commonly based upon the World Health Organization (WHO) or Response Evaluation in Solid Tumors (RECIST). On the other hand, the European Organization for Research and Treatment of Cancer (EORTC) Response Criteria incorporates FDG uptake and tumor metabolic response based upon SUV calculations and is broken down into categories of complete metabolic response (complete resolution of FDG uptake in the tumor), partial metabolic response (15 to > 25% SUV reduction), progressive metabolic disease (increase of tumor SUV of > 25%), and stable metabolic disease (increase in SUV of < 25% or decrease of < 15%). A more recent approach to response assessment is the Hopkins criteria, which assign a score of 1 through 5 based upon the visual assessment of tumor FDG uptake pattern and intensity. A score of 1, 2, or 3 is considered negative for residual disease and scores of 4 or 5 are considered positive for residual disease.

15.6.3 Radiation Therapy Planning

Methods

There are two methods for incorporating FDG-PET data into radiation treatment planning: (1) PET images are fused with

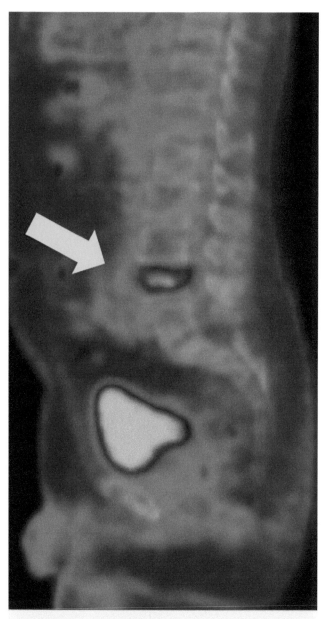

Fig. 15.2 Distant metastatic disease was detected on initial staging FDG-PET/CT in the L4 vertebral body (*arrow*). The primary tumor was head and neck squamous cell carcinoma.

separately acquired radiotherapy planning CT images or (2) acquired integrated PET/CT images are used directly. When integrated PET/CT images are to be used directly for radiotherapy, images are acquired with the patient in the planned treatment position (frequently with the patient positioned on a flat radiotherapy treatment bed mounted to the PET/CT bed) and allows for more accurate target volume delineation. Automatic delineation of the tumor can be performed by using a specified SUV cutoff value to separate target from background uptake. In order to minimize motion caused by patient respiration, "4D" PET/CT (which incorporates respiratory motion correction) can be utilized, or, when possible, the patient can be instructed to inhale deeply and then hold his/her breath during the acquisition over the thoracic field of view ("breath-hold" technique).

Effect of FDG-PET/CT on Radiation Therapy Planning

For H&N cancer patients, FDG-PET/CT has been shown to modify radiation treatment planning in up to 55% of cases, owing primarily to significant differences in tumor volume delineation between PET/CT and CT alone. In addition, PET/CT outperforms CT in identification of nodal metastases.[16]

15.7 Prognostic Information

15.7.1 Staging

Adding FDG-PET/CT routinely to a staging protocol for patients with H&N cancer (especially SCC) improves management and prognostic stratification, changing the TNM classification in about 32% of cases. FDG-PET/CT is also more sensitive and accurate than conventional imaging ($p < 0.001$) for this purpose. FDG-PET/CT can also upstage disease—positive findings on FDG-PET/CT are associated with significantly worse progression-free survival (PFS) and overall survival (OS) as compared to conventional imaging (3-year PFS = 56.8 vs. 74.5%, $p = 0.043$; 3-year OS = 61.3 vs. 85.3%, $p = 0.006$).[17]

In untreated patients, there is a linear relationship between SUV and clinical outcomes (i.e., higher SUV = worse clinical outcome). In particular, Torizuka et al demonstrated a poorer outcome in patients with lesion SUVs greater than 7.0. The primary tumor SUV especially is an independent predictor for local control and disease-free survival in H&N cancer patients.[18]

15.7.2 Posttherapy Evaluation

Pertaining to posttreatment, FDG-PET/CT has high prognostic utility regarding PFS and OS given the high NPV it offers. It is very useful in predicting therapeutic response[19] (▶ Fig. 15.3).

15.8 Selected Tumor Types

15.8.1 Squamous Cell Carcinoma

SCC is the most common type of H&N malignancy and is typically very FDG-avid. Although FDG-PET/CT has a high sensitivity (> 95%) for detecting primary SCC in the H&N, its primary role to date has been for the evaluation of possible cervical neck node involvement prior to treatment. There is strong evidence that FDG-PET/CT outperforms anatomic imaging in this arena as well as in the detection of distant metastatic disease. In fact, there is an approximately 13% frequency of change in management when FDG-PET/CT is utilized for distant disease detection.[20] Specific to clinically N0 H&N SCC patients, preliminary data from the ACRIN 6885 trial showed FDG-PET/CT to have a high NPV for node negativity in these patients, obviating the need for neck dissection.[21]

15.8.2 Salivary Gland Malignancies

Most studies thus far on salivary gland malignancies and PET imaging have enrolled only small numbers of patients. However, there is general agreement among these studies that FDG-PET/CT is clinically useful for staging and monitoring of treatment for these types of malignancies.

Degree of Fluorodeoxyglucose Uptake

Higher-grade salivary gland malignancies tend to have higher SUVs as compared to those that are intermediate- or low-grade. Cystic or mucinous tumors (such as mucoepidermoid or adenoid cystic carcinomas) tend to have lower uptake and SUVs. Hadiprodjo et al looked specifically at parotid gland tumors and demonstrated by ROC analysis that a cutoff maximum SUV greater than 4.2 was 88.9% sensitive and 80.2% specific for malignancy

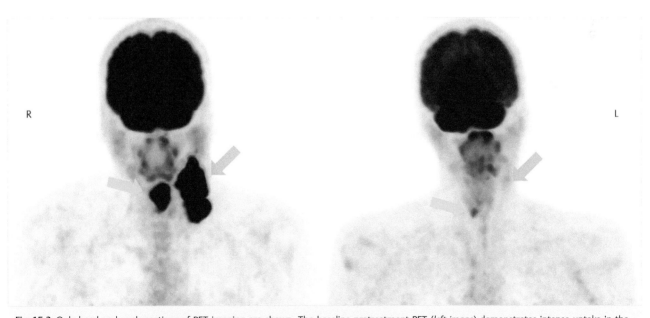

Fig. 15.3 Only head and neck portions of PET imaging are shown. The baseline pretreatment PET (*left image*) demonstrates intense uptake in the laryngeal malignancy (*green arrow*) and left-sided metastatic neck nodes (*blue arrow*). The posttreatment PET (*right image*) shows near complete resolution of the hypermetabolic primary laryngeal malignancy and left-sided neck nodes.

rather than a benign entity. A maximum SUV cutoff of greater than 11.6 was 100% specific for malignant parotid gland tumor.[22] FDG-PET/CT is particularly useful for higher-grade salivary gland malignancies in its ability to detect possible distant metastatic disease, which is more common in these types of tumors. As such, it has been suggested that PET imaging is more useful in general for higher-grade salivary gland tumors than for lower-grade tumors.[23] Pleomorphic adenoma, the most common salivary gland tumor, tends to have high FDG uptake. Mention must also be made of Warthin's tumors in the parotid glands, as they are also typically very FDG-avid and can mimic malignancy (such as pleomorphic adenoma) with a similar degree of uptake and SUVs.

15.8.3 Melanoma

Melanoma is also usually very FDG-avid. For nodes measuring over 6 mm in size, FDG-PET/CT detects about 83% of metastatic melanomatous lymph nodes. FDG-PET/CT also outperforms whole-body MRI for detection of cutaneous or subcutaneous metastases. Findings on FDG-PET/CT result in a change in management about 48.6% of the time in patients with melanoma with an overall accuracy of 98.7% as compared to FDG-PET alone (88.8%) or CT alone (69.7%).

15.8.4 Merkel Cell

Merkel cell tumors localize to the H&N in close to 50% of cases. Regarding nodal involvement, CT has a sensitivity of approximately 47%, while FDG-PET/CT has a much greater sensitivity of 83% and can also detect additional nodal metastases not seen on CT.[24] MRI outperforms both of these modalities when evaluating for central nervous system involvement in patients with Merkel cell tumors. A study by Siva et al included 102 patients from a 15-year period and demonstrated a significant impact of staging FDG-FDG/PET, which changed management in 37% of cases. Upstaging occurred in most of these cases due to localization of distant metastatic disease.[25]

15.8.5 Low Fluorodeoxyglucose-Avidity Tumors

In general, FDG uptake is low to moderately increased in lower-grade, well-differentiated, or mucinous-type tumors.[26] There may also be little FDG uptake in a necrotic node or tumor of any cell type.

15.8.6 Thyroid Carcinoma

Incidental Thyroid Uptake

Incidental thyroid uptake on FDG-PET/CT imaging may be characterized generally as either diffuse or focal. Diffuse uptake is most commonly benign such as that due to thyroiditis, most often Hashimoto's in the context of hypothyroidism.[27] Focal uptake is more concerning, given that focal uptake represents thyroid malignancy in approximately 30% of cases—most commonly papillary thyroid carcinoma.[28] When focal uptake is seen, additional evaluation should follow, such as thyroid ultrasound.

Dedifferentiated Thyroid Cancer

FDG-PET/CT has been most useful for detection of post-thyroidectomy residual thyroid cancer that has dedifferentiated after radioiodine ablation, no longer showing uptake on radioiodine scans but resulting in a rising thyroglobulin level. The "flip-flop phenomenon" refers to this loss of radioiodine accumulation in thyroid carcinoma that has become dedifferentiated and accumulates radioactive glucose (FDG) instead of radioiodine. A 2012 meta-analysis revealed a pooled sensitivity of FDG-PET/CT in cases of flip-flop phenomenon of 93 to 95% with PET/CT having a higher diagnostic accuracy than PET alone. Note is also made that the diagnostic accuracy of FDG-PET/CT is higher with elevated thyroglobulin levels.[29]

Aggressive Thyroid Cancer

FDG-PET/CT is also useful for staging and posttreatment follow-up in those patients with aggressive histological subtypes such as Hurthle cell carcinoma, which typically does not concentrate radioiodine well. The sensitivity and specificity of FDG-PET/CT for Hurthle cell thyroid carcinoma is on the order of 90 +%. Conversely, FDG-PET/CT does not perform as well in patients with recurrent medullary thyroid carcinoma, having a detection rate of only about 59%; this increases to nearly 75% when the calcitonin level is 1,000 ng/mL or more. Detection of anaplastic thyroid carcinoma is somewhat more complicated, as these tumors typically are not very radioiodine-avid and may not be associated with elevated thyroglobulin levels. On the other hand, all anaplastic thyroid cancer lesions (primary tumor, nodes, and distant disease) tend to be extremely FDG-avid. Therefore, FDG-PET/CT is used in patients with anaplastic thyroid tumors for staging, treatment monitoring, and follow-up, and has also been shown to have a direct impact on patient management in about 50% of cases[30] (▶ Fig. 15.4, ▶ Fig. 15.5).

15.8.7 Parathyroid Carcinoma

Brief mention is made of parathyroid carcinoma and FDG-PET. In general, FDG-PET/CT can be considered a complementary technique to conventional imaging for parathyroid carcinoma. FDG-PET/CT has been shown to be a sensitive modality for parathyroid carcinoma initial staging, tumor recurrence detection, and posttreatment evaluation, although small lesion size may limit evaluation in some cases.[31]

15.9 Potential FDG-PET/CT Imaging Pitfalls in the Head and Neck Region

Recognition of normal benign versus pathologic patterns of increased uptake in the H&N region is necessary when interpreting PET scans.[32] Consequently, it is of utmost importance to have an experienced reader perform this task.

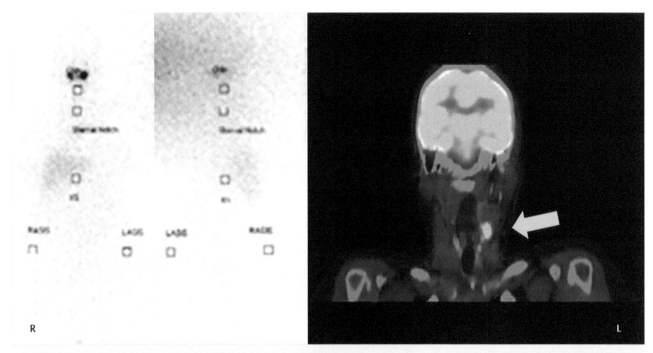

Fig. 15.4 Flip-flop phenomenon. Radioiodine scan on the left (whole-body posterior and anterior images) demonstrates only physiologic uptake. FDG-PET/CT image on the right demonstrates FDG-avid dedifferentiated malignancy in the left neck (*arrow*).

15.9.1 Physiologic Fluorodeoxyglucose Uptake

Brown Fat

One of the most common causes of false-positive uptake in the neck is physiologic brown fat activation, which can potentially obscure abnormal FDG uptake in neck nodes. At some imaging centers, valium is administered or warming techniques are employed (such as warmed towels placed around the neck) prior to FDG administration to prevent potential brown fat uptake.

Muscular Uptake

Another common confounding source of physiologic activity in the H&N is muscular uptake, which can also obscure abnormal findings in the adjacent small, complicated H&N structures. To minimize muscle uptake, the patient is asked to not chew (including gum and mints) or talk prior to FDG administration and during the uptake period.

Other Causes

Physiologic uptake can be seen in the vocal cords and arytenoid cartilages due to phonation. Physiologic uptake can also be seen in the salivary glands and diffusely in the thyroid gland.

15.9.2 Posttreatment Changes

Knowledge of any prior treatment and date of this treatment is vital information prior to imaging the patient.

Paralyzed or Injected Vocal Cord

Iatrogenic nerve injury can result in seemingly increased focal uptake in the contralateral, nonparalyzed vocal cord. In contrast, injections, including Teflon, into a paralyzed vocal cord can cause increased focal inflammatory uptake in the area of injection (i.e., within the paralyzed vocal cord itself; ▶ Fig. 15.6).[33]

Radiation and Surgery

Radiation or surgery can cause asymmetrically increased uptake to the treated side (usually in a diffuse pattern). In general, it is recommended that FDG-PET/CT imaging be performed 10 to 12 weeks after these treatments in order to minimize associated inflammatory uptake when evaluating for any residual disease.[32]

Technical and Artifactual Limitations

The spatial resolution of PET/CT has been previously addressed. Lesions below 4 mm may not be reliably detected on PET. In addition, excessive patient motion or misaligned PET and CT images may obscure findings. Finally, artifacts related to dental hardware can significantly limit evaluation of the neck.

Lesions with Low FDG-Avidity

As previously mentioned, mucinous or cystic lesions may not demonstrate significant FDG uptake. Necrotic nodes/lesions or neuroendocrine and spindle cell tumors may yield false-negative FDG uptake, also.

15.9.3 FDG-PET/MR Imaging

There is now a small volume of literature examining FDG-PET/MR for H&N malignancies. However, much more research needs to be conducted in this area to determine the clinical impact FDG-PET/MR may or may not have for these tumors. Current literature does state, however, that PET/MR does not

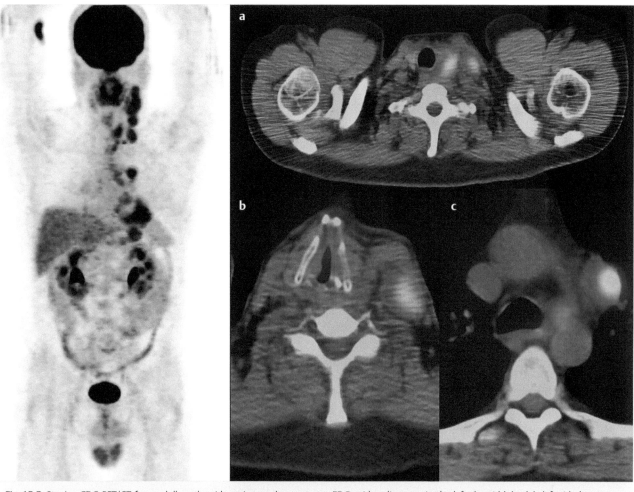

Fig. 15.5 Staging FDG-PET/CT for medullary thyroid carcinoma demonstrates FDG-avid malignancy in the left thyroid lobe **(a)**, left-sided neck **(a,b)**, and mediastinal nodal metastases **(c)**.

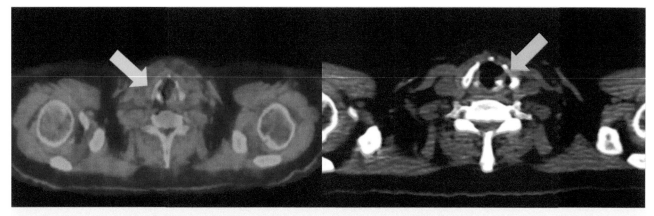

Fig. 15.6 The patient has left vocal cord paralysis due to recurrent laryngeal cord injury. The left vocal cord appears flaccid on the CT part of PET (*blue arrow*). The contralateral normal right-sided vocal cord demonstrates physiologic focal uptake (*green arrow*).

offer incremental value for initial staging as compared to MR alone. PET/MR is, however, more sensitive (with similar accuracy) than FDG-PET/CT when evaluating for recurrent tumor. Platzek et al performed a prospective study in a small sample of patients (*n* = 38), demonstrating that FDG-PET/MR did not significantly improve diagnostic accuracy for nodal metastases in the neck as compared to MR or PET alone.[34]

15.10 Conclusion

Obtaining a baseline FDG-PET/CT imaging study prior to therapy is not only useful regarding prognostication, but also aids in determining whether there has been a positive treatment response and/or whether there should be a change in management (via no response, upstaging, or downstaging). FDG-PET/CT imaging has proven to be most valuable for patients with H&N cancer in (1) detecting distant disease and (2) providing confidence regarding the absence of residual malignancy given its high NPV, frequently changing management in this patient population. Finally, it is important that PET/CT images be interpreted by an experienced reader to avoid misinterpretation of findings in the H&N region given the various pitfalls and intricate anatomy of the region.

References

[1] Hustinx R, Smith RJ, Benard F, et al. Dual time point fluorine-18 fluorodeoxyglucose positron emission tomography: a potential method to differentiate malignancy from inflammation and normal tissue in the head and neck. Eur J Nucl Med. 1999; 26(10):1345–1348

[2] Fukui MB, Blodgett TM, Snyderman CH, et al. Combined PET-CT in the head and neck: part 2. Diagnostic uses and pitfalls of oncologic imaging. Radiographics. 2005; 25(4):913–930

[3] Kinahan PE, Fletcher JW. PET/CT standardized uptake values (SUVs) in clinical practice and assessing response to therapy. Semin Ultrasound CT MR. 2010; 31:496–505

[4] Hess S, Hoilund-Carlsen PF. Contribution of FDG to Modern Medicine, Part I. Philadelphia, PA: Elsevier Health Sciences; 2004

[5] Al-Ibraheem A, Buck A, Krause BJ, Scheidhauer K, Schwaiger M. Clinical applications of FDG PET and PET/CT in head and neck cancer. J Oncol. 2009; 2009:208725

[6] Demirkan A, Kara PO, Ozturk K, et al. The role of 18F-FDG-PET/CT in initial staging and re-staging of head and neck cancer. J Biomed Graph Comput. 2014; 4:57–66

[7] Plaxton NA, Brandon DC, Corey AS, et al. Characteristics and limitations of FDG PET/CT for imaging of squamous cell carcinoma of the head and neck: a comprehensive review of anatomy, metastatic pathways, and image findings. AJR Am J Roentgenol. 2015; 205(5):W519–W531

[8] Rudmik L, Lau HY, Matthews TW, et al. Clinical utility of PET/CT in the evaluation of head and neck squamous cell carcinoma with an unknown primary: a prospective clinical trial. Head Neck. 2011; 33(7):935–940

[9] Subramaniam RM, Truong M, Peller P, Sakai O, Mercier G. Fluorodeoxyglucose-positron-emission tomography imaging of head and neck squamous cell cancer. AJNR Am J Neuroradiol. 2010; 31(4):598–604

[10] Bernier J. Head and Neck Cancer: Multimodality Management. Switzerland: Springer International Publishing; 2016

[11] Hassan O, Hamdy RA, Medany MM. The role of FDG PET in the diagnosis of occult primary with cervical lymph node metastases: a meta-analysis study. Egyptian J Ear, Nose. Throat and Allied Sciences. 2014; 15:7–16

[12] Nguyen A, Luginbuhl A, Cognetti D, et al. Effectiveness of PET/CT in the preoperative evaluation of neck disease. Laryngoscope. 2014; 124(1):159–164

[13] Yongkui L, Jian L, Wanghan, Jingui L. 18FDG-PET/CT for the detection of regional nodal metastasis in patients with primary head and neck cancer before treatment: a meta-analysis. Surg Oncol. 2013; 22(2):e11–e16

[14] Roh JL, Park JP, Kim JS, et al. 18F fluorodeoxyglucose PET/CT in head and neck squamous cell carcinoma with negative neck palpation findings: a prospective study. Radiology. 2014; 271(1):153–161

[15] Rohde M, Nielsen AL, Johansen J, et al. Head-to-head comparison of chest x-ray/head and neck MRI, chest CT/head and neck MRI, and 18F-FDG-PET/CT for detection of distant metastases and synchronous cancer in oral, pharyngeal, and laryngeal cancer. J Nucl Med. 2017; 58(12):1919–1924

[16] Li J, Xiao Y. Application of FDG-PET/CT in radiation oncology. Front Oncol. 2013; 3:80

[17] Ryu IS, Roh JL, Kim JS, et al. Impact of (18)F-FDG PET/CT staging on management and prognostic stratification in head and neck squamous cell carcinoma: A prospective observational study. Eur J Cancer. 2016; 63:88–96

[18] Torizuka T, Tanizaki Y, Kanno T, et al. Prognostic value of 18F-FDG PET in patients with head and neck squamous cell cancer. AJR Am J Roentgenol. 2009; 192(4):W156–60

[19] Kim R, Ock CY, Keam B, et al. Predictive and prognostic value of PET/CT imaging post-chemoradiotherapy and clinical decision-making consequences in locally advanced head & neck squamous cell carcinoma: a retrospective study. BMC Cancer. 2016; 16:116

[20] Castaldi P, Leccisotti L, Bussu F, Miccichè F, Rufini V. Role of (18)F-FDG PET-CT in head and neck squamous cell carcinoma. Acta Otorhinolaryngol Ital. 2013; 33(1):1–8

[21] Stack BC, Duan F, Sicks J, et al. The negative predictive value (NPV) of FDG-PET/CT I the head and neck squamous cell carcinoma (HNSCC) N0 patient, the first report of the ACRIN 6685 trial. J Clin Oncol. 2017; 6041:25

[22] Hadiprodjo D, Ryan T, Truong MT, Mercier G, Subramaniam RM. Parotid gland tumors: preliminary data for the value of FDG PET/CT diagnostic parameter. Am J Roentgenol. 2012; 198(2):W185:W90

[23] Murphy G, Hussey D, Metser U. Non-cutaneous melanoma: is there a role for (18)F-FDG PET-CT? Br J Radiol. 2014; 87(1040):20140324

[24] Colgan MB, Tarantola TI, Weaver AL, et al. The predictive value of imaging studies in evaluating regional lymph node involvement in Merkel cell carcinoma. J Am Acad Dermatol. 2012; 67(6):1250–1256

[25] Siva S, Byrne K, Seel M, et al. 18F-FDG PET provides high-impact and powerful prognostic stratification in the staging of Merkel cell carcinoma: a 15-year institutional experience. J Nucl Med. 2013; 54(8):1223–1229

[26] Sherry S, Mercier G, Kompel A, et al. FDG PET/CT and MR imaging in non-squamous cell tumors of head and neck with pathological correlation. J Nucl Med. 2009; 50 Suppl 2:1037

[27] Rothman IN, Middleton L, Stack BC, Jr, et al. The incidence of diffuse fluorodeoxyglucose positron emission tomography (PET) uptake in the thyroid of patients with autoimmune thyroiditis. Europ Archives Otolaryngol. 2011; 268:1501–1504

[28] Boeckmann J, Bartel T, Siegel E, Bodenner D, Stack BC, Jr. Can the pathology of a thyroid nodule be determined by positron emission tomography uptake? Otolaryngol Head Neck Surg. 2012; 146(6):906–912

[29] Salvatori M, Biondi B, Rufini V. Imaging in endocrinology: 2-[18F]-fluoro-2-deoxy-D-glucose positron emission tomography/computed tomography in differentiated thyroid carcinoma: clinical indications and controversies in diagnosis and follow-up. Eur J Endocrinol. 2015; 173(3):R115–R130

[30] Marcus C, Whitworth PW, Surasi DS, Pai SI, Subramaniam RM. PET/CT in the management of thyroid cancers. AJR Am J Roentgenol. 2014; 202(6):1316–1329

[31] Evangelista L, Sorgato N, Torresan F, et al. FDG-PET/CT and parathyroid carcinoma: Review of literature and illustrative case series. World J Clin Oncol. 2011; 2(10):348–354

[32] Blodgett TM, Fukui MB, Snyderman CH, et al. Combined PET-CT in the head and neck: part 1. Physiologic, altered physiologic, and artifactual FDG uptake. Radiographics. 2005; 25(4):897–912

[33] Chadwick JL, Khalid A, Wagner H, Stack BC, Jr. Teflon granuloma results in a false positive second primary on FDG-PET in a patient with history of nasopharyngeal cancer. Am J Otolaryngol. 2007; 28:251–253

[34] Platzek I, Beuthien-Baumann B, Schneider M, et al. FDG PET/MR for lymph node staging in head and neck cancer. Eur J Radiol. 2014; 83(7):1163–1168

16 Neck Management in Skin Cancer

William Harris, Mauricio A. Moreno, and Brian Moore

Abstract

This chapter examines the risk factors and clinical approach to regional management of aggressive skin cancer of the head and neck. Initially, the chapter touches on the epidemiology, patient evaluation, and role of imaging in head and neck cutaneous cancer. As the chapter progresses, the workup and management of aggressive cutaneous lesions is discussed, including the role of sentinel lymph node biopsy and the technique involved. Management of the N0 neck is also discussed as well as a comprehensive overview of posterolateral neck dissection technique and indications. Finally, the current recommendations on adjuvant therapy and the treatment of systemic disease are explored.

Keywords: neck dissection, sentinel lymph node biopsy, NMSC, posterolateral neck dissection, adjuvant therapy, cutaneous squamous cell cancer, Merkel cell carcinoma, lymphoscintigraphy

16.1 Introduction

Skin cancer of the head and neck is a heterogeneous and common malignancy. The vast majority of cases are nonmelanoma skin cancer (NMSC), especially basal cell carcinoma (BCC) and squamous cell carcinoma (SCC), followed by melanoma and Merkel cell carcinoma (MCC). Melanoma, cutaneous squamous cell cancer (cSCC), and MCC may be aggressive diseases that frequently require a multidisciplinary approach. Such cutaneous malignancies are at increased risk of regional metastases, with increased morbidity and an increased risk of disease-specific death. This chapter discusses the risk factors for and clinical approach to regional management of aggressive skin cancer of the head and neck.

16.2 Epidemiology

Approximately 5.4 million NMSCs are diagnosed yearly in the United States.[1] BCC and SCC account for about 99% of cases, while MCC, rare adnexal carcinomas, and sarcomas comprise about 1%. NMSC is not typically reported to cancer registries, such as the Surveillance, Epidemiology, and End Results (SEER) Program database, so the true incidence is difficult to assess—such data are extrapolated from procedural claims and longitudinal health cohorts. Health care expenditures related to NMSC in the United States were estimated at $4.8 billion between 2007 and 2011, with the majority attributed to office-based visits.[2]

Similarly, the incidence of cutaneous melanoma has been increasing over the past three to four decades and currently accounts for an estimated 65% of all deaths from skin cancer.[3] While melanoma is historically acknowledged as an aggressive and potentially lethal diagnosis, with 9,730 U.S. deaths estimated for 2017, the mortality risk for aggressive NMSC, particularly cSCC, has been more difficult to quantify.[4] At least 4,000 deaths annually in the United States were attributed to cSCC in 2012, with that number continuing to rise.[5]

Skin cancer is associated with prolonged exposure to ultraviolet (UV) radiation, with 75% of NMSC arising on the head and neck because of the increased sun exposure of these areas and nearly 65% of all melanomas attributed to prolonged exposure.[6,7] NMSC and melanoma are increasing in frequency, with a trend toward younger patients.[8,9] The risk factors associated with the various cutaneous malignancies are denoted in ▶ Table 16.1.

Table 16.1 Risk factors for developing skin cancer of the head and neck[3,10,11]

Risk factors	Melanoma	BCC and SCC	Merkel cell
Skin types	Fair skin, freckling, light hair	Fair skin, freckling, light hair	Fair skin, freckling, light hair
History	Family or personal history of melanoma Immunosuppression Elderly Male	Psoriasis treatment (PUVA and psoralen) Smoking HPV Prior BCC or SCC lesions Male Lymphoma Albinism Genodermatoses Xeroderma pigmentosum Bazex syndrome Epidermodysplasia verruciformis Chronic irritation	Psoriasis treatment (PUVA and psoralen) HIV/AIDS; CLL (immunosuppression) Elderly Male Merkel cell polyomavirus
Preexisting skin lesions	Atypical moles Congenital melanocytic nevi Dysplastic nevus syndrome	Basal cell nevus syndrome Actinic keratosis Bowenoid papulosis Epidermodysplasia verruciformis	
Environmental exposures	UV light	UV light Arsenic exposure Polycyclic hydrocarbons Coal tar	UV light

Abbreviations: AIDS, acquired immunodeficiency syndrome; BCC, basal cell carcinoma; CLL, chronic lymphocytic leukemia; HIV, human immunodeficiency virus; HPV, human papillomavirus; PUVA, psoralen and ultraviolet A therapy; SCC, squamous cell carcinoma; UV, ultraviolet.

16.3 Patient Evaluation

16.3.1 History

Cutaneous lesions of the head and neck must be addressed with a comprehensive and methodical approach, coupled with a high index of suspicion. A detailed history of potential recreational or occupational exposures, use of sun-protective behaviors (if any), past history of skin lesions and type, a family history of skin cancer, and comorbid conditions, especially transplant status and immunosuppression, must be obtained. The presence of formication (the sense that insects are crawling under the skin), facial pain, or cranial nerve paralysis should raise concern for perineural invasion (PNI), triggering anatomic imaging studies. PNI often presents as progressively worsening severe pain in one branch of the trigeminal nerve or as a slowly evolving paresis of one branch of the facial nerve that progresses over time to complete facial paralysis. This evolving paralysis is often misdiagnosed as Bell's palsy.

Patients with a neck or parotid mass should be queried as to their history of benign or malignant skin lesions in the region, particularly the cheek, zygomatic-temporal region, or temporoparietal scalp, as the parotid serves as the primary nodal basin for these anatomic areas.[12] This inquiry is essential, because skin cancer of the head and neck is often treated in the office setting, so patients (and providers) may underestimate the disease and its metastatic potential.[13]

16.3.2 Physical Examination

A patient's propensity to develop skin cancer can be generalized by the skin phenotype, with a determination of the Fitzpatrick scale: types I and II skin (light skin, light eyes, and a propensity to burn rather than tan) have historically been associated with the development of skin cancer, although this disease can affect all skin types.[14] Lesions found within the H-zone of the face, including the midface, upper lip, nose, medial canthus, eyelids, temples, lateral forehead, malar eminences, preauricular cheek, and periauricular tissues, are considered more difficult to treat due to a high risk of local recurrence and a tendency for deep invasion.[15] Suspicious lesions should be measured and palpated to estimate depth of invasion. Intranasal and intraoral examinations, including nasal endoscopy, are imperative to identify full-thickness involvement of the nose, cheek, or lip. Dermoscopy can be also be used as an instrument to aid in noninvasive diagnosis of NMSC and pigmented lesions, and has been shown to be useful in the preoperative evaluation of tumor margins, monitoring outcomes of topical treatments, as well as in posttreatment follow-up.[8]

In order to initially assess for evidence of potential PNI, a detailed cranial nerve examination is imperative. This is especially crucial in SCC, where 5 to 10% of individuals present with this feature, and where PNI is frequently associated with regional lymph node metastases and has a significantly negative impact on local control and survival.[16] The trigeminal nerve and the facial nerve are most commonly involved when PNI is present, and a thorough assessment of sensation and motor function in all branches, respectively, is required.[17]

Palpation of the parotid glands and cervical lymphatics, including those in the posterior triangle and suboccipital regions, is indicated as well. The lymphatic drainage system is notably complex, and not always reliable in regard to anatomical course.[12] In patients presenting with a parotid or neck mass, a thorough inspection should be performed for a potential synchronous skin primary, with particular focus paid to the temporoparietal scalp and periauricular region. In addition, examination of the upper aerodigestive tract (UADT) should be performed to rule out an unknown mucosal primary—level II adenopathy and metastatic parotid-area adenopathy are often difficult to distinguish clinically.

16.3.3 Biopsy

Suspicious cutaneous lesions of the head and neck warrant incisional or narrow-margin excisional biopsy. Incisional biopsy with a 2-, 3-, or 4-mm punch may be performed for a full-thickness assessment. Adequate shave biopsy that allows depth measurement is an acceptable technique in NMSC, and fine-needle aspiration biopsy is indicated for evaluating neck and parotid masses. Ideally, the resulting report will provide not only a pathologic diagnosis, but also information about depth of invasion, differentiation, and vascular or PNI. Synoptic reporting (▶ Table 16.2) of surgical specimens is more commonly used in melanoma evaluation, and has yet to be widely adopted in cSCC.[18]

Table 16.2 Synoptic report comparison for cutaneous squamous cell carcinoma (cSCC) and melanoma[19,20]

cSCC	Melanoma
Procedure	Procedure
Tumor site	Specimen laterality
Tumor size	Tumor site
Histologic type	Tumor size
Histologic grade	Macroscopic satellite nodules
Maximum tumor thickness	Histologic type
Anatomic level	Maximum tumor (Breslow) thickness
Margins (peripheral and deep)	Ulceration
Lymphovascular invasion	Mitotic rate
Perineural invasion	Lymphovascular invasion
Lymph nodes (number examined and number involved by metastatic carcinoma)	Neutropism
Pathologic staging (pTNM, AJCC, 8th ed.)	Tumor regression
	Regional lymph nodes (number of sentinel nodes involved, lymph nodes involved, matted nodes, lymph nodes examined, and sentinel lymph nodes examined)
	Pathologic stage classification (pTNM, AJCC 8th ed.)
	Presence of S-100, MARTI, HMB-45

Abbreviations: AJCC, American Joint Committee on Cancer; pTNM, pathological tumor-node-metastasis.

16.3.4 Imaging

The role of imaging in skin cancer depends on patient symptoms as well as clinical findings and the biopsy report. The majority of cutaneous malignancies do not require imaging in their initial workup and management. Larger lesions, and clinically thick or fixed lesions of the cheek and preauricular region, have the potential to involve the parotid gland or Stensen's duct, and a contrasted CT scan of the neck may identify parotid extension and facilitate adequate preoperative planning and comprehensive resection. CT imaging may also identify invasion into underlying bone, cartilage, muscle, and fascia, as well as bony remodeling, enlargement of neural foramina and canals, or widening of the pterygopalatine fossa in cases of suspected PNI. MRI remains the more sensitive modality as compared with CT in detecting early perineural spread, manifest as subtle nerve enhancement.[16] MRI and CT often provide complementary information in patients with deep scalp lesions, as the CT scan may demonstrate bony destruction and the MRI may depict the extent of intracranial spread. Clinically suspicious parotid masses or cervical lymph nodes also benefit from anatomic imaging with MRI, CT scan, or comprehensive neck ultrasound to permit accurate nodal staging. Nodes larger than 1.5 cm in levels I and II and those larger than 1 cm in other neck levels may warrant additional evaluation with fine-needle aspiration biopsy.

Routine use of PET-CT in head and neck NMSC is currently not recommended, except in MCC, where PET scans have been shown to alter staging in up to 33% of cases and change disease management in 43% of cases.[10,21] Alternatively, although it is integral to the clinical staging of stage III and IV melanoma, it is not recommended in stage I and II melanoma due to its low yield.[22] Approximately 60% of patients with palpable or macroscopic melanoma nodal metastasis will develop distant metastases. In addition, PET-CT has been shown to be 83% sensitive and 85% specific when evaluating deep soft tissue, lymph node, and visceral metastasis in patients with stage III or IV melanoma.[23,24] PET-CT imaging is also valuable in assessing response to immunotherapy, and for detection of recurrence in the follow-up period in late-stage disease.[23] The recent development of selective PET probes capable of detecting melanoma more specifically is being studied in small animal models with some promise as well.[25]

16.4 Patterns of Lymphatic Spread

Compared to other anatomic regions, lymphatic drainage from cutaneous sites in the head and neck exhibits marked complexity and variability. The lymphatic drainage patterns for the skin of the head and neck are depicted in ▶ Fig. 16.1.[26] In general, lesions anterior to a vertical line extending toward the vertex from the auricle will drain to the ipsilateral parotid gland and upper cervical lymph nodes, including lymph nodes along the external jugular chain in the parotid region. More posteriorly located lesions will drain to the postauricular, occipital, and posterior cervical nodes.[27] Lesions of the midface and lower lip may drain to the bilateral anterior cervical nodes, including the superficially located perifacial nodes, submental nodes, and

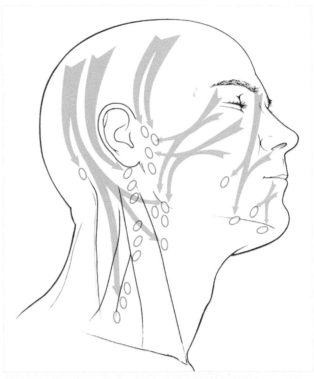

Fig. 16.1 Patterns of head and neck lymphatic spread.[26]

submandibular nodes. Lesions on the neck will likely drain to the closest underlying lymph nodes and those along the external jugular vein, but they are unlikely to involve the parotid gland. Within this general framework, there is significant variability, as is evidenced by studies that reveal a discordance of up to 34% between the clinical prediction and lymphoscintigraphy, making this imaging modality invaluable in depicting bilateral drainage (▶ Fig. 16.2).[28]

16.5 Management of Aggressive Lesions

16.5.1 Identification of High-Risk Lesions

Although the vast majority of NMSCs are curable through multiple different treatment modalities, aggressive lesions are capable of nodal metastases. Although aggressive variants of BCC exist (infiltrative/morpheaform and micronodular subtypes), they are associated with local recurrence rather than regional metastases and will not be discussed here.[29] There is a growing awareness of the clinical features of aggressive cSCC, which is leading to an appreciation of the need for a multidisciplinary, more proactive approach to the regional lymphatics.[30] Characteristics of aggressive cSCC, as noted by the American Joint Committee on Cancer (AJCC) eighth edition, and risk factors for regional metastases in both cSCC and melanoma are depicted in ▶ Table 16.3 and ▶ Table 16.4, respectively.

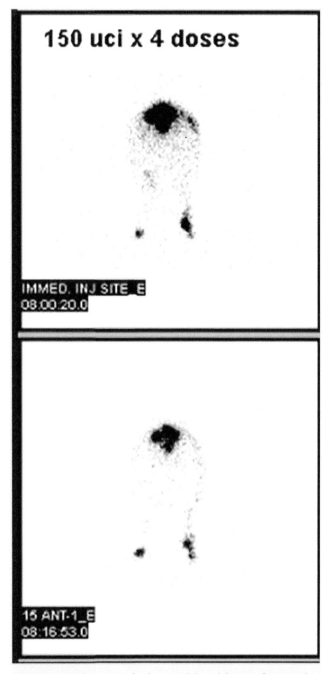

150 uci x 4 doses

IMMED. INJ SITE_E
08.00.20.0

15 ANT-1_E
08:16:53.0

Fig. 16.2 Lymphoscintigraphy depicting bilateral drainage from a scalp vertex lesion.

Table 16.3 Aggressive features for cutaneous squamous cell carcinoma[31]

High-risk histologic feature	Description	Affects T staging
Tumor size (cm)	≥2	Yes
Tumor thickness (mm)	>6	Yes
Level of invasion	Beyond dermis	Yes
Perineural invasion	Large caliber (≥0.1 mm diameter)	Yes
Differentiation	Poor differentiation	No
Growth pattern	Desmoplastic and spindle cell	No
Lymphovascular invasion	Tumor cells within vascular spaces	No
Anatomical location	Hair-bearing (lip and ear)	No
Immunosuppression	Organ transplant recipients (heart and lung especially), CLL, CML, AIDS	No

Abbreviations: AIDS, acquired immunodeficiency syndrome; CLL, chronic lymphocytic leukemia; CML, chronic myelogenous leukemia.

Table 16.4 Risk factors for regional metastases in skin cancer of the head and neck[3,12,32,33]

Nonmelanoma skin cancer	Melanoma
Recurrent lesion size >2.0 cm	Breslow thickness (continuous variable)
Depth >4.0 mm	Clark level >III
Clark levels IV–V	Ulceration of primary
Invasion to subcutaneous tissues	Patient age <60 y
Poor histologic differentiation	Histologic type other than superficial spreading
Preexisting scar	Lymphovascular invasion
Ear or lip location	Vertical growth phase present
Perineural invasion	Infiltrative tumor strands
Lymphovascular invasion	Single cell infiltration
Inflammation	Acantholysis

16.5.2 Impact of Regional Metastases

The reported rate of metastatic cSCC ranges from 0.1 to 21% in the literature, and these metastases are often delayed by several months from diagnosis of the primary lesion.[11,12] The range of variance in the literature is partly due to the aforementioned issue that NMSC is not routinely reported by cancer registries, or followed by SEER. Patients with nodal metastases of cSCC exhibit diminished overall survival (OS; 46.7 vs. 75.7%), disease-free survival (DFS; 40.9 vs. 65.2%), and disease-specific survival (DSS; 58.2 vs. 91.5%) at 5 years, compared with patients without nodal metastases.[12] As a result, there is a growing appreciation that nodal

metastases in cSCC demand aggressive treatment, predicated on the early identification of high-risk features in the primary lesion or, perhaps, early detection of regional metastases through sentinel lymph node biopsy (SLNB). Increasing depth of invasion and the histologic presence of lymphovascular invasion have exhibited the strongest correlation with nodal metastases.[12]

As in NMSC, the presence of nodal metastases in cutaneous melanoma portends a worse prognosis. Patients with subclinical lymphatic involvement detected on sentinel lymph node biopsy have a 3-year DFS of roughly 56%; in contrast, patients with comparable primary lesions but with negative sentinel nodes have a

3-year DFS of more than 88%. In fact, the presence of lymph node metastases has emerged as a stronger predictor of diminished DFS and DSS than Clark's level, Breslow's thickness, and ulceration status.[34] Much of the recent data on high-risk features for nodal metastases in melanoma have been gleaned from prospective trials evaluating SLNB. Historically, the depth of the primary melanoma was the most significant determinant of regional metastases, as lesions less than 1.0 mm thick have less than a 5% rate of nodal metastases, and lesions greater than 4.0 mm thick have a 30 to 50% rate of nodal metastases.[35] Erman et al found that a positive SLNB was the strongest factor for a decreased recurrence-free survival (RFS) and decreased OS. Other factors, such as an increased Breslow thickness of the primary lesion and presence of ulceration, were both found to decrease RFS and OS.[36]

16.5.3 Staging

Although the importance of clinical staging in melanoma has been well established, clinical staging, particularly of the regional lymph nodes, in cSCC continues to evolve. O'Brien et al helped describe that higher "P" and "N" stages correlate with larger or more numerous nodal metastases in either the parotid gland or cervical lymph nodes, and thus have adverse effects on locoregional control and survival, validating the parotid gland as a nodal basin for cutaneous malignancy of the head and neck. Further updates have been made to the eighth edition of the AJCC staging system for cSCC of the head and neck.[37] High-risk features such as location, size, depth, and differentiation are highlighted in cSCC, as depicted in ▶ Table 16.5.

Table 16.5 Staging of skin cancer of the head and neck

	Primary tumor (T)		
Melanoma		**cSCC**	
TX	Primary tumor cannot be assessed	Primary tumor cannot be assessed	
T0	No evidence of primary tumor	No evidence of primary tumor	
Tis	Melanoma in situ	Carcinoma in situ	
T1	Tumor ≤ 1.0 mm in thickness	Tumor < 2 cm	
a	< 0.8 mm without ulceration		
b	< 0.8 mm with ulceration or 0.8–1.0 mm with or without ulceration		
T2	Tumor > 1.0–2.0 mm in thickness	Tumor ≥ 2 cm but < 4	
a	1–2 mm without ulceration		
b	1–2 mm with ulceration		
T3	Tumor > 2.0–4.0 mm thick in thickness	Tumor ≥ 4 cm or minor bone erosion or PNI or deep invasion	
a	2.0–4.0 mm without ulceration		
b	2.0–4.0 mm with ulceration		
T4	Tumor > 4.0 mm in thickness	See below	
a	> 4.0 mm without ulceration	Tumor with gross cortical bone/marrow invasion	
b	> 4.0 mm with ulceration	Tumor with skull base invasion and/or skull base foramen involvement	
	Regional lymph nodes (N)		
Melanoma			**cSCC**
		Presence of in-transit, satellite, and/or microsatellite metastases	
NX	Regional lymph nodes not assessed	No	Regional lymph nodes not assessed
N0	No regional lymph node metastases	No	No regional lymph node metastases
N1	One positive lymph node or in-transit, satellite, and/or microsatellite metastases with no tumor-involved nodes		Metastasis in a single ipsilateral lymph node ≤ 3 cm and ENE (−)
a	One clinically occult (i.e., detected with SLNB)	No	
b	One clinically detected	No	
c	No regional lymph node disease	Yes	

Continued

N2	Two or three positive lymph nodes or in-transit, satellite, and/or microsatellite metastases with one tumor-involved node		See below	
a	Two or three clinically occult (i.e., detected with SLNB)	No		Metastasis in single ipsi- or contralateral lymph node ≤ 3 cm and ENE (+) or a single ipsilateral node > 3 cm but ≤ 6 cm and ENE (−)
b	Two or three, at least one that was clinically detected	No		Metastasis in multiple ipsilateral lymph nodes ≤ 6 cm and ENE (−)
c	One clinically occult or clinically detected	Yes		Metastasis in bilateral or contralateral lymph nodes ≤ 6 cm and ENE (−)
N3	Four or more positive nodes, or in-transit, satellite, and/or microsatellite metastases with two or more positive nodes, or any number of matted nodes with/without in-transit, satellite, and/or microsatellite metastases		See below	
a	Four or more clinically occult (i.e., detected with SLNB)	No		Metastasis in a single lymph node > 6 cm and ENE (−)
b	Four or more, at least one of which was detected clinically, or presence of matted nodes	No		Metastasis in a single lymph node > 3 cm and ENE (+) or multiple ipsilateral, contralateral, or bilateral nodes, any with ENE (+)
c	Two or more clinically occult or clinically detected and/or presence of matted nodes	Yes		N/A

Distant metastases (M)		
Melanoma		**cSCC**
M0	No distant metastases	No distant metastases
M1	Distant metastases	Distant metastases
a	Distant metastasis to skin, soft tissue (muscle and/or nonregional lymph node). M1a (0): LDH not elevated; M1a (1): LDH elevated	N/A
b	Lung metastasis. M1b (0): LDH not elevated; M1b (1): LDH elevated	N/A
c	Distant metastasis to non-CNS visceral sites with/without M1a or M1b sites of disease. M1c (0): LDH not elevated; M1c (1): LDH elevated	N/A
D	Distant metastasis to CNS with/without M1a, M1b, or M1c sites of disease. M1d (0): LDH normal; M1d (1): LDH elevated	N/A

Abbreviations: CNS, central nervous system; ENE, extranodal extension; LDH, lactate dehydrogenase; PNI, perineural invasion; SLNB, sentinel lymph node biopsy.
Source: Adapted from Amin et al.[31]

Given the challenges in identifying aggressive cSCC, alternative systems have recently been proposed that may offer increased prognostic accuracy by dividing T2 tumors based on the number of identified risk factors, incorporating other risk factors such as soft-tissue metastases, and modifying the nodal classification. Ideally, this evolution of staging systems and appreciation of high-risk features will drive changes in pathology reports to facilitate proactive treatment of at-risk nodal basins. One alternative staging system has demonstrated increased accuracy for predicting local recurrence, nodal metastases, and disease-specific death, compared to the AJCC or Union for International Cancer Control (UICC) systems.[38]

16.5.4 Management of the Primary Lesion

Because it is so common and enjoys a generally accepted favorable prognosis, cutaneous malignancy of the head and neck is treated by a variety of both practitioners and modalities. In general, treatments may be destructive or excisional in nature. For premalignant—or early low-risk lesions—destructive therapies may be appropriate, but multidisciplinary evaluation (including dermatologists, dermatologic surgeons, head and neck surgeons/surgical oncologists, radiation oncologists, and reconstructive surgeons) prior to excision, with comprehensive margin assessment, is the

Table 16.6 Recommendations for surgical margins according to the histology of the primary

Lesion	Surgical margin
Malignant melanoma	5 mm: pTis melanoma (in situ)
	1 cm: pT1 melanoma (< 1.0 mm)
	1–2 cm: pT2 melanoma (1.0–2.0 mm)
	1–2 cm: pT3 melanoma (2.0–4.0 mm)
	2 cm: pT4 melanoma (>4.0 mm)
Squamous cell carcinoma	4 mm in low-risk lesions
	6 mm in high-risk lesions
Basal cell carcinoma	3 mm in small lesions (< 2 cm)
	5–15 mm in morpheaform type or >2 cm

standard of care for aggressive lesions. Although traditional wide local excision is typically performed in advanced or aggressive lesions—at risk for, or associated with, nodal metastases—it should be noted that evaluation and treatment of regional lymph nodes can be performed with both wide local excision and Mohs' micrographic technique. Typical margins of excision are depicted in ▶ Table 16.6.

16.6 Management of Regional Metastases

16.6.1 The N0 Neck

Traditionally, regional metastases of head and neck NMSC have been approached in a reactive fashion, after a period of observation has occurred following primary treatment; melanoma was approached more aggressively because of a higher rate of lymph node metastasis (roughly 20%). The reported rate of regional lymph node metastases in cSCC is generally accepted as 4 to 5%, but it may reach as high as 20% in select populations.[39,40] Options for managing the N0 neck include watchful waiting, SLNB, and elective neck dissection (END) or radiation. Watchful waiting is recommended for patients with low-risk NMSC, and for patients with thin (< 0.8 mm) melanoma.

Elective Neck Dissection

The current literature does not support routine END for cutaneous malignancy in the clinically and radiographically negative neck (cN0); however, recent studies have shown it may be beneficial in specific situations. END has been advocated in the presence of isolated parotid metastasis, since occult microscopic disease is identified in the cervical lymph nodes (levels II and III) in 42% of patients. As the understanding of the role of the parotid gland as the primary lymphatic basin for the majority of the head and neck has evolved, the concurrent neck dissection is less viewed as "elective" but rather "therapeutic," since the first echelon nodes are already involved.[41] This is a reciprocal relationship, as occult parotid disease was identified in a comparable number of patients with anterior cervical lymph node metastases from cSCC of anterior/lateral scalp and facial primaries.

There are certain clinical situations when END for skin cancer is justified. Patients with skull base invasion by cSCC who underwent END demonstrated a significant difference in 5-year DFS versus those whose lymphatics were observed (57 vs. 32%, respectively). This was an orphan benefit for another indication for END: the need to identify and isolate recipient vessels for free tissue transfer as part of managing the primary tumor.[42] These findings all support the basis for including an END if the parotid gland is involved and an elective parotidectomy if the cervical nodal bundle is involved (site dependent) and, potentially, when there is skull base involvement by the primary lesion.

Sentinel Lymph Node Biopsy

SLNB has become increasingly important in the management of cutaneous malignancy. First introduced in 1992 by Morton et al, sentinel lymph node (SLN) mapping and biopsy is predicated on the premise that metastasizing tumor cells will spread first to the draining lymphatic basin, and an identifiable node within that basin accurately represents the status of the entire basin in both melanoma and cSCC.[43] The identification of a positive SLN has emerged as the most important prognostic factor for recurrence and survival in cutaneous melanoma, and is increasingly performed for MCC.[34] Increasing clinical primary tumor size (without a lower threshold of benefit), increasing tumor thickness, increasing mitotic rate, and an infiltrative growth pattern of primary MCC have been associated with positive SLNB, with reported positivity rates of 11 to 57%.[44] Although SLNB for MCC has been accompanied by false-negative results in up to 20% of cases, a negative SLNB has been associated with improved 5-year DSS (84.5 vs. 64.6%).[45,46]

With the increased acceptance of high-risk features in cSCC, there is growing interest in SLNB for cSCC—the technique has been shown to be reliable and feasible, with a false omission (false negative/false negative + true negative) rate of 5% that mirrors melanoma.[36,47] Unfortunately, specific risk factors have not been universally reported, and the low overall rate of regional metastases discourages routine SLNB in all cSCC patients. A recent meta-analysis identified positive sentinel nodes in 12.3% of reported patients with cSCC, noting the majority of positive results in AJCC stage T2 lesions and alternative stage T2a and T2b lesions, but additional prospective trials are required.[48] Schmitt et al have suggested that T2 tumors > 2 cm according to the AJCC-7 guidelines and T2b tumors in the alternative staging guideline proposed by Jambusaria-Pahlajani et al may warrant SLNB, as they were found to have 11.9 and 29.4% positive SLNB findings, respectively.[48]

Sentinel Lymph Node Biopsy Technique

According to current clinical practice, SLNB requires both preoperative lymphoscintigraphy and intraoperative lymphatic mapping. Preoperative lymphoscintigraphy involves the intradermal injection of 1.0 to 4.0 µCi of ^{99m}Tc sulfur colloid or ^{99m}Tc antimony trisulfide colloid in the four quadrants of the lesion periphery.[49,50] Looking forward, a newly Food and Drug Administration (FDA) approved receptor-binding molecular imaging agent, ^{99m}Tc-tilmanocept, has shown unique advantages over the colloid versions in its ability to rapidly clear injection site, yield high sentinel node extraction, and propensity for low distal node accumulation.[51] Immediate and delayed images are then performed to identify the draining lymphatic basins. More recently, fused single-photon emission CT/CT (SPECT/CT) has shown promise for these imaging studies in large part due to the clarity achieved through increased three-dimensional detail and superior resolution. One large prospective study comparing the modality to planar lymphoscintigraphy found it to be not only superior but also instrumental in changing surgical planning in 22% of cases (▶ Fig. 16.3).[52] Intraoperatively, the radiolabeled dye may be augmented by the intradermal injection of isosulfan blue dye, or methylene blue to increase the accuracy of the procedure.[34] Evidence supporting the use of one blue agent over another is limited in the head and neck literature, but a case-control study comparing the use of isosulfan blue to methylene blue showed no significant difference in the success rate of sentinel lymph node biopsy in those undergoing mapping for breast cancer.[53]

After obtaining baseline radioactivity levels with a gamma counter, the primary lesion is excised, and the previously identified basins are inspected with the gamma counter to locate areas of increased radioactivity. The frequent close proximity of the primary lesion to the primary nodal basin may create a phenomenon called "shine-through," whereby the different sites are not discernible or the proximate location of the primary falsely elevates the counts in the basin. It is for this reason that the primary lesion is typically excised first, but the sentinel lymph node biopsy may be performed first when the locations are farther apart. The sentinel nodes are accessed through small incisions that can be incorporated into a definitive nodal basin dissection incision if needed. Each SLN is identified and removed based on increased radioactivity counts and bluish discoloration (▶ Fig. 16.4). Some authors routinely monitor the facial nerve in the cases in which the SLNs map to the parotid basin, although this is not a universal practice.[49] Identified SLNs are then analyzed with routine hematoxylin and eosin (H&E)

staining, as well as immunohistochemical staining for proteins such as S-100, MARTI, Melan-A, and HMB-45 for melanoma, cytokeratin for cSCC, and CK-20 in MCC. Patients with positive sentinel nodes are often returned to the operating room within 2 to 3 weeks for comprehensive neck dissections (completion lymph node dissection [CLND]).[55]

Identification of the SLN allows the detection of occult regional metastases, promotes accurate staging, and facilitates appropriate delivery of adjuvant therapies. Meticulous serial sectioning of the lymph nodes, augmented by routine analysis and immunohistochemical staining, has identified more patients with positive nodes than END.[56] Limiting formal neck dissections to those patients with positive sentinel nodes spares unnecessary surgical morbidity for the roughly 80% of patients with intermediate-thickness melanoma, and the roughly 95% of patients with cSCC who do not have regional metastases. Subsequently, systemic therapy may be targeted to those patients who are at the greatest risk of metastases.[34]

Increasing experience with sentinel lymph node biopsy in the head and neck, however, has led to widespread acceptance, after a prolonged period of equipoise.[49] Because lymphatic drainage in the head and neck may be highly variable, discordant drainage basins should be anticipated and investigated. SLNB in the head and neck remains challenging, because of the variability in lymphatic drainage, the proximity of the basins to the primary (shine-through), and the higher number of sentinel nodes per basin.[50]

Complications are uncommon, and they include seroma, hematoma, sialocele formation, cranial nerve injury to the spinal accessory nerve or the facial nerve, and adverse reactions to the blue dye that range from erythema to anaphylaxis.[57] Although there is an acknowledged learning curve for sentinel lymph node biopsy, false-negative results have been documented in up to 10% of cases, and have been attributed to surgical failure or insufficient histopathologic detection.[49,50] By adhering to the "10% rule"

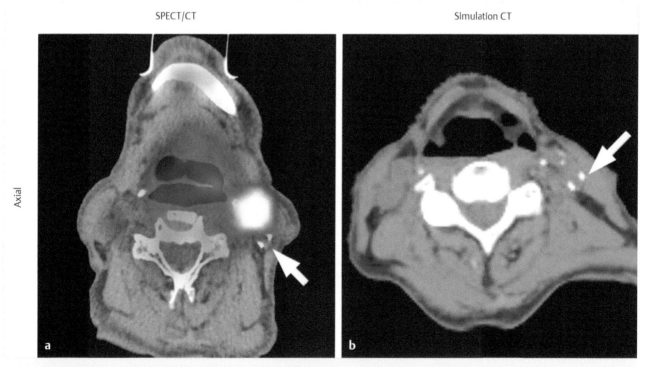

SPECT/CT   Simulation CT

Axial

Fig. 16.3 (a,b) SPECT/CT axial image demonstrating left sided level III positive lymph node.[54]

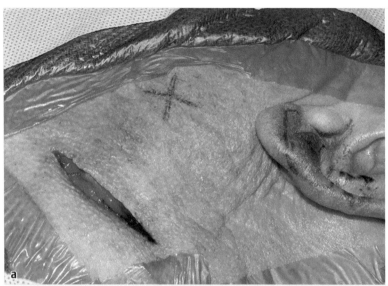
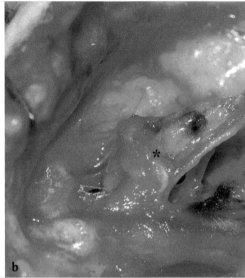

Fig. 16.4 Sentinel lymph node biopsy performed for a T1a melanoma of the left ear lobe. Preoperative lymphoscintigraphy mapped to the tail of parotid/level II region **(a)**, and this was marked with an "X" in the nuclear medicine suite. Because the primary site and sentinel node basin were distinct, sentinel lymph node biopsy was performed prior to wide local excision of the melanoma through an incision that would accommodate a parotidectomy with neck dissection. Intraoperative use of blue dye augments the preoperative radionucleotide, yielding a "hot" blue sentinel node immediately adjacent to the external jugular vein in the tail of parotid **(b)**.

proposed by McMasters et al, detection of occult metastases may be optimized by removing all blue lymph nodes, all clinically suspicious nodes, and all nodes that are ≥ 10% of the ex vivo radioactive count of the most radioactive sentinel node.[58] A false-negative result may lead to delayed detection and treatment of regional metastases, which could negatively impact survival.[59]

16.6.2 The N + Neck

The parotid gland constitutes a lymphatic basin for metastatic skin cancer, and occult cervical lymph node metastases are likely in over 40% of patients with cSCC parotid metastases.[12,60] Regional metastases of cSCC typically present within 6 to 12 months after the primary, and only 20 to 65% of lymphatic metastases present concurrently with the primary lesion.[61] Once identified, regionally metastatic NMSC or melanoma often merits multimodality therapy, with an appropriate lymphadenectomy, followed by adjuvant therapy.

In cSCC, disease-free intervals of ≤ 9 months presage a two-fold elevated risk of locoregional failure, and a threefold increased risk of disease-specific death, despite best current therapies.[62] The type of lymphadenectomy performed depends on the location (if known) of the primary malignancy and the history (if any) of prior treatment, especially radiation therapy (RT). The surgical principles for clinical nodal metastases are common for both NMSC and melanoma. If the parotid is involved with a functioning facial nerve, a superficial parotidectomy with facial nerve preservation may be performed followed by RT without adversely impacting disease control and survival in cSCC, even in the setting of microscopic residual disease.[63] Because the presence of nodal metastases in melanoma indicates more aggressive disease and a greater likelihood of distant metastases, every effort should be made to save a functioning facial nerve in melanoma as well. There is no difference in OS or DFS in patients undergoing a selective neck dissection

compared to a modified radical neck dissection, although a comprehensive neck dissection or modified radical neck dissection may be required in previously radiated patients.[64] When the parotid is involved and the neck is clinically negative, a selective neck dissection of at least levels II and III is sufficient for many cases in cSCC, although dissection of levels I to III is indicated for facial primaries, and levels II to V for posterior scalp and neck primaries.[12,62] The posterolateral neck dissection (PLND), described in the following section, is indicated for patients with posterior triangle metastases, or those with watershed or more posteriorly located primary lesions.

Posterolateral Neck Dissection: Technique

PLND has become the mainstay treatment for patients with metastatic lymphadenopathy from the posterior scalp and neck, which primarily includes two distinct groups of nodes (retroauricular and suboccipital).[65] Metastases from melanoma or NMSC originating posterior to a coronal plane made at the anterior border of the ears are thought to typically exclusively drain to the nodes in the parotid gland, postauricular nodes, or the suboccipital nodes.[66] It has been demonstrated by Lengele et al that the posterior scalp and retroauricular cutaneous regions primarily follow the superficial lateral and posterior accessory pathways. More specifically, drainage is thought to travel via the suboccipital and retroauricular nodes, and then most reliably enters the jugulodigastric nodes of level IIB, superficial jugular nodes, and finally the deep nodes of levels VA and VB. Due to the extent of this pathway, PLND, including removal of levels II to V as well as the retroauricular and suboccipital nodes, is generally considered an accepted approach in the setting of metastasis from a primary in this region.[67] Certain clinical situations may dictate that a parotidectomy be performed with the PLND, but routine, elective concurrent performance of parotidectomy with PLND is not required.

As with any patient, a thorough historical timeline, physical examination, and appropriate imaging as described earlier should be obtained prior to proceeding with PLND. Counseling should cover the risks of injury to the facial, spinal accessory, hypoglossal, and phrenic nerves, as well as the brachial and cervical plexuses, potential chyle leak, numbness (due to sacrifice of the supraclavicular plexus), and shoulder dysfunction (related to extensive dissection of and around cranial nerve [CN] XI and brachial plexus).

The surgical approach for a PLND is commonly performed through an S-shaped incision, or through a half-apron incision with a posterior limb (▶ Fig. 16.5). The skin is marked and injected with 1% lidocaine with 1:100,000 epinephrine. Subplatysmal flaps can be elevated over the mandible superiorly and the clavicles inferiorly; care should be taken to expose to nearly the midline posteriorly in the subcutaneous plane, beyond the anterior edge of the trapezius (▶ Fig. 16.6). Depending on the location of the primary lesion and the extent of adenopathy, levels IA and IB can be removed with the focus then turning to

dissection of levels II to IV, including the retroauricular and suboccipital nodes. In order to aid in the access to these nodes, the head of the trapezius can be reflected posteriorly, and the nodal packet delivered from the extreme posterior aspect of the dissection (▶ Fig. 16.7). Alternatively, the superior aspect of the trapezius muscle may be removed en bloc with the suboccipital nodes, as these structures are dissected off the splenius muscle (▶ Fig. 16.8). The spinal accessory nerve may first be identified entering the anterior border of the trapezius muscle, two fingerbreadths above the clavicle, or by using Erb's point as a reference. This nerve is then dissected and skeletonized along its course in the posterior triangle (▶ Fig. 16.9). The transverse cervical vessels may then be identified as the inferior limit of dissection. The fibrofatty tissue is then released from the posterior border of sternocleidomastoid muscle (SCM) for preparation, and to pass underneath this muscle as the external jugular vein is divided and included with the specimen due to the potential for adjacent nodal involvement.

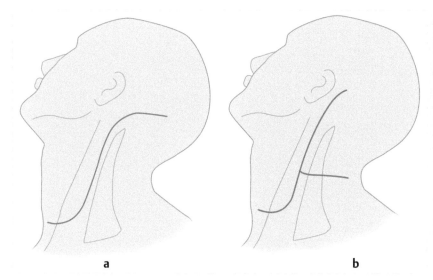

Fig. 16.5 Common surgical approaches for a posterolateral neck dissection. **(a)** S-shaped incision. **(b)** Apron or half-apron incision with posterior limb.

a

b

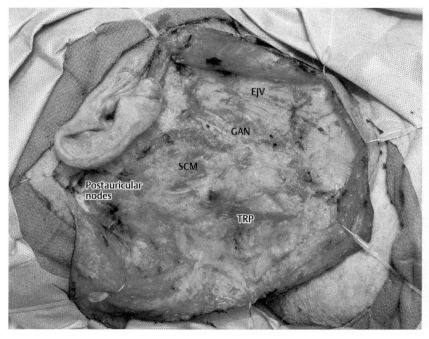

Fig. 16.6 Superficial anatomy of the posterior neck triangle following elevation of skin flaps. EJV, external jugular vein; GAN, greater auricular nerve; SCM, sternocleidomastoid muscle; TRP, trapezius muscle.

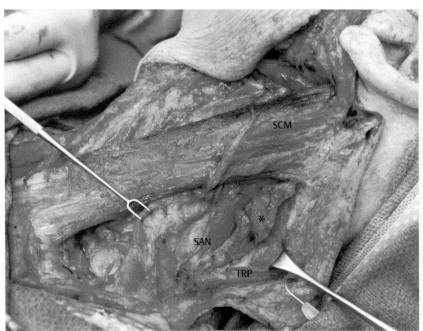

Fig. 16.7 Approach to the suboccipital nodes (*) by posterior retraction of the superior aspect of the trapezius muscle. SAN, spinal accessory nerve; SCM, sternocleidomastoid muscle; TRP, trapezius muscle.

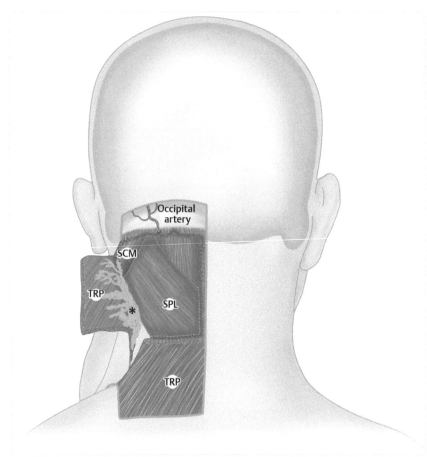

Fig. 16.8 Diagram of the posterior neck illustrating en bloc resection of the superior trapezius muscle with suboccipital nodes (*). SCM, sternocleidomastoid muscle; SPL, splenius capitis muscle; TRP, trapezius muscle;

Subsequently, attention is turned to the SCM where the fascia was released, thus allowing for elevation along with the fibrofatty contents of levels II to IV off the SCM moving from superior to inferior. With release of this fascia from the medial edge of the muscle, the segmental blood supply to the SCM can be divided. The proximal aspect of the spinal accessory nerve is then identified and dissected superiorly, to the point where it transitions lateral to the internal jugular vein, but deep to the posterior belly

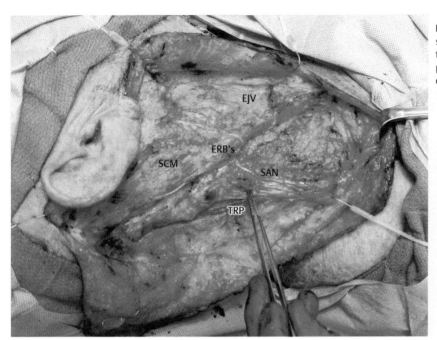

Fig. 16.9 Identification and dissection of the spinal accessory nerve through the posterior neck triangle. EJV, external jugular vein; ERB's, Erb's point; SAN, spinal accessory nerve; SCM, sternocleidomastoid muscle; TRP, trapezius muscle.

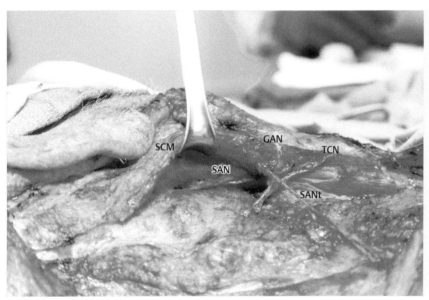

Fig. 16.10 Exposure of the proximal trunk of the spinal accessory nerve though a posterior neck approach. The nerve can be seen as it enters the SCM on its medial aspect, while its distal branch emerges from its posterior aspect in direction to the trapezius. GAN, greater auricular nerve; SAN, spinal accessory nerve; SANt, trapezius branch of the spinal accessory nerve; SCM, sternocleidomastoid muscle; TCN, transverse cervical nerve.

of digastric at the level of the transverse process of C1 (▶ Fig. 16.10). Using C1 as a landmark at this point in the dissection has been shown helpful in identifying not only the spinal accessory nerve and internal jugular vein but also the internal carotid artery.[68] The proximal spinal accessory nerve should then be skeletonized, and the contents exenterated off of the SCM in the floor of the neck. If performing an anterior approach, this allows for this to be passed underneath CN XI, and then brought forward with the remainder of the neck dissection specimen.

In a similar fashion, the dissection can be continued medially along the SCM allowing for identification of the cervical rootlets, thereby preserving the cervical contribution to the spinal accessory nerve. In moving more inferiorly, the contents of levels II to IV are dissected off the internal jugular vein. The plane of dissection is superficial to the deep cervical fascia with visual identification and preservation of the phrenic nerve. The omohyoid

muscle may then be divided to allow for easier access to the inferior aspect of level IV, with no appreciable functional deficit. The inferior limit of the internal jugular vein is exposed bluntly, allowing for the dissection to progress laterally to connect with the posterior limit of the dissection. Finally, the carotid sheath is opened and the fibrofatty contents of levels II to IV elevated off the carotid artery, vagus nerve, and internal jugular vein in sequence. The facial vein and superior thyroid vein are best identified and preserved if possible. Multiple branches of the external carotid system may be similarly identified and preserved. In this manner, the neck dissection specimen is then detached from the strap muscles and sectioned into levels ex vivo to be sent for permanent pathologic analysis.

Alternatively, the contents of levels II to IV may be approached through the posterior neck by retracting the SCM anteriorly. In this setting, once the proximal trunk of the spinal accessory nerve has been identified and dissected, the fibrofatty contents of the lateral neck are dissected off the lateral aspect of the internal jugular vein, maintaining the continuity of the specimen with the contents of the posterior triangle (▶ Fig. 16.11). The specimen is subsequently dissected off the floor of the neck musculature, divided, and sent for permanent pathologic analysis (▶ Fig. 16.12, ▶ Fig. 16.13, ▶ Fig. 16.14).

Completion Neck Dissection in SLN (+) Patients

The appropriate treatment pathway for head and neck melanoma patients with sentinel node positive (SN-positive) neck diagnoses remains undetermined. The combination of discordant drainage patterns, and the potential for bilateral drainage raise the specter of regional failure outside of the dissected beds. Recent findings noted in the Multicenter Selective Lymphadenectomy Trial II (MSLT-II) and DeCOG-SLT (complete lymph node dissection versus no dissection in patients with sentinel lymph node biopsy positive melanoma) trials have shown that neck CLND did not offer a melanoma-specific survival benefit compared with observation in SN-positive patients.[69,70] The MSLT-II trial did show, however, that CLND offered more comprehensive staging information by demonstrating additional lymph node metastases in 11.5% of the patients, potentially leading to the use of systemic therapy, and delivered improved regional control. A smaller study of 140 stage IIIa melanoma patients found a similar rate of 11.6% positive nonsentinel nodes on CLND, but the additional information led to a stage change in only 5.8% of cases.[71] The decision to proceed with

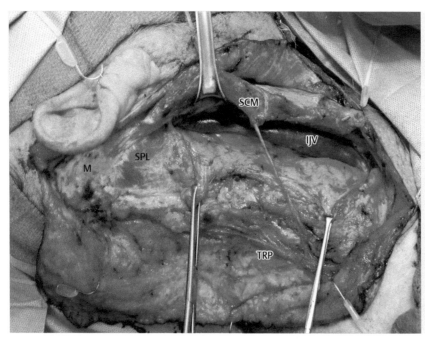

Fig. 16.11 The jugular nodes (levels II–IV) are addressed throughout the posterior neck. The specimen is dissected off the internal jugular vein and kept in continuity with the posterior neck contents. IJV, internal jugular vein; M, mastoid; SCM, sternocleidomastoid muscle; SPL, splenius capitis muscle; TRP, trapezius muscle.

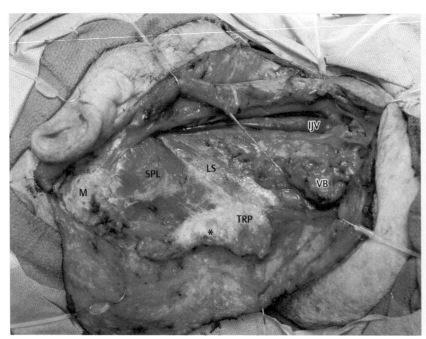

Fig. 16.12 The superior aspect of the trapezius muscle is reflected inferiorly to reveal the presence of a pathological suboccipital lymph node (*). The specimen is in continuity with normal-appearing postauricular lymph nodes. IJV, internal jugular vein; LS, levator scapulae muscle; M, mastoid; SPL, splenius capitis muscle; TRP, trapezius muscle; VB, nodal group Vb.

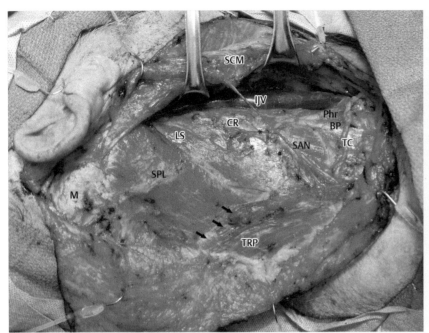

Fig. 16.13 View of the surgical field upon completion of the posterolateral neck dissection. Note that the trapezius muscle was transected (*arrows*), and its superior portion removed en bloc with the suboccipital lymph nodes. The spinal accessory nerve expresses branching pattern distally and receives a contribution from the cervical rootlets (*). BP, brachial plexus; CR, transected cervical rootlets; IJV, internal jugular vein; LS, levator scapulae muscle; M, mastoid; Phr, phrenic nerve; SAN, spinal accessory nerve; SCM, sternocleidomastoid muscle; SPL, splenius capitis muscle; TC, transverse cervical vessels; TRP, trapezius muscle.

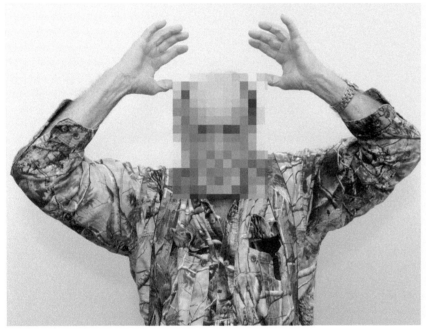

Fig. 16.14 Shoulder function of the same patient at 2 weeks postoperatively.

CLND depends on patient- and tumor-related factors, such as the number of sentinel nodes involved, the tumor burden within the nodes, and patient preference, but additional studies are certainly needed to answer this question.

Management of the Unknown Primary with Neck Metastases

In NMSC, the development of regional metastases in the absence of a primary lesion presents a clinical challenge. Patients should be queried as to their history of skin cancer, or skin lesions that have been removed previously. Often, an index lesion can be identified, but an exhaustive search for potential lesions should be undertaken in the absence of a clear history. Importantly, patients

with parotid or cervical involvement by SCC should be evaluated for UADT primary lesions. Patients with regional metastases and no identifiable primary should be treated aggressively with neck dissection followed by XRT for cSCC. Concurrent chemotherapy may be beneficial in SCC with adverse features.

16.6.3 Radiation Therapy in Regionally Metastatic Skin Cancer of the Head and Neck

When judiciously applied as a primary treatment modality in select patients who are poor surgical candidates, in anatomic regions that are difficult to reconstruct, or for those who refuse surgery, RT exhibits local control rates comparable to surgery for smaller lesions, BCC (vs. SCC), and for primary (vs. recurrent) tumors. RT has also been demonstrated to achieve local control in inoperable patients with MCC at a mean dose of 50 Gy, and there is also demonstrated efficacy in elective neck irradiation (without neck dissection or SLN biopsy) in MCC.[72] As with surgery, the clinical treatment volume is determined by the clinical and histologic features of the tumor. Larger margins are required for SCC and lesions larger than 2 cm; fields can be extended to the skull base along the course of involved cranial nerves.[73]

Adjuvant Therapy

Postoperative RT is commonly recommended in patients with parotid or cervical metastases from cSCC after either comprehensive or therapeutic selective neck dissection. At-risk, undissected levels are included in the radiation portals, thereby minimizing potential surgical morbidity in levels with a low likelihood of involvement.[12] Patients with lymphatic metastases from cSCC have demonstrated significant improvements in locoregional control (80 vs. 57%), and 5-year DFS (74 vs. 54%) with surgery and radiation compared with neck dissection alone.[74] Adjuvant RT has been included in a prognostic scoring model (Immunosuppression, Treatment, Extranodal spread, and Margin status [ITEM] score) as a favorable variable, in contradistinction to other components (immunosuppression, extranodal spread, and margin status) that accurately stratify patients into low-, moderate-, and high-risk categories for disease-specific death.[75] Adjuvant RT has demonstrated similar improvements in locoregional control and survival after SLN biopsy or regional lymphadenectomy in MCC.[76] The role of RT after a positive SLB biopsy in cSCC has not been explored, but may be an option for patients who refuse CLND.[77]

Postoperative RT has gained favor in cutaneous melanoma because of improved locoregional control rates up to 85 to 90% in high-risk patients, without an attendant impact on survival. High-risk patients are those individuals who are unable or unwilling to undergo re-excision for recurrent primary disease, those with surgical margins that are close (≤ 1 cm) or frankly positive, and patients with multiple positive lymph nodes or extracapsular extension.[78] The lack of correlation with survival benefit is important, however, as increasing nodal melanoma burden is associated with poorer regional control and distant metastases up to 70% within 1 year. The locoregional benefit of RT must be balanced against the limited impact on distant metastases and melanoma-specific survival and significantly higher rates of RT-related complications in such patients.[79]

16.6.4 Treatment of Advanced and Systemic Disease

At the present time, surgery with or without postoperative RT remains the mainstay for managing regionally metastatic cSCC, and surgery followed by systemic therapy is typically pursued for regionally metastatic melanoma. Applications of chemotherapy in cSCC of the head and neck continue to evolve, with the emergence of targeted molecular therapies and immunotherapy to supplement and supplant traditional cytotoxic agents, but there is no consensus on the indications and regimens. Vismodegib, a hedgehog signaling pathway inhibitor, has been approved by the

FDA for the treatment of locally advanced or metastatic BCC, and it has demonstrated efficacy in controlling disease in patients with basal cell-nevus syndrome.[80] Because of the frequent expression of the epidermal growth factor receptor in cSCC of the head and neck, there is significant interest in the use of monoclonal antibodies against its extracellular domain (cetuximab) or the internal tyrosine kinase component (erlotinib, gefitinib).[81,82,83] Additional randomized controlled trials should be undertaken, but targeted therapy holds great promise.

The addition of chemotherapy to adjuvant RT for metastatic cSCC is supported by the experience with UADT SCC. However, there is a paucity of data to support its routine use. A recent retrospective study reported an improvement in median RFS to 40.3 months in patients receiving adjuvant, platinum-based chemoradiation therapy versus 15.4 months in patients receiving radiation alone.[84] Despite a tendency to regard MCC as similar to other neuroendocrine tumors such as small cell lung cancer, it is a distinct disease, and the role of chemotherapy remains undefined. MCC tends to be initially chemosensitive, but treatment-related toxicities to the commonly used agents and early relapse limit its use as definitive therapy. The roles of adjuvant chemoradiation and targeted therapy also remain unclear.[85]

Adjuvant therapy use in melanoma is more well defined, but the emergence of newer targeted agents and immunotherapy has altered treatment regimens and provided hope to patients and clinicians. The decision for adjuvant therapy is based on risk stratification by established guidelines. High-risk, node-negative (stage IIb or IIc) patients are generally not recommended to undergo adjuvant therapy due their typically favorable prognosis, treatment toxicity, and lack of inclusion in recent immunotherapy trials.[86] Stage III (lymph node involvement without distant metastases) and stage IV (presence of distant metastases) have historically been shown to benefit from adjuvant therapy with interferon-alpha following complete resection, with slight improvements in OS. However, checkpoint inhibitor immunotherapies (nivolumab, ipilimumab, and pembrolizumab) and more targeted therapies (dabrafenib, trametinib, and vemurafenib) have demonstrated modest superiority to interferon.[87,88] Current literature points toward the use of adjuvant nivolumab for stage III and stage IV disease, with improved RFS at 12 and 18 months when compared to ipilimumab.[89] As a result of these recent innovations, systemic therapy for melanoma is dynamic, and patients should be treated on a clinical trial or according to established guidelines.

16.7 Conclusion

Head and neck skin cancer represents a heterogeneous group of malignancies with numerous treatment challenges related to the aesthetic and functional aspects of the head and neck, its variable lymphatic drainage, and a potential for underestimating the morbidity and mortality of the disease. Appropriate multidisciplinary management of head and neck cutaneous malignancy is predicated on early identification of aggressive lesions with metastatic potential. SLNB has emerged as the standard for assessing regional lymph node status in patients with intermediate-thickness melanoma, and this technique has additional applications in cSCC and MCC. When performed, selective neck dissections may be dictated by the lymphoscintigraphic mapping of the primary lesion, and augmented with adjuvant RT to improve outcomes in cSCC and locoregional control in melanoma. Whether reactive or proactive, neck dissection and sentinel lymph node biopsy in cutaneous malignancy of the head and neck provide valuable information that completes staging, contributes to prognosis, and determines the need for radiation or an evolving array of systemic therapies, making familiarity with these foundational techniques essential in managing these emerging epidemics.

References

[1] American Cancer Society. About Basal And Squamous Cell Skin Cancer. 2016. Available at: https://www.cancer.org/cancer/basal-and-squamous-cell-skin-cancer/about/key-statistics.html. Accessed October 2017

[2] Guy GP, Jr, Machlin SR, Ekwueme DU, Yabroff KR. Prevalence and costs of skin cancer treatment in the U.S., 2002–2006 and 2007–2011. Am J Prev Med. 2015; 48(2):183–187

[3] Ali Z, Yousaf N, Larkin J. Melanoma epidemiology, biology and prognosis. EJC Suppl. 2013; 11(2):81–91

[4] Surveillance, Epidemiology, and End Results Program. Cancer Stat Facts: Melanoma of the Skin. Bethesda, MD: National Institute of Health; 2017

[5] US Department of Health and Human Services. The Surgeon General's Call to Action to Prevent Skin Cancer. Washington, DC: Office of the Surgeon General; 2014

[6] Iannacone MR, Wang W, Stockwell HG, et al. Patterns and timing of sunlight exposure and risk of basal cell and squamous cell carcinomas of the skin: a case-control study. BMC Cancer. 2012; 12:417

[7] Armstrong BK, Kricker A. How much melanoma is caused by sun exposure? Melanoma Res. 1993; 3(6):395–401

[8] Lallas A, Argenziano G, Zendri E, et al. Update on non-melanoma skin cancer and the value of dermoscopy in its diagnosis and treatment monitoring. Expert Rev Anticancer Ther. 2013; 13(5):541–558

[9] Reed KB, Brewer JD, Lohse CM, Bringe KE, Pruitt CN, Gibson LE. Increasing incidence of melanoma among young adults: an epidemiological study in Olmsted County, Minnesota. Mayo Clin Proc. 2012; 87(4):328–334

[10] Porceddu SV, Veness MJ, Guminski A. Nonmelanoma cutaneous head and neck cancer and Merkel cell carcinoma: current concepts, advances, and controversies. J Clin Oncol. 2015; 33(29):3338–3345

[11] Brougham ND, Dennett ER, Cameron R, Tan ST. The incidence of metastasis from cutaneous squamous cell carcinoma and the impact of its risk factors. J Surg Oncol. 2012; 106(7):811–815

[12] Moore BA, Weber RS, Prieto V, et al. Lymph node metastases from cutaneous squamous cell carcinoma of the head and neck. Laryngoscope. 2005; 115 (9):1561–1567

[13] Lai SY, Weinstein GS, Chalian AA, Rosenthal DI, Weber RS. Parotidectomy in the treatment of aggressive cutaneous malignancies. Arch Otolaryngol Head Neck Surg. 2002; 128(5):521–526

[14] Fitzpatrick TB. The validity and practicality of sun-reactive skin types I through VI. Arch Dermatol. 1988; 124(6):869–871

[15] Yalcin O, Sezer E, Kabukcuoglu F, et al. Presence of ulceration, but not high risk zone location, correlates with unfavorable histopathological subtype in facial basal cell carcinoma. Int J Clin Exp Pathol. 2015; 8(11):15448–15453

[16] Penn R, Abemayor E, Nabili V, Bhuta S, Kirsch C. Perineural invasion detected by high-field 3.0-T magnetic resonance imaging. Am J Otolaryngol. 2010; 31 (6):482–484

[17] Frunza A, Slavescu D, Lascar I. Perineural invasion in head and neck cancers - a review. J Med Life. 2014; 7(2):121–123

[18] Sluijter CE, van Lonkhuijzen LR, van Slooten HJ, Nagtegaal ID, Overbeek LI. The effects of implementing synoptic pathology reporting in cancer diagnosis: a systematic review. Virchows Arch. 2016; 468(6):639–649

[19] Hale C. Skin: melanocytic tumor. Miscellaneous: melanocytic tumor. Features to Report. PathologyOutlines.com; 2017. Available at: http://www.pathologyoutlines.com/topic/skintumormelanocyticfeatures.html. Accessed May 5, 2018

[20] College of American Pathologists. Cancer Protocol Templates. 2018. Available at: http://www.cap.org/ShowProperty?nodePath=/UCMCon/Contribution%20Folders/WebContent/pdf/cp-skin-melanoma-17protocol-4001.pdf

[21] Concannon R, Larcos GS, Veness M. The impact of (18)F-FDG PET-CT scanning for staging and management of Merkel cell carcinoma: results from Westmead Hospital, Sydney, Australia. J Am Acad Dermatol. 2010; 62 (1):76–84

[22] Mirk P, Treglia G, Salsano M, Basile P, Giordano A, Bonomo L. Comparison between F-fluorodeoxyglucose positron emission tomography and sentinel lymph node biopsy for regional lymph nodal staging in patients with melanoma: a review of the literature. Radiol Res Pract. 2011; 2011:912504

[23] Perng P, Marcus C, Subramaniam RM. (18)F-FDG PET/CT and melanoma: staging, immune modulation and mutation-targeted therapy assessment, and prognosis. AJR Am J Roentgenol. 2015; 205(2):259–270

[24] Krug B, Crott R, Lonneux M, Baurain JF, Pirson AS, Vander Borght T. Role of PET in the initial staging of cutaneous malignant melanoma: systematic review. Radiology. 2008; 249(3):836–844

[25] Fuster D, Rubello D. PET imaging in melanoma. PET Clinics. 2011; 6:ix–x

[26] Klein JD, Myers JN, Kupferman ME. Posterolateral neck dissection: preoperative considerations and intraoperative technique. Oper Tech Otolaryngol: Head Neck Surg. 2013; 24(1):24–29

[27] Lentsch EJ, Myers JN. Melanoma of the head and neck: current concepts in diagnosis and management. Laryngoscope. 2001; 111(7):1209–1222

[28] O'Brien CJ, Uren RF, Thompson JF, et al. Prediction of potential metastatic sites in cutaneous head and neck melanoma using lymphoscintigraphy. Am J Surg. 1995; 170(5):461–466

[29] Vico P, Fourez T, Nemec E, Andry G, Deraemaecker R. Aggressive basal cell carcinoma of head and neck areas. Eur J Surg Oncol. 1995; 21(5):490–497

[30] Lai SY, Weber RS. High-risk non-melanoma skin cancer of the head and neck. Curr Oncol Rep. 2005; 7(2):154–158

[31] Amin MB, Edge SB, Greene FL, Byrd DR, Brookland RK. AJCC Cancer Staging Manual. 8th ed. New York, NY: Springer; 2017:1024

[32] Rowe DE, Carroll RJ, Day CL, Jr. Prognostic factors for local recurrence, metastasis, and survival rates in squamous cell carcinoma of the skin, ear, and lip. Implications for treatment modality selection. J Am Acad Dermatol. 1992; 26 (6):976–990

[33] Shashanka R, Smitha BR. Head and neck melanoma. ISRN Surg. 2012; 2012:948302

[34] Gershenwald JE, Thompson W, Mansfield PF, et al. Multi-institutional melanoma lymphatic mapping experience: the prognostic value of sentinel lymph node status in 612 stage I or II melanoma patients. J Clin Oncol. 1999; 17 (3):976–983

[35] Balch CM, Soong SJ, Gershenwald JE, et al. Prognostic factors analysis of 17,600 melanoma patients: validation of the American Joint Committee on Cancer melanoma staging system. J Clin Oncol. 2001; 19(16):3622–3634

[36] Erman AB, Collar RM, Griffith KA, et al. Sentinel lymph node biopsy is accurate and prognostic in head and neck melanoma. Cancer. 2012; 118(4):1040–1047

[37] O'Brien CJ, McNeil EB, McMahon JD, Pathak I, Lauer CS, Jackson MA. Significance of clinical stage, extent of surgery, and pathologic findings in metastatic cutaneous squamous carcinoma of the parotid gland. Head Neck. 2002; 24(5):417–422

[38] Jambusaria-Pahlajani A, Kanetsky PA, Karia PS, et al. Evaluation of AJCC tumor staging for cutaneous squamous cell carcinoma and a proposed alternative tumor staging system. JAMA Dermatol. 2013; 149(4):402–410

[39] Johnson TM, Rowe DE, Nelson BR, Swanson NA. Squamous cell carcinoma of the skin (excluding lip and oral mucosa). J Am Acad Dermatol. 1992; 26(3)(,)(Pt 2):467–484

[40] Czarnecki D, Staples M, Mar A, Giles G, Meehan C. Metastases from squamous cell carcinoma of the skin in southern Australia. Dermatology. 1994; 189 (1):52–54

[41] Jol JA, van Velthuysen ML, Hilgers FJ, Keus RB, Neering H, Balm AJ. Treatment results of regional metastasis from cutaneous head and neck squamous cell carcinoma. Eur J Surg Oncol. 2003; 29(1):81–86

[42] Cannon RB, Dundar Y, Thomas A, et al. Elective neck dissection for head and neck cutaneous squamous cell carcinoma with skull base invasion. Otolaryngol Head Neck Surg. 2017; 156(4):671–676

[43] Morton DL, Wen DR, Wong JH, et al. Technical details of intraoperative lymphatic mapping for early stage melanoma. Arch Surg (Chicago, Ill.: 1960). 1992; 127(4):392–399

[44] Schwartz JL, Griffith KA, Lowe L, et al. Features predicting sentinel lymph node positivity in Merkel cell carcinoma. J Clin Oncol. 2011; 29(8):1036–1041

[45] Howle J, Veness M. Sentinel lymph node biopsy in patients with Merkel cell carcinoma: an emerging role and the Westmead hospital experience. Australas J Dermatol. 2012; 53(1):26–31

[46] Kachare SD, Wong JH, Vohra NA, Zervos EE, Fitzgerald TL. Sentinel lymph node biopsy is associated with improved survival in Merkel cell carcinoma. Ann Surg Oncol. 2014; 21(5):1624–1630

[47] Durham AB, Lowe L, Malloy KM, et al. Sentinel lymph node biopsy for cutaneous squamous cell carcinoma on the head and neck. JAMA Otolaryngol Head Neck Surg. 2016; 142(12):1171–1176

[48] Schmitt AR, Brewer JD, Bordeaux JS, Baum CL. Staging for cutaneous squamous cell carcinoma as a predictor of sentinel lymph node biopsy results: meta-analysis of American Joint Committee on Cancer criteria and a proposed alternative system. JAMA Dermatol. 2014; 150(1):19–24

[49] Schmalbach CE, Nussenbaum B, Rees RS, Schwartz J, Johnson TM, Bradford CR. Reliability of sentinel lymph node mapping with biopsy for head and neck cutaneous melanoma. Arch Otolaryngol Head Neck Surg. 2003; 129(1):61–65

[50] de Wilt JHW, Thompson JF, Uren RF, et al. Correlation between preoperative lymphoscintigraphy and metastatic nodal disease sites in 362 patients with cutaneous melanomas of the head and neck. Ann Surg. 2004; 239 (4):544–552

[51] Surasi DS, O'Malley J, Bhambhvani P. 99mTc-Tilmanocept: a novel molecular agent for lymphatic mapping and sentinel lymph node localization. J Nucl Med Technol. 2015; 43(2):87–91

[52] Schmalbach CE, Bradford CR. Is sentinel lymph node biopsy the standard of care for cutaneous head and neck melanoma? Laryngoscope. 2015; 125 (1):153–160

[53] Eldrageely K, Vargas MP, Khalkhali I, et al. Sentinel lymph node mapping of breast cancer: a case-control study of methylene blue tracer compared to isosulfan blue. Am Surg. 2004; 70(10):872–875

[54] Daisne JF, Installé J, Bihin B, et al. SPECT/CT lymphoscintigraphy of sentinel node(s) for superselective prophylactic irradiation of the neck in cN0 head and neck cancer patients: a prospective phase I feasibility study. Radiat Oncol. 2014; 9(121):121

[55] Ross AS, Schmults CD. Sentinel lymph node biopsy in cutaneous squamous cell carcinoma: a systematic review of the English literature. Dermatol Surg. 2006; 32(11):1309–1321

[56] Doubrovsky A, De Wilt JH, Scolyer RA, McCarthy WH, Thompson JF. Sentinel node biopsy provides more accurate staging than elective lymph node dissection in patients with cutaneous melanoma. Ann Surg Oncol. 2004; 11 (9):829–836

[57] Shpitzer T, Segal K, Schachter J, et al. Sentinel node guided surgery for melanoma in the head and neck region. Melanoma Res. 2004; 14(4):283–287

[58] McMasters KM, Noyes RD, Reintgen DS, et al. Sunbelt Melanoma Trial. Lessons learned from the Sunbelt Melanoma Trial. J Surg Oncol. 2004; 86(4):212–223

[59] Cascinelli N, Morabito A, Santinami M, MacKie RM, Belli F. Immediate or delayed dissection of regional nodes in patients with melanoma of the trunk: a randomised trial. WHO Melanoma Programme. Lancet. 1998; 351 (9105):793–796

[60] O'Brien CJ. The parotid gland as a metastatic basin for cutaneous cancer. Arch Otolaryngol Head Neck Surg. 2005; 131(7):551–555

[61] Veness MJ, Porceddu S, Palme CE, Morgan GJ. Cutaneous head and neck squamous cell carcinoma metastatic to parotid and cervical lymph nodes. Head Neck. 2007; 29(7):621–631

[62] Ebrahimi A, Clark JR, Ahmadi N, et al. Prognostic significance of disease-free interval in head and neck cutaneous squamous cell carcinoma with nodal metastases. Head Neck. 2013; 35(8):1138–1143

[63] Ahmed MM, Moore BA, Schmalbach CE. Utility of head and neck cutaneous squamous cell carcinoma sentinel node biopsy: a systematic review. Otolaryngol Head Neck Surg. 2014; 150(2):180–187

[64] Wang JT, Palme CE, Wang AY, Morgan GJ, Gebski V, Veness MJ. In patients with metastatic cutaneous head and neck squamous cell carcinoma to cervical lymph nodes, the extent of neck dissection does not influence outcome. J Laryngol Otol. 2013; 127 Suppl 1:S2–S7

[65] Rouviere M. Anatomy of the Human Lymphatic System. Ann Arbor, MI: Edward Brothers Inc.; 1938:5–83

[66] Goepfert H, Jesse RH, Ballantyne AJ. Posterolateral neck dissection. Arch Otolaryngol. 1980; 106(10):618–620

[67] Lengele B, Hamoir M, Scalliet P, et al. Anatomic basis for the radiological delineation of lymph node areas. Major collecting trunks, head and neck. Radiother Oncol. 2007; 85:146–155

[68] Sheen TS, Chung TT, Snyderman CH. Transverse process of the atlas(C1): an important surgical landmark of the upper neck. Head Neck. 1997; 19 (1):37–40

[69] Faries MB, Thompson JF, Cochran AJ, et al. Completion dissection or observation for sentinel-node metastasis in melanoma. N Engl J Med. 2017; 376 (23):2211–2222

[70] Leiter U, Stadler R, Mauch C, et al. German Dermatologic Cooperative Oncology Group (DeCOG). Complete lymph node dissection versus no dissection in patients with sentinel lymph node biopsy positive melanoma (DeCOG-SLT): a multicentre, randomised, phase 3 trial. Lancet Oncol. 2016; 17(6):757–767

[71] Madu MF, Franke V, Bruin MM, et al. Immediate completion lymph node dissection in stage IIIA melanoma does not provide significant additional staging information beyond EORTC SN tumour burden criteria. Eur J Cancer. 2017; 87:212–215

[72] Koh CS, Veness MJ. Role of definitive radiotherapy in treating patients with inoperable Merkel cell carcinoma: the Westmead Hospital experience and a review of the literature. Australas J Dermatol. 2009; 50(4):249–256

[73] Khan L, Choo R, Breen D, et al. Recommendations for CTV margins in radiotherapy planning for non melanoma skin cancer. Radiother Oncol. 2012; 104 (2):263–266

[74] Veness MJ, Morgan GJ, Palme CE, Gebski V. Surgery and adjuvant radiotherapy in patients with cutaneous head and neck squamous cell carcinoma metastatic to lymph nodes: combined treatment should be considered best practice. Laryngoscope. 2005; 115(5):870–875

[75] Oddone N, Morgan GJ, Palme CE, et al. Metastatic cutaneous squamous cell carcinoma of the head and neck: the Immunosuppression, Treatment, Extranodal spread, and Margin status (ITEM) prognostic score to predict outcome and the need to improve survival. Cancer. 2009; 115(9):1883–1891

[76] Hruby G, Scolyer RA, Thompson JF. The important role of radiation treatment in the management of Merkel cell carcinoma. Br J Dermatol. 2013; 169(5):975–982

[77] Mojica P, Smith D, Ellenhorn JD. Adjuvant radiation therapy is associated with improved survival in Merkel cell carcinoma of the skin. J Clin Oncol. 2007; 25 (9):1043–1047

[78] Mendenhall WM, Amdur RJ, Grobmyer SR, et al. Adjuvant radiotherapy for cutaneous melanoma. Cancer. 2008; 112(6):1189–1196

[79] Guadagnolo BA, Myers JN, Zagars GK. Role of postoperative irradiation for patients with bilateral cervical nodal metastases from cutaneous melanoma: a critical assessment. Head Neck. 2010; 32(6):708–713

[80] Tang JY, Mackay-Wiggan JM, Aszterbaum M, et al. Inhibiting the hedgehog pathway in patients with the basal-cell nevus syndrome. N Engl J Med. 2012; 366(23):2180–2188

[81] Wollina U. Update of cetuximab for non-melanoma skin cancer. Expert Opin Biol Ther. 2014; 14(2):271–276

[82] Heath CH, Deep NL, Nabell L, et al. Phase 1 study of erlotinib plus radiation therapy in patients with advanced cutaneous squamous cell carcinoma. Int J Radiat Oncol Biol Phys. 2013; 85(5):1275–1281

[83] Lewis CM, Glisson BS, Feng L, et al. A phase II study of gefitinib for aggressive cutaneous squamous cell carcinoma of the head and neck. Clin Cancer Res. 2012; 18(5):1435–1446

[84] Tanvetyanon T, Padhya T, McCaffrey J, et al. Postoperative concurrent chemotherapy and radiotherapy for high-risk cutaneous squamous cell carcinoma of the head and neck. Head Neck. 2015; 37(6):840–845

[85] Miller NJ, Bhatia S, Parvathaneni U, Iyer JG, Nghiem P. Emerging and mechanism-based therapies for recurrent or metastatic Merkel cell carcinoma. Curr Treat Options Oncol. 2013; 14(2):249–263

[86] Eggermont AM, Suciu S, MacKie R, et al. EORTC Melanoma Group. Post-surgery adjuvant therapy with intermediate doses of interferon alfa 2b versus observation in patients with stage IIb/III melanoma (EORTC 18952): randomised controlled trial. Lancet. 2005; 366(9492):1189–1196

[87] Kirkwood JM, Strawderman MH, Ernstoff MS, Smith TJ, Borden EC, Blum RH. Interferon alfa-2b adjuvant therapy of high-risk resected cutaneous melanoma: the Eastern Cooperative Oncology Group Trial EST 1684. J Clin Oncol. 1996; 14(1):7–17

[88] Mocellin S, Pasquali S, Rossi CR, Nitti D. Interferon alpha adjuvant therapy in patients with high-risk melanoma: a systematic review and meta-analysis. J Natl Cancer Inst. 2010; 102(7):493–501

[89] Weber J, Mandala M, Del Vecchio M, et al. CheckMate 238 Collaborators. Adjuvant nivolumab versus ipilimumab in resected stage III or IV melanoma. N Engl J Med. 2017; 377(19):1824–1835

17 Melanoma

Shivangi Lohia and Eric J. Lentsch

Abstract

Cutaneous malignant melanoma (CMM) is an aggressive neoplasm, known for its ability to spread to regional lymphatics as well as distant sites. Although it is less common than basal cell and squamous cell carcinomas, the mortality rates associated with CMM far outstrip those of its less aggressive counterparts. When CMM is detected early, the chance of cure is very high; however, a significant number will have regional or distant spread, and the diagnostic and treatment rationale for these is complex. Herein we describe the diagnosis and treatment of regionally metastatic melanoma of the head and neck—with a focus on the differences in treatment of node-positive (N+) and node-negative (N0) patients. We will describe the central role of neck dissection in the treatment of the N+ neck, and the importance of sentinel lymph node biopsy as a diagnostic/therapeutic procedure in patients with N0 disease.

Keywords: melanoma, metastatic, neck dissection, sentinel node, MSLT-1, MSLT-2

17.1 Introduction

Cutaneous melanoma of the head and neck accounts for up to 20% of all cutaneous malignant melanomas (CMMs). It is aggressive, and in this region the overall prognosis has been reported to be poorer than in other sites.[1] During the last 30 years, incidence rates of CMM have increased steadily. Currently, it is estimated that in the United States 87,110 new melanomas will be diagnosed (about 52,170 in men and 34,940 in women) and 9,730 people are expected to die of melanoma.[2] Although this is only 10% of all cutaneous malignancies, CMM accounts for more than 75% of all deaths from skin cancer. Despite the advances made for early primary disease, the prognosis for regional metastatic melanoma remains dismal, with overall 5-year survival of 62%.[3]

17.1.1 Risk Factors for Metastasis

There are several well-known risk factors for spread of melanoma (▶ Table 17.1), the most important of which is the Breslow thickness of the primary tumor. Thicker tumors are more likely to gain access to vascular and lymphatic channels, and therefore to metastasize. Also, since facial skin is often thin, there is also a subgroup of thin melanomas (< 1 mm deep), which have invaded to Clark level IV or beyond, and behave more aggressively as well.

Multiple studies have reported the prognostic significance of anatomic site of the primary on survival rates. In general, patients with head and neck primaries are thought to have a worse prognosis than patients with extremity tumors.[4] Several studies have reported that tumors arising in the so-called BANS region (upper **b**ack, upper **a**rm, posterior **n**eck and **s**calp) have worse survival rates than in the non-BANS regions, though this remains controversial.[5,6] Within the head and neck, a review from the MD Anderson Cancer Center showed that lesions located on the scalp do significantly worse than lesions on the ear, face, or neck.[7] This finding has been corroborated by other investigators.[8]

Table 17.1 Risk factors for metastatic spread in cutaneous malignant melanoma

Sex:

- Male

Depth:

- Breslow's depth (and Clark's level in thin facial skin)
- ±Clark's level in thin facial skin

Primary site:

- Scalp or neck

Histological findings:

- Presence of histological ulceration
- Mitotic rate $\geq 1\ mm^2$
- Lympho/vascular invasion
- Immunosuppression

Histologic factors that increase the risk for metastatic spread include ulceration, mitotic rate greater than 1, and lymphovascular invasion. It is felt that these characteristics enable melanoma cells to invade small vessels or cause ulceration that may be closely tied to the factors that enable it to undergo lymph node metastasis. These factors have been shown to be associated not only with lymph node metastasis, but also with survival. Callery et al found that among clinical and histological node-positive patients, the prognosis was worse for patients with an ulcerated primary tumor, satellitosis, or a high mitotic rate.[9] Others have duplicated those findings,[10,11] the implication being that the presence of one or more histological risk factors is an important biological tumor marker that can be used in addition to tumor thickness to predict the probability of a primary tumor's metastatic potential.

17.1.2 Patterns of Spread

The clinical course of cutaneous melanoma is highly variable. Cutaneous melanomas can spread locally through dermal lymphatic channels to form cutaneous satellite lesions (within 2 cm of the primary lesion), as well as in-transit lesions along the course of the draining lymphatics. Most commonly, however, metastatic tumor progression presents as metastasis to draining regional lymph nodes.

The pattern of these lymph node metastases is important to understand as they will greatly affect treatment (▶ Fig. 17.1). In general, tumors located anteriorly on the face and neck generally spread to the facial, submental, submandibular, and deep cervical nodes. Tumors arising on the scalp and forehead, anterior to a coronal line drawn through the external auditory canal, most commonly spread to the parotid/periparotid lymph nodes, and upper jugular lymph nodes. Conversely, tumors arising on the scalp and occiput posterior to this line most commonly spread to the postauricular, suboccipital, and posterior

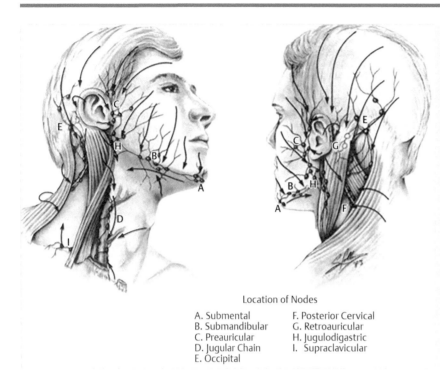

Fig. 17.1 Predicted patterns of lymphatic drainage from primary sites in the head and neck. (Adapted from Byers RM. Cervical and parotid node dissection. In: Balch CM, Houghton AN, Milton GW, et al, eds. Cutaneous Melanoma. 2nd ed. Philadelphia, PA: JB Lippincott; 1992.)

Location of Nodes

A. Submental
B. Submandibular
C. Preauricular
D. Jugular Chain
E. Occipital

F. Posterior Cervical
G. Retroauricular
H. Jugulodigastric
I. Supraclavicular

triangle lymph nodes. These drainage patterns have important ramifications for treatment: with facial and anterior scalp lesions requiring a neck dissection addressing those nodes (usually a supraomohyoid or lateral neck dissection) as well as consideration of a parotidectomy, while tumors of the posterior scalp and neck would require a neck dissection that addresses different nodal groups such as a posterolateral neck dissection.

17.2 Staging of the Neck in Melanoma

In 2017, the American Joint Committee on Cancer (AJCC) Melanoma Task Force revised the staging system for cutaneous melanomas based upon the most current data from multiple trials and studies.[12] Staging adheres to the traditional tumor–node–metastasis (TNM) classification system. This system classifies melanomas on the basis of their local, regional, and distant characteristics, as summarized in ▶ Fig. 17.2.

17.3 Treatment of Melanoma of the Neck

Surgery remains the mainstay of treatment for CMM. Primary lesions are surgically excised to achieve negative margins based on tumor thickness. The size of surgical margins has been disputed with some authors advocating for narrow margins (1 cm) and others for wide margins (4–5 cm). However, multiple studies have demonstrated comparable rates of local control and survival with 2-cm margins (for intermediate-thickness melanoma) and 1-cm margins (for thinner lesions).[13,14] Of course, primary surgical resection must also be balanced with its cosmetic and functional impacts with adequate understanding of

head and neck anatomy. Importantly, appropriate treatment of cutaneous melanoma must include consideration of the neck.

17.4 Management of the Neck

17.4.1 The Node-Positive Neck

Current management of the neck in CMM is guided by the presence or absence of clinically positive neck disease. Nodal disease is associated with poorer disease-specific outcomes; therefore, evidence of regional spread necessitates treatment. Though the decision to treat the neck is not controversial in patients with neck disease, there is some controversy regarding the type of treatment needed.

Traditionally, management of clinically evident nodal disease consisted of a radical neck dissection (RND). Unfortunately, this was associated with significant comorbidities and functional deficits due to sacrifice of key structures. With the advent of more conservative procedures, it became apparent that more aggressive surgical management did not appear to decrease recurrence rates. Thus, surgeons treating melanoma followed the lead of surgeons treating head and neck cancer in becoming more conservative in their neck dissections.

In the 1990s, various authors reported modifications to the RND by limiting lymphadenectomies to nodal groups at highest risk for metastases. O'Brien et al[15] observed this trend when they evaluated outcomes for 397 neck dissections performed for malignant melanoma. They noted increasing use of the modified radical neck dissections (MRND) and selective neck dissection (SND), and use of adjuvant radiation therapy. They found an overall regional recurrence rate of 24% regardless of which type of neck dissection was performed. Likewise, Turkula and Woods[16] described their experience with 58 patients, all of whom had clinically positive neck disease. Among this group, 34 were

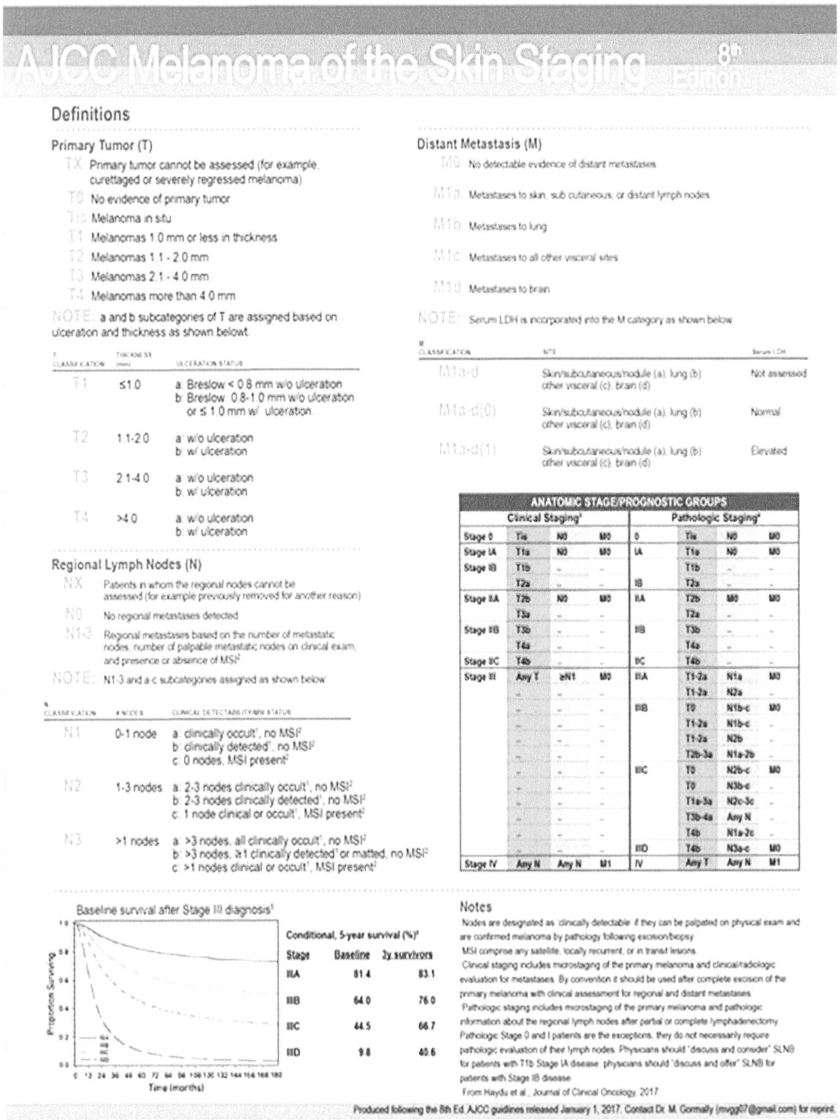

Fig. 17.2 Melanoma staging as described in the AJCC Staging Manual, eighth edition. (This image is provided courtesy of Dr. M. Gormally.)

treated with RND, 7 underwent MRD, and 17 were treated with SND. There were no significant differences in recurrence or survival rates between the three groups. More recently, these data were confirmed by Andersen et al,[17] who retrospectively evaluated a series of 57 patients treated for regional metastases and compared the extent of neck dissection in regard to nodal recurrence and survival. Overall, the rate of recurrence was not statistically different between the groups. Five-year melanoma-specific survival was also similar between the RND, MRND, and SND. The rates of failure or recurrence within the neck were similar to those previously reported within the literature. Finally, a retrospective review sought to evaluate the extent of lymphadenectomy among patients with regional metastases. Supriya et al[18] evaluated 97 patients with pathologically proven melanoma nodal metastases. From this group, 18 patients underwent comprehensive neck dissection (CND) and 79 were treated with SND. Analysis of the outcomes revealed no significant improvement in regional control or 5-year survival with CND.

Taken together, these findings support a more conservative approach to the management of the clinically positive neck in head and neck melanoma. Specifically, MRND and SND decrease morbidity and risk of functional deficits compared to RND, without adversely affecting risk of regional recurrence or overall survival. Importantly, in SNDs, the extent of lymphadenectomy must be tailored to the disease. As described earlier, consideration must be given to the location of the primary lesion when deciding what nodal groups to remove. Also for certain primary sites, a parotidectomy should be performed in conjunction with the neck dissection. Finally, consideration of adjuvant neck radiation should be given for patients who have multiple positive nodes or extracapsular extension.

17.4.2 The Node-Negative Neck

Management of the clinically negative neck is more controversial than the clinically positive neck. In the case of a patient with known melanoma in the head and neck and no regional lymph node involvement, three strategies have been utilized. The first is observation with treatment of the neck reserved for cases where regional disease manifests later. The second is the use of elective neck dissection (END). The third is the use of sentinel lymph node biopsy (SLNB).

Observation: For stage I disease (thin melanomas: ≤ 1 mm), the risk of occult metastases is relatively low, and management of the neck beyond observation is usually not considered. As the risk of regional metastases increases with increasing stage of the primary, most clinicians would consider some form of treatment; however, observation remains a viable option for some patients, especially those with severe comorbid conditions. Many clinicians argue that few, if any, studies have shown that END improves survival over expectant management of the neck. However, a large preponderance of the evidence suggests a survival benefit for node-positive patients undergoing SLNB as opposed to observation.[19]

END: Historically, if observation was not chosen, then END was commonly performed. END addresses nodal compartments at highest risk of metastases based on lymphatic drainage pathways. Thus—in the same fashion as treatment of the node-positive neck—a patient with a temporal scalp primary would need to have a parotidectomy and dissection of at least levels I, II, and III, or an MRND.

However, as described earlier, there is no evidence that END improves survival (vs. observation) among patients with CMM. Furthermore, ENDs are associated with functional and cosmetic risks, and increase treatment-related morbidity in patients who are ultimately found to be without occult metastases. For these reasons, ENDs have largely been replaced by the use of SLNB.

SLNB: It is performed with the use of dyes, radiographic contrast, or radioactive tracers to identify the first echelon of nodes receiving lymphatic drainage from the primary lesion. Once identified, these nodes are excised and evaluated for the presence of microscopic metastases, and can guide the decision to perform a more extensive neck dissection (▶ Fig. 17.3).

SLNB provides clinically valuable information regarding treatment and staging. In their landmark paper, Gershenwald et al[20] undertook a retrospective review of patients who underwent SLNB, and found sentinel nodal status to be the most important factor in predicting disease-free survival in patients with melanoma. A similar study verified these results in patients with head and neck melanoma.[21] While these studies confirmed the validity of SLNB as a diagnostic method, head and neck surgical oncologists were slow to adopt this new diagnostic technique. The complex lymphatic drainage often requires excision of nodes from areas of "danger," such as the parotid gland where the facial nerve is at risk. However, as later studies showed, there is a high success rate (95%) in identifying the sentinel node(s), with relatively low false-negative rates (< 5%) and very low complication rates with SLNB.[22,23]

Over the last 20 years, SLNB has shown to be a reliable diagnostic modality to determine which patients had nodal disease, and might be appropriate for completion lymphadenectomy (CND) and/or other adjuvant treatments. However, there has been a question as to whether we are improving the disease course of patients by using SLNB. Though some authors have shown that the use of SLNB and CND could decrease the rate of regional recurrence,[24,25,26] whether or not this technique improves survival in melanoma patients remained controversial. This was the question that the Multicenter Selective Lymphadenectomy Trial 1 (MSLT-1) was designed to answer. Published in 2014, it revealed that patients with intermediate-thickness melanomas with positive SLNB who underwent CND had a disease-free survival advantage compared to patients undergoing observation.[19] These data bolstered the clinicians who believed in the efficacy of SLNB and made it the preferred option in patients with intermediate-thickness melanoma.

However, other studies found contradictory evidence in regard to survival following SLNB and CND. In a large SEER database study performed by Sperry et al,[27] no survival benefit was seen

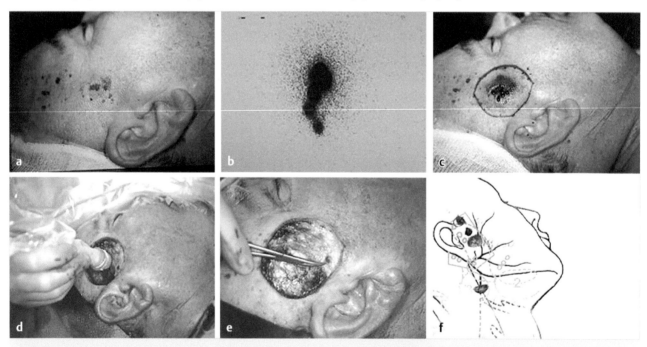

Fig. 17.3 Sentinel node biopsy for cutaneous malignant melanoma of the head and neck. A 50-year-old patient with a 2.7-mm Clark level IV melanoma of the right cheek. **(a)** Primary lesion. **(b)** Preoperative lymphoscintigraphy. **(c)** Intraoperative blue dye injection. **(d)** Intraoperative localization of a sentinel-node with hand-held gamma probe. **(e)** Intraoperative blue dye localization. **(f)** Identification of four sentinel lymph nodes, one of which was positive for nodal metastasis.

with SLNB when compared to observation. And most recently, the Multicenter Selective Lymphadenectomy Trial 2 (MSLT-2)[26] sought to evaluate the impact of immediate CND on melanoma-related survival. In this large-scale study, patients were randomized to CND or observation following SLNB. Analysis of the results showed no significant difference in melanoma-related death in patients who underwent immediate CND compared to those who underwent observation following positive SLNB. Findings from this study indicate that the performance of CND does not impart a survival advantage to patients beyond any survival the SLNB imparts. Thus, the counseling of patients who have a positive SLNB should include the option of both CND and observation. Currently, however, most national guidelines—including the National Comprehensive Cancer Network (NCCN) guidelines for melanoma—recommend a CND in the context of a positive SLNB.

One important caveat should be noted for head and neck melanoma patients in regard to the data supplied by the MSLT-2. In this trial, head and neck patients comprised only 13% of the study subjects. No subgroup analysis was performed on head and neck patients, yet the hazard ratios were very different for head and neck patients as compared to truncal and extremity, in that they appeared to favor CND. Of course, this cannot be inferred unless a subgroup analysis of the head and neck patients is performed; at this time, that appears unlikely (personal communication with author).

Thus, at the time of this writing, SLNB remains the preferred method to evaluate (and perhaps treat) the node-negative neck. Sentinel-node biopsy has a high value for staging clinically localized, intermediate-thickness melanoma, and provides a more accurate basis for formulating a prognosis than do standard demographic and histopathological factors. The presence or absence of tumor cells in the sentinel node is critical to both accurate AJCC staging and decisions regarding lymphadenectomy and adjuvant therapy. Current NCCN guidelines recommend CND at this time, though that recommendation may weaken as the data from the MSLT-2 are considered.

17.5 Conclusion

Treatment of patients with melanoma of the head and neck must take into account the possibility of regional metastatic spread of the disease. The clinician must be able to process the risk factors for this disease as well as the patterns of spread in forming a diagnostic and treatment plan. Treatment should be based on the clinical findings—with clinically positive patients treated with neck dissection, usually in the form of an SND or an MRND. In patients with clinically negative necks, consideration should be given to SLNB, and when this is positive a discussion of CND versus observation should be had with the patient.

References

[1] Lachiewicz AM, Berwick M, Wiggins CL, Thomas NE. Survival differences between patients with scalp or neck melanoma and those with melanoma of other sites in the Surveillance, Epidemiology, and End Results (SEER) program. Arch Dermatol. 2008; 144(4):515–521

[2] Siegel RL, Miller KD, Jemal A. Cancer Statistics, 2017. CA Cancer J Clin. 2017; 67(1):7–30

[3] Howlader N, Noone AM, Krapcho M, et al, eds. SEER Cancer Statistics Review, 1975–2014. Bethesda, MD: National Cancer Institute; 2016. Available at: https://seer.cancer.gov/csr/1975_2014/

[4] Balch CM, Soong S, Shaw HM, et al. An analysis of prognostic factors in 8,500 patients with cutaneous melanoma. In: Balch CM, Houghton AN, Milton GW, et al, eds. Cutaneous Melanoma. 2nd ed. Philadelphia, PA: JB Lippincott; 1992

[5] Wong JH, Wanek L, Chang LJ, Goradia T, Morton DL. The importance of anatomic site in prognosis in patients with cutaneous melanoma. Arch Surg. 1991; 126(4):486–489

[6] Garbe C, Büttner P, Bertz J, et al. Primary cutaneous melanoma. Prognostic classification of anatomic location. Cancer. 1995; 75(10):2492–2498

[7] Ballantyne AJ. Malignant melanoma of the skin of the head and neck. An analysis of 405 cases. Am J Surg. 1970; 120(4):425–431

[8] Close LG, Goepfert H, Ballantyne AJ, Jesse RH. Malignant melanoma of the scalp. Laryngoscope. 1979; 89(8):1189–1196

[9] Callery C, Cochran AJ, Roe DJ, et al. Factors prognostic for survival in patients with malignant melanoma spread to regional lymph nodes. Ann Surg. 1982; 196(1):69–75

[10] Johnson OK, Jr, Emrich LJ, Karakousis CP, Rao U, Greco WR. Comparison of prognostic factors for survival and recurrence in malignant melanoma of the skin, clinical Stage I. Cancer. 1985; 55(5):1107–1117

[11] Sagebiel RW. The pathology of melanoma as a basis for prognostic models: the UCSF experience. Pigment Cell Res. 1994; 7(2):101–103

[12] Gershenwald JE, Scolyer RA, Hess KR, et al. Melanoma of the skin. In: Amin MB, Edge SB, Greene FL, et al, eds. AJCC Cancer Staging Manual. 8th ed. New York, NY: Springer International Publishing; 2017:563–585

[13] Veronesi U, Cascinelli N, Adamus J, et al. Thin stage I primary cutaneous malignant melanoma. Comparison of excision with margins of 1 or 3 cm. N Engl J Med. 1988; 318(18):1159–1162

[14] Balch CM, Soong SJ, Smith T, et al. Investigators from the Intergroup Melanoma Surgical Trial. Long-term results of a prospective surgical trial comparing 2 cm vs. 4 cm excision margins for 740 patients with 1–4 mm melanomas. Ann Surg Oncol. 2001; 8(2):101–108

[15] O'Brien CJ, Gianoutsos MP, Morgan MJ. Neck dissection for cutaneous malignant melanoma. World J Surg. 1992; 16(2):222–226

[16] Turkula LD, Woods JE. Limited or selective nodal dissection for malignant melanoma of the head and neck. Am J Surg. 1984; 148(4):446–448

[17] Andersen PS, Chakera AH, Thamsborg AK, et al. Recurrence and survival after neck dissections in cutaneous head and neck melanoma. Dan Med J. 2014; 61 (12):A4953

[18] Supriya M, Narasimhan V, Henderson MA, Sizeland A. Managing regional metastasis in patients with cutaneous head and neck melanoma: is selective neck dissection appropriate? Am J Otolaryngol. 2014; 35(5):610–616

[19] Morton DL, Thompson JF, Cochran AJ, et al. MSLT Group. Final trial report of sentinel-node biopsy versus nodal observation in melanoma. N Engl J Med. 2014; 370(7):599–609

[20] Gershenwald JE, Thompson W, Mansfield PF, et al. Multi-institutional melanoma lymphatic mapping experience: the prognostic value of sentinel lymph node status in 612 stage I or II melanoma patients. J Clin Oncol. 1999; 17(3):976–983

[21] Leong SP, Accortt NA, Essner R, et al. Sentinel Lymph Node Working Group. Impact of sentinel node status and other risk factors on the clinical outcome of head and neck melanoma patients. Arch Otolaryngol Head Neck Surg. 2006; 132(4):370–373

[22] Schmalbach CE, Nussenbaum B, Rees RS, Schwartz J, Johnson TM, Bradford CR. Reliability of sentinel lymph node mapping with biopsy for head and neck cutaneous melanoma. Arch Otolaryngol Head Neck Surg. 2003; 129(1):61–65

[23] Chao C, Wong SL, Edwards MJ, et al. Sunbelt Melanoma Trial Group. Sentinel lymph node biopsy for head and neck melanomas. Ann Surg Oncol. 2003; 10 (1):21–26

[24] Gutzmer R, Al Ghazal M, Geerlings H, Kapp A. Sentinel node biopsy in melanoma delays recurrence but does not change melanoma-related survival: a retrospective analysis of 673 patients. Br J Dermatol. 2005; 153(6):1137–1141

[25] Leiter U, Eigentler TK, Häfner H-M, et al. Sentinel lymph node dissection in head and neck melanoma has prognostic impact on disease-free and overall survival. Ann Surg Oncol. 2015; 22(12):4073–4080

[26] Faries MB, Thompson JF, Cochran AJ, et al. Completion dissection or observation for sentinel-node metastasis in melanoma. N Engl J Med. 2017; 376 (23):2211–2222

[27] Sperry SM, Charlton ME, Pagedar NA. Association of sentinel lymph node biopsy with survival for head and neck melanoma: survival analysis using the SEER database. JAMA Otolaryngol Head Neck Surg. 2014; 140(12):1101–1109

18 Neck Dissection for Salivary Gland Malignancies

Vincent Vander Poorten

Abstract

A minority of patients with salivary gland carcinomas presents with clinically or radiologically obvious cervical lymph node metastasis. These patients' prognosis following treatment is significantly worse than that of patients with a clinically uninvolved neck. Adequate management of this aspect of the disease is thus of vital importance. There is little controversy on the management of clinically evident metastases. Primary surgery aiming at removal of all obvious suspected nodal disease will almost invariably result in pathological confirmation of the preoperative suspicion, and then entail postoperative radiotherapy, which, for all sites, improves locoregional control and survival. The optimal treatment of the clinically and radiologically uninvolved neck does continue to provoke discussion. It is not the question of whether or not to treat the neck that is the problem, as there is wide agreement on the tumor and the patient factors that make it more likely that the lymph nodes harbor occult metastases. When these factors are present, the neck should be electively treated. The major discussion, however, revolves around the best treatment strategy to use once the decision to proceed with neck treatment is made. On the one hand, there are the clinicians who prefer to treat those patients with an elective neck dissection, followed by postoperative radiotherapy on indication. On the other hand, others favor radiotherapy over elective neck dissection in this scenario. The rationale behind these two strategies is summarized.

Keywords: salivary gland carcinoma, clinically negative neck, elective neck dissection, elective radiotherapy, clinically positive neck, therapeutic neck dissection, neck metastasis

18.1 Introduction

Globally, the incidence of salivary gland carcinomas is 0.4 to 13.5 cases per 100,000 people per year; in the United States, the incidence rate is 1 per 100,000 people per year. The European incidences appear to be lower, with Belgium, the Netherlands, the United Kingdom, and Finland reporting around 0.6 to 0.7 cases per 100,000 people per year. A Danish population-based study reported a crude incidence of 1.1 per 100,000 people per year.[1]

Around 70% of these carcinomas arise in the largest gland, the parotid,[2] and 10 to 25% of salivary carcinomas arise in the minor salivary glands.[3] The rest are submandibular carcinomas, with sublingual carcinomas being very rare.

Prognostic indicators explaining the observed variability in chance of cure following treatment include patient, tumor, and treatment characteristics. Tumor characteristics with prognostic impact include anatomic site of the affected salivary gland, histotype of the tumor (22 malignant types in the most recent 2017 WHO classification),[4] TNM stage,[5] and specific growth characteristics (perineural/intraneural invasion, lymphatic invasion, surgical margins, extraglandular extension), which can be observed histopathologically following resection. One of the tumor-related factors with a strong independent prognostic impact is regional metastasis, as reflected in the clinical and pathological N-classification.[6]

Evaluation of the neck is mandatory whenever a salivary malignancy is suspected on clinical grounds. Available options, both for the primary and the neck, are ultrasound, which allows for ultrasound-guided fine-needle aspiration, CT scanning (▶ Fig. 18.1), which is superior for bone detail, and MR imaging, which is strongly advised when tumor mobility is impaired, and which has a superior soft-tissue detail, including visualization of perineural extension (▶ Fig. 18.2).

In clinically suspected or fine-needle aspiration cytology (FNAC) proven malignancy, before embarking on locoregional therapy, positron emission tomography (PET) with or without CT co-localization (PET-CT) is mainly important for detecting disease recurrence and to exclude (gross) distant disease. It is important to note that this modality fails in differentiating benign from malignant disease, as Warthin's tumors and pleomorphic adenomas show an increased uptake (high false-positive rate), and not infrequently, malignant tumors are not fluorodeoxyglucose-avid (high false-negative rate).[1,3,7]

18.2 Treatment of the Neck According to the Gland of Origin of the Primary Tumor

18.2.1 Parotid Carcinoma

The Clinically Positive Neck

Regional metastasis is clinically and/or radiologically evident at presentation (clinically positive [cN +] disease) in 14 to 29% of

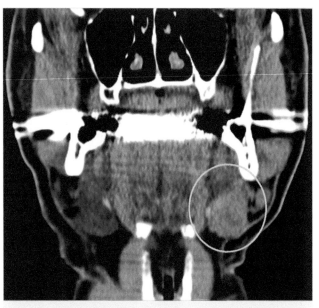

Fig. 18.1 Coronal contrast-enhanced CT scan image of a patient with a left submandibular gland adenoid cystic carcinoma, with invasion of the platysma muscle, but without bone invasion. (This image is provided courtesy of Prof. R. Hermans, MD, PhD, Radiology, University Hospitals Leuven, Leuven, Belgium.)

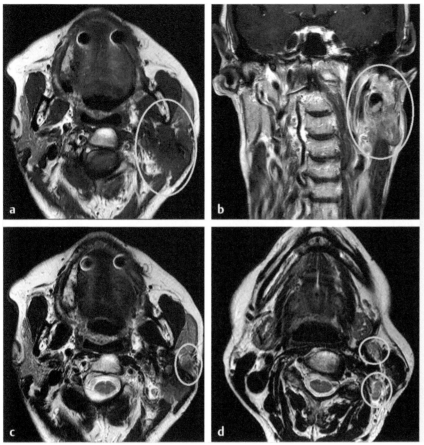

Fig. 18.2 **(a)** Axial T1-weighted MR image of a salivary duct parotid carcinoma with fixation to the deep tissues, invading the deep neck muscles, and involving the expected course of the seventh cranial nerve (CN VII), although function is intact. **(b)** Coronal T1-weighted MR image of the same patient. This leads to counseling about the need of a radical parotidectomy with sacrifice and reconstruction of CN VII. **(c)** Axial T2-weighted MR images showing intraparotid lymph node metastasis. **(d)** Axial T2-weighted MR image of the ipsilateral neck showing multiple nodal metastasis in level II. (These images are provided courtesy of Prof. R. Hermans, MD, PhD, Radiology, University Hospitals Leuven, Leuven, Belgium.)

patients.[6,8] This percentage increases in high-grade tumors and advanced T-status tumors.[9,10] The lymph node levels most frequently involved are levels II, III, and IV.[8,11] Parotid cancer–related cN + disease requires a (modified) radical neck dissection, removing levels I to V.[12] This therapeutic comprehensive neck dissection implies radicality toward nonlymphatic structures (nerve XI, jugular vein, or sternocleidomastoid muscle) depending on proximity of or involvement by lymph node metastases[13] (▶ Fig. 18.3a, ▶ Fig. 18.4). Recent studies confirmed this "old knowledge"; rates of pathologically positive (pN +) involvement in a recent study from Memorial Sloan Kettering Cancer Center were 52% in level I, 77% in level II, 73% in level III, 53% in level IV, and 40% in level V.[14] In a comparable study from Korea, rates of pN + involvement were 43% in level I, 90% in level II, 40% in level III, 57% in level IV, and still 43% in level V.[15]

As such, clinical neck disease implies a well-accepted negative prognostic value,[6,16] but recent reports revealed the independent negative prognostic impact of an increasing "lymph-node density," which is the ratio of the number of metastatic nodes to the total number of lymph nodes removed.[17,18]

A sometimes-overlooked problem is the deep lobe intraparotid lymph nodes. A significant proportion (53–65%) of patients with pN + disease on neck dissection will also have metastatic deposits in the "first echelon" intraparotid lymph nodes.[8,11] When a neck dissection is needed for removal of cN + disease, it seems logical and consequent that a deep lobe parotidectomy is performed to address this problem. There is usually no discussion on performing this type of "total parotidectomy" for large tumors, deep lobe tumors, or tumors that have already caused a

seventh cranial nerve (CN VII) paralysis (▶ Fig. 18.4), but the controversy surrounds the early-stage tumors with normal facial nerve function that need a therapeutic neck dissection[19] (▶ Fig. 18.3a). Authors from Mayo Clinic recommend performing a deep-lobe parotidectomy in high-grade tumors, especially if an intraparotid node in the specimen of the initially performed superficial parotidectomy is positive on frozen section[20] (▶ Fig. 18.3 a, b). The practical problem here is that preoperative grading (based on FNAC) is infrequently available for parotid cancer patients. The Köln group published a series of 142 patients in 2008, where, in their total parotidectomy specimens, 1 to 11 parotid lymph nodes were retrieved. Eighty percent of these parotid nodes were involved in cN0/ pN + patients.[11] While there is no direct evidence that resection of these nodes increases locoregional control in salivary gland cancer, this evidence is available in skin cancer, metastatic to the parotid. In this disease, a 20% local recurrence rate—the majority of which occurred in the parotid bed—was observed in patients treated with superficial parotidectomy (the deep lobe remaining in situ), despite being treated with postoperative radiotherapy.[21,22]

It is well accepted that pN + patients with salivary gland cancer need postoperative radiotherapy to the parotid bed and the ipsilateral neck. In this setting, adjuvant radiation not only doubles the rate of locoregional control, but also improves survival.[23,24] Two recent reports documented the benefit of a postoperative, platinum-based, concomitant chemoradiation scheme for high-risk major salivary gland carcinomas, and the approach certainly merits further research.[25]

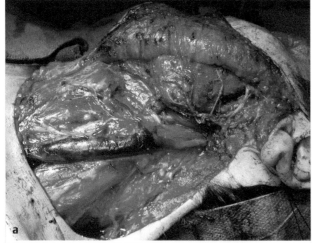

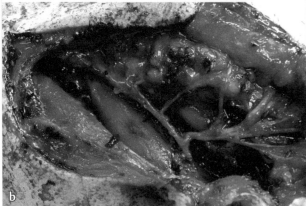

Fig. 18.3 (a) The same patient as in ▶ Fig. 18.2, following a retrograde cranial nerve (CN) VII dissection. Intraoperatively, the facial nerve found to be displaced anterosuperiorly, but ultimately uninvolved. A total conservative parotidectomy was possible, including a deep lobe parotidectomy, in conjunction with a therapeutic neck dissection (ND I–V, sternocleidomastoid, CN XI).[12] This picture was taken before removal of the last part of the deep lobe from underneath the main trunk of the facial nerve. (b) Another patient with total conservative parotidectomy in conjunction with a selective neck dissection of level II.

The Clinically Negative Neck

Observation, Elective Neck Dissection with or without Postoperative Radiation, or Elective Neck Irradiation

The rates of pN + disease, in patients who are defined as cN0 following clinical examination and high-quality imaging, are between 12 and 49%. This variation between series derives from the different tendency to regional metastasis of the plethora of salivary gland cancer histotypes, within which there even exist different grades, again determining metastatic behavior.[8,10,11,26,27,28]

For patients presenting with a cN0 parotid carcinoma, we usually try to estimate the theoretical risk of pN + disease, from the presence of established risk factors for occult neck disease. We then decide to treat the cN0 neck when the combined presence of different risk factors implies a probability that exceeds the threshold of 15 to 20%.

Among identified risk factors that predict micrometastatic disease in cN0 patients are clinical and histopathological factors. Clinical factors are age in the sixth decade or older, presence of pain, seventh nerve dysfunction, and locally advanced disease as reflected in the T-status. Histological factors include histotype and grade, extraglandular soft-tissue invasion, and lymphatic invasion.[8,26,28,29,30]

Histotypes that imply a high prevalence (> 50%) of occult nodal disease are salivary duct carcinoma (SDC), undifferentiated carcinoma (UC), adenocarcinoma not otherwise specified (AC-NOS), high-grade mucoepidermoid carcinoma (HG-MEC), and squamous cell carcinoma (SCC).[8,10] Textbook knowledge classically teaches that parotid adenoid cystic carcinoma (AdCC) has a low tendency to regional metastasis. Recently, however, a scrutinized analysis of the available literature revealed a 14.5% lymph node metastasis rate in parotid cN0 AdCC.[31] The same authors identified a high-grade subgroup in parotid AdCC (AdCC-HGT) that implies a pN + rate of up to 57%.[32] Acinic cell carcinoma (AcCC) and low-grade MEC are generally considered to have a low rate of pN + disease; nevertheless, authors routinely performing elective neck dissection (END) in patients with these subtypes also report higher-than-expected rates of

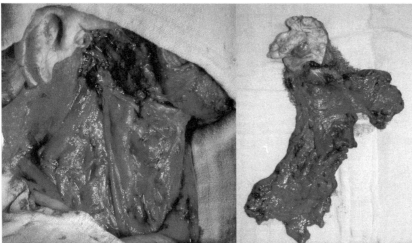

Fig. 18.4 Total radical parotidectomy including resection of involved skin and inferior half of auricle as well as masseter muscle (to the right) and a radical neck dissection (ND I-V, SCM, IJV, CNXI; to the left).[12] In the same procedure a static CN VII correction as well as a free anterolateral thigh muscle/skin flap is used for reconstruction. Postoperative radiotherapy is mandatory.

occult nodal disease.[10,11] Furthermore, also in AcCC, nowadays there is a high-grade subtype, which implies a higher risk.[33] To complicate the matter, early-stage cancers and low-grade cancers can also present with cN0pN + disease.[14,28,34] Stenner et al performed END in T1N0 and T2N0 patients and found a pN + rate of 21%.[14,28,34]

Available management options for the cN0 neck include observation, END with or without postoperative radiation on indication, and elective neck irradiation (ENI).

When a decision has been made to treat the neck, the first possible option is by elective neck surgery. Some authors propose a routine END for every patient with suspected or known parotid cancer.[10,27,34,35] Zbären et al substantiate this recommendation by their reporting of a 22% occult rate in operated patients. These END patients then had an improved 5-year rate of locoregional control when compared to the observation group. These findings have to be interpreted in the context that only a minority of the patients in this series (14/83) received radiotherapy; as such, it is plausible to argue that similar oncologic outcomes could have been obtained by systematic use of ENI in all of these patients.[9,27,36] Nobis et al report a 39% occult nodal disease rate, and Stennert et al report even a 45% rate in a series where all patients underwent neck dissection.[10,35] A Brazilian group reported a 37% rate of occult nodal disease, heralded by advanced T-status, severe desmoplasia, and histologic type (UC, HG-MEC, ACNOS, SDC, and SCC had a combined occult rate of 68%).[26] The problem here is that, of these factors, T-status is frequently the only one available in the preoperative setting.

A second effective option is ENI in patients who are defined "high risk" based on definitive histopathology of the resected primary.[24,29,30,36,37] This strategy is appealing to many clinicians, because many of the factors that imply a "high-risk" status only become clear following pathological examination of the resected primary (exact histotype, exact grade, extraparenchymal extension, lymphovascular invasion). As already stated, pre- and perioperative histotyping and grading of salivary carcinomas are frequently problematic (accuracy 51–62%),[13,29,38] whereas this information is much more reliable in the postoperative setting. When there is an indication for postoperative radiotherapy to the primary (based on final histopathology of the resected specimen), it parallels the indications for ENI of the unoperated cN0 neck. In the series of Herman et al,[36] the cN0 patients selected for ENI had a 100% regional control at a median follow-up of more than 5 years, as opposed to 10% regional recurrence in patients treated with END. Another supportive study is the one by Chen et al, who reported a 0% 10-year regional recurrence rate in patients with a salivary gland cancer and a cN0 neck having undergone ENI, as opposed to a 26% failure rate in operated patients.[39] While this sounds convincing, a selection bias in these data is not unlikely. Another argument in favor of ENI is the fact that patients who undergo END still need radiotherapy when a cN0 neck turns out to be pN + .[24,36,37]

The question of which approach to the cN0 neck in patients with parotid carcinoma is the best one, END with—on indication—postoperative radiation therapy, or immediate ENI, can only be answered reliably by conducting a prospective randomized trial. Given the rarity of the disease, such a trial can only be organized on a multicenter level.

Until that moment, different authors have tried different strategies to fine-tune the choice between the two modalities.

Preoperative ultrasound-guided FNAC of the neck and generous use of perioperative frozen section pathology have been advocated. The author's policy is to perform a standard, selective level II dissection in all preoperatively known carcinomas with a cN0 neck, before starting the parotidectomy. Frozen section analysis of the level II nodes is then available by the time the parotidectomy is finished, and if micrometastases are revealed, the neck is upstaged to pN + and a comprehensive neck dissection follows.[1] Similarly, other authors have promoted the concept of "level I and II node sampling" in high-risk patients.[40]

Which Levels to Address in Elective Neck Treatment of Parotid Carcinoma Patients?

The analysis of END specimens has given us an indication of which levels to address with either surgery or radiotherapy. The pivotal MSKCC study from Armstrong et al in 1992 concludes that the neck levels to be addressed are levels II, III, and IV. These findings are corroborated by recent studies confirming that, in cN0 necks, disease is rather rarely found in levels I and V.[8,14,30]

Practical Approach to the cN0 Neck in Parotid Carcinoma Patients: A Proposal of Options

We recently published an overview of three possible scenarios that can be encountered in the clinical reality in dealing with the cN0 neck in salivary gland cancer[19]:

- Scenario 1: There is a low risk of occult nodal disease (T1–T2 tumors, low-grade tumor, young patients):
  - A "wait-and-see" management can be justified.[14]
  - Alternatively, a selective level II dissection and frozen section can be performed at the beginning of the procedure, followed by a modified radical neck dissection in the rare cases where disease is present.[1]
  - A minority of authors would recommend a systematic END.[10,11,27,34]
- Scenario 2: Risk factors for occult nodal disease are discovered only after final histopathology of the primary is available (high grade and/or high stage):
  - ENI is recommended.[29,36]
- Scenario 3: High risk of occult nodal disease preoperatively certain:
  - END (II–IV or Ib–IV) and postoperative neck radiotherapy based on the histopathological findings in the primary and the neck specimen.
  - ENI, especially if adjuvant radiotherapy for the primary tumor is already likely.[29,36,37,41]
  - Superselective level II dissection with extension to a comprehensive neck dissection if disease is found in level II (▶ Fig. 18.3b). If no pathologically positive nodes are found on frozen section, then radiotherapy to the neck is indicated based on the histopathological findings on the primary.[1,13]

We consider extending the dissection to levels I and V in specific anatomical situations, such as primary tumors located anteriorly in the parotid, where metastases to level I are more likely, or large tumors in the parotid tail, where there is increased risk of spread to level V. Other authors systematically dissect levels I and II[40] or levels I to III.[35] They also perform frozen sections and convert to comprehensive neck dissection in the presence of occult nodal disease. We consider the rationale behind systematic dissection of level I to be inconsistent, given the low incidence of disease in level I in cN0 necks, as described in the landmark study by Armstrong et al.[8] Furthermore, in this study, all of the few patients with positive level I nodes also had positive level II nodes, which would also have been detected if limiting the dissection for frozen section to level II. Recent studies also confirm a low rate of cN0pN + in level I.[14,30]

18.2.2 Submandibular Gland Carcinoma

Reported rates of lymph node metastasis in submandibular gland cancer vary. A Japanese study reported pN + status as a function of T-status of the primary (T1: 0%; T2: 33%; T3: 57%; and T4: 100%).[42] In our own series, cN + disease at diagnosis was observed in 17% of the patients, but in cN0 patients treated with END, an occult rate of a further 22% was found. Survival decreased when comparing patients without clinically palpable regional metastases (5-year survival rate, 56%) to patients who presented with regional metastases (5-year survival rate, 14%; $p = 0.003$).[43] A recent study from Korea described similar findings, with a drop in 5-year overall survival from 40% for cN0 to 9% for cN + patients.[44]

The Clinically Positive Neck

The standard treatment for a preoperatively known submandibular gland cancer has shifted from a universally applied (both for cN0 and cN +) aggressive and extended surgery as monotherapy,[45] to a more functional procedure, tailored to the locally involved anatomy, followed by postoperative radiotherapy.[43,46,47,48] The standard operation in the past included the submandibular gland in a radical neck dissection, often with en bloc excision of the floor of mouth and lower rim of the mandible.[45] Given the reported rates of 40% pN + in level IV and 25% in level V, there is no discussion that for obvious cN + disease, a comprehensive levels I to V neck dissection preserving the nonlymphatic structures (internal jugular vein, sternomastoid muscle, and spinal accessory nerve), whenever possible, remains the standard of care.[13,48]

The Clinically Negative Neck

For the preoperatively known submandibular gland cancer with otherwise cN0 neck (▶ Fig. 18.1, ▶ Fig. 18.5, ▶ Fig. 18.6) in recent decades, there has been a shift toward conservative surgery (functional END). The MSKCC group[47] documented a rise in the use of levels I to III (supraomohyoid) neck dissection from none of the surgeries from 1939 to 1965, to 38% in the study period 1966 to 1982. Similarly, in the Netherlands' Cancer Institute, the levels I to III dissection comprising the submandibular gland accounted for 66% of operative procedures in the period 1973 to 1983, and for 71% of the procedures between 1984 and 1994.[43] The point these rather old studies make, that is, including the submandibular gland in an SND levels I to III being the minimal procedure, continues to stand. The occult rates found (21% in a recent American study,[49] 22% in our Amsterdam study, and 23% for AdCC—the most frequent malignant neoplasm of the submandibular gland—in a recent review)[31] justify performing more than a simple gland excision. The extent of the neck dissection (levels I–III) was again justified by a contemporary Japanese study that reported only levels I, II, and III being involved in cN0pN + patients (▶ Fig. 18.5, ▶ Fig. 18.6). Recently, it has been suggested that END can be omitted for T1 cancers, but T1 cancers are rare, so we believe it is safer have to have a standardized approach, and recommend elective management of the neck in all cN0 cases. From our perspective, more data are required to change this recommendation.[49]

18.2.3 Sublingual Gland Cancer

These are very rare tumors that are malignant in over 80% of the cases.[50] In over 80% again, they present in an advanced stage

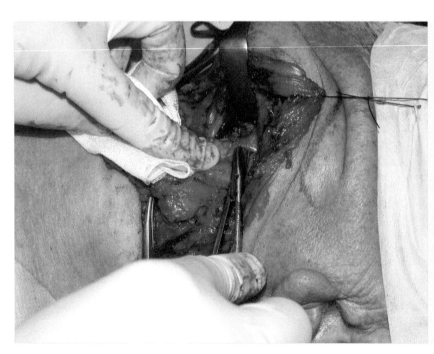

Fig. 18.5 Same patient as in ▶ Fig. 18.1. Procedure performed for cT3N0 adenoid cystic carcinoma of the left submandibular gland. Dissection of level I, including skin and platysma. Snapshot of the cutting of the lingual nerve branch to the submandibular ganglion.

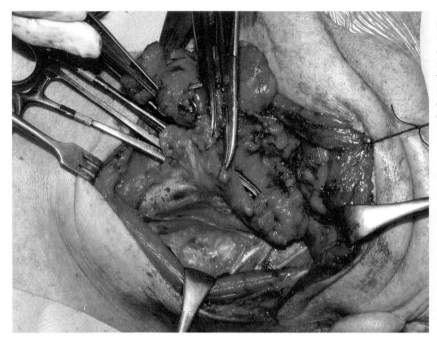

Fig. 18.6 Same patient as in ▶ Fig. 18.1 and ▶ Fig. 18.5. Additionally, levels II and III were dissected (ND I–III)[12] and the final pathological stage was pT3pN0. Postoperative radiotherapy of the neck was indicated (intensity-modulated radiation therapy of 66 Gy) and the patient has completed 10 years of follow-up without evidence of recurrence.

(III or IV, based on the T3/T4a classification of the primary) at diagnosis.[51] Most authors recommend holding the same rule as for submandibular cancer, that is, the minimal procedure for a cN0 neck being an SND levels I to III, including resection of the floor of mouth and the sublingual gland. This seems to be substantiated by a recent thorough literature review focusing on AdCC—again the most frequently encountered histotype in this site—reporting an occult nodal disease rate of 25%.[31]

18.2.4 Minor Salivary Gland Cancer

The Clinically Positive Neck

Clinical or radiological evidence of regional lymph node metastasis exists in about one in six minor salivary gland cancer (MiSGC) patients, and then obviously surgical treatment of the neck, that is, a comprehensive levels I to V neck dissection is indicated.[3]

The Clinically Negative Neck

END is indicated when the risk of subclinical disease in a cN0 neck exceeds 15 to 20%. When the neck is surgically entered as an approach to the primary, it is logical to also address the neck surgically. Generally, the attitude among surgeons is that the occult metastatic rate, as estimated from the appearance of regional disease in the untreated cN0 neck, is too low to justify END.[3] This has been recently substantiated for laryngeal, sinonasal, external acoustic meatus, and lacrimal gland origin.[52] In patients with oral cavity and oropharyngeal MiSGC,[53] however, and in patients with high-grade cancers such as high-grade MEC[3] or high-grade AdCC,[32] the occult rates largely exceed 20% and END is indicated. One remarkable study revealed a high rate of occult disease (47%) in a series of cN0 nasopharyngeal MiSGC patients where the primary was amenable to surgery.[54]

In MiSGC patients in general, if neck dissection reveals metastatic disease, postoperative radiotherapy improves locoregional control and survival.[24]

References

[1] Vander Poorten V, Bradley PJ, Takes RP, Rinaldo A, Woolgar JA, Ferlito A. Diagnosis and management of parotid carcinoma with a special focus on recent advances in molecular biology. Head Neck. 2012; 34(3):429–440

[2] Van Eycken L. Head and neck cancer. In: Van Eycken L, ed. Cancer Incidence in Belgium 2004-2005. Saint-Josse-ten-Noode: Belgian Cancer Registry; 2008:41

[3] Vander Poorten V, Hunt J, Bradley PJ, et al. Recent trends in the management of minor salivary gland carcinoma. Head Neck. 2014; 36(3):444–455

[4] El-Naggar AK, John KC, Grandis JR, Takata T, Slootweg PJ, eds. WHO classification of tumours of salivary glands. In: WHO classification of Head and Neck Tumours. 4th ed. Lyon: IARC; 2017:160–184

[5] UICC. Major salivary glands. In: Brierley JD, Gospodarowicz M, Wittekind C, eds. TNM Classification of Malignant Tumours. 8th ed. Oxford: Wiley-Blackwell; 2017;47–51

[6] Vander Poorten V, Hart A, Vauterin T, et al. Prognostic index for patients with parotid carcinoma: international external validation in a Belgian-German database. Cancer. 2009; 115(3):540–550

[7] Razfar A, Heron DE, Branstetter BF, IV, Seethala RR, Ferris RL. Positron emission tomography-computed tomography adds to the management of salivary gland malignancies. Laryngoscope. 2010; 120(4):734–738

[8] Armstrong JG, Harrison LB, Thaler HT, et al. The indications for elective treatment of the neck in cancer of the major salivary glands. Cancer. 1992; 69(3):615–619

[9] Zbären P, Schüpbach J, Nuyens M, Stauffer E, Greiner R, Häusler R. Carcinoma of the parotid gland. Am J Surg. 2003; 186(1):57–62

[10] Stennert E, Kisner D, Jungehuelsing M, et al. High incidence of lymph node metastasis in major salivary gland cancer. Arch Otolaryngol Head Neck Surg. 2003; 129(7):720–723

[11] Klussmann JP, Ponert T, Mueller RP, Dienes HP, Guntinas-Lichius O. Patterns of lymph node spread and its influence on outcome in resectable parotid cancer. Eur J Surg Oncol. 2008; 34(8):932–937

[12] Ferlito A, Robbins KT, Shah JP, et al. Proposal for a rational classification of neck dissections. Head Neck. 2011; 33(3):445–450

[13] Medina J, Zbären P, Bradley PJ. Management of regional metastases of malignant salivary gland neoplasms. Adv Otorhinolaryngol. 2016; 78:132–140

[14] Ali S, Palmer FL, DiLorenzo M, Shah JP, Patel SG, Ganly I. Treatment of the neck in carcinoma of the parotid gland. Ann Surg Oncol. 2014; 21(9):3042–3048

[15] Yoo SH, Roh JL, Kim SO, et al. Patterns and treatment of neck metastases in patients with salivary gland cancers. J Surg Oncol. 2015; 111(8):1000–1006

[16] Ali S, Palmer FL, Yu C, et al. A predictive nomogram for recurrence of carcinoma of the major salivary glands. JAMA Otolaryngol Head Neck Surg. 2013; 139(7):698–705

[17] Hong HR, Roh JL, Cho KJ, Choi SH, Nam SY, Kim SY. Prognostic value of lymph node density in high-grade salivary gland cancers. J Surg Oncol. 2015; 111 (6):784–789

[18] Suzuki H, Hanai N, Hirakawa H, Nishikawa D, Hasegawa Y. Lymph node density is a prognostic factor in patients with major salivary gland carcinoma. Oncol Lett. 2015; 10(6):3523–3528

[19] Lombardi D, McGurk M, Vander Poorten V, et al. Surgical treatment of salivary malignant tumors. Oral Oncol. 2017; 65:102–113

[20] Olsen KD, Moore EJ. Deep lobe parotidectomy: clinical rationale in the management of primary and metastatic cancer. Eur Arch Otorhinolaryngol. 2014; 271(5):1181–1185

[21] O'Brien CJ, McNeil EB, McMahon JD, Pathak I, Lauer CS, Jackson MA. Significance of clinical stage, extent of surgery, and pathologic findings in metastatic cutaneous squamous carcinoma of the parotid gland. Head Neck. 2002; 24(5):417–422

[22] Thom JJ, Moore EJ, Price DL, Kasperbauer JL, Starkman SJ, Olsen KD. The role of total parotidectomy for metastatic cutaneous squamous cell carcinoma and malignant melanoma. JAMA Otolaryngol Head Neck Surg. 2014; 140 (6):548–554

[23] Armstrong JG, Harrison LB, Spiro RH, Fass DE, Strong EW, Fuks ZY. Malignant tumors of major salivary gland origin. A matched-pair analysis of the role of combined surgery and postoperative radiotherapy. Arch Otolaryngol Head Neck Surg. 1990; 116(3):290–293

[24] Terhaard CH, Lubsen H, Rasch CR, et al. Dutch Head and Neck Oncology Cooperative Group. The role of radiotherapy in the treatment of malignant salivary gland tumors. Int J Radiat Oncol Biol Phys. 2005; 61 (1):103–111

[25] Vander Poorten V, Meulemans J, Delaere P, Nuyts S, Clement P. Molecular markers and chemotherapy for advanced salivary cancer. Curr Otorhinolaryngol Rep. 2014; 2(2):85–96

[26] Régis De Brito Santos I, Kowalski LP, Cavalcante De Araujo V, Flávia Logullo A, Magrin J. Multivariate analysis of risk factors for neck metastases in surgically treated parotid carcinomas. Arch Otolaryngol Head Neck Surg. 2001; 127 (1):56–60

[27] Zbären P, Schüpbach J, Nuyens M, Stauffer E. Elective neck dissection versus observation in primary parotid carcinoma. Otolaryngol Head Neck Surg. 2005; 132(3):387–391

[28] Kawata R, Koutetsu L, Yoshimura K, Nishikawa S, Takenaka H. Indication for elective neck dissection for N0 carcinoma of the parotid gland: a single institution's 20-year experience. Acta Otolaryngol. 2010; 130 (2):286–292

[29] Frankenthaler RA, Byers RM, Luna MA, Callender DL, Wolf P, Goepfert H. Predicting occult lymph node metastasis in parotid cancer. Arch Otolaryngol Head Neck Surg. 1993; 119(5):517–520

[30] Lau VH, Aouad R, Farwell DG, Donald PJ, Chen AM. Patterns of nodal involvement for clinically N0 salivary gland carcinoma: refining the role of elective neck irradiation. Head Neck. 2014; 36(10):1435–1439

[31] Silver CE, Bradley PJ, Barnes L, et al. International Head and Neck Scientific Group. Cervical lymph node metastasis in adenoid cystic carcinoma of the major salivary glands. J Laryngol Otol. 2017; 131(2):96–105

[32] Hellquist H, Skálová A, Barnes L, et al. Cervical lymph node metastasis in high-grade transformation of head and neck adenoid cystic carcinoma: a collective international review. Adv Ther. 2016; 33(3):357–368

[33] Vander Poorten V, Triantafyllou A, Thompson LD, et al. Salivary acinic cell carcinoma: reappraisal and update. Eur Arch Otorhinolaryngol. 2016; 273 (11):3511–3531

[34] Stenner M, Molls C, Luers JC, Beutner D, Klussmann JP, Huettenbrink KB. Occurrence of lymph node metastasis in early-stage parotid gland cancer. Eur Arch Otorhinolaryngol. 2012; 269(2):643–648

[35] Nobis CP, Rohleder NH, Wolff KD, Wagenpfeil S, Scherer EQ, Kesting MR. Head and neck salivary gland carcinomas–elective neck dissection, yes or no? J Oral Maxillofac Surg. 2014; 72(1):205–210

[36] Herman MP, Werning JW, Morris CG, Kirwan JM, Amdur RJ, Mendenhall WM. Elective neck management for high-grade salivary gland carcinoma. Am J Otolaryngol. 2013; 34(3):205–208

[37] Chen AM, Garcia J, Lee NY, Bucci MK, Eisele DW. Patterns of nodal relapse after surgery and postoperative radiation therapy for carcinomas of the major and minor salivary glands: what is the role of elective neck irradiation? Int J Radiat Oncol Biol Phys. 2007; 67(4):988–994

[38] Westra WH. The surgical pathology of salivary gland neoplasms. Otolaryngol Clin North Am. 1999; 32(5):919–943

[39] Chen AM, Granchi PJ, Garcia J, Bucci MK, Fu KK, Eisele DW. Local-regional recurrence after surgery without postoperative irradiation for carcinomas of the major salivary glands: implications for adjuvant therapy. Int J Radiat Oncol Biol Phys. 2007; 67(4):982–987

[40] Korkmaz H, Yoo GH, Du W, et al. Predictors of nodal metastasis in salivary gland cancer. J Surg Oncol. 2002; 80(4):186–189

[41] Frankenthaler RA, Luna MA, Lee SS, et al. Prognostic variables in parotid gland cancer. Arch Otolaryngol Head Neck Surg. 1991; 117(11):1251–1256

[42] Beppu T, Kamata SE, Kawabata K, et al. Prophylactic neck dissection for submandibular gland cancer. Nippon Jibiinkoka Gakkai Kaiho. 2003; 106(8):831–837

[43] Vander Poorten VL, Balm AJ, Hilgers FJ, et al. Prognostic factors for long term results of the treatment of patients with malignant submandibular gland tumors. Cancer. 1999; 85(10):2255–2264

[44] Roh JL, Choi SH, Lee SW, Cho KJ, Nam SY, Kim SY. Carcinomas arising in the submandibular gland: high propensity for systemic failure. J Surg Oncol. 2008; 97(6):533–537

[45] Conley J, Myers E, Cole R. Analysis of 115 patients with tumors of the submandibular gland. Ann Otol Rhinol Laryngol. 1972; 81(3):323–330

[46] Weber RS, Byers RM, Petit B, Wolf P, Ang K, Luna M. Submandibular gland tumors. Adverse histologic factors and therapeutic implications. Arch Otolaryngol Head Neck Surg. 1990; 116(9):1055–1060

[47] Spiro RH, Armstrong J, Harrison L, Geller NL, Lin SY, Strong EW. Carcinoma of major salivary glands. Recent trends. Arch Otolaryngol Head Neck Surg. 1989; 115(3):316–321

[48] Han MW, Cho KJ, Roh JL, Choi SH, Nam SY, Kim SY. Patterns of lymph node metastasis and their influence on outcomes in patients with submandibular gland carcinoma. J Surg Oncol. 2012; 106(4):475–480

[49] Pohar S, Venkatesan V, Stitt LW, et al. Results in the management of malignant submandibular tumours and guidelines for elective neck treatment. J Otolaryngol Head Neck Surg. 2011; 40(3):191–195

[50] Sun G, Yang X, Tang E, Wen J, Lu M, Hu Q. The treatment of sublingual gland tumours. Int J Oral Maxillofac Surg. 2010; 39(9):863–868

[51] Zdanowski R, Dias FL, Barbosa MM, et al. Sublingual gland tumors: clinical, pathologic, and therapeutic analysis of 13 patients treated in a single institution. Head Neck. 2011; 33(4):476–481

[52] Bishop JA, Barnes EL, Slootweg PJ, et al. International Head and Neck Scientific Group. Cervical lymph node metastasis in adenoid cystic carcinoma of the sinonasal tract, nasopharynx, lacrimal glands and external auditory canal: a collective international review. J Laryngol Otol. 2016; 130(12):1093–1097

[53] Suárez C, Barnes L, Silver CE, et al. Cervical lymph node metastasis in adenoid cystic carcinoma of oral cavity and oropharynx: a collective international review. Auris Nasus Larynx. 2016; 43(5):477–484

[54] Schramm VL, Jr, Imola MJ. Management of nasopharyngeal salivary gland malignancy. Laryngoscope. 2001; 111(9):1533–1544

19 Neck Dissection for Thyroid Carcinoma

Michael Kubala and Brendan C. Stack, Jr.

Abstract

Cervical metastasis in thyroid carcinoma is a common occurrence which needs to be addressed by the head and neck surgeon. This chapter will outline a comprehensive approach to treating neck disease in thyroid carcinoma. Thyroid carcinoma represents approximately 3.4% of all new cancers diagnosed in the United States. Up to 50% of patients with differentiated and 70% with medullary thyroid carcinoma present with nodal disease. In addition to a thorough history and physical examination, ultrasonography with fine needle aspiration of suspicious lymph nodes is the initial choice of imaging to evaluate the central and lateral neck compartments. The current management of thyroid carcinoma is hemi or total thyroidectomy with or without addressing the neck based on characteristics of the primary lesion and lymph nodes status. For differentiated thyroid carcinoma, prophylactic central neck dissection, but not lateral neck dissection, may be advocated for a clinically negative neck in advanced primary cancer. For medullary thyroid carcinoma, prophylactic central neck dissection is recommended in all patients, whereas prophylactic lateral neck dissection is recommended in certain patients. All patients presenting with pathologic cervical disease must have at least a central neck dissection and possible lateral neck dissection if the nodes appear in this compartment. Knowledge of the central and lateral neck compartment is essential to completing any surgical procedure in these areas, communicating in a multidisciplinary team approach to treatment, and minimizing complications.

Keywords: Differentiated thyroid carcinoma, medullary thyroid carcinoma, central neck compartment, central neck dissection, lateral neck compartment, lateral neck dissection

19.1 Introduction

Thyroid carcinoma arises from the thyroid gland, an endocrine organ located in the anterior neck responsible primarily for the regulation of body metabolism. According to Surveillance, Epidemiology, and End Results (SEER) estimates, there will be an estimated 56,870 new cases of thyroid cancer diagnosed in 2017, representing 3.4% of all new cancer cases within the United States. Most new patients are diagnosed during the fifth and sixth decades of life, with a predilection for females and the Caucasian race. The rate of new thyroid cancers has been rising on an average of 3.8% over the past 10 years, seemingly due to increased awareness and detection. Current 5-year survival rates for all comers with thyroid cancer is 98.2%, representing one of the highest survival rates among cancers.[1]

There are five defined types of thyroid carcinoma: papillary thyroid carcinoma (PTC), follicular thyroid carcinoma (FTC), Hürthle cell (oncocytic), medullary thyroid carcinoma (MTC), and anaplastic. Differentiated thyroid carcinoma (DTC), papillary and follicular, makes up more than 90% of all thyroid cancers. Within DTC, papillary accounts for about 85% of cases.[2] PTC is known to spread primarily through the lymphatic system. This usually begins within the first echelon nodes in the central neck compartment (level VI) before spreading to the

lateral neck (levels II-IV) or into the superior mediastinum (level VII). FTC, on the other hand, primarily spreads hematogenously with common local invasion of the primary tumor.

It has been established that DTC involves cervical lymph node metastases in 20 to 50% of patients. Cervical lymph node metastasis is a known risk factor for significantly predicted poorer overall survival outcomes.[2] MTC is categorized separately from DTC because it develops from a different cell type within the thyroid, the parafollicular C cells. It has been well established that MTC behaves more aggressively than DTC, and therefore, should be treated differently. In the sporadic type of MTC, 70% of patients who present with a palpable thyroid nodule have cervical metastases.[3] Because of this high rate of metastases, MTC has a different staging system and recommendations for initial surgical treatment.

The current standard of treatment for all types of thyroid carcinoma is surgical excision in the form of hemi or total thyroidectomy with or without neck dissection at the same time. The need for surgical removal of the lymph nodes of the central and lateral neck, therefore, comes into question during the surgical planning for the treatment of thyroid cancer. Evaluation of the neck for metastases should begin with a cervical ultrasound, preferably at the time of initial diagnosis. Anatomy of the central neck compartment should be completely understood to weigh the risks and benefits of a prophylactic central neck dissection in the clinically negative neck, and to prevent complications during a therapeutic central neck dissection. Lateral neck dissection, commonly done with minimal patient morbidity, should only be done in the presence of confirmed lateral neck pathologic disease.

19.2 Preoperative Evaluation of the Neck for Thyroid Carcinoma

Once the diagnosis of thyroid carcinoma has been established, the neck needs to be evaluated for the presence of locoregional metastasis. The pattern of lymph node metastasis is somewhat predictable for all types of thyroid carcinoma based on location of the tumor within the gland, as seen in ▶ Fig. 19.1. Upper third tumors have almost a 3.3 times increased incidence of lateral neck spread (level III/IV) compared to middle or lower third tumors. Likewise, middle third and lower third tumors have about a 3 to 13.5 times increased incidence of central neck spread (level VI/VII) compared to upper third tumors.[4] Initial screening of the central and lateral neck compartments of all patients should be done via cervical ultrasound followed by additional imaging studies (usually CT) for advanced, bulky, or invasive disease.[2]

If, after physical examination and preoperative imaging studies, the patient does not have pathologic appearing lymph nodes, they are classified as a clinically negative neck (cN0). Any lymphadenopathy found should be further investigated. The most common way to diagnose suspicious thyroid nodules and lymph nodes is to perform ultrasound-guided fine needle aspiration (USGFNA). In a high-volume, multispecialty center, FNA

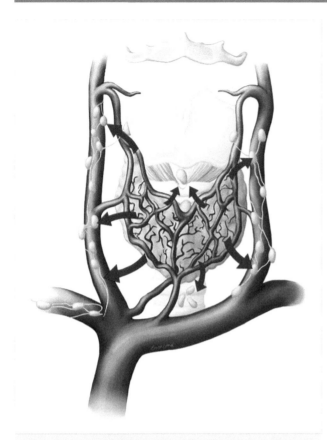

Fig. 19.1 Lymphatic drainage of the thyroid gland. Superior third tumors have a higher propensity to spread to the lateral neck compared to middle and lower third tumors, which tend to metastasize to the central neck first. (Reproduced from Tang AL, Steward DL. Developmental and surgical anatomy of the thyroid compartment. In: Terris DJ, Duke WS, eds. Thyroid and Parathyroid Diseases: Medical and Surgical Management. New York, NY: Thieme; 2016:11.)

can be performed and interpreted by a pathologist during the same clinic visit, expediting the diagnosis, surgical planning, and initiation of treatment. Incisional biopsy is not recommended because this commonly requires entering into or near the thyroid, causing scarring and possibly increasing the difficulty of the subsequent thyroidectomy and/or neck dissection. Once metastasis has been confirmed in either the central or lateral neck, the patient is classified as a clinically positive neck (cN1a or cN1b, respectively).

19.2.1 Cervical Ultrasound

Cervical ultrasound of the central and lateral neck should be completed at the time of initial evaluation and FNA of suspected thyroid carcinoma. Preoperative ultrasound identifies suspicious cervical adenopathy in 20 to 31% of cases. Features suspicious for metastatic cancer involvement include enlargement, loss of fatty hilum, round shape, hyperechogenicity, cystic changes, microcalcifications, and increased peripheral vascularity.[2] No single feature is absolute for malignancy; so, the decision to perform an FNA should be based on the totality of patient risk factors, imaging characteristics, and size greater than 10 mm.

If initial evaluation of an FNA from a lymph node is indeterminate (Bethesda class II), thyroglobulin washout can be completed on the specimen. The addition of thyroglobulin washout is helpful in lymph nodes which are cystic, inadequate, or have indeterminate cytologic evaluation, or inconsistent sonographic characteristics. Currently, studies show that a thyroglobulin level less than 1 ng/mL indicates a benign node.[2] No level has been established to indicate malignancy and current research into the ratios of FNA thyroglobulin to serum thyroglobulin may increase predictive accuracy.[5]

19.2.2 Additional Imaging

The American Thyroid Association (ATA) advocates for the use of cervical ultrasound as the first-line imaging for evaluation of nodal metastasis, followed by cross-sectional imaging such as computed tomography (CT) or magnetic resonance imaging (MRI) if needed. Indications for further imaging would include invasive primary tumor, advanced disease, inability to fully assess nodal extent on ultrasound, posterior location of the thyroid tumor (adjacent to trachea or esophagus), and multiple or bulky lymph node involvement. Invasive disease can be clinically evident with hoarseness, shortness of breath, dysphagia, hemoptysis, or airway obstruction. Findings consistent with laryngeal, tracheal, and/or esophageal involvement will prompt the surgeon to prepare accordingly.

19.2.3 TNM and Staging

The most commonly used staging system for thyroid cancer was developed by the American Joint Committee on Cancer (AJCC). Unlike other cancers of the head and neck, age is an important prognostic factor in this staging system. There are also separate classifications for differentiated, medullary, and anaplastic histologic diagnoses. ▶ Table 19.1 and ▶ Table 19.2 outline the 7th edition of the AJCC classification for differentiated and medullary thyroid cancer, respectively. Updates to the classification system are expected to take effect in the near future, with the most significant change being increasing the age of poorer prognosis from 45 to 55 years of age. Furthermore, after further studies on survivability, the stages have been shifted down, requiring more advanced disease for higher classification.

19.3 The Central Neck

19.3.1 Surgical Definition of Central Neck Levels

Effective communication of preoperative planning, intraoperative dissection, pathologic reporting, and administration of adjuvant treatment is based on the uniformity of terminology by defining the relevant anatomy of the central neck compartment. Collaboration of multiple surgical societies has led to the definition of the central neck compartment and how it relates to thyroid surgery. The central neck compartment can be defined as levels VI and VII and shown in ▶ Fig. 19.2, and includes all of the neurovascular, lymphatic, and visceral components contained within its boundaries.[6,7]

Table 19.1 American Joint Committee on Cancer TMN Classification for Differentiated and Medullary Thyroid Cancer.

Primary tumor (T)

TX	Primary tumor cannot be assessed
T0	No evidence of primary tumor
T1	Tumor 2 cm or less in greatest dimension limited to the thyroid
• T1a	Tumor 1 cm or less limited to the thyroid
• T1b	Tumor between 1 and 2 cm limited to the thyroid
T2	Tumor between 2 and 4 cm in greatest dimension limited to the thyroid
T3	Tumor greater than 4 cm in the greatest dimension limited to the thyroid, or any tumor with minimal extrathyroidal extension (limited to sternothyroid muscle or perithyroidal soft tissue)
T4	Advanced disease
• T4a	Tumor of any size extending beyond the thyroid capsule to invade the soft tissues, larynx, trachea, esophagus, or recurrent laryngeal nerve
• T4b	Tumor invades paravertebral fascia or encases carotid artery or mediastinal vessel

Regional lymph nodes (N)

NX	Regional lymph nodes cannot be assessed
N0	No regional lymph node metastasis
N1	Regional lymph node metastasis
• N1a	Metastasis to level VI
• N1b	Metastasis to unilateral, contralateral, or bilateral cervical, retropharyngeal, or superior mediastinal lymph nodes

Distant metastasis (M)

M0	No distant metastasis
M1	Distant metastasis

Source: Data from Edge SB. AJCC Cancer Staging Manual, 7th ed. New York, NY: Springer; 2010.

Table 19.2 American Joint Committee on cancer staging for differentiated and medullary thyroid carcinoma

Differentiated thyroid carcinoma		Medullary thyroid carcinoma	
Under 45 y old			
• Stage I: Any T Any N M0			
• Stage II: Any T Any N M1			
45 y and older		All ages	
Stage I	T1 N0 M0	Stage I	T1 N0 M0
Stage II	T2 N0 M0	Stage II	T2–3 N0 M0
Stage III	T3 N0 M0 T1–3 N1a M0	Stage III	T1–3 N1a M0
Stage IVa	T4a N0–1a M0 T1–4a N1b M0	Stage IVa	T4a N0–1a M0 T1–4a N1b M0

Table 19.2 continued

Differentiated thyroid carcinoma		Medullary thyroid carcinoma	
Stage IVb	T4b Any N M0	Stage IVb	T4b any N M0
Stage IVc	Any T Any N M1	Stage IVc	Any T any N M1

Source: Data from Edge SB. AJCC Cancer Staging Manual, 7th ed. New York, NY: Springer; 2010.

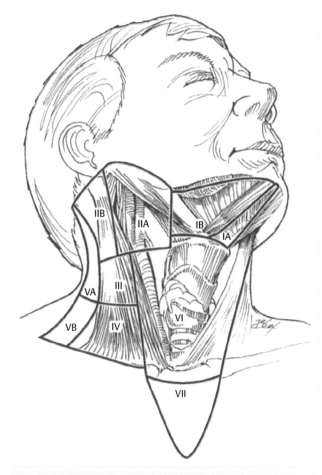

Fig. 19.2 Anatomical neck levels. The central neck compartment is defined as levels VI and VII. The lateral neck compartment is defined as levels I through V. (Reproduced with permission from Genden EM, Kao J, Packer SH, Jacobson AS. Carcinoma of unknown primary site. In: Genden EM, Varvares MA, eds. Head and Neck Cancer: An Evidence-Based Team Approach. New York, NY: Thieme; 2008:181.)

Boundaries of the Central Neck

The level VI compartment is bounded superiorly by the inferior border of the hyoid bone, laterally by the medial border of the carotid arteries, anteriorly by the superficial layer of the deep cervical fascia, posteriorly by the deep layer of the deep cervical fascia, and inferiorly by the plane of the sternal notch. The level VII compartment, or anterior superior mediastinal compartment, is bounded superiorly by the plane of the sternal notch, laterally by the mediastinal pleura, anteriorly by the posterior border of the manubrium, posteriorly by the deep layer of the deep cervical fascia, and inferiorly by the innominate artery on the right and corresponding axial plane on the left.[7]

Lymph Nodes

Within the central neck compartment, the lymph node groups are further defined based on location. The prelaryngeal, or Delphian, nodes are located anterior to the thyroid cartilage and superior to the thyroid gland. The pretracheal nodes are located anterior to the tracheal and between the thyroid gland and the sternal notch. The right and left paratracheal nodal groups are located on either side of the trachea, but have important differences based on the course of their respective recurrent laryngeal nerves (RLNs). In the left paratracheal region, lymphatic tissues generally lie anterior to the RLN. However, since the right RLN courses more ventrally within the paratracheal region because of the innominate artery, lymphatic tissue lies both anterior and posterior to the nerve. Bilaterally, the remaining borders of the paratracheal region are the trachea medially, the common carotid artery laterally, and the retropharyngeal and retroesophageal regions posteriorly.[7]

Vascular Structures

As described earlier, many vascular structures are present in the central neck compartment. The surgeon needs to be aware not only these vessels but also of their branching vessels. The brachiocephalic, or innominate artery, is the first branch of the arch of the aorta and gives rise to the right subclavian and common carotid arteries. It also determines the more ventral and lateral course of the right RLN. The left common carotid artery is the second branch of the arch of the aorta and defines the left lateral border of the central compartment. The superior thyroid artery is commonly the first branch of the external carotid artery and supplies the superior pole of the ipsilateral thyroid lobe. The inferior thyroid artery is a branch of the thyrocervical trunk from the subclavian artery and supplies the inferior pole of the ipsilateral thyroid lobe. It also supplies the ipsilateral inferior and superior parathyroid glands. The inferior thyroid artery travels posterior to the common carotid artery, but has a highly variable relationship with the RLN.[8]

The superior and middle thyroid veins drain into the internal jugular vein. The superior vein accompanies its paired artery; however, the middle vein does not have a paired artery. The inferior thyroid veins are variable in number and location, draining most commonly into the brachiocephalic veins, and also into the internal jugular vein. Although the internal jugular vein does not by definition lie in the central neck compartment, it is worth noting that its intimate association with the common carotid artery can bring it into the surgical field if tissue is dissected and retracted into the surgical field.

Nerves

Several nerves lie within the central neck compartment and have significant clinical importance. The RLN is a branch of the tenth cranial nerve (Vagus) and is derived from the sixth branchial arch. It innervates all of the intrinsic muscles of the larynx with the exception of the cricothyroid muscle and provides sensation to the larynx below the glottis, along with portions of the trachea and esophagus. During embryologic development, the RLN courses around the arteries of the sixth branchial arch. On the left, this is the ductus arteriosus, which *ex utero* becomes the ligamentum arteriosum. On the right,

the sixth branchial artery is obliterated. The RLN then migrates cranial to the next remaining branchial artery, the right subclavian artery. Therefore, the course of the RLN varies between the right and left sides of the body.

The right subclavian artery lies more anterior and lateral compared to the aortic arch and ligamentum arteriosum on the left. This results in the nerve traveling more lateral to medial and anterior to posterior on the right when it comes back to the larynx, as opposed to simply traveling superior in the tracheoesophageal groove as it on the left. The motor fibers of the nerve enter the larynx posterior to the cricothyroid joint underneath the inferior constrictor muscle.

Although rare, the head and neck surgeon must be aware of the possibility of a non-RLN (NRLN). This anomaly occurs almost exclusively on the right, with a prevalence of 0.7% in the general population. The most common cause of an NRLN is failure of the embryologic development of the right fourth branchial arch, the subclavian artery. It has been found that 86.7% of right NRLNs are associated with an aberrant subclavian artery pattern. These nerves can originate either above or below the laryngotracheal junction and track with the superior thyroid artery, branch directly off the Vagus, or display a looping trajectory into the laryngotracheal junction.[9]

The external branch of the superior laryngeal nerve (EBSLN) branches from the Vagus nerve high in the neck and accompanies the superior thyroid vasculature as it courses toward the cricothyroid muscle. It inserts directly into the muscles, which acts as a laryngeal tensor. Classification schemes have been proposed to describe the location of the EBSLN for better identification and preservation during thyroid or central neck dissection. They focus on several aspects of the nerve's course, including the intersection with the superior thyroid vessels, location on the nerve above a horizontal plane of the superior border of the superior thyroid pole, location of the cricothyroid–inferior constriction junction, and distance between the nerve and the superior thyroid vessels.[10,11,12,13,14] Complete discussion of these schemes is beyond the scope of this chapter.

Parathyroid Glands

The parathyroid glands are endocrine glands located on the posterior aspect of the thyroid gland and secrete parathyroid hormone, which regulates calcium homeostasis in the circulation. The inferior parathyroid glands migrate caudally in the anterior neck in association with the thymus gland. The final location of the inferior parathyroid glands is wherever the glands separate from the thymus. This can be anywhere from the hyoid bone to the lower mediastinum. In approximately 50% of patients, the inferior parathyroid glands can be found within 1 cm inferior, lateral, or posterior to the inferior pole of the thyroid. They are located typically anterior to the coronal plane drawn along the vertical axis of the RLN.

The superior parathyroid glands migrate attached to the posterior midportion of the thyroid lobe and, therefore, have a more predictable location in the central neck. In 85% of cases, the superior gland may be located on the posterior aspect of the thyroid lobe in a 2-cm diameter circle centered 1 cm above the crossing of the inferior thyroid artery and the RLN. The superior parathyroid glands lie posterior to the coronal plane drawn along the RLN.[15]

19.3.2 Central Neck Dissection

In patients diagnosed with PTC, 35% present with clinically evident regional nodal metastasis. Furthermore, up to 80% of patients presenting with no clinical evidence of nodal disease will have microscopic evidence of metastasis following elective neck dissection.[16] Zhang et al found in a retrospective study of more than 1,000 patients that male gender, age younger than 45 years, multifocal lesions, extrathyroidal extension, and primary tumors greater than 6 mm were risk factors for central neck metastasis.[4]

Uniformity in the reporting of nodal regions dissected, the surgical procedure performed, and the exact location of disease is crucial for the complete treatment of thyroid carcinoma. The American Head and Neck Society Endocrine Committee recently published guidelines for reporting central neck dissections. The procedure should be defined as either prophylactic (elective) or therapeutic. Distinguishing the differences between these two categories is important for the preoperative counseling of the patient. For prophylactic neck dissections, the surgeon must explain the risk, benefits, and alternatives to patients as well as why, if they have no apparent disease within the lymph nodes, he or she would advise for the removal of the lymph nodes.

Defining the extent of the central neck dissection is important for staging, adjuvant treatment, and, if necessary, revision operations. The term "central neck dissection" implies the surgeon removed the entire contents of the pretracheal and prelaryngeal lymph nodes, which is rarely the case in practice. The designation of the procedure is completed by including laterality or bilateral. By including right, left, or bilateral, the surgeon indicates removing the paratracheal lymph nodes on that respective side. Therefore, a complete description of a central neck dissection should be [prophylactic/therapeutic] [right/left/bilateral] central neck dissection.[16]

Complete dissection and removal of compartmental lymph nodes provide the best initial surgical management of disease. Previous methods of "berry picking," or choosing pathologic appearing lymph nodes intraoperatively, can miss microscopic disease within the remaining lymph nodes. It can also lead to increased complications from inadequate dissection of critical structures. Therefore, berry picking lymph nodes is not recommended for central neck dissections.[16]

19.3.3 Prophylactic Central Neck Dissection

A thorough discussion must take place between the patient and the multidisciplinary team before proceeding with a prophylactic neck dissection in a cN0 neck. The goals of the procedure are to improve disease-free survival, decrease the risk of local recurrence, improve the accuracy of posttreatment thyroglobulin level, determine the need for postoperative radioactive iodine therapy, and guide the long-term management of disease. Best evidence for determining the need for prophylactic central neck dissection in the cN0 neck would be a prospective, randomized control trial; however, one does not currently exist in the literature.

The ATA addressed the issue of neck dissections in the 2015 American Thyroid Association Guidelines Task Force on Thyroid Nodules and Differentiated Thyroid cancer. From this, they developed guidelines for prophylactic central neck dissections. Since approximately 14% of T1 DTC patients present with central compartment metastasis, prophylactic central neck dissection is not recommended in carcinomas less than 2 cm without extrathyroidal extension without clinical or sonographic lymphadenopathy.[2] No improvement was shown in long-term patient outcome, while increasing the likelihood of temporary morbidity.

Prophylactic central neck dissection should be offered to patients who have advanced (T3/4) primary tumors or clinically involved lateral compartment neck nodes, that is, clinical metastases that skip level VI. In patients with T4 cancer, approximately 86 and 93% will have metastasis to the central and lateral compartments, respectively.[2] Prophylactic neck dissection is also advocated in patients who show aggressive disease characteristics, such as older or very young age, multifocal disease, or aggressive pathologic variants (tall cell, diffuse sclerosing, insular variants). The current evidence also shows that the presence or absence of molecular markers are not independent prognostic indicators of survival, and should therefore not be considered when deciding to undergo a prophylactic neck dissection.[16]

The management of prophylactic central neck dissection is somewhat different in children, seemingly due to two specific factors. First, the vast majority of children present with some form of regional lymph node metastasis. Second, decreased disease-free survival is most strongly correlated with the presence of persistent or recurrent locoregional disease. Extent of dissection is based on consideration of focality, size, and experience of surgeon as compared to the risks of the procedure. Ipsilateral dissection should occur for ipsilateral thyroid disease, and contralateral dissection can be based on size and intraoperative findings.[17]

Management of the central neck in MTC tends to be more aggressive when compared to DTC. Overall metastasis of MTC to the central or lateral neck compartments can be greater than 75%. Disease spread to the ipsilateral central and lateral neck is approximately 80% and spread to the contralateral neck is approximately 45%. Because of the significant tendency for MTC to spread to adjacent neck lymph nodes, all patients with diagnosed MTC with a cN0 neck may be considered for a bilateral central neck dissection.[18]

19.3.4 Therapeutic Central Neck Dissection

A therapeutic central neck dissection should be performed in any patient who presents with clinically apparent central compartment lymphadenopathy on physical examination or imaging. This should be performed at the same time as total thyroidectomy, since dissection of the central neck after thyroidectomy will have the added challenge of scarring and destruction of tissue planes.[2] The recommendation for therapeutic central neck dissection also applies to children with proven gross extrathyroidal and/or locoregional metastasis.[17]

The extent of therapeutic neck dissection needs to address the distribution of disease while taking into account the risks of bilateral central compartment surgery. If central neck lymphadenopathy is unilateral on preoperative evaluation, the ipsilateral paratracheal lymph nodes should be removed. The patient should also be informed of the possibility of contralateral paratracheal dissection based on intraoperative examination of lymph nodes.[16]

Bilateral therapeutic central neck dissection should be recommended to patients with bilateral central neck lymphadenopathy on initial presentation. Bilateral dissection for unilateral central neck disease remains an area of controversy with need for further research. Currently, it has been noted that bilateral dissection may be associated with higher morbidity, primarily RLN palsy, and hypoparathyroidism, with no reduction in the rate of recurrence. Therefore, the decision to proceed with contralateral dissection for single-sided disease should be based on pathologic characteristics of the initial biopsy, intraoperative findings, and patient risk factors as described previously.[16] Any patient with MTC who presents with positive central neck nodes should undergo a bilateral central neck dissection.[18]

19.3.5 Central Neck Complications

As with any surgical procedures, there exists risks to the anatomical structures of the surgical field that can result in morbidity and possibly mortality to the patient. Mortality from central neck dissection is extremely rare; however, morbidity, including hypoparathyroidism, injury to the RLN, or injury to the external branch of the superior laryngeal nerve, is not uncommon. These morbidities are most commonly transient, but permanent adverse consequences are certainly a reality after a central neck dissection. The most significant possible morbidity would be the need to place a tracheotomy tube.

Hypoparathyroidism

Transient or permanent hypoparathyroidism is a common morbidity following central neck dissection caused by either the direct removal of parathyroid tissue or devitalization of parathyroid tissue in situ. Hypoparathyroidism leads to hypocalcemia causing symptoms such as numbness or tingling around the mouth or in the fingers and toes, muscle cramps, carpopedal spasm, fatigue, irritability, altered mental status, or abnormal ECG findings. Permanent hypoparathyroidism is defined as requiring therapeutic vitamin D and/or calcium replacement at 6 months postoperatively or a fasting albumin-corrected serum calcium below 8.0 mg/dL. Incidental parathyroidectomy during central neck dissection for thyroid carcinoma has been found to be between 28 and 41%.[19,20] Central neck dissection in the setting of total thyroidectomy is an independent risk factor for incidental parathyroidectomy with an odds ratio of 9.6.[20] The overall rate of transient and permanent hypoparathyroidism in central neck dissection for thyroid carcinoma is difficult to determine due to variations between prophylactic and therapeutic dissections, ipsilateral and bilateral dissections, and dissections done with or without concurrent thyroidectomy. Transient hypoparathyroidism ranges from 9 to 52%, whereas permanent hypoparathyroidism ranges from 2.6 to 16.2%.[21,22,23]

Dissection of the parathyroid glands should proceed in an atraumatic manner with preservation of the blood supply from the inferior thyroid artery. The superior parathyroid glands are more easily identified and dissected from the surgical specimen based on their more reliable location posterior to the superior pole of the thyroid gland. Consequently, the superior glands are most likely preserved during central neck dissection. The locations for the inferior parathyroid glands within the central neck are more variable, which put them at higher risk for incidental parathyroidectomy during dissection.[24] If the parathyroid glands are not identified and preserved in situ, the surgical specimen should be examined for potential parathyroid candidates. Biopsy and frozen specimen are used to confirm parathyroid tissue, and not tumor or thyroid tissue, before autotransplantation is performed. The resected parathyroid tissue should be minced into small 1- to 2-mm pieces and inserted into an ipsilateral strap or sternocleidomastoid muscle. Routine autotransplantation of the inferior parathyroid glands has been shown to reduce the rate of permanent hypoparathyroidism if the gland was devascularized or if incidental parathyroidectomy occurred.[25]

Unilateral Recurrent Laryngeal Nerve Injury

Damage to the RLN is arguably the most feared complication during thyroidectomy or central neck dissection. The RLN innervates the intrinsic muscles of the larynx, including the only abductor muscle, the posterior cricoarytenoid muscle. Transient or permanent injury to the nerve can result in dysfunction of the ipsilateral side of the larynx with limited or no mobility of the vocal cord. This can cause considerable morbidity to the patient, including hoarseness, shortness of breath, activity intolerance, and aspiration leading to pneumonia. Transient nerve injury is commonly defined as evidence of nerve dysfunction from the immediate postoperative period to 6 months. Permanent nerve injury is diagnosed once dysfunction has persisted for 6 months, with a definitive diagnosis at 1 year.

Jeannon et al did a systematic review of more than 25,000 patients undergoing thyroid surgery to determine the incidence of RLN injury. They found a 9.3% incidence of temporary injury and a 2.3% incidence of permanent injury. Furthermore, they investigated the most common methods to evaluate the larynx, including indirect laryngoscopy, fiberoptic nasolaryngoscopy, and video stroboscopy. Although videostroboscopy evaluation discovered the lowest incidence of nerve palsy, it requires specialized equipment that may not be available in all offices. Therefore, they recommended that patients presenting with postoperative symptoms of RLN palsy be evaluated with fiberoptic nasolaryngoscopy.[26]

Extralaryngeal branching (ELB) of the RLN is a known risk to the nerve during dissection. A systematic review of more than 28,000 nerves found the prevalence of ELB to be 60%. Interestingly, the prevalence was 73% in cadaveric studies and only 39% in intraoperative studies, suggesting that ELB is significantly underreported from the operating room since it is not routinely examined. There are several patterns of branching, with bifurcation being the most common and branching occurring within 2 cm of the cricothyroid joint. When branching occurs, it is almost certain that the anterior branch will have positive motor response.[27] The presence of ELB has been found to increase unilateral temporary nerve palsy approximately 7 times and permanent nerve palsy 13 times compared to nonbranching nerves.[28] Therefore, it is imperative that the surgeon be aware of possible branching of the nerve during identification.

The traditional method to prevent damage to the RLN is through meticulous dissection and preservation. However, even the most minute trauma to the nerve can result in clinical symptoms. In order to decrease the likelihood of nerve trauma, intraoperative nerve monitoring (IONM) has been developed to aid in the identification of the RLN. IONM consists of electrophysiological measurements of the intrinsic muscle of the larynx by electrodes on specialized endotracheal tubes. Responses to stimulus of the nerve before and after removal of the thyroid gland and central neck contents can theoretically predict potential nerve palsy. Use of IONM can aid in the identification of the RLN in between 98 and 100% of cases.[16] IONM has not become a universal standard in all cases, as a systematic meta-analysis comparing visualization alone to IONM found no statistical significance in RLN palsy in all cases.[29] However, there does seem to be an advantage of using IONM for high-risk, reoperative, complex, or bilateral thyroid surgery.[2] Unfortunately, difficult RLN dissections cannot always be anticipated, and argument exists for universal monitoring. In the unlikely scenario of nerve transection, primary reanastomosis is strongly recommended.

Bilateral Recurrent Laryngeal Nerve Injury

This very rare, but extremely serious, complication occurs as a result of injury to the bilateral RLNs during either total thyroidectomy or bilateral central neck dissection. The vocal cords will become fixed in the median, paramedian, or lateral position in the glottis, resulting in a varying degree of airway obstruction. It is difficult to determine the exact incidence of this complication due to its rarity, but estimates of permanent paralysis range from 0.01 to 0.6%.[30]

Injury to the External Branch of the Superior Laryngeal Nerve

Injury to the external branch of the superior laryngeal nerve will cause ipsilateral paresis or paralysis to the cricothyroid muscle. Clinically, this can result in a spectrum of voice changes such as a hoarse/breathing voice, vocal fatigue and diminished vocal performance (especially in high pitch and singing voices), decreased loudness, and vocal fatigue. The rate of EBSLN injury varies between 0 and 58% seemingly due to limited data, variability of vocal symptoms, and difficulty identifying changes in postoperative laryngoscopic exams.[31] As with the RLN, IONM has become more common with the external branch of the superior laryngeal nerve. Several studies have shown that the use of IONM identifies the EBSLN in up to 98.5% of cases, which can decrease the rate of nerve injury during dissection.[14]

19.4 The Lateral Neck

19.4.1 Surgical Definitions of Lateral Neck Levels

Starting from the radical neck dissections in the early 20th century to the selective neck dissections of the modern era, the classification of surgical lymph node groups in the lateral neck have developed as a way to better understand head and neck cancer. The ATA has developed a consensus statement for lateral neck dissection anatomy, terminology, and rationale to better facilitate treatment of thyroid carcinoma.[32] The lateral neck is defined by levels II, III, IV, and V in ▶ Fig. 19.2.

Boundaries of the Lateral Neck

This is reviewed here for thyroid nodal disease, but is addressed in greater detail in Chapter 2. Level I, otherwise known as the submandibular and submental nodal groups, is defined by the body of the mandible superiorly, stylohyoid muscle posteriorly, and the digastric muscle anteriorly and posteriorly. This level is further subdivided into Ia and Ib. The submental nodal group, Ia, does not carry a laterality and is bounded by the anterior bellies of the digastric muscles and the hyoid bone. The submandibular nodal group, Ib, is bounded by the anterior and posterior bellies of the ipsilateral digastric muscle along with the mandible. It also contains the submandibular gland.

Level II, the upper jugular nodal group, extends from the skull base inferiorly to the inferior border of the hyoid bone. The anterior border is the stylohyoid muscle, and the posterior border is the posterior border of the sternocleidomastoid muscle. The deep border is the fascia overlying the levator scapulae muscle. The spinal accessory nerve traverses obliquely in an anterosuperior to inferolateral fashion to divide this level into IIa, the anteroinferior contents, and IIb, the posterosuperior contents.

Level III, the midjugular nodal group, lies between the lower border of the hyoid bone and a horizontal plane from the lower border of the cricoid cartilage. The anterior border is the sternohyoid muscle, and the posterior border is the posterior border of the sternocleidomastoid muscle. The deep border is the deep cervical fascia overlying the anterior scalene muscle.

Level IV, the lower jugular nodal group, lies between the lower border of the cricoid cartilage and the superior border of the clavicle. The anterior and posterior borders are the same as level III. The deep border is the fascia overlying the cervical plexus. The thoracic duct, the largest vessel of the lymphatic system, is most commonly found near the junction of the left internal jugular subclavian veins. A systematic review of scientific literature determined that the thoracic duct most commonly enters the internal jugular vein (46%), followed by the jugulo-venous angle (32%), and the subclavian vein (18%). Other sites of termination include the external jugular vein, brachiocephalic vein, transverse cervical vein, suprascapular vein, and a right-side termination.[33] It is important to know that the thoracic duct lies superficial to the fascia of the anterior scalene muscle, putting it at risk during dissection of the inferior portion of level IV.

Level V, the posterior neck triangle, has its apex at the convergence of the sternocleidomastoid and the trapezius muscle, and base at the superior border of the clavicle. The anterior border is the posterior border of the sternocleidomastoid. The posterior border is the anterior border of the trapezius. This level is subdivided by a horizontal plane continuous with the inferior border of the cricoid cartilage. Superiorly is Va, containing the nodes around the spinal accessory, and inferiorly is Vb, containing the transverse cervical and supraclavicular nodes.

Vascular Structures

The lingual artery, the second branch of the external carotid artery, is present briefly in level I deep to the submandibular gland before running deep to the hypoglossal muscle. The facial artery branches off the external carotid artery posterior to the posterior belly of the digastric muscle. It runs on the deep surface of the submandibular gland before emerging near the inferior border of the mandible deep to the marginal mandibular nerve. The Hayes Martin Maneuver can be performed to protect the marginal mandibular nerve by ligating the facial pedicle at the inferior margin of the mandible and reflecting the soft tissue, along with the nerve, superiorly out of the surgical field. The submental artery branches from the facial artery deep to the submandibular gland and runs anteriorly superficial to the mylohyoid muscle. The facial vein originates in the lower portion of the face, joining the facial artery, as it crosses superficial to the inferior border of the mandible. Unlike the facial artery, the facial vein runs superficial to the submandibular gland before joining the anterior division of the retromandibular vein to form to common facial vein, which then drains into the internal jugular vein.

Few arterial structures are present in levels II, III, and IV. The occipital artery, a branch of the external carotid artery, may be encountered in the superior portion of level IIb as it crosses superficial to the internal jugular vein and cranial nerve XI. Here, it will branch to supply the superior portion of the sternocleidomastoid muscle. The inferior thyroid artery, from the thyrocervical trunk, is present in level IV and courses medially deep to the common carotid artery on its way to the inferior pole of the thyroid gland. The common, internal, and external carotid arteries are found at the medial boundary spanning the lateral neck, and, as a general rule, should be minimally manipulated during dissection unless there is gross involvement by primary or metastatic disease.

The internal jugular vein is present at the medial aspect of levels II to IV, beginning at the skull base, deep to the posterior belly of the digastric muscle, and terminating in the brachiocephalic vein after joining with the subclavian vein. The vein does not typically have lateral branches. The thyrolinguofacial trunk arises medially from the internal jugular vein and will be encountered as the jugular lymph nodes are dissected off the vein.

Arteries encountered within level V include the first part of the subclavian artery, giving rise to the thyrocervical trunk and then to the transverse cervical artery. The transverse cervical artery courses in a medial to lateral fashion superficial to the anterior scalene muscle but deep to the omohyoid muscle before it divides into its superficial and deep branch at the anterior border of the trapezius. The external jugular vein is formed from the confluence of the posterior division of the retromandibular vein and the posterior auricular vein. It crosses superficially to the sternocleidomastoid muscle to empty into the subclavian vein within level V.

Nerves

Several cranial nerves, nerves of the cervical plexus, the brachial plexus, and the sympathetic cervical chain are found in multiple levels within the lateral neck compartment. The marginal mandibular branch of cranial nerve VII exits the parotid gland in the lower lateral part of the face and crosses the mandible twice before innervating the nerves of the lower lip and chin. The lower extent of the nerve is commonly 1 to 2 cm below the angle of the mandible within level I. The lingual nerve is a sensory nerve from the mandibular division of the trigeminal nerve which provides sensation and taste to the anterior two-thirds of the tongue. It is

found during removal of the submandibular gland, when the mylohyoid is reflected to expose the lingual nerve superficial to the submandibular duct.

Cranial nerve X, the vagus nerve, contains sensory, motor, and autonomic branches innervating multiple areas of the body. Regarding the head and neck, it provides sensation and motor control of skeletal muscles to the pharynx and the larynx via the superior and RLNs. Traveling through the neck in the carotid sheath between the internal jugular vein and carotid arteries, it is present in levels II to IV and should not be extensively manipulated during routine lateral neck dissection.

Cranial nerve XI, the spinal accessory nerve, is a motor nerve innervating the sternocleidomastoid and trapezius muscles. It travels in a mediolateral and superoinferior direction from the jugular foramen, anterior to the vagus nerve, to the sternocleidomastoid muscle, dividing level II into two sections. After piercing the sternocleidomastoid muscle, it continues through level V to enter the trapezius. The two muscles combined to help tilt and rotate the head, elevate the shoulder, and abduct the arm.

Cranial nerve XII, the hypoglossal nerve, is a motor nerve innervating the extrinsic, except for the palatoglossal, and intrinsic muscles of the tongue. After it leaves the skull base through the hypoglossal canal, the nerve passes between the internal jugular vein and the carotid arteries as it arches toward the tongue. It reaches the posterior aspect of the greater cornu of the hyoid bone before traveling anteriorly deep to the submandibular duct. Therefore, its importance is the dissection of levels I and II.

The cervical plexus is a syncytium of the anterior rami of the first four cervical spinal nerves. It gives rise to the ansa cervicalis, the greater auricular nerve, and the phrenic nerve. The ansa cervicalis, arising from C1 to C3, provides motor control to the strap muscles, except for the thyrohyoid, and sits superficial to the carotid sheath. The greater auricular is formed from C2 and C3, providing sensation to the skin overlying the parotid gland and the ear lobule. It courses around the posterior border of the sternocleidomastoid muscle as it travels superiorly toward the parotid gland. It is often encountered while defining the lateral border of level II. The phrenic nerve is both a sensory and motor nerve to the diaphragm formed from C3 to C5. It lies deep to the prevertebral layer of the deep cervical fascia over the anterior scalene muscle deep to level IV.

The second neurologic plexus of the neck is the brachial plexus. It is formed by the anastomoses of anterior rami of the spinal nerves C5 to C8 and T1. It provides both sensory and motor control to the chest and ipsilateral upper extremity. It is found within level V in the fascia between the anterior and medial scalene muscles.

The cervical sympathetic chain is part of the sympathetic nervous system providing vasoconstrictive innervation to involuntary smooth muscles of the head and neck along with secretory control to the lacrimal and salivary glands. It is located within the deep portion of the prevertebral fascia anterior to the transverse process of the vertebral bodies. The cervical sympathetic chain commonly consists of three ganglia: the superior, middle, and inferior (stellate). The superior ganglion is consistently located near the skull base at the opening of the carotid canal. The middle ganglion lies near the inferior thyroid artery. The inferior ganglion is typically fused with the first thoracic ganglion to form the stellate ganglion just posterior to the origin of the vertebral artery.

19.4.2 Lateral Neck Dissection

As with the central neck dissection, having a uniform system to describe the extent of a lateral neck dissection is essential to operative planning, pathologic reporting, and arranging adjuvant therapy.[6,32] The terms radical and modified radical neck dissections are inadequate to describe the extent of a dissection in the modern era. Selective neck dissection has become the most widely accepted terminology and refers to the removal of less than all five nodal levels with the preservation of the spinal accessory nerve, internal jugular vein, and sternocleidomastoid muscle. The procedure should be reported with the side and level/sublevels dissected.[32]

Lateral neck dissection for DTC is dependent on the most common pathways of nodal drainage. Risk factors for spread to the lateral neck include extrathyroidal extension, multifocal lesions, and central neck disease.[4] It has been shown that skip metastasis to the lateral neck compartment can occur in up to 18% of papillary thyroid carcinoma.[16] Skip metastasis is defined as spread of metastatic disease past the first echelon nodes of the central neck to the second echelon nodes of the lateral neck (VI or III). The ATA advocates that a routine selective lateral neck dissection for thyroid carcinoma should include levels IIa, III, IV, and Vb. Dissection in level IIb is undertaken only if there is preoperative evidence of disease in this level or suspicious appearing nodes in upper level IIa which lie in close proximity to IIb. This also applies to level Va, which should only be explored with preoperative evidence of suspicious lymphadenopathy.[2]

MTC tends to have about the same chance of skip metastasis when compared to DTC, about 25%. Furthermore, the rate of lateral neck metastasis tends to be directly related to the frequency of central neck spread.[18] In patients with minimal central neck disease, the rate of ipsilateral and contralateral lateral neck disease was found to be 77 and 38%, respectively. The same study found that advanced central neck disease had a 98% chance of ipsilateral and 77% chance of contralateral lateral neck disease.[34] Preoperative serum calcitonin also has a predictive value for the extent of metastatic spread, with increasing levels indicating more distant spread with a less likely chance of a biochemical cure.[18]

19.4.3 Prophylactic Lateral Neck Dissection

When considering a lateral neck dissection in a patient with DTC and a cN0, the surgeon must consider the possible rate of metastasis and the potential morbidity of the procedure. As determined by the ATA and supported by the American Head and Neck Society, prophylactic neck dissection is not considered appropriate in any DTC patient with a clinically negative neck. This is also true for children.[2,17]

As previously described, the rate of metastasis in MTC is higher when compared to DTC and can be directly related to the serum calcitonin level. It has been advocated that a serum calcitonin level of greater than 20 pg/mL be used as a cutoff to proceed with a prophylactic lateral neck dissection in cN0.[18] No consensus was made for this number, and further investigations are needed to support this decision. Prophylactic contralateral lateral neck dissection is recommended in patients with serum calcitonin levels of greater than 200 pg/mL, central compartment disease, and

positive preoperative imaging of the ipsilateral lateral neck compartment.[18]

19.4.4 Therapeutic Lateral Neck Dissection

For DTC and MTC, therapeutic lateral neck dissection should only be performed for biopsy-proven metastasis in levels II to V. When metastasis is present on the initial presentation, lateral neck dissection should take place at the same time as total thyroidectomy.[2]

Metastasis or recurrence of disease may occur several years or even decades after initial presentation. Surveillance of the lateral neck with ultrasound should occur every 6 to 12 months after completion of initial treatment, depending on the risk category of the patient. If suspicious lymph nodes appear as described previously, they should be biopsied and treated with lateral neck dissection if pathologic.[32]

Preoperative confirmation of recurrent disease can be achieved with a second set of imaging, typically a CT scan of the neck with contrast. However, localization of disease intraoperatively in a previous surgical field can be difficult because of scar tissue. Radioguided surgery has been shown to be effective for localization in other head and neck procedures, such as parathyroidectomy and sentinel lymph node biopsy. First developed after using residual therapeutic radioactive iodine 131, radioguided surgery using 99m-technetium, 18F-fluorodeoxyglucose, or 131-iodine is useful and can be a valuable tool for recurrent PTC.[35,36,37]

Therapeutic lateral neck dissection in children should be performed only after cytologic confirmation of metastasis. As with adults, this should proceed in a compartment-oriented fashion, typically consisting of levels II, III, IV, and Vb. There has been no evidence to support contralateral dissection without proven disease.[17]

19.4.5 Lateral Neck Complications

Marginal Mandibular Nerve

Injury to the marginal mandibular nerve can occur during level Ib and high level IIa neck dissections. As described earlier, the nerve can be found within the fascia superficial to the facial pedicle along the inferior border of the mandible. Reflecting the fascia out of the surgical plane after ligation of the pedicle can theoretically protect the nerve during dissection. Insult to the marginal mandibular nerve will cause weakness or paralysis to the depressor labii inferioris, depressor anguli oris, and mentalis muscles, resulting in an asymmetric smile and oral incompetency particularly with liquids. The incidence rates of temporary paresis and permanent paralysis have been found to be 14% and 4 to 7%, respectively, following level I neck dissection. However, the same study found that dissection of level IIa without level Ib resulted in no cases of marginal mandibular nerve weakness.[38]

Spinal Accessory Nerve

Injury or sacrifice of the spinal accessory nerve will lead to the painful and debilitating shoulder syndrome. Patients will often present with excruciating pain (anesthesia, neuropathic pain) to the neck, upper back, and affected shoulder. The paralyzed sternocleidomastoid and trapezius will cause limited abduction of the arm, shoulder droop, scapular winging, and internal rotation of the arm. Much of our knowledge of the shoulder syndrome comes from the morbidity of treating head and neck squamous cell cancer in the past with radical neck dissections. Over time, with further studies into the drainage patterns of head and neck cancers and the survivability after neck dissection, modifications to the radical neck dissection were made to spare the spinal accessory nerve. In the current era of treatment, intentional resection of the spinal accessory nerve is only indicated with gross tumor involvement of the nerve found intraoperatively or inability to remove the tumor without removing the nerve. Injury to the spinal accessory nerve is relatively uncommon, with transient and permanent paresis estimated to be about 1 and 0.3%, respectively.[39] Treatment of spinal accessory deficit is primarily physical therapy focused on strengthening the surrounding muscles to compensate for the deficiencies.

Hypoglossal Nerve

The hypoglossal nerve is the sole innervating nerve for the extrinsic and intrinsic muscles of the tongue, except for the palatoglossus. Therefore, damage to the nerve during dissection of level Ib or IIa can lead to weakness and atrophy of one side of the tongue affecting speech and the oral phase of swallowing. Iatrogenic injury has been estimated to be less than 1% in lateral neck dissections for thyroid cancer.[39]

Brachial Plexus

Injury to the brachial plexus during lateral neck dissection is a rare occurrence, with only a handful of case reports published. Most involve an anatomic variant of the superior trunk, C5 and C6, traveling over the supraclavicular fat pad before diving posteriorly behind the clavicle. Injury to the superior root will cause an Erb-Duchenne palsy with the arm rotated medially by the patient's side and the forearm in an extended and pronated position.[40,41] There have been no reported cases of injury to the middle or inferior trunk. The anterior scalene muscle covers these trunks of the brachial plexus, making injury to these extremely difficult without any reported cases.

Cervical Sympathetic Chain

Damage to the cervical sympathetic chain is an extremely rare complication of neck dissections, reported as less than 1% of all neck dissections.[42] No literature has been published examining the incidence of this complication specifically in lateral neck dissection for thyroid carcinoma. Most common situations which put the cervical sympathetic chain at risk during dissection are inadvertent dissection beyond the carotid sheath into the prevertebral fascia and tumor and/or metastatic extensive into the prevertebral space. Injury to the chain will result in Horner's syndrome, resulting in ipsilateral eyelid ptosis, miosis with anisocoria, facial anhydrosis, and enophthalmos.

Cervical Plexus

The location of the great auricular nerve puts it at risk during level II dissection primarily in two situations. First, the nerve can be easily transected during the raising of skin flaps because of its superficial location lateral to the border of the platysma in the subcutaneous tissue. Secondly, the nerve commonly runs through the superior aspect of level II, limiting or obstructing the removal of tissue from IIb. Sacrifice of the nerve may be necessary in order for the dissection to be completed in its entirety. Dysesthesia can occur as a result of injury to the great auricular nerve, with patients describing the sensation of burning, itching, electrical shock, or pins and needles to the skin overlying the parotid gland and ear lobule. Shaving, talking on the phone, and putting in earrings can turn from an everyday process to a painful activity. Many patients experience recovery of the majority of their anesthesia 9 to 12 months postoperatively. Studies on the incidence of great auricular nerve injury after neck dissection are lacking and could be determined with further research.

The phrenic nerve lies underneath the prevertebral fascia of the deep cervical plexus and is not encountered during lateral neck dissection unless the surgeon goes beyond the boundaries of level IV. Injury to the phrenic nerve can result in elevation of the ipsilateral hemidiaphragm causing reduction in lung capacity, shortness of breath, and fatigue. Polistena et al found an incidence of 0.14% injury to the phrenic nerve in a retrospective institutional review of 675 lateral neck dissections for thyroid cancer. This occurred in a patient with direct metastatic infiltration of tumor into the nerve.[39]

Chyle Leak

Chyle leak, or chyle fistula, occurs when there is damage to the thoracic duct or lymphatic vessels leading to the accumulation of lymphatic fluid within the surgical bed. The location of the thoracic duct is highly variable not only in its terminal location but also in the path which it takes to get there, making it highly susceptible to injury. Incidence of chyle leak during lateral neck dissection for thyroid cancer is between 1 and 8%.[43] A prospective study for the identification of chyle leak during lateral neck dissection found an intraoperative leak rate of 5.2%, all of which occurred on the left side. Interestingly, the same study had a postoperative chyle leak rate of 8.3%, with 62.5% of those occurring in the right neck.[44] Therefore, it is pertinent for the surgeon to be diligent within the right neck during dissection, as careless dissection can lead to transection of an aberrant thoracic duct or large lymphatic duct. An extremely rare, but potentially major, complication involving the thoracic duct is a chylothorax, or accumulation of chyle within the pleural cavity. A systematic review of the literature calculated the incidence of chylothorax in thyroidectomy with neck dissection to be 1.85%, with 20 total cases reported.[45]

Vascular Injury

The internal jugular vein serves as the medial border during lateral neck dissection. Because of this, it is encountered and manipulated in every level of the lateral, putting it at risk during the procedure. Potential injuries to the vein include hematoma following inadequate ligation of feeding vessels, puncture of the side wall, thrombosis, and complete resection due to tumor invasion. Thrombosis can occur as a reaction from manipulation of the vessel wall or prolonged compression of the vein during surgery. Early postoperative thrombosis can occur in approximately 25% of patients within the first week; however, after at least 3 months from the procedure, only 5% of the thromboses remained.[46] Complications from an internal jugular vein thrombosis include septic emboli, pulmonary embolism, and intracranial propagation of the clot. Complete resection of a single internal jugular vein does not typically have morbidity for the patient. The morbidity of resecting both internal jugular veins simultaneously is significant causing severely elevation of intracranial pressure leading to altered level of consciousness, headaches, blindness, and stroke.[46]

Complications with the common and internal carotid arteries are uncommon intraoperatively, as these vessels are not extensively manipulated during routine dissection. Any intraoperative injury, that is, puncture or inadvertent ligation, should be corrected immediately with a vein patch or reconstruction. Intraoperative consultation with a vascular surgery may be necessary if repair is unsuccessful. Patients must be monitored in the immediately postoperative period for cerebrovascular accident. The most feared long-term complication of any neck dissection is the carotid artery blowout, which occurs in less than 5% of all head and neck cancer patients undergoing surgical resection. Risk factors associated with carotid artery blowout in head and neck cancers include body mass index less than 22.5, open wound to the neck requiring dressing changes, radical neck dissection, and total external beam radiation dose greater than 70 Gy.[47] Mortality of this complication can be as high as 60%.[48]

References

[1] SEER Cancer Stat Facts. Thyroid Cancer. National Cancer Institute. Bethesda, MD. Available at: http://seer.cancer.gov/statfacts/html/thyro.html. Accessed May 5, 2018

[2] Haugen BR, Alexander EK, Bible KC, et al. 2015 American Thyroid Association Management Guidelines for Adult Patients with Thyroid Nodules and Differentiated Thyroid Cancer: The American Thyroid Association Guidelines Task Force on Thyroid Nodules and Differentiated Thyroid Cancer. Thyroid. 2016; 26(1):1–133

[3] Moley JF. Medullary thyroid carcinoma: management of lymph node metastases. J Natl Compr Canc Netw. 2010; 8(5):549–556

[4] Zhang L, Wei WJ, Ji QH, et al. Risk factors for neck nodal metastasis in papillary thyroid microcarcinoma: a study of 1066 patients. J Clin Endocrinol Metab. 2012; 97(4):1250–1257

[5] Jeon MJ, Kim WG, Jang EK, et al. Thyroglobulin level in fine-needle aspirates for preoperative diagnosis of cervical lymph node metastasis in patients with papillary thyroid carcinoma: two different cutoff values according to serum thyroglobulin level. Thyroid. 2015; 25(4):410–416

[6] Carty SE, Doherty GM, Inabnet WB, III, et al. Surgical Affairs Committee Of The American Thyroid Association. American Thyroid Association statement on the essential elements of interdisciplinary communication of perioperative information for patients undergoing thyroid cancer surgery. Thyroid. 2012; 22(4):395–399

[7] Carty SE, Cooper DS, Doherty GM, et al. American Thyroid Association Surgery Working Group, American Association of Endocrine Surgeons, American Academy of Otolaryngology-Head and Neck Surgery, American Head and Neck Society. Consensus statement on the terminology and classification of central neck dissection for thyroid cancer. Thyroid. 2009; 19(11):1153–1158

[8] Yalçin B. Anatomic configurations of the recurrent laryngeal nerve and inferior thyroid artery. Surgery. 2006; 139(2):181–187

[9] Henry BM, Sanna S, Graves MJ, et al. The non-recurrent laryngeal nerve: a meta-analysis and clinical considerations. PeerJ. 2017; 5:e3012

[10] Cernea CR, Ferraz AR, Nishio S, Dutra A, Jr, Hojaij FC, dos Santos LR. Surgical anatomy of the external branch of the superior laryngeal nerve. Head Neck. 1992; 14(5):380–383

[11] Kierner AC, Aigner M, Burian M. The external branch of the superior laryngeal nerve: its topographical anatomy as related to surgery of the neck. Arch Otolaryngol Head Neck Surg. 1998; 124(3):301–303

[12] Friedman M, LoSavio P, Ibrahim H. Superior laryngeal nerve identification and preservation in thyroidectomy. Arch Otolaryngol Head Neck Surg. 2002; 128(3):296–303

[13] Selvan B, Babu S, Paul MJ, Abraham D, Samuel P, Nair A. Mapping the compound muscle action potentials of cricothyroid muscle using electromyography in thyroid operations: a novel method to clinically type the external branch of the superior laryngeal nerve. Ann Surg. 2009; 250(2):293–300

[14] Wang K, Cai H, Kong D, Cui Q, Zhang D, Wu G. The identification, preservation and classification of the external branch of the superior laryngeal nerve in thyroidectomy. World J Surg. 2017; 41(10):2521–2529

[15] Hinson AM, Stack BC. Applied embryology, molecular genetics, and surgical anatomy of the parathyroid glands. In: Stack BC, Bodenner D, eds. Medical and Surgical Treatment of Parathyroid Diseases: An Evidence-Based Approach. Springer; 2017:20–21

[16] Agrawal N, Evasovich MR, Kandil E, et al. Indications and extent of central neck dissection for papillary thyroid cancer: an American Head and Neck Society Consensus Statement. Head Neck. 2017; 39(7):1269–1279

[17] Francis GL, Waguespack SG, Bauer AJ, et al. American Thyroid Association Guidelines Task Force. Management guidelines for children with thyroid nodules and differentiated thyroid cancer. Thyroid. 2015; 25(7):716–759

[18] Wells SA, Jr, Asa SL, Dralle H, et al. American Thyroid Association Guidelines Task Force on Medullary Thyroid Carcinoma. Revised American Thyroid Association guidelines for the management of medullary thyroid carcinoma. Thyroid. 2015; 25(6):567–610

[19] Cavanagh JP, Bullock M, Hart RD, Trites JR, MacDonald K, Taylor SM. Incidence of parathyroid tissue in level VI neck dissection. J Otolaryngol Head Neck Surg. 2011; 40(1):27–33

[20] Zhou HY, He JC, McHenry CR. Inadvertent parathyroidectomy: incidence, risk factors, and outcomes. J Surg Res. 2016; 205(1):70–75

[21] Caliskan M, Park JH, Jeong JS, et al. Role of prophylactic ipsilateral central compartment lymph node dissection in papillary thyroid microcarcinoma. Endocr J. 2012; 59(4):305–311

[22] Kwan WY, Chow TL, Choi CY, Lam SH. Complication rates of central compartment dissection in papillary thyroid cancer. ANZ J Surg. 2015; 85(4):274–278

[23] Giordano D, Valcavi R, Thompson GB, et al. Complications of central neck dissection in patients with papillary thyroid carcinoma: results of a study on 1087 patients and review of the literature. Thyroid. 2012; 22(9):911–917

[24] Sitges-Serra A, Gallego-Otaegui L, Suárez S, Lorente-Poch L, Munné A, Sancho JJ. Inadvertent parathyroidectomy during total thyroidectomy and central neck dissection for papillary thyroid carcinoma. Surgery. 2017; 161 (3):712–719

[25] Wei T, Li Z, Jin J, et al. Autotransplantation of inferior parathyroid glands during central neck dissection for papillary thyroid carcinoma: a retrospective cohort study. Int J Surg. 2014; 12(12):1286–1290

[26] Jeannon JP, Orabi AA, Bruch GA, Abdalsalam HA, Simo R. Diagnosis of recurrent laryngeal nerve palsy after thyroidectomy: a systematic review. Int J Clin Pract. 2009; 63(4):624–629

[27] Henry BM, Vikse J, Graves MJ, et al. Extralaryngeal branching of the recurrent laryngeal nerve: a meta-analysis of 28,387 nerves. Langenbecks Arch Surg. 2016; 401(7):913–923

[28] Casella C, Pata G, Nascimbeni R, Mittempergher F, Salerni B. Does extralaryngeal branching have an impact on the rate of postoperative transient or permanent recurrent laryngeal nerve palsy? World J Surg. 2009; 33(2):261–265

[29] Pisanu A, Porceddu G, Podda M, Cois A, Uccheddu A. Systematic review with meta-analysis of studies comparing intraoperative neuromonitoring of recurrent laryngeal nerves versus visualization alone during thyroidectomy. J Surg Res. 2014; 188(1):152–161

[30] Sarkis LM, Zaidi N, Norlén O, Delbridge LW, Sywak MS, Sidhu SB. Bilateral recurrent laryngeal nerve injury in a specialized thyroid surgery unit: would routine intraoperative neuromonitoring alter outcomes? ANZ J Surg. 2017; 87(5):364–367

[31] Barczyński M, Randolph GW, Cernea CR, et al. International Neural Monitoring Study Group. External branch of the superior laryngeal nerve monitoring during thyroid and parathyroid surgery: International Neural Monitoring Study Group standards guideline statement. Laryngoscope. 2013; 123 Suppl 4:S1–S14

[32] Stack BC, Jr, Ferris RL, Goldenberg D, et al. American Thyroid Association Surgical Affairs Committee. American Thyroid Association consensus review and statement regarding the anatomy, terminology, and rationale for lateral neck dissection in differentiated thyroid cancer. Thyroid. 2012; 22(5):501–508

[33] Phang K, Bowman M, Phillips A, Windsor J. Review of thoracic duct anatomical variations and clinical implications. Clin Anat. 2014; 27(4):637–644

[34] Machens A, Hauptmann S, Dralle H. Prediction of lateral lymph node metastases in medullary thyroid cancer. Br J Surg. 2008; 95(5):586–591

[35] Scurry WC, Lamarre E, Stack B. Radioguided neck dissection in recurrent metastatic papillary thyroid carcinoma. Am J Otolaryngol. 2006; 27(1):61–63

[36] Francis CL, Nalley C, Fan C, Bodenner D, Stack BC, Jr. 18F-fluorodeoxyglucose and 131I radioguided surgical management of thyroid cancer. Otolaryngol Head Neck Surg. 2012; 146(1):26–32

[37] Bellotti C, Castagnola G, Tierno SM, et al. Radioguided surgery with combined use of gamma probe and hand-held gamma camera for treatment of papillary thyroid cancer locoregional recurrences: a preliminary study. Eur Rev Med Pharmacol Sci. 2013; 17(24):3362–3366

[38] Møller MN, Sørensen CH. Risk of marginal mandibular nerve injury in neck dissection. Eur Arch Otorhinolaryngol. 2012; 269(2):601–605

[39] Polistena A, Monacelli M, Lucchini R, et al. Surgical morbidity of cervical lymphadenectomy for thyroid cancer: a retrospective cohort study over 25 years. Int J Surg. 2015; 21:128–134

[40] Gacek RR. Neck dissection injury of a brachial plexus anatomical variant. Arch Otolaryngol Head Neck Surg. 1990; 116(3):356–358

[41] Monteiro MJ, Altman K, Khandwala A. Injury to the brachial plexus in neck dissections. Br J Oral Maxillofac Surg. 2010; 48(3):197–198

[42] Prim MP, De Diego JI, Verdaguer JM, Sastre N, Rabanal I. Neurological complications following functional neck dissection. Eur Arch Otorhinolaryngol. 2006; 263(5):473–476

[43] Glenn JA, Yen TW, Fareau GG, Carr AA, Evans DB, Wang TS. Institutional experience with lateral neck dissections for thyroid cancer. Surgery. 2015; 158(4):972–978, discussion 978–980

[44] Roh JL, Kim DH, Park CI. Prospective identification of chyle leakage in patients undergoing lateral neck dissection for metastatic thyroid cancer. Ann Surg Oncol. 2008; 15(2):424–429

[45] Merki V, Pichler J, Giger R, Mantokoudis G. Chylothorax in thyroid surgery: a very rare case and systematic review of the literature. J Otolaryngol Head Neck Surg. 2016; 45(1):52

[46] Quraishi HA, Wax MK, Granke K, Rodman SM. Internal jugular vein thrombosis after functional and selective neck dissection. Arch Otolaryngol Head Neck Surg. 1997; 123(9):969–973

[47] Chen YJ, Wang CP, Wang CC, Jiang RS, Lin JC, Liu SA. Carotid blowout in patients with head and neck cancer: associated factors and treatment outcomes. Head Neck. 2015; 37(2):265–272

[48] Bond KM, Brinjikji W, Murad MH, Cloft HJ, Lanzino G. Endovascular treatment of carotid blowout syndrome. J Vasc Surg. 2017; 65(3):883–888

20 Elective Neck Dissection for Upper Aerodigestive Tract Cancers

Anil K.D. Cruz, Harsh Dhar, and Manish Mair

Abstract

Neck metastasis is an important prognostic factor in head and neck cancers. Elective neck dissection implies prophylactic removal of lymph nodes at the highest risk of metastasis. Incidence and patterns of spread are unique to the different subsites of the upper aerodigestive tract and this has influenced management for decades. There has been a shift in the philosophy with regard to the elective treatment of the neck in upper aerodigestive tract cancers in the recent past with the development of transoral surgical procedures, recognition of a change in the epidemiology of oropharyngeal cancers, but more importantly the emergence of new evidence. This chapter discusses the indications and extent of elective neck dissection in light of the available literature. Issues specific to each subsite are alluded to in distinct sections.

Keywords: neck dissection/methods, mouth neoplasms, laryngeal neoplasms/surgery, pharyngeal neoplasms/surgery

20.1 Introduction

Neck metastasis is one of the most important prognostic factors in head and neck cancers. Its presence even with the smallest of primary cancer upstages the disease to stage III, impacting survival and necessitating the addition of adjuvant therapy. Prognosis worsens with increasing size, number of lymph nodes, as well as the presence of extracapsular spread (ECS).[1] Early detection and appropriate treatment of the neck is therefore of paramount importance. When the primary modality of treatment is surgery, management of the neck could be elective or therapeutic. Elective neck dissection (END) is a nodal dissection procedure performed in a clinico-radiologically node-negative neck. Surgery is usually a selective procedure which entails removal of nodes at the highest risk of metastasis for the index cancer. Nodes harvested at surgery, if they contain metastases, are usually occult in nature. A therapeutic neck dissection (TND) in contrast is a procedure performed when nodal metastases are clinico-radiologically manifested. A TND entails a comprehensive dissection of the neck which usually is a modified neck dissection with removal of all levels of nodes (levels I–V) while preserving nonlymphatic structures (sternocleidomastoid, internal jugular vein, and spinal accessory nerve) unless involved by disease.

The role of END has been a contentious issue in the management of early oral cancers where surgery is the primary treatment modality. With an increasing role of transoral robotic surgery (TORS) and transoral laser microsurgery (TOLM) in oro- and laryngopharyngeal cancers, the role of END has gained attention in recent years.

20.2 Elective Neck Dissection in Oral Cancers

20.2.1 Background

The role of END for early oral cancer has been a debate that has plagued the head and neck community worldwide for over five decades. The primary cancer is usually treated by excision via per-oral route. Controversy surrounds the appropriate management of the neck in this clinical scenario. There are two schools of thought—one in favor of END and the other which proposes a wait and watch (WW) policy followed by TND in patients who develop a nodal relapse.

The proponents of the WW group cite a lack of robust evidence for disease control or survival in favor of performing an END. Furthermore, they state that up to 70% of patients who are true node negative undergo unnecessary surgery with associated morbidity and costs. They believe that intensive follow-up will ensure early detection of nodal relapse and timely salvage without compromise in disease control.

Proponents of END, on the other hand, cite a definite advantage in terms of locoregional control and survival. They allude to the fact that both the neck and the primary tumor are treated at a single stage. Moreover, neck dissection in this scenario is usually a selective procedure and not associated with significant morbidity or prolonged hospitalization. Being a staging procedure, nodal metastasis is identified at an occult stage in contrast to a WW approach, where recurrences are known to present at a higher N stage with possible ECS, necessitating larger surgery, and an increased need for adjuvant treatment with resultant worsening of overall prognosis. Given the fact that published studies had small sample sizes and were predominantly retrospective in nature, the management of the neck in this situation remained in the state of clinical equipoise. This in turn resulted in gross variability in practice across the globe.

Elective neck treatment was generally recommended in patients in whom the probability of occult metastasis was greater than 20%. This was based on the findings of Weiss et al[2] who using a decision tree analysis suggested 20% as the threshold for elective neck treatment. Clinicians therefore attempted to identify patients who were node positive using advances in imaging or at an increased propensity to nodal metastasis using adverse tumor factors as a surrogate. This guided treatment philosophy for the elective treatment of the neck.

20.2.2 Imaging to Predict Nodal Metastasis

Multiple imaging modalities in the form of ultrasonography (USG; with or without guided fine needle aspirate cytology

[FNAC]), computed tomography (CT), magnetic resonance imaging (MRI), and positron emission tomography (PET) have been used in an attempt to accurately stage the neck prior to surgery. The diagnostic accuracy of these various imaging modalities was assessed in a meta-analysis by Liao et al[3] who looked at 32 studies specifically in the node-negative situation. This meta-analysis showed no significant difference in sensitivity and specificity across the various imaging modalities, with the sensitivity ranging between 52 and 66% and the specificity between 78 and 83%. Although CT was seen to be more specific than USG, the overall diagnostic accuracy of the various imaging techniques was more or less similar and no single modality stood out as being the most reliable imaging tool for occult neck metastasis. Similarly, Kyzas et al[4] in a meta-analysis looking at the role of 18 FDG PET concluded that the sensitivity was just 50% in the clinically node-negative neck. In this context, it is pertinent to note that in the recently published Sentinel European Node Trial (SENT)[5] of 415 patients labeled as node negative following an extensive preoperative workup that included either CT and/or MRI with or without USG-guided FNAC, 23% of nodes still turned out to be positive when the sentinel node was examined. This was despite a rigorous workup in a trial setting which would be definitely more intense than in routine clinical practice. Given, therefore, the low sensitivity of imaging in the preoperative setting, this approach did not seem reliable in identifying patients with occult nodal metastasis.

20.2.3 Tumor Characteristics

Various histological factors associated with the primary tumor were used to identify patients at a higher risk for metastasis. While increasing tumor size logically would be the most practical and easiest to use, this often does not hold true with a number of smaller tumors exhibiting biological aggressiveness and an increased risk of metastasis. Tumor grade, thickness, and aggressive histological factors (lymphovascular embolism, perineural invasion) have been described as predictors of occult metastasis in early oral cancers. Among them, the most extensively studied is tumor thickness. Spiro et al[6] conducted a study on tongue and floor of the mouth cancers to look at the predictive value of the tumor thickness. The results showed that the risk of occult nodal metastasis in tumors ≤ 2 mm, 3 to 8 mm, and > 8 mm was 7, 26, and 41%, respectively. They also concluded that disease-related death increases with the increase in tumor thickness. Subsequent studies from different authors corroborated these findings but used different depths as cutoff. In a meta-analysis of 16 studies with 1,136 patients from the published literature, Huang et al[7] looked at the nodal metastasis rates at sequential cutoff points of tumor thickness and found that there was a statistically significant increase in the risk of occult nodal metastasis between 4 and 5 mm (4.5 vs. 16.6%, $p = 0.007$). They thus concluded that the neck should be electively addressed at tumor thickness 4 mm and beyond. The association of PNI and grade with increased risk of nodal metastasis has also been extensively researched. While these pathological features were helpful in identifying patients at risk of metastasis, they were available only on postoperative histopathology, thus limiting their application in preoperative planning.

20.2.4 Previous Attempts to Address the Issue

There have been attempts to address this issue through numerous retrospective studies, as well as prospective randomized controlled trials (RCT). However, all these studies had serious limitations such as small number of patients and varying endpoints to draw meaningful conclusions. In an attempt to overcome these shortcomings, Fasunla et al[8] conducted a meta-analysis on the four RCTs that had been published to date. The findings were in favor of END reducing the risk of disease-specific death. However, even this meta-analysis when critically analyzed seemed to have statistical limitations which included small numbers (283 patients) and wide variations with respect to time periods of accrual, analysis, end points, as well as gross heterogeneity of these studies. Moreover, the findings of one study seemed to be at variance with the others and could have thus influenced results. Given these limitations, therefore, there was still a need for generation of robust level I evidence to address the issue.

20.2.5 Current Evidence in the Management of the N0 Neck

Recently, results of a large single institutional RCT[9] (NCT00193765) with adequate statistical power published by our group demonstrated the benefit of END. The trial initiated in 2004 was designed to demonstrate a 10% increase in overall survival (OS) by an END over the WW policy assuming a baseline 5-year OS of 60%. A total of 596 patients were randomized from trial initiation till June 2014 at which point the Data and Safety Monitoring Committee observing a difference in event rate in the two arms ordered an interim analysis. Out of the 596 patients, 500 who had undergone a minimum of 9 months of follow-up at that point in time were included in the final analysis. The arms were equally balanced for both stratification factors (site, sex, preoperative imaging, and T size) as well as grade, LVE and/or PNI, depth of invasion, and the receipt of adjuvant RT, all factors known to influence outcomes in these patients. The median depth of invasion of patients included was 6 mm indicative of the early nature of patients included in the trial. There was a highly significant difference in the OS (80 vs. 67.5%; $p = 0.014$) and in disease-free survival (DFS; 69.5 vs. 45.9%; $p < 0.001$) in favor of elective neck treatment. This translated into one life being saved for every eight patients (OS difference of 12.5%) and one less recurrence for every four patients (DFS difference of 23.6%) electively operated in this setting. After adjusting for covariates in a cox proportional hazard model for multivariate analysis, the study intervention of END showed a significantly improved OS.

The findings of our study were corroborated in an updated meta-analysis[10] that included the findings of five RCTs of 779 patients. Adjusting for heterogeneity between the trials, this meta-analysis suggested that END at the time of resection of the primary tumor confers an improved DFS and OS in patients with clinically node-negative oral cancer. Thus, with strong level I evidence in favor of END, it should become the standard of care for early-stage node-negative oral cancers. A WW approach results in a statistically significant detriment in OS as well as DFS.

20.2.6 Is the Benefit Seen in all Groups of Patients?

While the OS benefit favors most subgroups, there was a suggestion[9] that patients with thinner tumors less than 3 mm may not benefit from an END. While it is known that thinner tumors would have a lower propensity for neck node metastasis,[6] and therefore fewer event rates, a study would need a very large sample size to conclusively confirm or disprove this issue. Moreover, at present there is no validated method of estimating depth of invasion of tumors preoperatively or at the time of primary surgery. Therefore, it would be safer to offer END to all patients irrespective of the tumor thickness. However, the only time it may seem logical against advocating an END is when a patient seeks opinion after surgery was performed elsewhere with tumor thickness on histopathology not more than 3 mm given the lack of definite evidence of support from published literature.

The other area of contention is whether the results of the benefit of END could be extrapolated to buccal and alveolar cancers, given that the majority of published literature is focused on tongue cancers. The findings of our RCT[9] did show a benefit in favor of buccal mucosa as well, although with lesser statistical power. This could be attributed to the smaller number of patients with buccal cancer randomized on the trial, despite the fact that these cancers are common in our part of the world. Buccal cancers usually need a cheek flap approach for excision or reconstruction, except for a small minority that require entry into the neck; therefore, the neck would be addressed.

20.2.7 Beyond Histopathology—The Use of Molecular Markers

Recently, there has been an interest in the use of gene expression signatures for predicting tumors at an increased risk of nodal metastasis. In a large multicentric cohort[11] using a diagnostic DNA microarray, the negative predictive value of the diagnostic signature on early stage oral cancers was 89%. This study also suggested that the rate of undetected nodal mets would decrease from 28 to 11%. This approach would decrease the rate of overtreatment and avoid the need of unnecessary neck dissections in a significant proportion of patients. While gene expression signatures do show promise, the findings of this initial observation need to be validated in larger patient cohorts and by others before they are incorporated into clinical practice.

20.2.8 Intensity of Follow-up

Nodal relapses in the WW approach are known to present at an advanced stage and are responsible for a poor outcome. This was shown in a study by Andersen et al[12] where despite a regular 3 monthly follow-up, 77% of the patients who were clinically node negative at initial observation had a pathologically adverse feature (N greater than N1 and ECS) at the time of neck dissection. The randomized trial conducted by our group[9] attempted to answer this question by way of a second randomization, as to whether intensifying follow-up by the addition of neck sonography to regular clinical follow-up would detect nodes earlier and impact salvage and survival. In the same cohort of 500 patients with a median follow-up of 39 months, 252 were randomized to clinical examination with USG and 244 to clinical examination alone. A significantly higher proportion of patients had N2–N3 nodes as well as presence of ECS in the WW arm. The findings of this study revealed that neck ultrasound confers no survival advantage over recommended clinical examination ($p = 0.89$). Cox regression analysis continued to demonstrate the overriding benefit of END ($p = 0.02$).[13]

20.2.9 Extent of Neck Dissection in the Elective Setting

Numerous publications have revealed that the highest risk of occult metastasis in oral cancers is at levels I to III. In a retrospective study of 967 patients who underwent a selective neck dissection, Byers[14] concluded that the supraomohyoid neck dissection (levels I–III) was adequate for all pN0 oral cancer patients and for selected p N1 in the absence of ECS. In a subsequent publication, the same group of authors[15] reported a 15.8% incidence of skip metastasis and advocated an extended supraomohyoid neck dissection encompassing levels I to IV particularly for tongue cancers. However, this publication had inherent flaws and the true incidence of isolated level IV metastasis was less than 5%. An RCT conducted by the Brazilian Head and Neck Group[16] showed the safety of a supraomohyoid neck dissection in the node-negative setting and there was no need to do more than a levels I to III clearance. Dissection of level IV as advocated by some is without evidence and unnecessary dissection, particularly when done in the left neck, runs the risk of chyle duct injury.

Supraomohyoid dissection is known to be associated with shoulder dysfunction. This has been attributed to excessive handling and clearance of the lymph nodes in and around the accessory nerve (level IIb). There has been interest in the recent past at attempts to avoid dissection of this nodal basin which in turn would result in safeguarding the accessory nerve and better shoulder function. Paleri et al[17] in a meta-analysis of 904 patients reported that metastasis to the level IIb was seen only in 3.4% of oral cancer patients.

To address these issues, our group conducted a study[18] evaluating the pattern of nodal metastasis in early oral cancers. This was a prospective study of 583 neck dissections, the surgical procedure performed by the same group of authors where nodal stations were harvested on table and sent in separate prelabeled containers for pathological assessment ensuring accuracy of reporting metastatic patterns. It was observed that 91% of nodal metastasis was concentrated at levels I to III, and 96% at levels I to IV. Skip metastasis was most commonly seen in tongue cancers at level III (17.5%). However, skip metastasis to levels IV and V were never observed in the absence of metastasis to levels I to III. Multivariate analysis identified the presence of level IIa as the single most important factor to predict metastasis at level IIb. The study also showed that positive levels IIb and III are statistically significant factors predicting level V metastasis. From this large prospective study, it would be reasonable to conclude that clearance of levels I to III is adequate in the clinically node-negative neck. Dissection in and around level IIb could be avoided in the absence of metastasis to level IIa.

20.2.10 Role of Sentinel Node Biopsy

Sentinel node biopsy (SNB) is a well-established procedure particularly for cancers of the breast and melanoma. It has been shown to be fairly accurate in these cancers avoiding the morbidity associated with nodal dissection of the axilla and groin. Conceptually extrapolating these findings to the elective management of the neck is attractive and would result in better function and cosmetic outcomes and therefore has been tried in head and neck cancers (see Chapter 21). Results of the largest multicenter, prospective (SENT) trial[5] which included 415 patients from 14 European centers showed a sensitivity of 86% with a high negative predictive value of 95%. In a subsequent meta-analysis by Liu et al[19] of 66 studies including data from the SENT trial composing of 3,566 patients with cT1–T2 N0 OSCC, the pooled sentinel node identification rate was 96.3% (95% CI: 95.3–97.0%). The pooled sensitivity was 0.87 (95% CI: 0.85 ± 0.89), pooled negative predictive value was 0.94 (95% CI: 0.93 ± 0.95), and AUC was 0.98 (95% CI: 0.97 ± 0.99). Thus, SNB is an efficient diagnostic tool to detect occult nodal metastasis with a high negative predictive value. Given that the failure rate of around 6% following a SNB is similar to that of an END, it is unlikely to be an RCT comparing the two. If such a trial is needed to be done with a noninferiority randomized controlled design, the minimum number of patients required would be over 1,000, with a conservative margin of 7%. Other endpoints would therefore have to be used such as function, costs, and time of procedure. Given that SNB has a steep learning curve, needs a nuclear medicine facility, and requires immunohistochemistry and serial step sectioning of the sentinel node and a second surgery if the node is positive, it is unlikely to replace selective neck dissection as standard of care. Performing an END with an appropriately placed scar in a skin crease and avoidance of excessive handling of the accessory nerve at level IIb seems to be a reasonable alternative rather than an SNB in light of its above limitations. However, the SNB continues to be an approach practiced by some centers in Europe.

20.2.11 Elective Management of the Contralateral Neck

Unilateral neck dissection is done for well lateralized lesions, while bilateral neck dissection is recommended for lesions that cross the midline. Debate surrounds the management of the contralateral neck in lesions that approach the midline. A study conducted by our group[20] consisting of 243 tongue cancer patients identified the involvement of the contralateral neck in this situation. The overall incidence of contralateral nodal metastasis was seen in 71 (29%) patients. Importantly 69 patients (97%) had ipsilateral nodal metastasis. The findings of this study confirm that contralateral nodal metastasis is extremely rare in a negative ipsilateral neck and therefore need not be treated electively.

20.3 Elective Neck Dissection for Pharyngeal and Laryngeal Cancers

While surgery forms the mainstay of treatment for oral cancers, radiation/chemoradiation is often the primary treatment modality in tumors of the larynx and pharynx, largely due to the impact on function and cosmesis associated with surgical procedures. Evolution of the minimally invasive techniques of TOLM and TORS resulted in many of these patients being considered for surgery. As the neck is not violated while addressing the primary tumor in these procedures, the role of elective management of the neck needs to be reviewed.

20.3.1 Oropharyngeal Cancers

Background

There has been a steep rise in the prevalence of oropharyngeal cancers in the last decade with the recognition of the human papilloma virus as a significant epidemiological risk factor.[21] Given the morbidity associated with open surgeries, management of oropharyngeal cancers has traditionally been nonsurgical (radiation/chemoradiation). However, there has been a recent recognition that these nonsurgical treatments were also associated with significant late toxicities in as high as 43% of patients.[22] These included pharyngeal dysfunction in 27%, laryngeal dysfunction in 12%, and 13% of patients being feeding tube dependent primarily due to the radiation effects on the pharyngeal constrictors and larynx. Simultaneously it was found that these cancers are biologically different and associated with a better prognosis raising the possibility of downstaging these cancers as well as decreasing the intensity of treatment.[23] It therefore seemed conceptually attractive to factor surgery into the treatment algorithm and decrease the dose of chemoradiation, thus avoiding serious consequences. The possibility of resection of these cancers, with the advent of TORS, with good oncological outcomes as well as preservation of swallowing function made this possible.[24] Given that these procedures were performed via the mouth without violation of the neck, appropriate management of the neck in the node-negative situation needed to be considered.

Incidence of Occult Neck Metastasis and Extent of Elective Neck Dissection

The oropharynx is a lymphatic-rich region with a high predilection for nodal spread. The incidence of occult nodal metastasis even in small T1–T2 tumors is as high as 25 to 30%.[25] This therefore necessitates addressing the neck electively for clinically node-negative tumors.

Extent of Elective Neck Dissection

Levels II to IV are the first echelon of nodal spread in oropharyngeal cancers.[25] Isolated skip metastasis to level IV is rare. In addition, the levels I and V were involved only in the presence of positive nodes at other levels. This finding is consistent across most reported series with isolated level I metastasis being negligible.[26] Thus, it would be logical to address levels II to IV when the neck is being addressed. Some centers advocate only dissection of levels II and III avoiding dissection of level IV if these stations are negative. This is done with the aim to prevent postoperative chyle leak, particularly in left neck dissection.[26] Both sides of the neck need to be addressed electively when the tumor approaches the midline as well as for centrally located tumors since the incidence of bilateral nodal metastasis is high. Moore et al have also recommended addressing the contralateral neck electively for posterior tonsillar involvement citing spread via the retropharyngeal route with the incidence of contralateral nodal metastasis to be as high as 22%.[27] The presence of occult contralateral nodal metastasis has also been reported to be high in the presence of multiple positive ipsilateral nodes. Therefore, addressing the contralateral neck electively is advised in the presence of midline tumors (base tongue, soft palate, and posterior pharyngeal wall), lesions crossing the midline or involving the posterior tonsillar pillar and in the presence of ipsilateral positive nodes.

Timing of Elective Neck Dissection in Oropharyngeal Cancers

Neck dissection at the time of the TORS procedure is known to be associated with pharyngocutaneous fistula, particularly when the submandibular triangle and level II are dissected. This has prompted some to suggest an interval neck dissection rather than simultaneously at the time of resection of the primary. In a meta-analysis of 12 series on TORS for oropharyngeal cancer, of 654 neck dissections, 61% were concurrent while 39% were staged neck dissections.[24] The overall rate of pharyngocutaneous fistulae in this meta-analysis was 2.5%. Moore et al in their series of 148 patients similarly reported intraoperative pharyngocutaneous communications in 29% of patients which were all addressed at the time of surgery with only 4% subsequently developing subcutaneous fluid accumulation in the postoperative period. Given that the incidence of pharyngocutaneous fistula after on-table repair is low, simultaneous neck dissection along with the primary may be safely performed. In a retrospective comparative analysis,[28] there was no reported difference in oncological outcomes or postoperative complications between those who underwent concurrent neck dissection and those who underwent staged neck dissection. Moreover, the duration of hospital stay was also significantly longer in the group that underwent staged neck dissection (median stay of 15 vs. 8 days). Given the lack of consensus in support of either approach, the timing of neck dissection with TORS for oropharyngeal cancers is still a matter of debate with the majority, however, favoring a simultaneous approach. Interestingly, those who recommend interval neck dissection cite that there is a potential logistical advantage of scheduling more robotic procedures per day in the operating room.[28]

20.3.2 Laryngeal and Hypopharyngeal Cancers

Background

The development of the TOLM procedure resulted in a shift in the treatment philosophy of early laryngopharyngeal cancers (particularly for glottic tumors) in the last two decades. The primary could be excised via the oral route and was shown to be oncologically safe in a number of reported series. Given the fact that surgery required a single sitting, without significant alteration in function and that radiation could be avoided, there was an increasing acceptance of TOLM procedures particularly among European centers. The need to electively address the neck thus became a consideration in a subset of these patients.

Treatment philosophy in the management of the neck in this situation is again dictated by the probability of the development of nodal metastasis. Given the fact that the glottis has sparse lymphatics and the incidence of neck metastasis is less than 5% for early lesions,[29] elective dissection is not recommended if the neck is clinically and radiographically negative. On the contrary, supraglottis and hypopharynx are lymphatic-rich areas with a high (30–40%) incidence of occult nodal metastasis even in early (T1, T2) cancers.[25,29] END is thus warranted for early cancers in these locations when the primary tumor is surgically addressed.

The Extent of Elective Neck Dissection in Laryngo-Hypopharyngeal Tumors

Neck metastasis in laryngo-hypopharyngeal cancers predominantly occurs to levels II to IV.[25,29] In contrast, the occurrence of metastasis to levels I and V was seen only in the presence of nodal metastasis at other levels and never in isolation. Thus, performing an END of the jugular group of nodes (II–IV) is considered oncologically safe in a cN0 neck.

The Contralateral Neck

The contralateral neck needs to be electively addressed in situations where the disease is proximal to or has crossed the midline. In well-lateralized lesions, the incidence of contralateral occult neck nodes is minimal (< 5%)[25,29] and need not be addressed if the ipsilateral neck is negative. However, the presence of metastasis to the ipsilateral neck is associated with a high risk of contralateral nodal disease, thus necessitating an elective contralateral neck dissection in these cases.

Timing of Neck Dissection in Laryngeal and Hypopharyngeal Cancers

As with oropharyngeal cancers, there is debate as to whether END should be simultaneous or as an interval procedure. Proponents of the staged procedure cite the possibility of in-transit metastasis within lymphatics which might not be addressed if the neck is addressed simultaneously resulting in a higher incidence of regional recurrence.[30] Performing a staged neck dissection, therefore, would ensure comprehensive clearance of these nodes and ensure better locoregional control. In addition, there is a possibility of an increased incidence of pharyngocutaneous fistula, particularly for resections of hypopharyngeal cancers. A theoretical possibility of improved healing of the raw surface with better swallowing outcomes has also been postulated if the neck is addressed in a staged manner. Given the lack of evidence in favor of either timing of neck dissection in this situation, it is usually dictated by individual treatment philosophies. Fortunately, the majority of these patients are treated by radiation/chemoradiation protocols given the complexity of resection of supraglottic and hypopharyngeal cancers and, therefore, timing of addressing the neck is a moot issue.

Addressing Level IIb in Oro- and Laryngopharyngeal Cancers

Recent recognition of shoulder morbidity associated with dissection of level IIb (supraspinal region) has raised the debate as to the need of dissection of this area in order to minimize handling of the accessory nerve. Paleri et al, in a systematic review of 14 studies, found a low incidence of isolated metastasis to level IIb (5.2% in oropharyngeal and 0.3% in laryngeal tumors).[17] They suggested that there appears to be no advantage in performing dissection in this area, particularly for laryngeal primaries. Thus, aggressive dissection in the region of level IIb may not be necessary in the elective setting for node-negative necks.

20.4 Conclusion

Elective dissection of the neck should be standard of care whenever surgery is preferred as the primary modality of treatment. This is because of the strong level I evidence in its favor and the limitations of identifying patients at a higher propensity of neck metastasis preoperatively in those with early oral cancers. For oropharyngeal and laryngopharyngeal cancers, END is safer, as these are lymphatic-rich areas with a high propensity to metastasis. Early glottis cancers are the only exception being devoid of lymphatics. The nodal levels needed to be addressed during an END are guided by the site of the primary tumor and nodal basins at the highest risk for metastasis. Debate still surrounds the decision between interval and simultaneous neck dissection at the time of transoral procedures for oro- and laryngopharyngeal cancers. Decision is based on individual institutional preference with the majority, however, performing neck dissection at the time of primary surgery.

References

[1] Wreesmann VB, Katabi N, Palmer FL, et al. Influence of extracapsular nodal spread extent on prognosis of oral squamous cell carcinoma. Head Neck. 2016; 38 Suppl 1:E1192–E1199

[2] Weiss MH, Harrison LB, Isaacs RS. Use of decision analysis in planning a management strategy for the stage N0 neck. Arch Otolaryngol Head Neck Surg. 1994; 120(7):699–702

[3] Liao L-J, Lo W-C, Hsu W-L, Wang C-T, Lai M-S. Detection of cervical lymph node metastasis in head and neck cancer patients with clinically N0 neck-a meta-analysis comparing different imaging modalities. BMC Cancer. 2012; 12:236

[4] Kyzas PA, Evangelou E, Denaxa-Kyza D, Ioannidis JPA. 18F-fluorodeoxyglucose positron emission tomography to evaluate cervical node metastases in patients with head and neck squamous cell carcinoma: a meta-analysis. J Natl Cancer Inst. 2008; 100(10):712–720

[5] Schilling C, Stoeckli SJ, Haerle SK, et al. Sentinel European Node Trial (SENT): 3-year results of sentinel node biopsy in oral cancer. Eur J Cancer. 2015; 51 (18):2777–2784

[6] Spiro RH, Huvos AG, Wong GY, Spiro JD, Gnecco CA, Strong EW. Predictive value of tumor thickness in squamous carcinoma confined to the tongue and floor of the mouth. Am J Surg. 1986; 152(4):345–350

[7] Huang SH, Hwang D, Lockwood G, Goldstein DP, O'Sullivan B. Predictive value of tumor thickness for cervical lymph-node involvement in squamous cell carcinoma of the oral cavity: a meta-analysis of reported studies. Cancer. 2009; 115(7):1489–1497

[8] Fasunla AJ, Greene BH, Timmesfeld N, Wiegand S, Werner JA, Sesterhenn AM. A meta-analysis of the randomized controlled trials on elective neck dissection versus therapeutic neck dissection in oral cavity cancers with clinically node-negative neck. Oral Oncol. 2011; 47(5):320–324

[9] D'Cruz AK, Vaish R, Kapre N, et al. Head and Neck Disease Management Group. Elective versus therapeutic neck dissection in node-negative oral cancer. N Engl J Med. 2015; 373(6):521–529

[10] Ren Z-H, Xu J-L, Li B, Fan T-F, Ji T, Zhang C-P. Elective versus therapeutic neck dissection in node-negative oral cancer: evidence from five randomized controlled trials. Oral Oncol. 2015; 51(11):976–981

[11] van Hooff SR, Leusink FKJ, Roepman P, et al. Validation of a gene expression signature for assessment of lymph node metastasis in oral squamous cell carcinoma. J Clin Oncol. 2012; 30(33):4104–4110

[12] Andersen PE, Cambronero E, Shaha AR, Shah JP. The extent of neck disease after regional failure during observation of the N0 neck. Am J Surg. 1996; 172 (6):689–691

[13] D'Cruz A, Vaish R, Gupta S, et al. Does addition of neck ultrasonography to physical examination, in follow-up of patients with early stage, clinically node negative oral cancers, influence outcome? A randomized control trial (RCT). J Clin Oncol. 2016; 34(15) Suppl:6020–6020

[14] Byers RM. Modified neck dissection. A study of 967 cases from 1970 to 1980. Am J Surg. 1985; 150(4):414–421

[15] Byers RM, Weber RS, Andrews T, McGill D, Kare R, Wolf P. Frequency and therapeutic implications of "skip metastases" in the neck from squamous carcinoma of the oral tongue. Head Neck. 1997; 19(1):14–19

[16] Brazilian Head and Neck Cancer Study Group. Results of a prospective trial on elective modified radical classical versus supraomohyoid neck dissection in the management of oral squamous carcinoma. Am J Surg. 1998; 176(5):422–427

[17] Paleri V, Kumar Subramaniam S, Oozeer N, Rees G, Krishnan S. Dissection of the submuscular recess (sublevel IIb) in squamous cell cancer of the upper aerodigestive tract: prospective study and systematic review of the literature. Head Neck. 2008; 30(2):194–200

[18] Pantvaidya GH, Pal P, Vaidya AD, Pai PS, D'Cruz AK. Prospective study of 583 neck dissections in oral cancers: implications for clinical practice. Head Neck. 2014; 36(10):1503–1507

[19] Liu M, Wang SJ, Yang X, Peng H. Diagnostic efficacy of sentinel lymph node biopsy in early oral squamous cell carcinoma: a meta-analysis of 66 studies. PLoS One. 2017; 12(1):e0170322

[20] Singh B, Nair S, Nair D, Patil A, Chaturvedi P, D'Cruz AK. Ipsilateral neck nodal status as predictor of contralateral nodal metastasis in carcinoma of tongue crossing the midline. Head Neck. 2013; 35(5):649–652

[21] Chaturvedi AK, Engels EA, Pfeiffer RM, et al. Human papillomavirus and rising oropharyngeal cancer incidence in the United States. J Clin Oncol. 2011; 29 (32):4294–4301

[22] Machtay M, Moughan J, Trotti A, et al. Factors associated with severe late toxicity after concurrent chemoradiation for locally advanced head and neck cancer: an RTOG analysis. J Clin Oncol. 2008; 26(21):3582–3589

[23] Ang KK, Harris J, Wheeler R, et al. Human papillomavirus and survival of patients with oropharyngeal cancer. N Engl J Med. 2010; 363(1):24–35

[24] de Almeida JR, Byrd JK, Wu R, et al. A systematic review of transoral robotic surgery and radiotherapy for early oropharynx cancer: a systematic review. Laryngoscope. 2014; 124(9):2096–2102

[25] Candela FC, Kothari K, Shah JP. Patterns of cervical node metastases from squamous carcinoma of the oropharynx and hypopharynx. Head Neck. 1990; 12 (3):197–203

[26] Van Abel KM, Moore EJ. Focus issue: neck dissection for oropharyngeal squamous cell carcinoma. ISRN Surg. 2012; 2012:547–017

[27] Moore EJ, Olsen KD, Martin EJ. Concurrent neck dissection and transoral robotic surgery. Laryngoscope. 2011; 121(3):541–544

[28] Möckelmann N, Busch C-J, Münscher A, Knecht R, Lörincz BB. Timing of neck dissection in patients undergoing transoral robotic surgery for head and neck cancer. Eur J Surg Oncol. 2015; 41(6):773–778

[29] Candela FC, Shah J, Jaques DP, Shah JP. Patterns of cervical node metastases from squamous carcinoma of the larynx. Arch Otolaryngol Head Neck Surg. 1990; 116(4):432–435

[30] Steiner W, Ambrosch P. Endoscopic Laser Surgery of the Upper Aerodigestive Tract: With Special Emphasis on Cancer Surgery. Thieme; 2000: (Expert Opinion-Book, 5)

21 Sentinel Node Dissection

Francisco Civantos and Samuel J. Trosman

Abstract

The technology and indications for sentinel node dissection have continued to expand over the last several years. It is used routinely for intermediate thickness melanoma and Merkel cell carcinoma, and has been used for cutaneous squamous cell carcinoma of the head and neck. Sentinel node biopsy has been shown to be a reliable staging technique for intermediate thickness oral cavity cancer, with sensitivity and negative predictive value rates mirroring those for melanoma. Its use in pharyngeal and laryngeal cancer continues to be investigated. The use of ⁹⁹ᵐTc tilmanocept, a CD206 receptor target, allows for more specificity for the first echelon sentinel lymph nodes and may result in improved accuracy and a lower false-negative rate. The widespread availability and accuracy of combined SPECT/CT imaging provides a scrollable three-dimensional analysis of the drainage basins, resulting in better targeted dissections and patient counseling. Despite these technological advances, the use of the gamma probe for sentinel node dissection is not always intuitive and requires specific training and expertise, especially in cutaneous lesions that show frequent metastases to the parotid gland. Serial step sectioning and immunohistochemistry analysis are critical to the detection of micrometastases. Intraoperative frozen section analysis has also shown great promise for identifying sentinel nodes in oral cavity squamous cell carcinoma, allowing for completion lymphadenectomy in the same setting. Sentinel node biopsy and dissection remains an intriguing prognostic and potentially therapeutic option for malignancies with an intermediate risk of regional metastases, with increased diagnostic information compared to watchful waiting with serial imaging but sparing the morbidity of a full elective neck dissection in patients who end up with microscopically negative lymphatic basins.

Keywords: melanoma, oral cavity squamous cell carcinoma, lymphoscintigraphy, gamma probe, tilmanocept, SPECT, immunohistochemistry

21.1 Introduction

Management of the clinically node-negative neck in patients with early-stage head and neck cancer remains controversial. A significant body of literature, culminating in a recent randomized trial, has proven there is significant risk of decreased survival and increased morbidity with a watchful waiting/observational approach for lesions with a relatively high (> 15%) rate of regional metastasis.[1] However, this must be balanced with the morbidity of systematic cervical lymphadenectomy, which may include temporary or permanent lower lip weakness, shoulder dysfunction, lymphedema, chyle leak, and a long list of rarer neurological and vascular complications. This dilemma is magnified for lesions that approximate the midline, where bilateral neck dissections are under consideration.

Sentinel node dissection and biopsy (SNB) involves the integration of radiologic and surgical techniques. While lymphoscintigraphy can be used alone for anatomic mapping of the

drainage pathways of a lesion, evaluation of the true histopathological status of the lymph node is the only strategy for detection of micrometastases. Cross-sectional imaging studies such as computed tomography (CT), magnetic resonance imaging (MRI), and fused positron emission tomography (PET)/CT continue to improve in their sensitivity for regional lymphatic spread; however, they generally will not reliably identify metastatic disease less than 1 cm in size, and will almost never detect micrometastases less than 5 mm in size.

Morton et al reintroduced the concept of sentinel node biopsy to surgical practice in publications describing the technical details and their early prospective clinical experience in patients with clinically N0 cutaneous malignant melanoma.[2,3] After injection of vital blue dye at the primary site, 259 sentinel nodes were identified in 194 of 237 lymphatic nodal basins, and the incidence of false-negative sentinel nodes (i.e., the identified sentinel node is found to be disease free when metastatic disease is present in the regional lymphatic vessels) was less than 1%. The model of initial sentinel node biopsy with detailed pathologic analysis followed by completion dissection if positive has been subsequently validated for multiple head and neck subsites.

Based on the work of Krag and Alex et al,[4,5] modern sentinel node biopsy has been performed using peritumoral intradermal injections of radiotracers such as unfiltered technetium 99 m (⁹⁹ᵐTc) sulfur colloid and intraoperative gamma detection probes. This combined modality allows placement of the biopsy incision directly over the radiolabeled sentinel node(s), with dissection aimed directly at the most radioactive node without disturbance of surrounding tissues. Sentinel node biopsy in melanoma using the gamma probe resulted in retrieval of sentinel nodes in over 80% of cases, with a very low incidence of false negatives.[6,7] Sentinel node retrieval has continued to improve to approximate 99% in more recent studies. In addition, nearly all authors have reported occasional unusual drainage patterns that would have been missed in standard cervical lymphadenectomy, particularly unexpected bilateral drainage for lateralized lesions, "skip" drainage to a more distant node in a group than might be anticipated, and drainage to multiple lymph node groups in the neck.

As has occurred in clinically node-negative melanoma, sentinel node biopsy ultimately offers the possibility of identifying those patients with clinically N0 carcinomas of the other head and neck subsites, including aerodigestive tract sites, who harbor occult metastases in the cervical lymphatics. At this point, it has primarily been applied in the more accessible oral cavity site. It is important that an established negative predictive value (NPV) and false-negative rate (FNR) be available for each tumor type before incorporating it into routine clinical practice. In particular, the NPV is an important value that might be used in the informed consent process for an appropriate patient who might truly not harbor disease in his neck. The NPV for a particular tumor type should estimate the risk that a patient would recur in the neck after a negative sentinel node biopsy. Since selective neck dissection is an excellent technique for staging the cervical lymphatics, with moderate but generally acceptable morbidity, it is important that quality data be generated before accepting the less invasive sentinel node biopsy approach. On the other hand, particularly for oral cancer, patients presenting with relatively superficial lesions, perhaps estimated to be 1 to 3 mm in thickness, for which the cervical lymphatics would often be observed, sentinel node biopsy may theoretically represent a more aggressive approach for those who desire a more intense evaluation of the lymph nodes relative to what is currently standard.

21.2 Sentinel Node Biopsy for Cutaneous Malignancies

21.2.1 Melanoma

Reports from multiple large-volume centers have shown the benefit of sentinel node biopsy for patients with invasive, intermediate-risk clinically node-negative melanoma. This led to the creation of a phase III prospective trial termed the "Multicenter Selective Lymphadenectomy Trial (MSLT-1)," which randomized 2,001 patients with cutaneous melanoma of all subsites to either (1) wide excision and observation, with lymphadenectomy for nodal recurrence, or (2) wide excision and sentinel node biopsy, with immediate lymphadenectomy for positive nodal disease. Among patients whose lymphatic basins turned out to harbor micrometastases, in those with intermediate thickness (Breslow depth: 1.2–3.5 mm) melanomas, sentinel node biopsy significantly improved mean 10-year disease-free survival (71.3 vs. 64.7%), as well as rates of 10-year distant disease-free survival (hazard ratio: 0.62) and melanoma-specific survival (hazard ratio: 0.56). In addition, again only for those who actually harbored lymphatic metastases, sentinel node biopsy improved mean 10-year disease-free survival in patients with thick (>3.5 mm) cutaneous melanoma (50.7 vs. 40.5%).[8] National Comprehensive Cancer Network (NCCN) guidelines currently recommend sentinel node biopsy for N0 patients with cutaneous melanoma thickness of 0.76 to 1 mm and either ulceration or mitotic rate of ≥ 1 per mm^2, and for all N0 patients with melanoma of thickness of greater than 1 mm.[9]

More recently, the second Multicenter Selective Lymphadenectomy Trial (MSLT-2) was performed in an effort to evaluate the utility of completion lymphadenectomy in patients with intermediate thickness cutaneous melanoma and positive SNB. A total of 1,934 patients with positive SNB were randomized to either (1) immediate completion lymphadenectomy or (2) observation with ultrasound. Patients with immediate lymphadenectomy had an increased rate of regional control (mean: 92 vs. 77%) and a slightly higher disease-free survival (mean: 68 vs. 63%), but had a nearly equivalent rate of melanoma-specific survival (86% in both groups). The authors suggest that any survival benefit from early surgery may occur in patients with disease limited to the sentinel nodes. The prognostic value of completion lymphadenectomy has to be weighed against the risk of complications, as MSLT-II showed a significant increase in the incidence of lymphedema (24.1 vs. 6.3%) in the lymph node dissection group.[10] No anatomic subsite data were provided in this study. However, given the importance of avoiding the local effects of regional recurrence in the head and neck, and to a lesser degree the lymphedema that occurs relative to

extremity melanoma, most authors still advocate completion lymphadenectomy for positive sentinel nodes in the head and neck region.

21.2.2 Merkel Cell Carcinoma

Merkel cell carcinoma is a rare, aggressive neuroendocrine cutaneous malignancy that frequently arises in the head and neck. While increasing tumor size appears to be the main risk factor for lymphatic spread, even small (< 2 cm) lesions have high rates of regional metastases. Although there is conflicting evidence regarding a survival benefit to sentinel node biopsy in Merkel cell carcinoma, NCCN guidelines currently recommend SNB for all clinical N0 tumors due to improved prognostic information on regional control.[11] Adjuvant radiation therapy appears to be associated with improved survival, and can be considered as an alternative to completion lymphadenectomy in sentinel node–positive patients.[12] For larger, deeper lesions, elective lymphadenectomy should be considered, as the rate of sentinel node positivity is exceedingly high.[13]

21.2.3 Cutaneous Squamous Cell Carcinoma

The role of sentinel node biopsy in the treatment of cutaneous squamous cell carcinoma remains unclear. The NCCN recommends the consideration of SNB in certain high-risk lesions, "although the benefit of and indication for this technique has yet to be proven."[14] Systematic reviews have shown positive and negative predictive values of over 90%, with similar FNRs to that of melanoma.[15,16] However, larger prospective trials are needed to validate the technique in this patient population. Most importantly, appropriate selection criteria delineating which squamous cell carcinomas are appropriate for the sentinel node procedure need to be identified.

21.3 Sentinel Node Biopsy in Oral Cavity and Aerodigestive Tract Malignancies

Aerodigestive tract malignancies show an increased propensity for regional metastases, especially lesions with high-risk features such as size greater than 2 cm, thickness greater than 3 to 4 mm, angiolymphatic invasion, and perineural invasion. Several analyses have shown a survival benefit to the prophylactic treatment of the N0 neck in early-stage head and neck squamous cell carcinoma (HNSCC), including a recent prospective trial that showed improved survival in patients with stage I/II lateralized oral cavity cancers who received unilateral elective neck dissection versus those who were observed and underwent therapeutic neck dissection if/when they developed N+ disease.[1] The risk of occult metastases must be weighed against the morbidity of neck dissections for patients, many of who will not have pathologic neck disease. Sentinel node biopsy offers a diagnostic technique to identify subclinical cervical metastases and is ideal for situations where the expected risk of metastases falls in the 5 to 15% range, which might be too high to feel comfortable with observation but too low to justify a full selective neck dissection. It also may be particularly useful for patients with stage 1 lesions of borderline size and thickness that approximate the midline, for whom the morbidity of bilateral neck dissection for clinically and radiologically negative cervical lymphatic basins is difficult to justify.

Multiple centers in the United States and Europe initiated single-institution trials of sentinel node biopsy for upper aerodigestive tract malignancies in the 1990s and 2000s, mostly for oral cavity cancer, as this is the most accessible subsite, though some included oropharyngeal lesions as well. Studies consistently reported NPVs of 95 to 100%, similar to the rates seen in cutaneous melanoma. They also described unexpected patterns of lymphatic drainage, including unexpected contralateral drainage, and upstaging made possible by the identification of micrometastases via fine sectioning and immunohistochemistry (IHC) in 10 to 20% of cases.[17]

The importance of appropriate step sectioning and IHC of sentinel nodes to the accuracy of the technique has been emphasized in nearly every study. Christensen et al in 2010 performed an exhaustive step sectioning and IHC at 150 µm of the numerous nonsentinel nodes in their completion neck dissections from their validation trial after initial SNB and subsequent lymphadenectomy showed extremely low rates of additional occult metastases. In no case, with the additional fine sectioning of nonsentinel nodes, did they find a micrometastasis in a nonsentinel node in a patient with negative sentinel nodes.[18] Only in one case with a positive sentinel node and positive nonsentinel node by routine technique was an additional micrometastasis found. This study validates the current algorithm of fine sectioning of sentinel nodes with IHC and routine analysis of nonsentinel nodes. In addition, in another review, Jefferson et al performed reexamination of 35 negative sentinel nodes from 10 patients and sectioned the nodes at 150 µm rather than the original 2-mm sections. In this study, they did not find any additional microcarcinomas, suggesting that the additional yield of finer than 2-mm sectioning is small.[19] Clearly an additional micrometastasis may occasionally be found, and this infrequent occurrence could make a major difference for a patient. Currently, 150 µm sectioning is standard practice in Europe, but in North America the labor intensity of this practice is felt unjustifiable by most pathology departments, and 2-mm thick sections are more common.

The first large European multicenter trial evaluating the accuracy of SNB for HNSCC was published in 2010. A total of 227 SNB procedures were carried out on 134 patients; 79 patients underwent SNB alone, while 55 underwent sentinel node-assisted neck dissection. The authors reported a 93% successful sentinel node identification rate, with a 95% NPV for sentinel node biopsy. Patients receiving SNB did not have significantly different long-term survival compared to patients receiving elective neck dissection, prompting the authors to conclude that SNB is a viable alternative to lymphadenectomy in N0 patients with early-stage HNSCC. There was concern that the technique was problematic for floor of the mouth tumors, as four of the five false negatives came from these patients.[20]

In order to formally validate sentinel node biopsy for oral cavity cancer, an NCI-funded trial was completed in North America under the auspices of the American College of Surgeons Oncology Group (ACOSOG). One-hundred forty patients with T1 or T2 clinically N0 oral cancer underwent

lymphoscintigraphy with [99mTc] sulfur colloid, nuclear imaging, and narrow-exposure SNB followed by immediate completion neck dissection. SNB with step sectioning and IHC had an NPV of 96% for all tumors, and an NPV of 100% for T1 tumors. The FNR was 9.8%. Investigators were categorized as experts who came in with significant numbers of cases versus intermediate users who took the animal course and were trained on the protocol. None of the false negatives occurred in the expert group of investigators on this study.[21]

Based on the strong validation data, it has been felt that it was appropriate to transition to sentinel node biopsy as primary neck management, in a research setting, for appropriately selected cases. A meta-analysis of 21 pooled validation studies and 847 patients showed an overall sensitivity of 93% for SNB.[22] Techniques have been reported for accurate SNB for squamous cell carcinoma in the floor of mouth, alleviating a prior concern. These techniques do involve more extensive level I dissection to separate the lymphatic basins from the primary tumor. In 2015, the results of the EORTC-approved Sentinel European Node Trial (SENT) with SNB as primary neck management in oral cancer, with neck dissection for positive sentinel nodes only, was published. This was the first prospective trial to use SNB as the sole staging procedure in oral cancer, without concurrent END. Four-hundred fifteen patients with T1–2N0 HNSCC underwent SNB followed by neck dissection within 3 weeks if positive. A sentinel node was detected in 99.5% of cases; 109 of the 415 patients (26%) had occult metastases. SNB showed a sensitivity of 86% and an NPV of 95%. The disease-free survival for the cohort was 92%, prompting the authors to confirm SNB as a safe oncologic procedure. Unexpected contralateral lymphatic drainage occurred in 12% of cases, with seven positive contralateral sentinel nodes that would have been missed with an en-bloc unilateral neck dissection. The FNR was higher than expected at 14%, which is likely related to technical issues in a multi-institutional trial consisting of a large group of surgeons with a variety of techniques and experience levels. The authors in their discussion imply that this number would come down with continued refinements in technique.[23]

Multiple single institution studies looking at SNB with completion neck dissection only for positive sentinel nodes have also been completed concurrent with this trial and are detailed in ▶ Table 21.1.[24,25,26,27] All studies report acceptable NPV, and several larger trials report significantly lower FNRs, in the range of 6 to 9%, indicating that technical factors may explain some of the variations in data. It should be mentioned that in smaller series with few positive sentinel nodes, one false negative could skew the FNR tremendously.

Table 21.1 Studies with sentinel nodes as primary neck management ($n > 50$ included)

Study	n	NPV (%)	FNR (%)
Pezier et al[24] (2012)	59	97.5	6
SENT trial[23] (2015)	415	95	14
Pedersen et al[25] et al (2016)	258	95	5
Flach et al[26] (2014)	62	88	20
Broglie et al[27] (2011)	51	96	6

Abbreviations: FNR, false-negative rate; NPV, negative predictive value.

21.4 Surgical Technique: Practical Guidelines

21.4.1 Patient Selection

An appropriate patient for sentinel node dissection is one with a small, injectable lesion that carries a significant risk of lymphatic micrometastases but a relatively low risk of distant metastases. In the head and neck region, SNB is standard for intermediate-thickness melanoma. It can be used for stage 1 melanoma, but the yield of micro metastases is low and it usually is not justified in this group without other risk factors. On the other hand, for deeply invasive melanoma with greater than 4 mm depth of invasion, the traditional concept is that high risk of distant disease makes prophylactic treatment of lymphatic micrometastases irrelevant. The MSLT-1 trial calls the latter concept into question, as significant benefits in terms of regional control, reduced morbidity, and increased disease-free survival may occur even in this group. For cutaneous lesions of other histologies, the criteria are less well defined in the literature, and surgeons tend to extrapolate from the experience in melanoma.

In cancer of the oral cavity, criteria for sentinel node biopsy remain controversial. The standard approach in 2017 is selective neck dissection for all significantly invasive lateralized lesions (stage 1 and above) and watchful waiting for extremely thin stage 1 lesions. Thickness estimates are based on physical examination and generous biopsy of the thickest appearing portion of the lesion. Management of midline stage 1 lesions of intermediate thickness may represent an area of continued controversy. The "most aggressive" advocates of sentinel node biopsy argue for SNB for all N0 patients, stages I and II. We believe a reasonable way to apply this technology is to use it in those situations where watchful waiting has been applied frequently, but where a reasonable argument could also be made for selective neck dissection. This would certainly include stage I and early stage II tumors with an intermediate depth of invasion, corresponding to estimates of 2 to 4 mm depth of invasion, and stage 1 midline lesions with even thicker depths. It could be offered as an alternative to neck dissection for lateralized lesions with estimated depths up to 8 mm, for patients who are concerned about the morbidity of neck dissection, with caveats related to small false omission rates (the NPV subtracted from 100), and the need to perform two stages of surgery when sentinel nodes are detected to be positive on final pathology. The bulk of patients in the ACOSOG validation trial were in this last group. With greater experience and larger published clinical trials on SNB, the proper group for selection will be better delineated.

Since early cancer of the oral cavity has a smaller risk of distant metastases than melanoma, the manner in which these patients need to be approached is somewhat different from the way we approach melanoma patients. We do not want to lose the opportunity for cure with timely lymphadenectomy, but need to balance this against the morbidity of formal neck dissection in numerous patients who do not harbor lymphatic metastases. Multiple series have confirmed that the technique is not appropriate for T3 and T4 primary tumors due to the significant volume of tissue that would need to be injected, the excessively large number of radioactive nodes generated, the

greater risk that grossly positive nodes exist, the potential for false negatives due to incomplete injection, and the technical futility of removing a large number of nodes in piecemeal fashion. Furthermore, since the risk of having a positive node increases with increasing stage, there comes a point where the percentage of patients who will convert to neck dissection is too large to justify the SNB procedure. To the contrary, the technique is best applied to T1 lesions and smaller T2 lesions. If a lesion is less than 3 cm in maximal diameter but has significant fixation of the tongue or other manifestation of deep invasion, then this lesion is truly a T4 lesion and results with sentinel node biopsy are unlikely to prove accurate and useful.

If the primary tumor meets criteria, the next issue is to determine whether the cervical lymph nodes are clinically involved. While SNB is an excellent technique for detecting micrometastases, it is less useful for detecting nonpalpable but grossly involved lymph nodes. This appears to be particularly true with squamous cell carcinoma. It is postulated that when a large percentage of the lymph node is replaced by cancer, physiologic obstruction can occur and alternative patterns of lymphatic drainage develop. It is important to detect the presence of such gross disease on preoperative imaging and physical exam and, as a last opportunity, at the time of intraoperative palpation. We should avoid applying SNB to this group of patients in order to avoid false positives. Generally, contrast-enhanced CT or MRI are the cross-sectional imaging modalities most commonly used. These should be strictly interpreted, and patients should be excluded if there are nodes greater than 1.2 to 1.5 cm in size with central necrosis, irregular enhancement, or a poorly defined or irregular capsular border, or with groups of three or more asymmetrically located lymph nodes with a minimal axial diameter of 8 mm or more in the suspected tumor drainage area. Fused PET/CT is also useful in ruling out regional metastases greater than 1 cm, but remains plagued by false positives and should be evaluated with some skepticism, particularly if the PET scan is performed shortly after an oral biopsy or if superinfection of the tumor is suspected. Inflammatory nodes can have elevated SUV values and patients may be inappropriately denied the opportunity for a SNB approach.

21.4.2 Injection of the Primary Tumor

The injection is performed prior to the surgical procedure, generally on the morning of surgery. Injection can also sometimes be performed late on the day before, although the effect of this on the success rate of sentinel node identification is still unclear. While awake injection and imaging in radiology is the most commonly used technique, as we extend this procedure to endoscopically accessible oropharyngeal, supraglottic, and hypopharyngeal lesions, it is likely that cooperative efforts with the nuclear radiologist and the use of portable cameras will allow for intraoperative endoscopic injection and gamma probe–guided sentinel node biopsy without the need for uncomfortable injections in an awake patient. Theoretical advantages of injecting under general anesthesia include better exposure of the primary and avoidance of motion of the patient related to discomfort. This may eventually increase the reliability of this method. Taking into account that the radio localization of the detected hot spots does not represent the drainage of the primary but rather the drainage of the tracer deposits, which act as a surrogate for the lymphatic drainage of the primary, the impact of a thorough and representative tracer injection is evident. Due to the density and direction of the head and neck lymphatics, the primary may drain into several alternative lymphatic pathways, all representing first echelon "sentinel" lymph nodes (▶ Fig. 21.1).

Nevertheless, due to regulatory issues related to the injection of radioactive substances and the scarcity of widely available portable nuclear imaging, awake injection remains the most commonly used technique. It is important to ensure that the patient is comfortable so that an adequate preoperative injection is obtained. We use topical anesthetic, mild oral sedation, and/or lingual, inferior alveolar, or sphenopalatine nerve blocks to ensure patient comfort during manipulation and injection of the primary tumor. Direct injection of the tumor with local anesthetic should not be performed as it may affect uptake of the radionuclide and reportedly may even cause it to precipitate in the tissues. The injection technique involves narrow injection with a fine 25-gauge needle on a tuberculin syringe, circumferentially encompassing the leading edge of the lesion and, for thicker lesions, an additional injection in the center of the lesion. Typically, we have used five tuberculin syringes with 1 mL aliquots of technetium 99 sulfur colloid, similar to doses used for melanoma, with a total radioactivity of 400 millicuries representing a standard dose for the morning of surgery. A higher dose would be used the night before.

More recently, we have begun using ^{99m}Tc tilmanocept, a CD206 receptor targeting pharmaceutical, instead of technetium sulfur colloid. The receptor targeting nature of tilmanocept eliminates

the shine-through effect that may be seen with radiolabeled colloids that are retained for long periods of time at the injection site. Also, tilmanocept appears to have greater retention in first echelon nodes with less movement downstream due to its receptor binding properties, and appears to have greater flexibility in the timing of imaging and surgery (same day vs. next day). One phase III multi-institutional trial has shown lower FNRs and greater accuracy with ^{99m}Tc tilmanocept when compared to ^{99m}Tc sulfur colloid.[28] Peritumoral injection with 50 µg of ^{99m}Tc-tilmanocept within 15 hours (same day) or between 15 and 30 hours of surgery (next day) is accomplished in a similar manner as described earlier.

We have used the aforementioned technique for visible oral lesions. For cutaneous lesions, it is well documented that a scar from a previous excisional biopsy can be injected to allow for accurate sentinel node biopsy. Whether a previously excised oral lesion could undergo sentinel node excision by injection of an intraoral scar is not proven, but logically similar principles should apply. It is important to inject narrowly, and not to inject the deep tissues. The radionuclide will diffuse more widely in the oral cavity around the site of injection than occurs in the skin and will usually go to the neck more quickly. There is no benefit to trying to inject a margin around the tumor, as this will lead to an unmanageable excess of radioactive nodes.

The use of blue dye concurrently with radionuclide particles has become popular in sentinel node biopsy for cutaneous lesions. This is a reasonable technique for skin, and certainly can help during the learning phase of the procedure, as the subtle blue dyed lymphatic vessels can be traced toward the sentinel node. Furthermore, reinjection of the blue dye can be performed in the operating room under anesthesia, and can provide a measure of security against inadequacy of preoperative injection due to patient discomfort. Particularly for oral cancer, our preference is to use the radionuclide alone. Numerous publications indicate that it is extremely unlikely to have blue sentinel nodes that are not radioactive. Anaphylactic allergic reactions to isosulfan blue dye, though rare, can occur. For oral lesions, we prefer to remove the primary first to eliminate radioactive background at the primary site. When the technique is performed in this sequence, the blue dye has usually run through to the distal lymphatics by the time the oral resection is completed and margins are sent, making the dye less useful. Finally, oral cavity resections have functional implications that force the surgeon to obtain adequate but closer margins compared to those obtained for cutaneous melanoma. Blue staining of the oral tissues can lead to loss of the visual cues the surgeon uses to guide decisions regarding whether there is tumor involvement at a margin. For all of these reasons, we prefer not to use adjunctive blue dye, particularly for oral lesions. However, other surgeons prefer to use adjunctive blue dye and obtain excellent results. The removal of sentinel nodes based solely on the blue dye technique is less accurate and should not be performed without also injecting radionuclide.

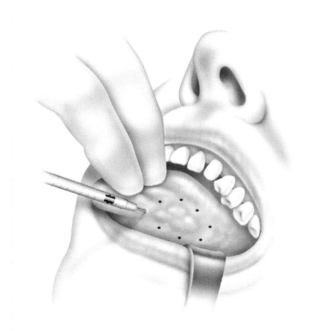

Fig. 21.1 A 1.5-inch needle and tuberculin syringe are used to inject gingerly, completely encompassing the lesion. Excess force should be avoided so that nonphysiologic drainage patterns will not be opened. Sedation, topical anesthetics, and nerve blocks can be used, but lidocaine should not be infiltrated into the bed of injection. Avoid injecting more widely or deeply than necessary, as the injected colloid will extravasate more widely than is apparent.

21.4.3 Radiologic Lymphatic Mapping

After injection, nuclear imaging of the lymphatics is obtained. We now routinely use fused single photon emission computed tomography–computed tomography (SPECT/CT) due to its superior three-dimensional localization ability and a potential to detect more sentinel nodes in unexpected drainage basins. Scrollable images allow for improved targeting and patient counseling prior to the sentinel node dissection (▶ Fig. 21.2).

A dynamic phase should be acquired with serial images for at least one-half hour following injection. These images should be acquired for 1 minute each. Transmission images should be acquired for 1 to 2 minutes in each new movement of the camera (transmission images are obtained using a flat source placed on the detector opposite the working detector. This is done to achieve better localization of any lymph nodes that take up the radiopharmaceutical by superimposing them on a body image). While it is possible to perform sentinel node biopsy with the intraoperative gamma probe alone, the radiologic image can be useful in providing a guide to the location of the sentinel node, allowing for a more complete informed consent process by predicting unexpected drainage to the contralateral neck or other areas that were not expected to be involved. It can also allow for greater surgical efficiency, and likely shorter surgery times, by more exactly delineating the anatomic location of sentinel nodes. In the modern practice of head and neck sentinel node biopsy, most surgeons advocate for the use of fused preoperative SPECT/CT.

21.4.4 Removal of the Primary Tumor

As mentioned earlier, we prefer to resect the primary tumor first. If the injection field is sufficiently narrow, this usually eliminates or greatly reduces background radioactivity at the primary site that can confound the sentinel node identification. The usual, appropriate surgical margins with frozen section control should be obtained. The sentinel node technique for aerodigestive tract malignancies can also be performed in conjunction with a mandibulotomy or other technique of exposure, as long as the primary tumor stage is T2 or less, and as we extend the procedure to the oropharynx this may become more common. In some situations, it may be necessary to perform the nodal biopsy prior to primary resection. However, for most appropriate oral and cutaneous lesions, the lesion will be accessible for resection prior to addressing the lymphatics. Removal of the primary tumor first is less important when the lymphatic basin is distant from the primary tumor, and is often less of an issue for skin lesions (i.e., auricular scalp or nasal lesions). However, this can be important for lesions of the neck or preauricular skin where the lymphatics are immediately deep to the primary tumor. It is especially important in cancer of the floor of the mouth due to the immediate proximity of the submandibular lymphatics.

21.4.5 Gamma Probe–Guided Sentinel Node Biopsy

The hand-held gamma probe is now used to confirm the location of the sentinel lymph nodes, which previously were determined by lymphoscintigraphy and subsequent SPECT-CT. The skin is marked with the location of the nodes. Background readings should be taken of the precordium (▶ Fig. 21.3) as a lower limit background measurement, as well as at the resected primary site as an upper limit of background. The latter is important in avoiding errors due to shine through from the primary injection site.

If the patient is to undergo sentinel node biopsy alone, with neck dissection planned only for positive findings intraoperatively or on permanent histopathology, the incision can be drawn narrowly over the node. However, the incision must be consistent with the possibility of subsequent neck dissection, and the planned incision for the formal lymphadenectomy should be considered. Alternatively, the incision can be drawn in the line of that to be used for neck dissection, although shorter in length, and flaps can be elevated. This latter approach is always used when immediate gamma probe–guided completion neck dissection is the plan, either due to patient preference for combined lymphatic mapping and selective neck dissection or as part of a validation trial. After the incision is made, subplatysmal flaps are

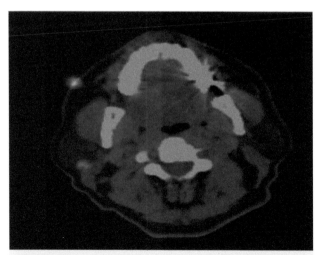

Fig. 21.2 SPECT CT showing lymph node over mandible in vicinity of facial artery, deep node on posterior parotid capsule, and parotid node medial to retromandibular vein. None of these nodes require dissection of main trunk of facial nerve to remove.

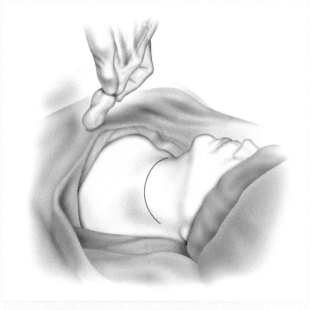

Fig. 21.3 Background reading is taken at the precordium.

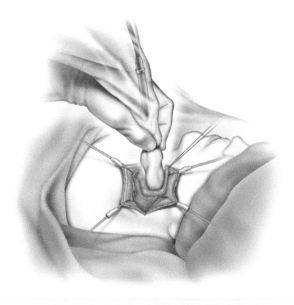

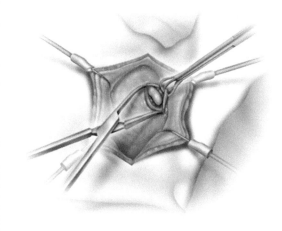

Fig. 21.5 The sentinel node is excised using a combination of blunt dissection and division of tissue using bipolar cautery. Unipolar cautery should be avoided when the proximity of neurovascular structures is not known.

Fig. 21.4 Blunt dissection towards the hotspot is followed by reinsertion of the gamma probe into the path of dissection and angulation in various directions, seeking the radioactively tagged lymph node.

elevated sufficiently to provide access to the hot area. The neck should first be carefully palpated in order to identify palpable gross lymphatic disease that may not be physiologically functional, and hence may not take up radioactivity. The finding of gross cancer involvement would, of course, contraindicate sentinel node biopsy and mandate formal lymphadenectomy.

If no gross disease is identified, the surgeon will now localize the sentinel node(s). Use of the probe to locate the nodes in a three-dimensional location is not intuitive and it is best learned through instruction by a surgeon with experience in the technique. Initial readings are taken of the precordium and back table in order to assess the level of hematogenous radioactivity. Readings are also obtained from the resected tumor specimen and the bed of resection. The probe is slowly passed over the neck at a steady rate, assessing the auditory input for radioactivity generated by the gamma probe. Care is taken to aim away from the primary resection bed. Since the probe measures radioactivity over time, rapid or unsteady movement will lead to higher readings and louder auditory input, and should be avoided. Using steady constant motion, the probe is moved radially across each hot spot allowing the surgeon to determine the direction in which to proceed, in three dimensions, in order to locate the sentinel node. The surgeon then bluntly dissects toward the sentinel node. Bipolar cautery can be used to divide the tissues to provide wider exposure. We recommend avoidance of paralysis and caution in using unipolar electrocautery as the neurovascular structures in the neck are not specifically identified, although the spinal accessory and marginal nerves may often be visualized during the course of the procedure.

As a dissection cavity is opened, the gamma probe is introduced into this space along the plane of dissection and angled in various directions in order to guide the surgeon to the sentinel node (▶ Fig. 21.4). The sentinel node is bluntly excised (▶ Fig. 21.5). Probe readings (counts per minute) are recorded

for initial readings taken while the node is in the patient, as well as for "ex vivo" readings of the extracted node, away from the patient (▶ Fig. 21.6). Repeat readings are taken of the resection bed to ensure that there are no adjacent hot nodes that also need to be removed. Any node exhibiting 10% or more of the radioactivity of the most radioactive node in the same anatomic area will be considered an additional sentinel node and will be harvested separately. If there are a large number of very radioactive nodes (i.e., more than six), this essentially represents a failure of the technique and piecemeal removal of a large number of nodes is illogical. The surgeon should remove the four most radioactive nodes or proceed to selective neck dissection if indicated. In the case where there is a very "hot" sentinel node in a specific area, there may be a relatively "hot" node in a completely separate anatomic region (i.e., submental region vs. level II jugular region) that does not reach 10% of the radioactivity of the hottest node. If this second node is truly in a separate area and is significantly greater than background (two or more times background readings), it should still be harvested as a sentinel node, as it may represent a separate drainage pattern from a different portion of the tumor. Review of the imaging and knowledge of basic anatomic principles will allow the surgeon to judge whether such additional areas of borderline radioactivity need to be excised. When the SLN dissections are performed prior to resection of an oral cavity cancer, or if significant radioactivity persists in the bed of resection, the use of intraoral lead shields can be helpful. The presence of a collimator on the gamma probe is recommended to reduce background signal from the primary tumor, and most modern probes have fine tips with collimators. With posterior tongue tumors, background activity can be avoided by using a transoral suture on the tongue to pull the primary bed away from the lymphatics.

The issue of dealing with background activity at the primary site is most marked for level I nodes with cancer of the floor of the mouth. In this situation, the surgeon may need to perform some initial dissection, below the level of the marginal mandibular nerve, transecting the tissues down to the level of the

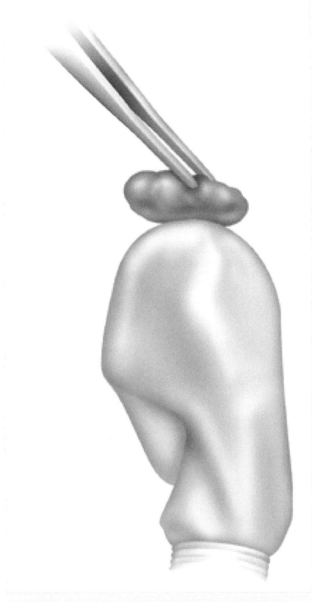

Fig. 21.6 Ex vivo readings pointing away from the patient should confirm whether this is the radioactive node.

mylohyoid muscle. In this manner, the lymph nodes are mobilized away from the oral cavity, allowing for more accurate identification of the SLN(s) by placing the gamma probe into the tunnel thus created and directing the probe inferiorly away from the background radioactivity at the floor of the mouth injection site. Each SLN is labeled, measured, described, and recorded separately as to location and total ex vivo counts per second.

Skin lesions of the periauricular region and scalp represent a unique technical challenge as they commonly drain to the parotid lymph nodes. The proximity of the facial nerve branches and the dense nature of parotid tissue often make blunt dissection problematic. In our experience, in many cases, nodes can be identified on the capsule of the parotid gland, which can be safely excised with a capsular dissection. These may be located on the tail of the parotid, anterior edge of the parotid, or region around the temporal vessels (for scalp lesions). Electromyographic intraoperative facial nerve monitoring is useful in such cases. If the gamma probe directs the surgeon to nodes deep within the parotid, then in many cases it is best to identify a distal branch of the facial nerve, or occasionally even the main trunk, and perform a localized excision of the hot portion of the parotid gland, with identification of the facial nerve. Such a procedure might be termed a "gamma probe–guided partial parotidectomy" and still simplifies the procedure relative to a formal lateral lobe parotidectomy with concurrent neck dissection. In this situation, it is particularly important to tag the tissue adjacent to facial nerve branches with permanent suture in order to provide for easy reexploration if the sentinel node is positive. In high-risk situations for metastasis, consider proceeding with formal parotidectomy, given the difficulties of reexploration in the parotid area. Similar marking of the location of the spinal accessory nerve would be advantageous if it is identified in the course of an upper jugular sentinel node biopsy.

21.4.6 Rigorous Histopathologic Assessment of the Sentinel Node

In any situation where sentinel node biopsy alone is performed, exhaustive histopathologic evaluation of the sentinel node with fine step sectioning as well as concurrent IHC should be performed to rule out microscopic foci of cancer and to allow for therapeutic neck dissection or radiation. While intraoperative frozen sections often prove difficult in cases of melanoma or neuroendocrine carcinomas, large-scale reviews have shown step-section frozen section analysis to be cost-effective and accurate in breast axillary lymph node biopsies.[29] At least one institutional review of frozen section analysis of sentinel nodes in oral cavity squamous cell carcinoma has shown a high degree of accuracy, with an NPV of 99% when compared to the permanent specimen analysis.[30] It is our practice to send intraoperative frozen sections on sentinel nodes suspicious for squamous cell carcinoma metastases, evaluating three- or four-step sections within the node.

It is also important for the pathologist to classify the type of metastatic lymph node involvement. Currently, the nomenclature used in sentinel lymph node pathologic examination is extrapolated from AJCC breast cancer staging: namely, the distinction between micrometastases (0.2–2 mm; ▸ Fig. 21.7) and macrometastases (> 2 mm). The discovery of isolated tumor cells in lymph node specimens by morphologic (IHC) or nonmorphologic (flow cytometry or PCR) means should be differentiated from micrometastases, as the prognostic implications of these clusters of cells in oral cavity cancer are unknown. Additionally, there may be mummified keratin positive or anucleate cells that are not considered a positive outcome for sentinel node analysis.

21.5 Risks and Complications of Sentinel Node Biopsy

Complications are relatively rare with the aforementioned technique, as the minimally invasive nature of the procedure

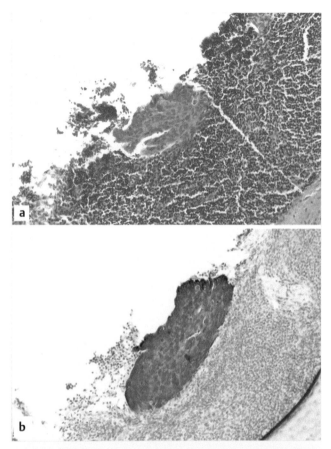

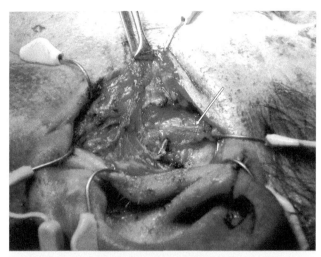

Fig. 21.8 Deep intraparotid sentinel node biopsy. The frontalis branch has been identified and is indicated by the arrow.

Fig. 21.7 Micrometastasis seen on hematoxylin and eosin stain (**a**) and immunohistochemistry (IHC) for cytokeratin (**b**). With IHC micrometastases are more easily identified.

relative to the moderate morbidity of neck dissection is the impetus for the development of the technique. Nonetheless, like any procedure, complications can occur. One concern with SNB in the head and neck region is the theoretical risk of injury to the facial and spinal accessory nerves during blunt dissection through a narrow exposure. It is also possible that surgeons employing this technique might leave behind sentinel nodes deep in the parotid gland, which allows the avoidance of facial nerve dissection but can imply an oncologic risk. It is important, once the procedure is initiated, to do what is necessary to make the most of the radionuclide injection and ensure that all sentinel nodes of appropriate radioactivity, representing real first echelon drainage pathways, are removed (▶ Fig. 21.8).

Although there remains a paucity of data on the exact complication rate of SNB, reported incidences of even minor complications are less than 1%. Theoretically in the hands of an inexperienced operator, the risk of injury to the facial or spinal accessory nerves may be greater with SNB than with formal parotidectomy and selective neck dissection. The SNB procedure in the head and neck should only be performed by surgeons who perform large volumes of neck dissections and parotidectomies and are comfortable with the anatomy.

Another issue is our frequent inability to achieve immediate diagnosis of positive sentinel nodes, especially in melanoma. Frozen section, while useful in squamous cell carcinoma, is absolutely not

accurate for melanoma, and tissue is often better preserved for permanent sections. The only exception to this is if gross clinically positive metastases are encountered, which rarely occurs. A touch preparation for cytology can be performed on the sectioned normal-appearing node.

Thus, for the minority of patients with micrometastases identified in the sentinel nodes, we are sometimes dealing with issues of reexploration and dissection in functionally delicate areas. The potential risk of nerve injury related to the reexploration of an inflamed, recently operated wound needs to be considered. Rushing the pathological analysis to allow for early reexploration and tagging adjacent to any visualized nerves with blue Prolene sutures at the time of the sentinel node procedure are steps that can make secondary lymphadenectomy easier.

21.6 Conclusion

Sentinel node biopsy offers a minimally invasive prognostic and potentially therapeutic surgical option for patients with intermediate risk, clinically node-negative disease. It has become the standard of care for intermediate thickness N0 melanoma of the head and neck, is recommended by the NCCN for all N0 Merkel cell carcinomas, and is an emerging technique for the staging of lymphatics in cutaneous squamous cell carcinoma. It is also an option to be considered in the NCCN guidelines for early oral cavity cancer as alternative to neck dissection for intermediate thickness lesions.

Selective neck dissection remains the standard approach for the majority of oral cancers, particularly for larger and significantly invasive T2, T3, and T4 lesions. Significant data already exist, however, to advocate SLNB as a reasonable alternative to selective neck dissection for smaller, thinner oral cancers, including those of the floor of the mouth albeit with a slightly modified technique, that fall in a category where watchful waiting might reasonably be chosen as an alternative but where the tumors are not so minimally invasive that the risk of metastases is negligible.

The sentinel node concept has been discarded by some based on the misconception that selective neck dissection has no significant morbidity. Coming from a tradition of more radical neck procedures, the selective neck dissection is generally viewed as an intervention with negligible morbidity by many head and neck surgeons. Although the morbidity of selective neck dissection is significantly less than that of modified radical and radical dissections, there is measurable morbidity in a variable percentage of patients, including issues with shoulder function secondary to temporary trapezius weakness followed by adhesive capsulitis of the shoulder, pain syndromes, contour changes, and lower lip mobility. There is associated visible neck asymmetry. This has been demonstrated in numerous quality-of-life studies and objective functional assessments. The moderate morbidity of selective neck dissection has led some to suggest watchful waiting as an alternative for patients of lower risk. SNB has developed as an intermediate option in response to this controversy, with all of the aforementioned complications observed much less frequently.

The sentinel node technique is likely to have an increasing role in the management of head and neck cancer in the future. Surgeons can gain experience in the use of this technique for cutaneous malignancies and early-stage oral cancers with minimal to intermediate invasiveness. The technique can also be practiced in the context of a gamma probe–guided neck dissection for more invasive cancers, preferably in the context of a clinical trial, allowing the patient to benefit from improved mapping of drainage patterns and more accurate staging through better identification of micrometastases. Pilot data on the use of this technique in the pharynx and larynx will continue to emerge. We hope to provide a guide to surgeons as they evaluate the neck both clinically and radiographically, and to describe the developing role of lymphoscintigraphy and sentinel node biopsy in detecting microscopic lymphatic metastases.

References

[1] D'Cruz AK, Vaish R, Kapre N, et al. Head and Neck Disease Management Group. Elective versus therapeutic neck dissection in node-negative oral cancer. N Engl J Med. 2015; 373(6):521–529

[2] Morton DL, Wen DR, Wong JH, et al. Technical details of intraoperative lymphatic mapping for early stage melanoma. Arch Surg. 1992; 127(4):392–399

[3] Morton DL, Wen DR, Foshag LJ, Essner R, Cochran A. Intraoperative lymphatic mapping and selective cervical lymphadenectomy for early-stage melanomas of the head and neck. J Clin Oncol. 1993; 11(9):1751–1756

[4] Alex JC, Krag DN. Gamma-probe guided localization of lymph nodes. Surg Oncol. 1993; 2(3):137–143

[5] Alex JC, Weaver DL, Fairbank JT, Rankin BS, Krag DN. Gamma-probe-guided lymph node localization in malignant melanoma. Surg Oncol. 1993; 2(5):303–308

[6] Krag DN, Meijer SJ, Weaver DL, et al. Minimal-access surgery for staging of malignant melanoma. Arch Surg. 1995; 130(6):654–658, discussion 659–660

[7] Glass LF, Messina JL, Cruse W, et al. The use of intraoperative radiolymphoscintigraphy for sentinel node biopsy in patients with malignant melanoma. Dermatol Surg. 1996; 22(8):715–720

[8] Morton DL, Thompson JF, Cochran AJ, et al. MSLT Group. Final trial report of sentinel-node biopsy versus nodal observation in melanoma. N Engl J Med. 2014; 370(7):599–609

[9] National Comprehensive Cancer Network (NCCN) Clinical Practice Guidelines in Oncology. Melanoma. Available at: https://www.nccn.org/professionals/physicians_gls/PDF/melanoma.pdf. Published 2016. Accessed September 30, 2017

[10] Faries MB, Thompson JF, Cochran AJ, et al. Completion dissection or observation for sentinel-node metastasis in melanoma. N Engl J Med. 2017; 376(23):2211–2222

[11] National Comprehensive Cancer Network (NCCN) Clinical Practice Guidelines in Oncology. Merkel Cell Carcinoma. Available at: https://www.nccn.org/professionals/physician_gls/PDF/mcc.pdf. Published 2017. Accessed September 30, 2017

[12] Mojica P, Smith D, Ellenhorn JD. Adjuvant radiation therapy is associated with improved survival in Merkel cell carcinoma of the skin. J Clin Oncol. 2007; 25(9):1043–1047

[13] Shnayder Y, Weed DT, Arnold DJ, et al. Management of the neck in Merkel cell carcinoma of the head and neck: University of Miami experience. Head Neck. 2008; 30(12):1559–1565

[14] National Comprehensive Cancer Network (NCCN) Clinical Practice Guidelines in Oncology. Squamous Cell Skin Cancer. Available at: https://www.nccn.org/professionals/physician_gls/pdf/squamous.pdf. Published 2017. Accessed September 30, 2017

[15] Ross AS, Schmults CD. Sentinel lymph node biopsy in cutaneous squamous cell carcinoma: a systematic review of the English literature. Dermatol Surg. 2006; 32(11):1309–1321

[16] Ahmed MM, Moore BA, Schmalbach CE. Utility of head and neck cutaneous squamous cell carcinoma sentinel node biopsy: a systematic review. Otolaryngol Head Neck Surg. 2014; 150(2):180–187

[17] Stoeckli SJ. Sentinel node biopsy for oral and oropharyngeal squamous cell carcinoma of the head and neck. Laryngoscope. 2007; 117(9):1539–1551

[18] Christensen A, Bilde A, Therkildsen MH, et al. The prevalence of occult metastases in nonsentinel lymph nodes after step-serial sectioning and immunohistochemistry in cN0 oral squamous cell carcinoma. Laryngoscope. 2011; 121(2):294–298

[19] Jefferson GD, Sollaccio D, Gomez-Fernandez CR, Civantos F, Jr. Evaluation of immunohistochemical fine sectioning for sentinel lymph node biopsy in oral squamous cell carcinoma. Otolaryngol Head Neck Surg. 2011; 144(2):216–219

[20] Alkureishi LW, Ross GL, Shoaib T, et al. Sentinel node biopsy in head and neck squamous cell cancer: 5-year follow-up of a European multicenter trial. Ann Surg Oncol. 2010; 17(9):2459–2464

[21] Civantos FJ, Zitsch RP, Schuller DE, et al. Sentinel lymph node biopsy accurately stages the regional lymph nodes for T1-T2 oral squamous cell carcinomas: results of a prospective multi-institutional trial. J Clin Oncol. 2010; 28(8):1395–1400

[22] Govers TM, Hannink G, Merkx MA, Takes RP, Rovers MM. Sentinel node biopsy for squamous cell carcinoma of the oral cavity and oropharynx: a diagnostic meta-analysis. Oral Oncol. 2013; 49(8):726–732

[23] Schilling C, Stoeckli SJ, Haerle SK, et al. Sentinel European Node Trial (SENT): 3-year results of sentinel node biopsy in oral cancer. Eur J Cancer. 2015; 51(18):2777–2784

[24] Pezier T, Nixon IJ, Gurney B, et al. Sentinel lymph node biopsy for T1/T2 oral cavity squamous cell carcinoma–a prospective case series. Ann Surg Oncol. 2012; 19(11):3528–3533

[25] Pedersen NJ, Jensen DH, Hedbäck N, et al. Staging of early lymph node metastases with the sentinel lymph node technique and predictive factors in T1/T2 oral cavity cancer: A retrospective single-center study. Head Neck. 2016; 38 Suppl 1:E1033–E1040

[26] Flach GB, Bloemena E, Klop WM, et al. Sentinel lymph node biopsy in clinically N0 T1-T2 staged oral cancer: the Dutch multicenter trial. Oral Oncol. 2014; 50(10):1020–1024

[27] Broglie MA, Haile SR, Stoeckli SJ. Long-term experience in sentinel node biopsy for early oral and oropharyngeal squamous cell carcinoma. Ann Surg Oncol. 2011; 18(10):2732–2738

[28] Agrawal A, Civantos FJ, Brumund KT, et al. [(99m)Tc]Tilmanocept accurately detects sentinel lymph nodes and predicts node pathology status in patients with oral squamous cell carcinoma of the head and neck: results of a phase III multi-institutional trial. Ann Surg Oncol. 2015; 22(11):3708–3715

[29] Lim J, Govindarajulu S, Sahu A, Ibrahim N, Magdub S, Cawthorn S. Multiple Step-section Frozen Section sentinel lymph node biopsy–a review of 717 patients. Breast. 2013; 22(5):639–642

[30] Terada A, Hasegawa Y, Yatabe Y, et al. Intraoperative diagnosis of cancer metastasis in sentinel lymph node of oral cancer patients. Oral Oncol. 2008; 44(9):838–843

22 Robotic Neck Dissection: The Retroauricular Approach

Estelle Eun Hae Chang, Yoon Woo Koh, and Kang Dae Lee

Abstract

Neck dissections are performed when cancer metastasis to cervical lymph nodes are diagnosed or suspected. Traditionally, neck dissections have been performed via an open transcervical incision. In order to avoid visible scars, remote-access robotic and endoscopic procedures for head and neck surgery have been developed. The first transaxillary robotic neck dissection was performed in 2009. Since the introduction of the transaxillary approach, various novel techniques of remote-access thyroid and head and neck surgery have been introduced and adopted by many head and neck and endocrine surgeons worldwide. One of the most commonly used methods is the retroauricular (facelift) robotic approach, which has become increasingly popular especially for head and neck surgeons who are already familiar with the facelift procedure. This approach has shown greater ease of access and lower complication profile when compared to the previously described remote-access robotic and endoscopic approaches. In 2011, Koh and his team successfully performed their first robotic lateral neck dissection via the retroauricular incision and have since published several studies to demonstrate the safety and comparable clinical and oncologic outcomes to traditional open neck dissections. This chapter describes the specific operative procedure of this novel robotic retroauricular modified lateral neck dissection. The preoperative considerations, including patient selection criteria, to surgical anatomy and steps of the robotic neck dissection are described. Postoperative management and surgical pearls to increase surgical success are also discussed.

Keywords: neck dissections, robotic, remote access, retroauricular, facelift

22.1 Introduction

Neck dissections are performed when cancer metastasis to cervical lymph nodes are diagnosed or suspected, which are frequently associated with malignancies of upper aerodigestive tract, skin of the head and neck region, salivary glands, and thyroid. First described by Crile in 1906, radical neck dissection was considered to be the standard procedure for surgical treatment of neck disease. There has been a shift over the past few decades toward less invasive surgical procedures, with an interest in preserving of nonlymphatic structures (i.e., sternocleidomastoid muscle, internal jugular vein [IJV], spinal accessory nerve [SAN]). The modified neck dissections with conservation of nonlymphatic structures have been shown to result in comparable oncologic outcomes with superior functional outcomes.

Traditionally, neck dissections have been performed via an open transcervical incision. Although useful in exposing the neck for adequate removal of cervical lymph nodes, these traditional cervical incisions invariably result in visible scars especially in young patient population. Over the past decade, advancement in technology and interest in avoiding visible cervical scars led to the development of remote-access robotic thyroidectomy. D.J. Terris

(Georgia Health Sciences University, United States) was the first to describe the retroauricular (facelift) robotic thyroidectomy approach in 2011. This approach showed promises with ease of access and lower complication profile when compared to the previously described remote-access robotic thyroidectomy approaches. This access is also appealing to head and neck surgeons most of who are already familiar with the facelift procedure. Although Terris has advocated this approach mainly for hemithyroidectomy, Y.W. Koh, a head and neck surgeon from South Korea, has quickly adapted the retroauricular approach and expanded its application to performing a variety of head and neck procedures, including but not limited to excision of benign head and neck tumors (lipomas, branchial cleft cysts, neurogenic tumor, etc.), total thyroidectomy with central neck dissection, and lateral neck dissections for thyroid and nonendocrine head and neck cancers. This chapter describes the specific operative procedures of this novel robotic retroauricular modified lateral neck dissection, including preoperative considerations and postoperative management.

22.2 Surgical Anatomy

It is important to note that the surgical anatomy and the structures involved in the procedure remain constant whether the neck dissection is performed via open traditional incision or via remote-access retroauricular incision. However, a surgeon needs to be accustomed to the surgical view and the axis of dissection when considering the retroauricular approach. Similar to the transaxillary approach, a good and safe working space creation is essential for successful outcomes. However, unlike the transaxillary thyroidectomy, the surgical view would be addressed in a superior to inferior manner; therefore, it is important for the operator to anticipate the local anatomical structures which would be visualized as the operation progresses. The details of working space formation are described below. The axis of dissection is superior to inferior and posterior to anterior. Similar to the conventional open approach, surgeons have options to perform level Vb dissection by either dissecting the posterior edge of SCM or by dissecting from underneath the SCM by pulling the level Vb content anteriorly. The details of both techniques will be described later.

22.3 Indications of the Procedure

1. Relatively limited, small, early-stage malignant carcinomas of the head and neck region with known or suspected metastasis to the neck.
2. Evidence of neck metastasis without gross, extensive extracapsular spread (ECS).
3. Patients who are willing to receive the robotic/endoscopic operation after having been informed of certain disadvantages of the robotic/endoscopic procedures, including relatively high medical costs and longer operation times and hospital stays.

22.4 Contraindications of the Procedure

1. Patients with previous head and neck surgery.
2. Patients with previous head and neck radiation.
3. Patients with unresectable neck nodal metastasis with ECS.
4. Large, bulky tumors requiring tracheostomy prior to neck dissection.

22.5 Preoperative Considerations

22.5.1 Choosing the Appropriate Candidate

The length and circumference of the patient's neck are two most important determinants for good exposure and safe surgical field. The best exposure for retroauricular neck dissection is usually achieved in slender necks with smaller neck circumference. The operation is also feasible and safe with obese necks but does require more expertise from the surgeon.

22.5.2 Preoperative Imaging Studies

Preoperative evaluation should be performed as per the standard and routine procedure by the local institution similarly to conventional open neck dissection surgery. The authors recommend CT and/or MRI with contrast for further evaluation of nodal metastasis. These imaging studies can help us evaluate and assess the presence of ECS in metastatic lymph nodes and the extent of disease, which are essential information in determining a patient's candidacy for retroauricular robotic approach.

22.5.3 Anesthetic Considerations

Similar to conventional open neck dissection procedures, orotracheal or nasotracheal intubation is performed. Nerve integrity monitor endotracheal tube can also be used depending on the surgeon's preference and if the lateral neck dissection is done in conjunction with total thyroidectomy.

22.6 Surgical Instruments

22.6.1 Instruments to Retract and Secure the Skin Flap

- Skin hook.
- Army–Navy retractor.
- Right angle "breast" retractor.
- Self-retaining retractor (L & C Bio, Seongnam-si, Korea).

22.6.2 Robotic Surgical System (Da Vinci Robotic System—Intuitive Surgical Inc., Sunnyvale, CA)

This procedure can be done using either the Si or the Xi robotic systems. In the authors' experience, it is easier to perform the procedure using the Xi system than the Si system for the following

reasons: greater rotation of patient side cart which allows easier docking and positioning of robotic arms, ability to use three instrument arms instead of two, and improved high-definition of the endoscope resolution.

- 30-degree face-down dual-channel endoscope (Intuitive Surgical Inc.).
- Instruments with the Si robotic system:
  - 5-mm Maryland forceps (Intuitive Surgical Inc.) or 8-mm Maryland bipolar forceps (Intuitive Surgical Inc.).
  - 8-mm monopolar curved scissors or 5-mm Harmonic curved shears (Intuitive Surgical Inc.).
  - 8-mm fenestrated bipolar forceps or 8-mm ProGrasp forceps (Intuitive Surgical Inc.).
- Instruments with the Xi robotic systems:
  - 8-mm Maryland bipolar forceps (Intuitive Surgical Inc.).
  - 8-mm monopolar curved scissors (Intuitive Surgical Inc.).
  - 8-mm fenestrated bipolar forceps or 8-mm ProGrasp forceps (Intuitive Surgical Inc.).
  - The instrument arms of the Xi system have the ability to accommodate the new Erbe-integrated energy device (Erbe USA Inc., Marietta, GA), which enables both monopolar and bipolar coagulation.

22.6.3 Other Instruments

- Bovie tip (electrocautery tip): conventional size of spatula type and also additional tips of various lengths.
- Hemoclip or Hem-o-lock: for ligation of large blood vessels or vessels that cannot be controlled through cautery.
- Debakey forceps/Russian forceps.
- Yankauer suctions (long metal tip).

22.7 Operative Procedure

22.7.1 Step 1: Patient Positioning

The patient is placed in supine position with the head rotated to the contralateral side of the dissection. Extra neck extension with a shoulder roll is considered to be unnecessary and therefore not recommended (▸ Fig. 22.1).

22.7.2 Step 2: Designing the Retroauricular Skin Incision

The retroauricular incision is designed around the earlobe and along the retroauricular sulcus. The tail of the incision is about 0.5 to 1 cm behind the hairline and thus completely hidden once the hair is fully grown back. The incision can also be extended anterior to the earlobe comparably to the standard face-lift incision if a greater skin flap height is required for adequate working space formation (▸ Fig. 22.1).

22.7.3 Step 3: Skin Flap Elevation and Working Space Creation

Once the retroauricular incision is made, the subplatysmal flap is carefully elevated, first exposing the sternocleidomastoid (SCM) muscle. Early anatomical landmarks such as the great auricular nerve and the external jugular vein are visualized and carefully

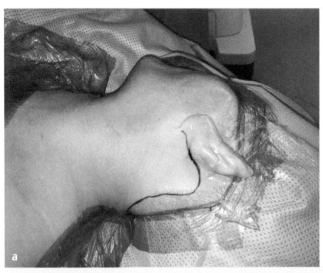
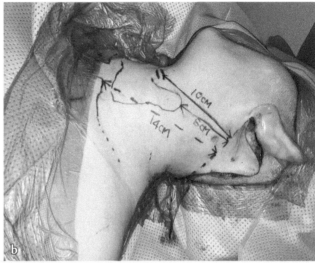

Fig. 22.1 (a,b) Skin incision for the retroauricular thyroidectomy combined with neck dissection.

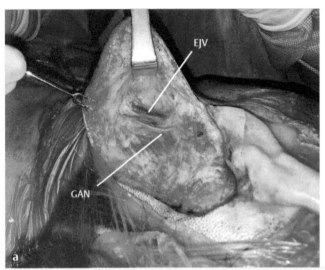
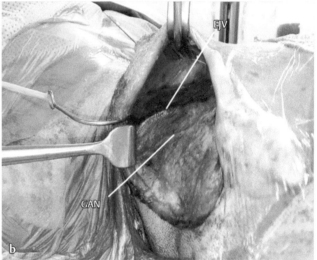

Fig. 22.2 (a,b) Skin flap elevation. After skin incision, subplatysmal flaps are elevated above the sternocleidomastoid (SCM) muscle. The great auricular nerve and external jugular vein should be preserved superficial to the SCM muscle. Elevation of skin flap for robotic retroauricular neck dissection is widely elevated to create adequate working space especially toward the posterior neck.

preserved (▶ Fig. 22.2a). For adequate level I exposure, it is important to carefully dissect the flap above the parotid tail and mandible by staying directly under the platysma in order not to injure the marginal mandibular nerve. The subplatysmal flap is elevated until the posterior border of SCM is exposed posteriorly, beyond the strap muscle raphe anteriorly and down to the suprasternal notch and the clavicle inferiorly (▶ Fig. 22.2b).

Creating a good working space is the key to successful operation. When compared to the retroauricular thyroidectomy, the area required for robotic neck dissection to create a proper working space is wider especially toward the posterior neck. This is to ensure that the level V lymph nodes can be accessed for complete and thorough posterior neck dissection (▶ Fig. 22.2b). During this procedure of the skin flap elevation, the role of the assistant surgeon is to hold the elevated skin flap with retractors to provide countertraction and facilitate flap dissection. Once sufficient

working space is established, a self-retaining retractor is inserted and secured to hold the subplatysmal flap into position. In order to improve the surgical field exposure and increase the efficiency of the dissection, an anchoring suture with black silk 2–0 can be applied to the skin flap and SCM (▶ Fig. 22.3). For adequate working space, the skin flap should be elevated until the parotid tail and the angle of mandible are exposed, while preserving the marginal mandibular nerve (▶ Fig. 22.3).

22.7.4 Step 4: Robotic Arms Docking

The da Vinci robotic surgical system (Intuitive Surgical Inc.), the Si or the Xi system, is introduced with a face-down 30-degree dual-channel endoscopic camera arm placed in the center. Given the configuration and design of the robotic systems, the senior author utilizes three instrument arms (Maryland forceps,

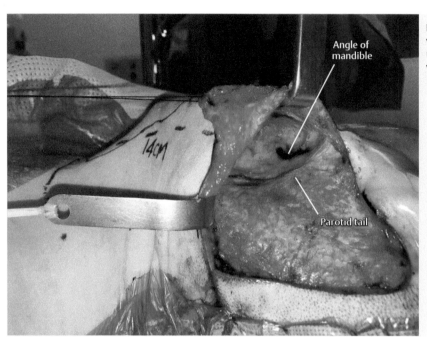

Fig. 22.3 Skin flap elevation. For adequate working space, the skin flap should be elevated until the parotid tail and the angle of mandible, while the marginal mandibular nerve is preserved.

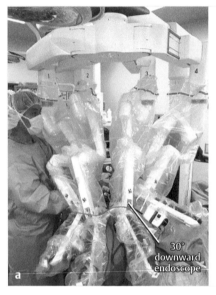
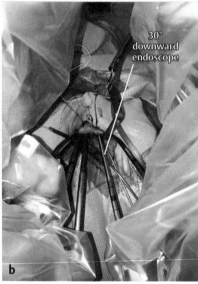

Fig. 22.4 (a,b) Docking of the robotic arms and its configuration. A face-down 30-degree dual-channel endoscopic arm is placed at the center, and three instrument arms are mounted with 8-mm Maryland bipolar forceps, 8-mm fenestrated bipolar forceps or 8-mm ProGrasp forceps, and 8-mm monopolar curved scissors at either side.

ProGrasp forceps, Harmonic curved shears or monopolar scissors) when using the Si system and even when using the Xi system (▶ Fig. 22.4).

The surgical steps taken for robotic retroauricular thyroidectomy with or without neck dissections are the same regardless of the robotic system used for the procedure. However, there are some distinct configurations when docking the instrument arms that are different between the two robotic systems. First, an additional third robotic instrument arm could be inserted through the RA port without collision of robotic instrument arms when using the Xi system (▶ Fig. 22.4). A face-down 30-degree dual-channel endoscopic arm is placed at the center, and three instrument arms are mounted with 8-mm Maryland bipolar forceps, 8-mm fenestrated bipolar forceps or 8-mm ProGrasp forceps, and 8-mm monopolar curved scissors at either side. The Maryland forceps is placed on the left side of the endoscope, and the Harmonic curved shears or Monopolar scissors is placed on the right side of the endoscope.

When using the ProGrasp forceps, it is placed between the endoscope and the Harmonic curved shears or Monopolar scissors for the right-sided neck surgery, and it is placed between the Maryland forceps and the endoscope when performing the surgery on the left side of the neck. An additional advantage of the Xi system is that its instrument arms can be combined with the new ERBE integrated energy device (Erbe USA Inc.), which allows both monopolar and bipolar coagulation with 8-mm instrumental arms.

22.7.5 Step 5: Robotic Dissection

Once the docking stage is complete, robotic neck dissection is ready to begin. An assistant surgeon is seated near the surgical field on the opposite side of the patient cart. The assistant's role is to offer countertraction and additional retraction to facilitate the dissection using two long Yankauer suctions or any other similar long suction tips. The use of suction is to suck out fume

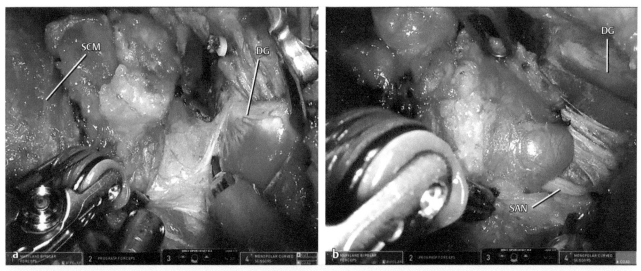

Fig. 22.5 (a,b) Identification of the posterior belly of the digastric muscle (DG) and the spinal accessory nerve (SAN). Dissecting the inferior border of submandibular gland reveals the posterior belly of the DG underneath. After meticulous but cautious dissection of the adjacent soft tissues, the SAN is skeletonized and its branches to sternocleidomastoid muscle and trapezius muscle can be identified.

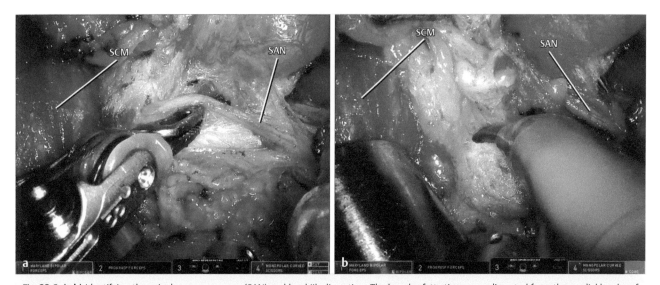

Fig. 22.6 (a,b) Identifying the spinal accessory nerve (SAN) and level IIb dissection. The lympho-fatty tissues are dissected from the medial border of the sternocleidomastoid (SCM) muscle and the SAN is traced in the inferior direction. For the level IIb dissection, the SAN is traced laterally and inferiorly toward the lateral border of the SCM muscle.

created by thermocoagulation which can fog the endoscope and obstruct the view. Retraction and countertraction offered by the assistant can greatly improve the efficiency and safety of the dissection procedure.

The initial dissection is made along the lower border of the submandibular gland and the tail of parotid gland, where the posterior belly of the digastric muscle is identified underneath these structures (▶ Fig. 22.5a). Dissecting along the posterior belly of the digastric muscle and retracting it superiorly allows the exposure of the internal jugular vein (IJV). The spinal accessory nerve (SAN) is then identified and preserved (▶ Fig. 22.5b). If the level IIb is to be performed, it can be done at this stage by dissecting the fibro fatty tissue superior to SAN up to the skull base. For the level IIb dissection, the SAN is traced laterally and inferiorly toward the lateral border of the SCM. The medial border of the SCM is dissected

from superior to inferior direction toward the clavicle. The SAN is skeletonized and followed until the posterior border of the SCM and toward its insertion onto the trapezius muscle (▶ Fig. 22.6). The SCM muscle is maintained in its retracted position so that levels IIb and the lateral aspect to the carotid sheath of IIa and upper III are dissected. Fibro fatty tissue underneath the SCM is dissected fully inferiorly to expose the carotid sheath. A second assistant surgeon is helpful to provide additional retraction of the SCM using Army-Navy retractors. If the second assistant surgeon is not available, suture on the SCM muscle with 2–0 Black silk can be repositioned underneath the SCM to provide further counterretraction. The dissected specimen of level IIb is retracted superiorly and medially to continue the dissection of the levels IIa and III in a superior to inferior fashion. The lympho-fatty tissue is carefully dissected from the IJV using monopolar scissors and harmonic curved

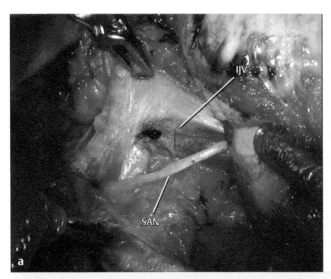

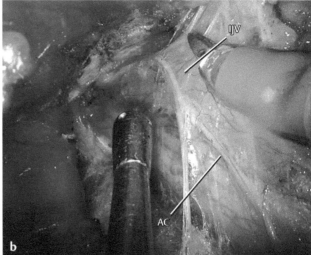

Fig. 22.7 (a,b) Dissection of levels II and III. The dissected specimen of level IIb is retracted superiorly and medially to commence the robotic dissection at levels IIa and III in a superior to inferior fashion. The lympho-fatty tissue is carefully dissected from the internal jugular vein using monopolar scissors.

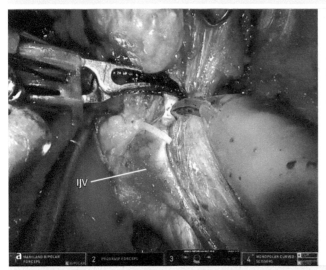

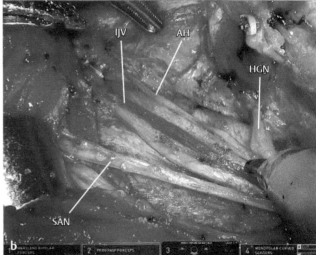

Fig. 22.8 (a,b) Completion of levels II and III dissection. The branches of the internal jugular vein can also be ligated using the Hem-o-lok Ligation System or using the Harmonic curved shears or bipolar cautery depending on the size of the vessel. The hypoglossal nerve and ansa hypoglossi are identified and preserved near the carotid bifurcation and the spinal accessory nerve and the superior thyroid artery are identified and preserved.

shears (► Fig. 22.7). The hypoglossal nerve and ansa hypoglossi are identified and preserved near the carotid bifurcation area and the superior thyroid and lingual arteries are identified and preserved. The branches of the IJV can also be ligated using the Hem-o-lok Ligation System or using the Harmonic curved shears or bipolar cautery depending on the size of the vessel (► Fig. 22.8).

To address the levels IV and V, the assistant surgeon may need to realign the axis of the robotic instrument arms toward the lower neck. Once the SCM is fully retracted, the dissection can continue inferiorly from levels IIb to V (► Fig. 22.9). The previously dissected levels II and III content is retracted medially, and the dissection of the lympho-fatty tissue is continued toward levels III and IV by exposing the carotid artery and the IJV medially (► Fig. 22.9). The dissected specimen is retracted superiorly for countertraction, as it is being dissected and lifted off the scalene muscles posteriorly (► Fig. 22.10). Once the specimen is dissected free from the great vessels and the vagus nerve medially down to

the clavicle, the attention can now be addressed to the posterior neck. The dissection is done from lateral to medial direction from level V toward the dissected specimen anteriorly. The omohyoid muscle can be preserved or transected if required as part of the specimen. The cervical plexus and the transverse cervical artery are identified and preserved (► Fig. 22.10). As the level IV dissection is performed, the phrenic nerve and the brachial plexus are also preserved. Extreme caution is given to carefully ligate lymphatic and thoracic ducts (► Fig. 22.11). To securely ligate the lymphatic ducts, Hemoclips or Hem-o-lok Ligation System can be used (► Fig. 22.11). Similarly, the branches of the IJV can also be ligated using the Hem-o-lok Ligation System or using the Harmonic curved shears or bipolar cautery depending on the size of the vessel. Once the neck dissection is completed, the specimen is delivered in one piece via the retroauricular incision by the assistant surgeon (► Fig. 22.12).

Once the final specimen is removed, the surgical bed is irrigated with copious amount of warm saline. Meticulous hemostasis

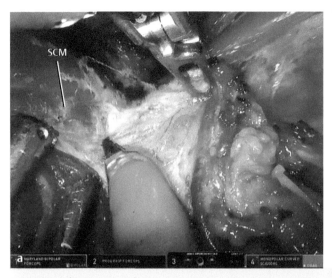
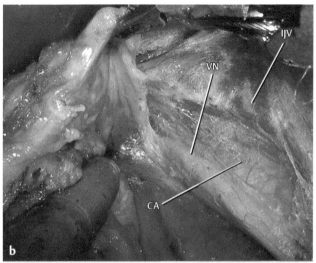

Fig. 22.9 (a,b) Dissection of the levels IV and V. Once the sternocleidomastoid muscle is fully retracted, the dissection can continue inferiorly from levels IIb to V. The previously dissected levels II and III content is retracted medially, and the dissection of the lympho-fatty tissue is continued toward levels III and IV by exposing the carotid artery and the internal jugular vein medially.

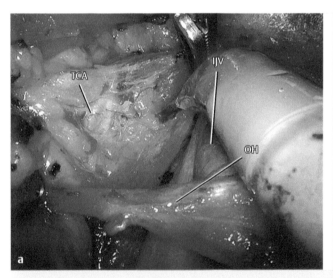
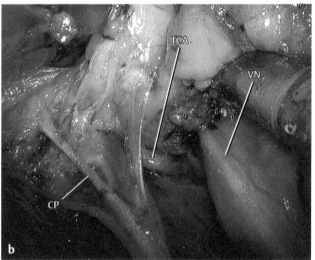

Fig. 22.10 (a,b) Dissection of levels IV and V. Once the specimen is dissected free from the great vessels and the vagus nerve medially down to the clavicle, the omohyoid muscle can be preserved and the cervical plexus and the transverse cervical artery are identified and preserved.

control and verification of chyle leak around the lymphatic duct ligation site are important final steps of the procedure. A closed suction drain is securely placed posterior to the retroauricular incision for optimal cosmetic results. The wound is closed with simple interrupted sutures, and skin glue material can be applied as well.

It is important to remember that the concept and the extent of robotic neck dissection is the same as in traditional open neck dissection. The surgical view and the direction of approach of the neck dissection, as well as the instruments used, are the only significant differences between the two approaches.

22.8 Postoperative Management

The principle of postoperative care is no different from conventional open neck dissection. The patient should be closely monitored for any signs of hemorrhage, hematoma, seroma, or chyle leakage. The drain is removed once the drainage amount

is below 30 mL over 24 hours. It is important to routinely check for any signs of skin discoloration or skin flap necrosis.

22.9 Postoperative Complications

Mouth corner deformity or asymmetry from marginal mandibular nerve injury can very occasionally occur, but a great majority of these cases are temporary and tend to resolve within 1 to 3 months following surgery. It tends to occur especially with level I dissections, and it is thought to be secondary to thermocoagulation or traction injury. Similarly to the conventional open neck dissections, ear lobe numbness secondary to the greater auricular nerve injury and postoperative hemorrhage or hematoma can infrequently occur. The ear lobe numbness is temporary if the nerve was preserved intact during surgery. It can be managed conservatively as the numbness tends to fade away, but this can take several months to resolve.

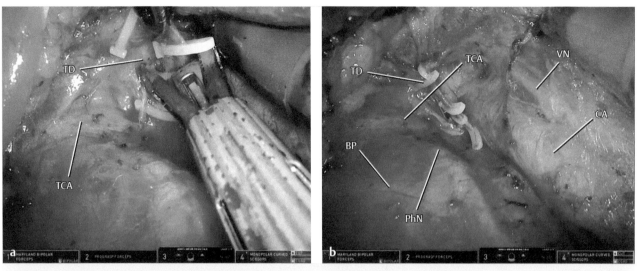

Fig. 22.11 (a,b) Ligation of the thoracic duct (TD). The transverse cervical artery and the phrenic nerve and the brachial plexus are well preserved. The TD is sealed with Hem-O-Lok to prevent a chyle leakage.

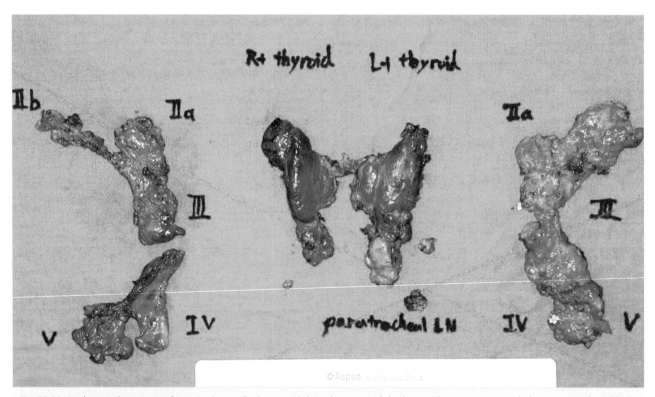

Fig. 22.12 Final surgical specimen after completion of robotic total thyroidectomy with both central compartment neck dissections and modified radical neck dissection levels II to V via retroauricular approach. The specimen can be separately removed with level-by-level strategy.

22.9.1 Possible Postoperative Complications

- Neurogenic injury (usually temporary):
  - Marginal mandibular nerve.
  - Greater auricular nerve.
- Seroma/hematoma/hemorrhage.
- Wound problems (extremely rare):
  - Hair loss along incision line within hairline.
  - Wound infection, dehiscence.
  - Skin flap discoloration, ischemic changes, necrosis.
  - Hypertrophic scar, keloid formation.

22.10 Further Comments

Careful patient selection, appropriate patient positioning in the operating room, and adequate working space formation are the key factors contributing to the safety, efficiency, and success of the procedure. The Xi system, if available, may be preferable to

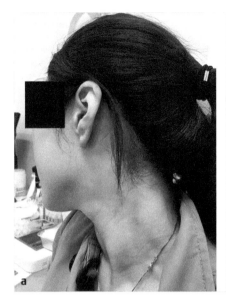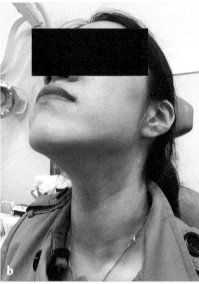

Fig. 22.13 (a,b) Postoperative photo of patients who received robotic retroauricular total thyroidectomy with both central compartment neck dissection and ipsilateral modified radical neck dissection levels II to V.

the Si system given the use of all three instrument arms and enhanced 3D HD vision.

The greatest advantage of robotic approach when compared to the traditional open neck surgery is not only the superior cosmetic outcome but also the possibility of extremely precise surgical dissection (▶ Fig. 22.13). Highly precise and fine plane dissection can be conducted with the application of the 10 times magnified 3D HD vision, the use of three instrument arms, and the tremor filtering system.

Transcervical incision used in open neck dissection surgery often leaves a very noticeable scar, which can be completely avoided by placing the surgical incision behind the auricle and within the hairline with the use of the retroauricular approach. When compared to other remote-access approaches to lateral neck, the lymph node compartments can be more easily reached and dissected given the direct and short distance of dissection. Additionally, a simple patient positioning negates the risk of intraoperative brachial plexus injury or any other physical sequelae resulting from patient positioning. This is an ideal and versatile approach for head and neck surgeons who wish to perform surgeries on both benign and malignant tumors of head and neck with superior cosmetic outcome when compared to the traditional open cervical approaches.

Suggested Readings

[1] Byeon HK, Holsinger FC, Duvvuri U, et al. Recent progress of retroauricular robotic thyroidectomy with the new surgical robotic system. Laryngoscope. 2017:[Epub ahead of print]

[2] Byeon HK, Kim H, Chang JW, et al. Comprehensive application of robotic retroauricular thyroidectomy: the evolution of robotic thyroidectomy. Laryngoscope. 2016; 126(8):1952–1957

[3] Byeon HK, Koh YW. The new era of robotic neck surgery: the universal application of the retro auricular approach. J Surg Oncol. 2015; 112 (7):707–716

[4] Koh YW, Choi EC. Robotic approaches to the neck. Otolaryngol Clin North Am. 2014; 47(3):433–454

[5] Lira RB, Chulam TC, de Carvalho GB, et al. Retroauricular endoscopic and robotic versus conventional neck dissection for oral cancer. J Robot Surg. 2017: [Epub ahead of print]

[6] Byeon HK, Holsinger FC, Tufano RP, et al. Robotic total thyroidectomy with modified radical neck dissection via unilateral retro auricular approach. Ann Surg Oncol. 2014; 21(12):3872–3875

[7] Kim WS, Byeon HK, Park YM, et al. Therapeutic robot-assisted neck dissection via a retro auricular or modified facelift approach in head and neck cancer: a comparative study with conventional transcervical neck dissection. Head Neck. 2015; 37(2):249–254

[8] Kim WS, Park JH, Byeon HK, et al. A study comparing free-flap reconstruction via the retro auricular approach and the traditional transcervical approach for head and neck cancer: a matched case-control study. Ann Surg Oncol. 2015; 22(3):S349–S354

[9] Koh YW, Chung WY, Hong HJ, et al. Robot-assisted selective neck dissection via modified face-lift approach for early oral tongue cancer: a video demonstration. Ann Surg Oncol. 2012; 19:1334–1335

[10] Kim WS, Koh YW, Byeon HK, et al. Robot-assisted neck dissection via a transaxillary and retroauricular approach versus a conventional transcervical approach in papillary thyroid cancer with cervical lymph node metastases. J Laparoendosc Adv Surg Tech A. 2014; 24(6):367–372

[11] Byeon HK, Holsinger FC, Koh YW, et al. Endoscopic supraomohyoid neck dissection via a retro auricular or modified facelift approach: Preliminary results. Head Neck. 2014; 36:425–430

[12] Lee HS, Kim WS, Hong HJ, et al. Robot-assisted supraomohyoid neck dissection via a modified face-lift or retroauricular approach in early-stage cN0 squamous cell carcinoma of the oral cavity: a comparative study with conventional technique. Ann Surg Oncol. 2012; 19:3871–3878

[13] Kim WS, Lee HS, Kang SM, et al. Feasibility of robot-assisted neck dissections via a transaxillary and retroauricular ("TARA") approach in head and neck cancer: preliminary results. Ann Surg Oncol. 2012; 19:1009–1017

[14] Kang SW, Lee SH, Ryu HR, et al. Initial experience with robot-assisted modified radical neck dissection for the management of thyroid carcinoma with lateral neck node metastasis. Surgery. 2010; 148:1214–1221

[15] Ahn D, Lee GJ, Sohn JH. Comparison of the retro auricular approach an transcervical approach for excision of a second branchial cleft cyst. J Oral Maxillofac Surg. 2017; 75(6):1209–1215

[16] Lin FC, Yang TL, Tung MC, et al. Robot-assisted excision of cervical cystic hygroma though a retroauricular hairline approach: a case report. J Med Case Reports. 2016; 10:154

[17] Singer MC, Seybt MW, Terris DJ. Robotic facelift thyroidectomy: I. Preclinical simulation and morphometric assessment. Laryngoscope. 2011; 121:1631–1635

[18] Terris DJ, Singer MC, Seybt MW. Robotic facelift thyroidectomy: II. Clinical feasibility and safety. Laryngoscope. 2011; 121:1636–1641

[19] Terris DJ, Singer MC, Seybt MW. Robotic facelift thyroidectomy: patient selection and technical considerations. Surg Laparosc Endosc Percutan Tech. 2011; 21(4):237:242

[20] Terris DJ, Singer MC. Robotic facelift thyroidectomy: facilitating remote access surgery. Head Neck. 2012; 34:746–747

[21] Terris DJ, Singer MC. Qualitative and quantitative differences between 2 robotic thyroidectomy techniques. Otolaryngol Head Neck Surg. 2012; 147:20–25

23 Radioguided Neck Dissection

Quinn A. Dunlap and Brendan C. Stack, Jr.

Abstract

Long-term survival for differentiated thyroid cancer (DTC) is greater than 90% with appropriate medical and surgical therapy as well as appropriate follow-up consisting of monitored thyroid-stimulating hormone (TSH)/thyroglobulin (Tg), neck ultrasonography, computed tomography, and radioactive iodine or [18]fluoro-fludeoxyglucose (^{18}F-FDG) uptake scanning (SPECT and PET, respectively), when indicated. However, a subset of treated patients experience a structural incomplete response to initial therapy, while an additional subset experience tumor recurrence. While surgery has been proven in the literature to provide the best treatment response in these patients, the presence of significant scarring and fibrosis may hinder the identification and complete excision of diseased tissue. For this reason, radioguided neck dissection has been created and progressively developed to facilitate localization and excision of malignant tissue in a real-time format. Within this chapter, we will cover the concept, clinical indications, methods, and procedural execution of radioguided neck dissection for excision of persistent or recurrent DTC.

Keywords: differentiated thyroid cancer, structural incomplete response, radioactive iodine 131, [18]fluoro-fludeoxyglucose, single-photon emission computed topography, positron emission topography, neck ultrasonography, computed topography, thyroglobulin, thyroid remnant

23.1 Introduction

Total thyroidectomy is indicated for patients who present with thyroid cancer that is greater than 4 cm, demonstrates gross extrathyroidal extension (clinical T3b and T4 disease), clinically apparent nodal metastasis (clinical N1 disease), and/or distant metastasis (clinical M1 disease). In addition, total thyroidectomy (vs. hemithyroidectomy) is still an option for patients presenting with thyroid cancer measuring 1 to 4 cm in size without extrathyroidal extension, nodal metastasis, or distant metastasis.[1] Therapeutic bilateral central compartment dissection is indicated in addition to total thyroidectomy if clinically involved central nodes are involved either preoperatively (on imaging) or intraoperatively; prophylactic central neck dissection (ipsilateral or bilateral) should be considered in patients presenting with clinical T3 or T4 disease or clinically involved lateral neck nodes; and therapeutic lateral neck dissection is indicated in patients with biopsy-proven metastatic lateral cervical lymphadenopathy.[1,2] The advantages of performing total thyroidectomy over hemithyroidectomy are well known and consist of a decreased risk of locoregional recurrence (LRR), ability for postsurgical radioactive iodine (RAI) ablation (see ▶ Table 23.1), and increased surveillance capability during follow-up through the utilization of Tg, thyroglobulin antibodies (anti-Tg), and RAI whole body scanning (WBS), [18]fluoro-fludeoxyglucose (^{18}F-FDG) positron emission tomography (PET), or either of these modalities in combination with computed tomography (PET or SPECT/CT).[3] This comes with a potential cost of the risks of postoperative bilateral vocal cord dysfunction (possible tracheotomy) and hypoparathyroidism. Increased sensitivity and specificity of surveillance modalities leads to earlier detection and treatment of recurrence or persistence of disease, and thus improved patient outcomes.

An aggressive initial management approach with regard to differentiated thyroid carcinoma has been proven to render an approximately 90% long-term survival rate[4,5,6] with recent data exhibiting annual death rates less than 2%.[7] However, studies also indicate that patients within this population possess LRR rates of up to 30%, depending on the initial treatment modality, and of this population, 30% recur and approximately 30% are never fully eradicated of disease with another 15% dying of disease,[5] also producing 10-year cumulative survival rates of 49.1, 89.3, and 32.5% for all patients, patients younger than 45 years, and patients older than 45 years, respectively. In addition, another subset within this population never fully achieves structural eradication of disease, with detected persistence of structural disease at follow-up known as structural incomplete response (SIR). This has been shown to occur in 2 to 6% of American Thyroid Association (ATA) low-risk patients, 19 to 28% of intermediate-risk patients, and 67 to 75% of high-risk patients (see ▶ Table 23.1). Within the SIR population, 50 to 85% have been shown to possess persistent disease despite additional therapy with disease-specific death rates as high as 11%. This population has the highest risk with regard to disease-specific mortality of any of the response to therapy categories[1] (see ▶ Table 23.2).

Table 23.1 Characteristics (ATA and AJCC/TNM) that impact postoperative radioiodine decision making

ATA risk staging (TNM)	Description	Body of evidence suggests RAI improves *disease-specific* survival	Body of evidence suggests RAI improves *disease-free* survival	Postsurgical RAI indication
ATA low-risk T1a N0, Nx M0, Mx	Tumor size < 1 cm (uni- or multifocal)	No	No	No
ATA low-risk T1b, T2 N0, Nx M0, Mx	Tumor size > 1–4 cm	No	Conflicting observational data	Not routine May be considered for patients with aggressive histology or vascular invasion (ATA intermediate risk)
ATA low to intermediate risk T3 N0, Nx M0, Mx	Tumor size > 4 cm	Conflicting data	Conflicting observational data	Consider the presence of other adverse features and age

Continued

Table 23.1 continued

ATA risk staging (TNM)	Description	Body of evidence suggests RAI improves *disease-specific* survival	Body of evidence suggests RAI improves *disease-free* survival	Postsurgical RAI indication
ATA low to intermediate risk T3 N0, Nx M0, Mx	Microscopic ETE, any tumor size	No	Conflicting observational data	Consider Generally favored; may not require in small tumor with microscopic ETE
ATA low to intermediate risk T1–3 N1a M0, Mx	Central compartment neck lymph node metastases	No, except possibly in patients > 45 y-o (NTCTCSG stage III)	Conflicting observational data	Consider Generally favored, especially with structural evidence of disease or increased age; insufficient evidence if < 5 microscopic nodal metastases without other adverse features
ATA low to intermediate risk T1–3 N1b M0, Mx	Lateral neck or mediastinal lymph node metastases	No, except possibly in sub-group of patients > 45 y-o	Conflicting observational data	Consider Generally favored, especially with structural evidence of disease or increased age
ATA high-risk T4 Any N Any M	Any size, gross ETE	Yes, observational data	Yes, observational data	Yes
ATA high risk M1 Any T Any N	Distant metastases	Yes, observational data	Yes, observational data	Yes

Abbreviations: AJCC, American Joint Committee on Cancer; ATA, American Thyroid Association; ETE, extra thyroid extension; RAI, radioactive iodine; TNM, tumor, node, metastasis.
Source: Data from 2015 American Thyroid Association Management Guidelines for Adult Patients with Thyroid Nodules and Differentiated Thyroid Cancer: The American Thyroid Association Guidelines Task Force on Thyroid Nodules and Differentiated Thyroid Cancer.

Table 23.2 Classifications of response to therapy (total thyroidectomy with radioiodine remnant ablation) in patients with differentiated thyroid cancer

Category	Definitions	Clinical outcomes	Management implications
Excellent response	Negative imaging *and* suppressed Tg < 0.2 ng/mL *or* stimulated Tg > 10 ng/mL *or* rising anti-Tg antibody levels	1–4% recurrence < 1% disease-specific death	Early decrease in intensity and frequency of follow-up and degrees of TSH suppression
Biochemical incomplete response	Negative imaging *and* suppressed Tg > 1 ng/mL *or* stimulated Tg > 10 ng/mL *or* rising anti-Tg antibody levels	At least 30% spontaneously evolve to NED 20% achieve NED following additional therapy < 1% disease-specific death	If stable/declining serum Tg, then continued observation with ongoing TSH suppression If rising Tg or anti-Tg antibody values, then additional investigation and potentially additional therapy
Structural incomplete response	Structural or functional evidence of disease With any Tg level With or without anti-Tg antibodies	50–85% continue to have persistent disease despite additional therapy Disease-specific death rates as high as 11% with locoregional metastases and 50% with structural distant metastases	Additional treatments (RAI/surgery) vs. ongoing observation depending on multiple clinicopathologic factors including size, location, rate of growth, RAI avidity, FDG avidity, and specific pathology of the structure lesions
Indeterminate response	Nonspecific findings on imaging studies Faint uptake in thyroid bed on RAI scanning Nonstimulated Tg detectable Stimulated Tg detectable, but < 10 ng/mL *or* anti-Tg antibodies stable or declining in the absence of structural or functional disease	15–20% will have structural disease identified during follow-up In the remainder, nonspecific changes are either stable or resolved < 1% disease-specific death	Continued observation with appropriate serial imaging of the nonspecific lesions and serum Tg monitoring. Nonspecific findings that become suspicious over time should be further evaluated with further imaging and/or biopsy

Abbreviations: FDG, fludeoxyglucose; NED, no evidence of disease; RAI, radioactive iodine; TSH, thyroid-stimulating hormone.
Source: Data from 2015 American Thyroid Association Management Guidelines for Adult Patients with Thyroid Nodules and Differentiated Thyroid Cancer: The American Thyroid Association Guidelines Task Force on Thyroid Nodules and Differentiated Thyroid Cancer.

Higher rates of disease remission (29–51%) have been demonstrated across studies following surgical intervention for persistent or LRR disease, and thus the development of nodal recurrence or residual macroscopic thyroid tissue is considered a surgical disease.[1,8,9] However, as recurrence or persistence of disease will virtually always present in a previously operated field, the unavoidable presence of significant fibrosis and scarring frequently hinders the surgeon's capability to identify and excise diseased tissue. For this reason, surgeons have begun using nuclear medicine technology in combination with CT for assistance in intraoperative localization, excision, and confirmation of cure with regard to persistent or recurrent differentiated thyroid cancer (DTC), which is today known as radioguided neck dissection (RGND). To clarify, DTC is the only thyroid malignancy demonstrated to uptake radionuclides, and thus radionuclide imaging studies and RGND cannot be utilized for detection or resection of anaplastic or medullary thyroid cancer. Radioguided surgery can be beneficial intraoperatively, even in cases of DTC which is scan negative because of the sensitivity of operative radiation detection equipment.

23.1.1 Target Specificity of a Radionuclide versus Background

Nuclear medicine imaging derives its utility from the capability to detect abnormal physiologic function in concordance with and in spite of significant anatomic or morphologic change. Clinical information is derived through the observation of the distribution pattern of a pharmaceutical agent labeled with a radioactive tracer administered to the patient, enabling qualitative and quantitative measurements of radiopharmaceutical distribution that can have a dramatic effect on patient management in diseases of the head and neck.[10]

Radiopharmaceuticals are designated into two parts: the pharmaceutical portion, which ultimately determines the distribution of the particle, and the radionuclide label, which enables detection of the distribution of the particles. The radionuclide label emits nonparticulate gamma rays that are waves of electromagnetic radiation capable of being detected externally utilizing scintillation camera(s) positioned close to the patient. By way of a complex programed algorithm, separate flashes of light produced by the scintillation camera(s) due to the detection of gamma rays are plotted as dots on a field spatially related to the gamma emissions from the patient. In accord, the higher the rate of gamma emissions from a particular area (i.e., an area with greater amount of radiopharmaceutical), the greater the density of dots present on the formulated spatially related image, thus enabling target specificity due to concentration of a radiopharmaceutical in comparison to the otherwise normal background. Of note, some radionuclides only emit gamma rays (technetium-99 m [Tc-99m], I123) while other possess multiple mechanisms of decay with emission of both beta and gamma emissions (I131, ^{18}F-FDG).

It is worth noting and imperative to the successful execution of RGND, these gamma rays can be detected not only by the use of a scintillation camera but also with a "gamma probe," which is utilized intraoperatively by the surgeon for assistance in identification and verification of successful excision of malignant disease within the neck.[8,11,12] In contrast to radioguided

parathyroid surgery, in which the gamma probe cannot be utilized for location of the diseased tissue, use of the gamma probe for intraoperative assistance in localization of diseased tissue is one of two fundamental benefits in RGND. The second of these benefits consists of ex vivo confirmation of target excision. In this regard, specimen radioactivity counts may only be meaningfully interpreted when expressed as a proportion of background radioactivity, with gamma probe measurement demonstrating a significant increase in radioactivity of the specimen in comparison to background as a reliable indicator of successful excision.[13]

23.1.2 Imaging Modalities

Multiple imaging modalities of progressive complexity and utility have been developed over the previous decades for diagnostic, surveillance, and intraoperative use with regard to head and neck pathology. Recently, nuclear medicine imaging has been combined with CT in order to correlate nuclear medicine imaging findings with anatomic location, thus better enabling localization of disease. These imaging modalities and their interrelation will be discussed later. Of importance, one should note that nuclear medicine imaging studies can be performed as either static or dynamic studies. Static studies are obtained after sufficient time has elapsed for the radiopharmaceutical to reach its final biodistribution, while dynamic imaging studies are taken at multiple points in time to assess the changes in biodistribution of radiopharmaceutical over time. While dynamic imaging studies are used for diagnostic and localization purposes within the head and neck (e.g., 4D CT for parathyroid adenoma localization), RGND studies are limited to static (planar or tomographic) imaging studies, and thus the discussion in this chapter will be limited to static scintigraphic nuclear medicine imaging studies.

Planar Imaging

For the performance of planar scintigraphy, images are obtained utilizing a standard low-energy parallel hole collimator, also known as pinhole collimation. As this was the first type of scintigraphic nuclear medicine imaging created, it possesses the most short and simple protocol with the least complex necessary equipment. In accord, the advantages of performing this type of imaging consist of not requiring patients to sit still for long periods without a break, the capability for the imaging to be performed with the use of a basic Anger camera, and the capability of performing in patients in whom SPECT can be challenging, such as obese or claustrophobic patients.[14] The advantages come at the expense of decreased sensitivity to what most consider an inadequate degree; therefore, this type of imaging is rarely used currently due to the availability of more sensitive and specific imaging modalities.

Single-Photon Emission Computed Tomography

Single-photon emission computed tomography (SPECT) was developed subsequent to planar imaging as a more complex method for utilizing the same radiopharmaceutical distribution principles as discussed above. Instead of utilizing a single Anger camera, SPECT utilizes two or more multihead Anger cameras that rotate 360 degrees around the patient, thereby enabling three-dimensional reconstruction within the head and neck region.[10] While this protocol does require more complex and thus more costly equipment (multihead Anger cameras and software for 3D reconstruction) as well as prolongation of the imaging protocol, it also overcomes the interpretation difficulties associated with the superimposition of tracer activity onto planar images, which in turn provides a significant increase in sensitivity.[14] Planar and SPECT imaging are performed utilizing I123, I131, or Tc-99 m radioisotopes, which will be discussed in detail later in the chapter.

Positron Emission Tomography

Positron emission tomography is so named due to the use of pharmaceutical compounds labeled with positron-emitting radioisotopes that function as molecular probes to image and measure biochemical processes in vivo.[15] As with SPECT and planar imaging, the amount of radiolabeled material administered is minimal and thus does not disrupt underlying molecular and biochemical processes, but enables the detection of the pharmaceutical's biodistribution through the utilization of scintigraphy. Unlike planar and SPECT imaging, however, PET utilizes the radiopharmaceutical ^{18}fluoro-fludeoxyglucose (^{18}F-FDG), and is used not only in head and neck imaging but also for the detection of oncologic pathology throughout the entire body.[16] PET finds its value in surveillance, perioperative, and intraoperative thyroid imaging in that the mechanism of ^{18}F-FDG uptake differs from that of I131 and I123, thus enabling detection of recurrent or persistent disease in radioiodine-negative DTC patients.[12,17,18,19]

SPECT/CT and PET/CT

Following the development of SPECT, PET, and CT, the idea was created to fuse either SPECT or PET with CT in order to enable increased accuracy of localization of detected disease. This addition of anatomic information (CT) to functional information (SPECT/PET) can be achieved either by using a hybrid SPECT/PET-CT scanner capable of the consecutive acquisition of SPECT/PET and multislice CT in one unit, or by software fusion of separately acquired diagnostic CT and SPECT/PET images. If a hybrid SPECT/PET-CT is to be performed, CT is often done in the absence of intravenous (IV) contrast, limiting the radiation dose as well as the diagnostic value of the CT scan. On the other hand, SPECT/PET-CT images (acquired separately) usually consist of CT with IV contrast with an increase in diagnostic value of the CT, but with the expense of a higher radiation dose to the patient as well as cost burden for the institution to fund high-accuracy software fusion of SPECT/PET and CT images. Therefore, in the literature and also clinically, SPECT/PET-CT (hybrid) is often performed and correlated with diagnostic (CT with contrast) images for operative planning.[14] In addition, the literature definitively demonstrates that SPECT/PET-CT possesses significantly increased sensitivity, specificity, localization, and lesion characterization than any of these modalities alone, and thus has become the standard of care with regard to surveillance and operative planning of recurrent or persistent DTC.[18,19,20,21,22]

23.1.3 Radionuclide Options

As previously described, radiopharmaceuticals are composed of two critical components consisting of the pharmaceutical portion and the radionuclide tracer. Several radionuclide tracers have been developed and used in nuclear medicine imaging throughout the years. The primary radionuclide tracers utilized in radioguided thyroid surgery are described below.

Technetium-99m

A number of elements other than iodine are selectively concentrated within the thyroid gland, one of which is technetium. However, technetium is not a naturally occurring element and only exists in radioactive form, with one of these isotopes being Tc-99 m. This radiotracer's physical characteristics make it an attractive option for use in scintillation scanning (planar or SPECT), particularly with regard to initial evaluation of possible presence of thyroid disease as well as in evaluation of thyroid disease in children. First, the particle is trapped within the thyroid gland but not organified, resulting in a relatively short 6-hour half-life that enables imaging acquisition approximately 15 to 20 minutes following IV administration. Second, the particle produces virtually no beta emissions and moderately low gamma emissions enabling administration with a minimal radiation dose and without local tissue ablation. Last, Tc99-m is readily available as well as inexpensive.[10,14,23] However, the necessity of radionuclide evaluation for initial evaluation of thyroid disease has become somewhat rare over the previous decade (i.e., limited to evaluation of thyroid nodule in the setting of hyperthyroid symptoms and a suppressed TSH), and even in necessary situations I123 has become the preferred radionuclide for this particular evaluation.[1] As such, Tc-99 m is rarely clinically utilized in radionuclide evaluation, surveillance, or intraoperative guidance in the management of DTC today.

Iodine 123

Thyroid hormone biosynthesis begins with the trapping of inorganic plasma iodide within the thyroid gland, followed by oxidation to iodide and subsequent organification. As a result, radioactive iodine uptake provides a means to detect and document the presence, size, shape, location, and functional characteristics of thyroid tissue. I123, unlike technetium, is administered orally and subsequently trapped and organified within the thyroid gland, producing a half-life of approximately 13 hours, and results in a delayed but extended optimal imaging window of 4 to 24 hours in comparison to Tc-99 m. I123 has also been proven to produce higher target-to-background images in comparison to Tc-99 m with a consequent increase in sensitivity and accuracy on scintigraphic studies. However, I123 is also less readily available, more expensive, and delivers a higher radiation dose to the patient. In light of the fact that the use of radionuclide imaging for initial evaluation of thyroid nodules in recent years has substantially decreased, I123 has become the study of choice if radionuclide studies do become necessary in the initial workup of a thyroid nodule(s) due to its higher target-to-background imaging characteristics.[1,10] Worth noting, neither Tc-99 m nor I123 (SPECT/CT) are routinely utilized in the evaluation of recurrent or persistent DTC due to decreased image quality and thus sensitivity and localization in comparison to I131 SPECT/CT and ^{18}F-FDG PET/CT.[14,17,22,24]

Iodine 131

As with I123, I131 is orally administered with subsequent trapping and organification within the thyroid gland, producing an excellent and highly specific mechanism to obtain information regarding presence, size, shape, and function of thyroid tissue. However, I131 is administered in doses ranging from 30 to 300 mCi in the literature (30–150 mCi in recent ATA guidelines), and is never utilized in initial diagnostic thyroid imaging studies due to its exertion of a significantly higher radiation dose to the patient, longer half-life (>8 days), and multiple different mechanisms of decay, including release of both beta and gamma emissions. The beta emissions released by I131 irradiates and induces ablation of the immediate local region of tissue in which the radiopharmaceutical concentrates during distribution, making it a valuable tool for therapeutic ablation of remnant thyroid tissue and distant metastatic disease in persistent or recurrent DTC, as well as nonsurgical treatment of Grave's disease[1,6,10,25] (see ▶ Table 23.1 for risk stratification and decision making regarding I131 RAI remnant ablation). In addition, since the advent of SPECT/CT the literature has shown that I131 SPECT/CT may be performed at either therapeutic (>30 mCi) or subtherapeutic (1–5 mCi) levels with increased ability in detection and thus guidance for resection of persistent or recurrent DTC in comparison to Tc-99 m and I123 SPECT/CT in iodine-avid tissues.[6,22,24,26] Furthermore, due to the radionuclides emission of gamma particles, it may also be administered preoperatively with subsequent use of a gamma probe. This enables intraoperative confirmation of successful excision of diseased tissue via both ex vivo detection of radioactivity following excision of the specimen as well as in vivo confirmation with return of the wound bed to background in iodine-avid persistence

or recurrence of DTC (which will be described in detail later in this chapter).[8,11,22,27] Of particular importance, review of the literature demonstrates a known "flip-flop" phenomenon in which radioiodine-avid tissues do not uptake ^{18}F-FDG and thus are not visible on PET/CT imaging with the converse also being true (see ▶ Fig. 23.1).[22]

[18]Fluoro-Fludeoxyglucose

Although multiple radioisotopes have been utilized in PET imaging (^{11}C, ^{15}O, ^{13}N, ^{68}Ga, ^{18}F), ^{18}F-FDG has by far exerted the most significant clinical impact on PET imaging. The amounts of radiolabeled material administered to the patient are exceedingly small (micrograms–nanograms), and thus produce no pharmacologic effects or risk of toxic radiation dose. In this manner, PET possesses the ability to assess molecular alteration associated with pathology disturbing the underlying biophysiologic processes. ^{18}F-FDG is a glucose analog, and thus is taken up by glucose transporters in tissues with a significantly increased metabolic demand. As malignant cells maintain a high metabolic rate secondary to unregulated growth and progression through the cell cycle, this radioisotope localizes and concentrates within malignant disease of multiple different types following uptake and trapping within these cells via conversion of FDG to FDG-6-phosphate by hexokinase.[28] Consequently, its use is currently widespread for the purposes of surveillance and detection of recurrent or persistent disease throughout the field of oncology.[16] Although PET/CT imaging was not initially considered for surveillance or detection of DTC due to the available, highly specific radionuclides already in use, it has proven to be an invaluable tool for surveillance, detection, and intraoperative guidance with regard to iodine-negative DTC thyroid cancer over the previous 15 years.[8,12,18,19] Persistent or recurrence of radioiodine-negative DTC is initially suspected in the setting of negative I131 SPECT/CT upon follow-up with

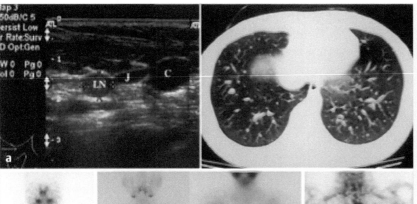

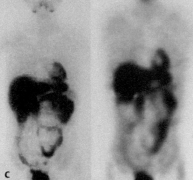
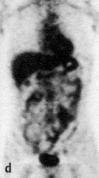

Fig. 23.1 A 38-year-old man with cervical LNs and lung metastases of differentiated thyroid cancer demonstrating "flip-flop phenomenon." **(a)** Neck ultrasonography and chest CT show mild cervical lymphadenopathy and multiple lung metastases, respectively. C, common carotid artery; J, internal jugular vein; LN, lymph node. **(b)** 131I scan shows cervical LNs and lung metastases. **(c)** 99mTc-MIBI planar and SPECT images show no significant accumulation at either site. **(d)** FDG-PET scan is also negative. (Adapted with permission of Iwata et al.[22])

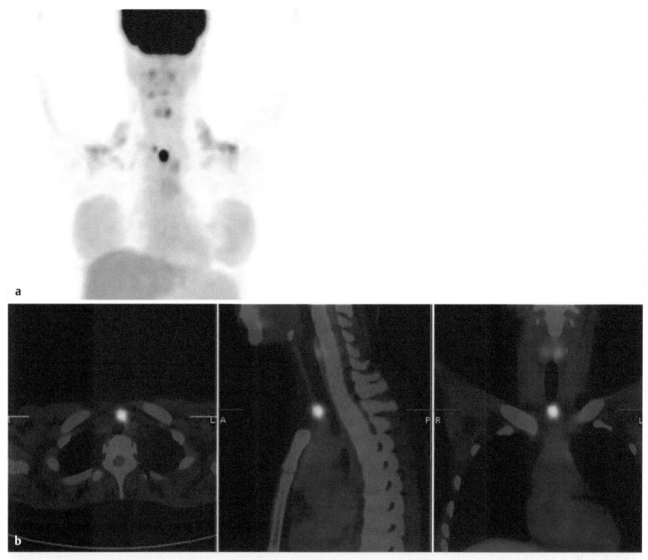

Fig. 23.2 **(a)** Preoperative PET and **(b)** preoperative fused PET/CT imaging, revealing isolated focal ^{18}F-FDG uptake involving the pretracheal region of the upper mediastinum. (Adapted with permission of Agrawal et al.[18])

persistently elevated or increasing Tg or anti-Tg levels. Further investigation is warranted in such a setting, consisting of neck ultrasonography (NUS) with possible fine needle aspiration (FNA) and ^{18}F-FDG PET/CT (see ▸ Fig. 23.2), as it has proven to have superior sensitivity in comparison to Tc-99 m SPECT/CT.[1,2,17,19,22] As with I131, concentrated areas of ^{18}F-FDG emit gamma rays during decay, which has an approximate half-life of 2 hours (unlike I131), that can be detected with a gamma probe and correlated with preoperative PET/CT. This was first successfully demonstrated in a series of patients with colorectal carcinoma.[28,29] Not long afterward, head and neck surgeons began developing and implementing protocols for utilizing TSH-stimulated PET/CT imaging and gamma probe RGND for intraoperative confirmation of successful identification and excision of persistent and recurrent DTC.[8,12,18,30]

23.1.4 Intraoperative Equipment

Fortunately, the unique additional requirements for performing RDNG within a head and neck practice consist only of a nuclear medicine department and radiodetection device. The type of radiodetection device used will depend on whether RGND is being performed utilizing I131 or ^{18}F-FDG, and several detectors of each type are commercially available through manufacturers. However, the importance of a nuclear medicine physician and department within the institution cannot be overemphasized. Their presence is absolutely necessary for handling of radionuclides and generation of reliable images (SPECT/PET-CT) that provide an essential road map for the surgeon as well as intraoperative confirmation of successful excision and cure of disease.[8,27] Additional equipment recommended for, but not unique to, RGND includes intraoperative recurrent laryngeal nerve (RLN) monitoring as well as monitoring for display of preoperative imaging studies (SPECT/PET-CT). The protocol for administration, dosing, and procedural execution of RGND will be discussed later in the chapter.

23.1.5 Radiation Safety

As the performance of RGND necessitates the utilization of radioisotopes for successful execution, radiation safety is somewhat of a concern for those that are routinely performing these procedures. The vast majority of this concern is with regard to the frequent utilization of ^{18}F-FDG for RGND due to its associated higher energy emission owing to two resulting high-energy (511 kV) annihilation photons.[16,31] To address this concern, studies have been completed to measure and quantify the relative risk of radiation exposure to the operating room staff, as the amount of radiation exposure for an individual is dependent on multiple variables including dose injected to the patient, time elapsed from injection to arrival in the operating suite, operative duration, and distance between each provider and the patient.[28] In consideration of all these variables, the largest deep dose equivalent per case appears to be received by the surgeon (164 ± 135 uSv), followed by the anesthetist, scrub technologist, postoperative nurse, circulating nurse, and preoperative nurse.[32] From the body doses measured, it has been calculated that a surgeon can perform approximately 150 to 260 hours of radioguided surgery annually without exceeding permissible limits for professional workers.[28,31] Therefore, one can reasonably conclude that radiation exposure to operating room personnel is well below the limits of the U.S. Nuclear Regulatory Commission. The concern for significant radiation exposure secondary to I131 RGND seems to be relatively nonexistent in consideration of its widespread use and concomitant paucity of evidence in the literature.[33]

Special consideration is required with regard to any administration of radiopharmaceuticals to the pregnant or lactating female patient. The fetus is known to be highly radiosensitive, particularly during the first trimester, and so the use of radiopharmaceuticals is best avoided in this population with immediate discontinuance of breast-feeding if radioisotopes are utilized on a postpartum lactating patient.[10]

23.2 Clinical Indications

The primary indication for the performance of RGND is the presence of recurrent or persistent DTC. Higher rates of disease remission (29–51%) have been demonstrated across studies following surgical intervention for persistent or locoregional recurrent disease, and thus the development or persistence of nodal involvement or macroscopic thyroid tissue is considered a surgical disease.[1,8,9] In the indicated population, RGND is an innovative means by which a surgeon may utilize highly specific radiopharmaceuticals to intraoperatively visualize a structure of interest for en bloc excision and potential cure, with this technology enabling increased localization, minimally invasive incisions, and reduction of patient morbidity and inpatient hospital utilization. This capability proves to be particularly important in the resection of persistent or recurrent DTC, as these lesions invariably occur within a previously operated field with a significant degree of fibrosis and scarring, thus muddying the anatomic planes and altering the original anatomy. These patients most often present in one of three ways, which will be covered in the following text.

23.2.1 Small Volume Disease

Those with persistent small volume disease most commonly present as a SIR or biochemical incomplete response (BIR) following treatment with persistence of disease detected on

laboratory testing (Tg/anti-Tg ab), I131 SPECT/CT, and/or NUS upon follow-up in clinic. If small volume disease is detected on NUS or laboratory evaluation (persistently elevated or rising Tg or anti-Tg levels) but not in I131 SPECT, the residual disease has possibly underwent dedifferentiation or "stunning" (following multiple I131 imaging studies) with transformation from iodine-avid to iodine-negative tissue, and thus should be evaluated with ^{18}F-FDG PET/CT.[1,8,17,22] If structural disease is successfully detected on PET/CT and/or NUS, FNA should be performed for diagnosis,[2] and if DTC returns, the patient then progresses to SIR status. The SIR group has been shown to compose the highest risk group with regard to mortality in those treated for DTC (see ► Table 23.1). Within the SIR population, 50 to 85% have been shown to possess persistent disease despite additional therapy with disease-specific death rates as high as 11%. Of the DTC patients who present with BIR following initial treatment (15–20%), approximately 30% spontaneously evolve to no evidence of disease (NED), and another 20% achieve NED status with additional (nonsurgical) therapy. The remaining 50% either remain in this category indefinitely or progress to SIR, warranting surgical intervention. Also worth noting, of those who initially present with indeterminate response (IR), 15 to 20% of patients progress to SIR status through continued follow-up and surveillance (see ► Table 23.2).[1] In the context of these findings, the detection and resection of structurally persistent DTC via RGND becomes of paramount importance for patient outcomes.

23.2.2 Recurrence in an Operated Field

A small fraction of patients who achieve the excellent response (ER) category following initial treatment experience recurrence (1–4%) with only 1% of these patients dying of disease[1]; therefore, those with complete cure and subsequent true recurrence compose only a small fraction of those who would benefit from RGND. However, risk of recurrence does vary based on ATA risk stratification so that higher risk patients who achieve NED status possess a higher risk of recurrence, and tumor recurrence has been shown to be more prevalent prior to the age of 20 years and dramatically increase after the age of 60 years.[4] As these patients achieve the ER category through negative RAI scanning and laboratory evaluation at follow-up, the mainstay for surveillance in this population is NUS. In the instance of biopsy-proven recurrence via NUS with FNA, the patient progresses to SIR status and radionuclide imaging studies are necessary for operative planning,[8] as delay in (surgical) therapy following initial manifestation of recurrence for greater than a year has been shown to have an adverse effect on patient outcomes.[4]

23.2.3 Thyroid Remnants

Total thyroidectomy with possible central compartment and lateral neck dissection (depending on tumor size nodal involvement) remains the treatment of choice for DTC greater than 4 cm and an optional treatment modality for DTC 1 to 4 cm. Completeness of surgical resection of the primary tumor, and thus successful performance of a an extracapsular total thyroidectomy, is one of the most important prognostic factors in determining recurrence risk, probability of disease progression, and disease-specific mortality.[1,26] Recent more selective use of RAI for postoperative thyroid remnant ablation (see ► Table 23.1) has even further increased the importance of surgically resecting all native thyroid tissue during initial total thyroidectomy not only for decreasing recurrence but also to decrease false-positive findings during routine postoperative surveillance. However, with the recent advancements in highly specific radionuclide imaging techniques (SPECT/CT), it has become apparent that even meticulous surgical dissection during total thyroidectomy rarely results in absolute removal of all thyroid tissue (1%; see ► Fig. 23.3). Furthermore, the locations of this remnant thyroid tissue have recently been demonstrated to appear in characteristic locations that are closely related to the surgical technique of executing a total thyroidectomy (see ► Fig. 23.4).[26]

Amputated Superior Lobe/Pyramidal Lobe

In the performance of a total thyroidectomy, the surgeon most often removes each lobe of the thyroid working in a superior to inferior direction along the lateral aspect (following division of the middle thyroid vein) before dividing Berry's ligament posteromedially. In accord, one of the initial steps is blunt dissection of the superior pole from the underlying structures to medialize this portion of the gland for identification of the superior parathyroid gland prior to working inferiorly. The external branch of the superior laryngeal nerve (SLN) is known to enter the thyrohyoid membrane just deep to the superior aspect of the superior lobe as well as superior thyroid artery (STA). The SLN is not routinely identified during the procedure, but instead the surgeon takes care to divide the STA as close to the thyroid parenchyma as possible to avoid damage to the SLN, separating the superior lobe from the underlying structures following STA ligation. As a result, a portion of the superior lobe may be amputated during this portion of the procedure, leaving remnant thyroid tissue in this location (79% per Zeuren et al).[26,34]

Although textbooks and scientific articles alike describe and validate the presence of a pyramidal lobe in the majority of patients (55–70%), the significant variability in its length when present is often underappreciated. Furthermore, a portion of the pyramidal lobe or other thyroglossal duct tract elements may reside outside of the thyroid capsule, and so often avoid detection despite a meticulous surgical dissection. Consequently, the superior aspect of the pyramidal lobe (or other extracapsular diminutive

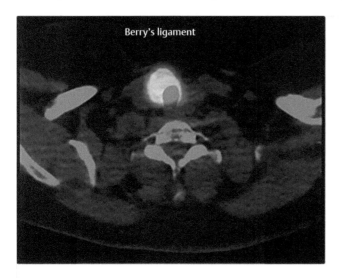

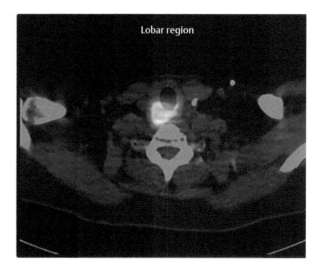

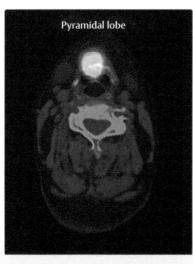

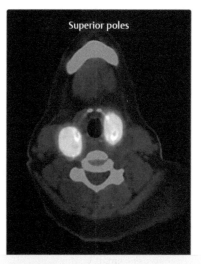

Fig. 23.3 SPECT/CT most commonly localized the specific uptake areas within the thyroid bed in the regions of Berry's ligament, lobar region, pyramidal lobe, and superior poles. (Adapted with permission of Zeuren et al.[26])

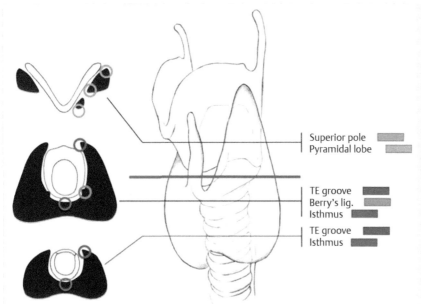

Fig. 23.4 Three-quarter view of thyroid and larynx with cross-sectional levels indicated. *Red line* indicates division between the upper and lower thyroid bed uptake regions. Upper cross-section depicts superior pole remnants from the anterior and the posterior margin of the superior pole (*yellow circles*) as well as midline/paramidline pyramidal lobe remnants (*blue circle*). Middle cross-section depicts Berry's ligament (*green circle*) and isthmus-related remnants (*purple circles*). Lower cross-section depicts tracheoesophageal (TE) groove remnants (*red circles*). (Adapted with permission of Zeuren et al.[26])

Superior pole
Pyramidal lobe

TE groove
Berry's lig.
Isthmus

TE groove
Isthmus

thyroid tissue) is often amputated despite the surgeon's diligent attempt to identify and resect all tissue in this region (46% per Zeuren et al).[26,34,35]

Berry's Ligament Remnant

The last portion of the procedure to be performed prior to delivery and thus excision of the thyroid lobe from the neck is the division of the ligament of Berry (LoB). This portion is reserved as the final step due to the ligament's posteromedial location on the lobe and thus difficult access, as well as its close proximity (< 3 mm) to the RLN. The RLN most often runs immediately deep to the LoB prior to entering the larynx at the cricothyroid joint, and the RLN should virtually always be identified prior to division of the ligament with careful attention to avoid nerve injury. Due to its close proximity to the RLN, extensive dissection is limited in this area, and previously performed autopsy studies demonstrate that normal thyroid tissue is often found in the LoB. Not surprisingly, remnant thyroid tissue can often be retained in this area even in the hands of the most experienced thyroid surgeons. Zeuren et al indicated this area as the most prevalent area of radionuclide uptake in postoperative SPECT/CT imaging studies (87%).[26,34,36]

Amputated Isthmus/Tracheoesophageal Groove Remnants

In the performance of a total thyroidectomy, the isthmus is most often cross-clamped and divided as an intermediate step before moving to resection of the contralateral lobe, and the exact same surgical technique is performed on the contralateral side. Prior studies have exhibited that in the area of the isthmus, as well as along the tracheoesophageal groove bilaterally, thyroid tissue is often present outside of the orthotopic lobar-isthmus thyroid body. Furthermore, close review of the anatomy of the thyroid gland reveals that the thyroid gland itself has no true defined anatomic fibrous capsule but rather a pseudocapsule that is derived

from the midline deep layer of cervical fascia; therefore, one can reasonably conclude that in several instances, it may not be possible to define discrete anatomical boundaries clearly delineating the normal thyroid from surrounding tissue, and so scant thyroid tissue on the trachea adjacent to the thyroid isthmus (57%) or deep within the tracheoesophageal groove (67%) may be left behind at several discrete anatomic locations despite the endeavor of an experienced surgeon to perform a meticulous extracapsular thyroidectomy.[26,34,37]

23.2.4 Sentinel Lymph Node Biopsy

Sentinel lymph node biopsy (SLNB) is routinely performed, recently with increasing frequency, for melanotic and squamous cell malignancies of the head and neck for assistance in determining appropriate treatment regimens (medical and surgical) as well as prognosis. However, with regard to DTC, due to the high false-negative rate demonstrated in recent studies, SLNB alone should not be performed in lieu of performance of RGND to guide lymphadenectomy in a specific neck compartment (central or lateral).[38]

23.2.5 Radionuclide Selection

Radionuclide selection in the performance of RGND largely depends on the avidity of the tissues with regard to iodine uptake. Native thyroid tissue, and therefore DTC in most cases, will uptake, trap, and organify iodine radionuclides as discussed earlier in the chapter. However, in the instance of recurrence or persistence of DTC, there is possibility that additional mutations and thus progressive dedifferentiation has occurred. In the interim since initial detection, the development of iodine-negative DTC that will not uptake iodine and thus produce false-negative findings on iodine-related radionuclide imaging studies is possible. Some have also described these tissues acquiring iodine negativity secondary to "stunning" of the tissue following multiple I131 radionuclide studies with higher administered doses of I131 (> 5 mCi).[1,12,22] This occurrence is suspected in the setting of negative iodine radionuclide imaging studies with positive finding on NUS (evidence of structural disease) and/or persistently elevated or rising Tg/anti-Tg levels. In these particular instances, the use of ^{18}F-FDG radionuclide imaging studies (PET/CT) is indicated, as iodine-negative tissues have been shown to possess affinity for ^{18}F-FDG, and thus uptake with positive findings on imaging studies.[1,8,17,22]

In summary, if the area of recurrence or persistence demonstrates iodine affinity, I131 should be utilized for preoperative imaging studies as well as intraoperative gamma probe detection, as I131 has been demonstrated to possess superior sensitivity to I123 in this regard.[24] If persistence or recurrence of iodine-negative DTC is suspected (as described earlier), ^{18}F-FDG should be utilized for possible detection and, if detected, intraoperatively for gamma probe guidance, as this radionuclide has been proven superior with regard to sensitivity to Tc-99 m.[17,22] In all instances, the radionuclide that was utilized for detection and thus preoperative imaging studies should also be used for intraoperative guidance.

23.3 Procedural Execution

Since utilization of RGND has been implemented, a variety of effective protocols have been described within the literature with high rates of success.[8,11,12,18,27] This text is by no means intended to serve as a substitute for formal training or clinical/surgical experience, which becomes of paramount importance in patient selection in consideration that in every case of RGND, the surgeon will be entering a previously operated field that may possess a high degree of scarring and fibrosis as well as possible anatomic alteration. In addition to developing a thorough understanding of the surgical anatomy within the central and lateral neck compartments, the technical aspects necessary for successful procedural execution are similar in concept to that of lymphoscintigraphy and sentinel lymph node dissection, which the literature indicates requires approximately 20 to 40 supervised cases for adequate proficiency.[13] The remainder of the chapter will cover the procedural execution of RGND from preoperative imaging to confirmation of excision of diseased tissue.

23.3.1 Preoperative Imaging with Demonstrated Affinity for a Given Radionuclide

Prior to any discussion regarding RGND for the treatment of persistent or recurrent DTC, persistence or recurrence must be proven. This may be detected by postoperative I131 scintigraphy (WBS or SPECT/CT), NUS, or ^{18}F-FDG PET/CT most often occurring along with elevated serum Tg or anti-Tg. Once disease is detected, FNA (CT or ultrasound guided) should be performed if possible for pathologic confirmation of disease prior to surgical intervention.[2] Refer to the discussion of imaging modalities, types of radionuclides, and radionuclide selection for additional details regarding preoperative imaging studies. In short, the patient will demonstrate either iodine-avid or iodine-negative persistent or recurrent disease, with I131 SPECT/CT being the imaging modality of choice for iodine-avid tissue and ^{18}F-FDG PET/CT being the imaging modality of choice for iodine-negative tissues.[22,24]

23.3.2 Day of Injection of Patient with Radionuclide

The timing of injection of radionuclide is dependent on the radionuclide selection, as I131 and ^{18}F-FDG possess significantly different half-lives (I131: approximately 8 days, ^{18}F-FDG: approximately 2 hours). See "Discussion" section regarding radionuclide selection for further details. Studies in the literature indicate that for I131, administration should be performed 3 to 7 days prior to surgery, whereas for ^{18}F-FDG it should be injected 1 to 3 hours prior to surgical intervention. Although administration of therapeutic doses of I131 (> 30 mCi) prior to radioguided surgery has been described in the literature, more commonly subtherapeutic doses (1–5 mCi) are administered, as the majority of these patients have either failed I131 medical therapy or possess disease too bulky (> 1 cm) to be treated with I131. Following administration of ^{18}F-FDG on the day of surgery (2–10 mCi), the patient should be kept in an isolated holding area prior to transport to the operating suite to minimize radiation exposure to hospital and operating room staff.[8,11,30,39] Either I131 or ^{18}F-FDG may be administered following administration of TSH to facilitate increased uptake within the tissue of interest, and virtually all patients who meet indication for RGND will also be treated with postoperative thyroid hormone suppression.[8,19]

23.3.3 Preoperative Interdisciplinary Communication/Operating Room Setup

If performing ^{18}F-FDG radioguided surgery, effective interdisciplinary communication between the surgical and anesthesia team, as well as the operating room staff, should be conducted prior to bringing the patient back to the operating room to ensure adequate timing of intervention as well as minimize time of intervention and thus radiation exposure. At our institution (University of Arkansas for Medical Sciences), the authors routinely request the use of a monitored endotracheal tube to provide intraoperative RLN monitoring, which requires visualized precise placement with assistance of the Glide Scope (Verathon, Bothell, WA) to ensure optimal lead positioning. An esophageal temperature probe is also placed (anesthesiologist's preference if the probe is actually used to monitor patient temperature) to assist with identification by palpation and avoidance of injury to the esophagus intraoperatively. A single dose of preoperative antibiotics and steroids is also given prior to all cases.

While multiple operating room setups are feasible and subject to change based on the basic design of the operating suite, an example of efficient operating room setup with necessary equipment is provided for reference in ▶ Fig. 23.5.

23.3.4 Determination of Background

Determination of background is performed by obtaining one to two background radiation counts at the start of the case; these measurements are most often obtained from neutral zones over

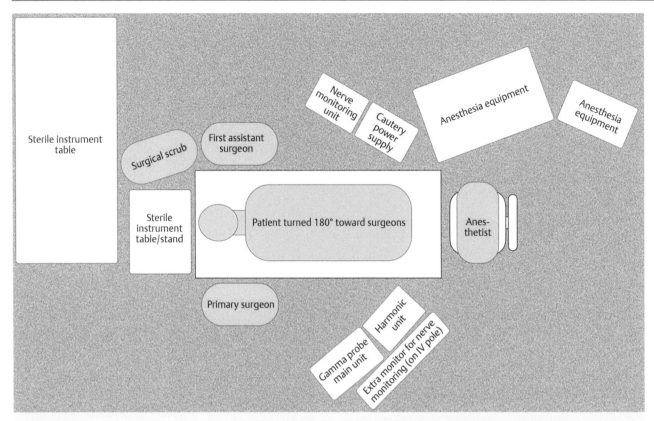

Fig. 23.5 Example of efficient operating room setup for radioguided neck dissection (RGND) with appropriate equipment. (Adapted with permission of Cox and Stack.[13])

the patient's right shoulder and right supraclavicular area. A dollop of fat is often excised immediately after creating the skin incision, and in this instance the dollop is utilized as a negative control. In order to facilitate adequate documentation and avoid confusion regarding the appropriate patient as well as gamma counts, a pre-printed 3 × 5″ index card is utilized for each case, scanned into the electronic medical record (EMR), and travels with the patient's physical chart (see ▶ Fig. 23.6). Gamma counts may be performed with a standard, commercially available gamma probe with its spectral window set for the I131 isotope for I131 intraoperative radioguidance, and ^{18}F-FDG gamma counts may be performed using a specially designed, shielded gamma probe. These devices have been shown to be comparable in sensitivity to detection of disease.[8]

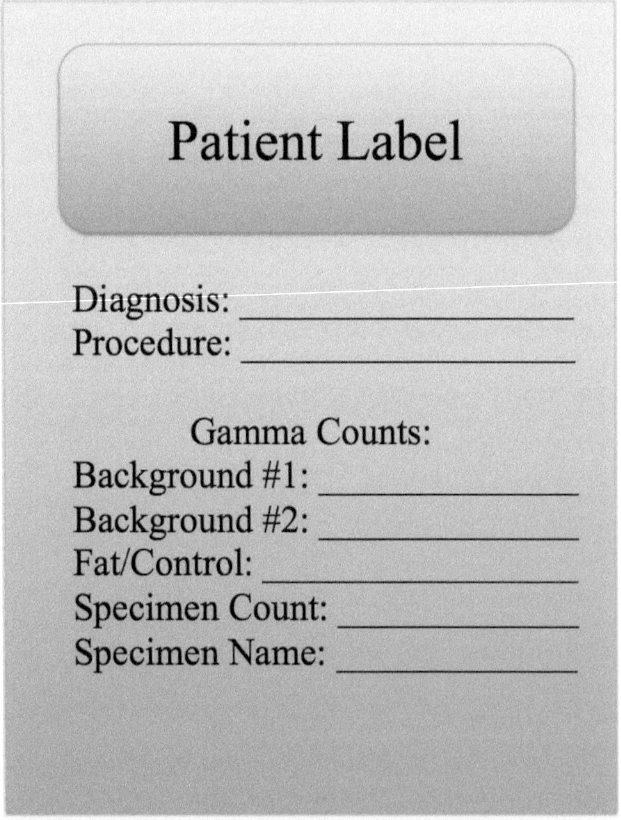

23.3.5 Incision Placement

The placement of the incision is determined based on the location of uptake, as well the presence of previous incisions. As virtually all patients meeting RGND criteria have previously undergone a total thyroidectomy, the midline neck incision created for performance of this procedure is most often used and simply reopened, provided this incision will enable adequate exposure of the persistent or recurrent disease within the neck. If the patient has previously undergone a selective lateral neck dissection (levels II–VI) for surgical treatment for lateral nodal involvement, this incision may be utilized for exposure. If there is concern that a previous incision will not adequately provide exposure of the diseased tissue, the surgeon may choose to either extend the previous incision to allow appropriate exposure

Patient Label

Diagnosis: _____
Procedure: _____

Gamma Counts:
Background #1: _____
Background #2: _____
Fat/Control: _____
Specimen Count: _____
Specimen Name: _____

Fig. 23.6 Example of layout for 3 × 5″ index card stamp or printout for documentation during radioguided neck dissection.

(most common), or simply create another 1 to 2 cm horizontal incision overlying the disease area as determined by preoperative imaging. If a new incision is created, the surgeon should attempt to place this in a skin crease of the neck to minimize appearance of the resultant scar.

23.3.6 In Situ Identification of Target of Interest

As previously delineated, operative intervention is timed so that the radionuclide being used for intraoperative guidance is maximally sequestered within the persistent or recurrent disease detected on preoperative imaging studies (NUS/PET/SPECT). However, the surgeon must rely on these preoperative studies in addition to direct visualization, palpation, and scanning of the field with the probe. This can be done in various ways. The skin over the area of maximum uptake may be marked by the nuclear medicine physician in his or her department. This area can be confirmed by scanning over and around the mark during surgery. Alternatively, the probe can be placed in the wound to identify the area of increased radionuclide uptake. By dragging the probe across the field in two passes at right angles to each other, the focus of maximum activity can be identified in two dimensions.[8,13,29]

23.3.7 Excision of Target of Interest

Once the diseased tissue has been successfully identified, the surgeon should attempt to resect disease tissue en block, rather than "berry-picking," as studies in the literature have demonstrated that undetected satellite tumors have been identified on pathology from en bloc excision performed with radioguidance, particularly if I131 is the radionuclide of choice.[8,11] Once the disease tissue has been excised en bloc, the gamma probe may then be utilized for ex vivo confirmation of radioactivity, which is recorded (see ▶ Fig. 23.6). In this manner, the surgeon may determine with a high degree of accuracy that the excised tissue is, in fact, the diseased tissue visualized on preoperative radionuclide imaging studies, as gamma probe readings are a far more accurate predictor of cure rather than size, mass, or cellularity.[13,40]

23.3.8 Basin Returns to Background

As a secondary means of confirmation of cure in the successful execution of RGND, the remaining wound bed should return to the previously measured background gamma readings (taken from the right shoulder/supraclavicular area) following complete excision of diseased tissue. False-positive readings can be obtained if the probe is directed toward the salivary glands or the heart. In the instance that the remaining wound bed does not return to background following excision despite ex vivo confirmation of excision of diseased tissue, the surgeon should carefully explore the wound bed for additional disease to be excised. Wound bed return to background is indicative of successful complete disease resection, and complete hemostasis should be ensured prior to wound closure. Drain placement is at the discretion of the surgeon and dependent on the extent of dissection and disease resection.

23.3.9 Mitigation of False Positive from Background (Salivary Glands, Heart)

Of fundamental importance in successful procedural execution of RGND and in order to avoid spurious or false-positive counts, due to background radioactivity, measurements of the negative control (fat dollop) and any specimens of interest are performed with the gamma probe held so that it is facing the ceiling. Particularly in the utilization of ^{18}F-FDG, the radionuclide is taken up in area of high glucose uptake, and thus characteristically concentrates in areas such as the salivary gland and heart.

References

[1] Haugen BR, Alexander EK, Bible KC, et al. 2015 American Thyroid Association Management Guidelines for Adult Patients with Thyroid Nodules and Differentiated Thyroid Cancer: The American Thyroid Association Guidelines Task Force on Thyroid Nodules and Differentiated Thyroid Cancer. Thyroid. 2016; 26(1):1–133

[2] Eng OS, Grant SB, Weissler J, et al. Operative bed recurrence of thyroid cancer: utility of a preoperative needle localization technique. Gland Surg. 2016; 5 (6):571–575

[3] Pacini F, Schlumberger M, Dralle H, Elisei R, Smit JW, Wiersinga W, European Thyroid Cancer Taskforce. European consensus for the management of patients with differentiated thyroid carcinoma of the follicular epithelium. Eur J Endocrinol. 2006; 154(6):787–803

[4] Mazzaferri EL. Long-term outcome of patients with differentiated thyroid carcinoma: effect of therapy. Endocr Pract. 2000; 6(6):469–476

[5] Mazzaferri EL. An overview of the management of papillary and follicular thyroid carcinoma. Thyroid. 1999; 9(5):421–427

[6] do Rosário PW, Borges MA, Alves MF, et al. [Follow-up of high-risk patients with differentiated thyroid cancer without persistent disease after initial therapy]. Arq Bras Endocrinol Metabol. 2006; 50(5):909–913

[7] Siegel RL, Miller KD, Jemal A. Cancer statistics, 2015. CA Cancer J Clin. 2015; 65(1):5–29

[8] Francis CL, Nalley C, Fan C, Bodenner D, Stack BC, Jr. 18F-fluorodeoxyglucose and 131I radioguided surgical management of thyroid cancer. Otolaryngol Head Neck Surg. 2012; 146(1):26–32

[9] Schuff KG, Weber SM, Givi B, Samuels MH, Andersen PE, Cohen JI. Efficacy of nodal dissection for treatment of persistent/recurrent papillary thyroid cancer. Laryngoscope. 2008; 118(5):768–775

[10] Noyek AM, Witterick IJ, Kirsh JC. Radionuclide imaging in otolaryngology-head and neck surgery. Arch Otolaryngol Head Neck Surg. 1991; 117 (4):372–378

[11] Travagli JP, Cailleux AF, Ricard M, et al. Combination of radioiodine (131I) and probe-guided surgery for persistent or recurrent thyroid carcinoma. J Clin Endocrinol Metab. 1998; 83(8):2675–2680

[12] Kraeber-Bodéré F, Cariou B, Curtet C, et al. Feasibility and benefit of fluorine 18-fluoro-2-deoxyglucose-guided surgery in the management of radioiodine-negative differentiated thyroid carcinoma metastases. Surgery. 2005; 138(6):1176–1182, discussion 1182

[13] Cox MD, Stack BC Jr. Minimally invasive radioguided parathyroidectomy. In: Stack BC Jr, Bodenner DL, eds. Medical and Surgical Treatment of Parathyroid Diseases. Switzerland: Springer International; 2017:187–190

[14] Yarbrough TL, Bartel TB, Stack BC Jr. Single-Photon scintigraphic imaging of the parathyroid glands: planar, tomography (SPECT), and SPECT-CT. In: Stack BC Jr, Bodenner DL, eds. Medical and Surgical Treatment of Parathyroid Diseases. Switzerland: Springer International; 2017:131–144

[15] Basu S, Kwee TC, Surti S, Akin EA, Yoo D, Alavi A. Fundamentals of PET and PET/CT imaging. Ann N Y Acad Sci. 2011; 1228:1–18

[16] Kwee TC, Torigian DA, Alavi A. Overview of positron emission tomography, hybrid positron emission tomography instrumentation, and positron emission tomography quantification. J Thorac Imaging. 2013; 28(1):4–10

[17] Wu HS, Huang WS, Liu YC, Yen RF, Shen YY, Kao CH. Comparison of FDG-PET and technetium-99 m MIBI SPECT to detect metastatic cervical lymph nodes in well-differentiated thyroid carcinoma with elevated serum HTG but negative I-131 whole body scan. Anticancer Res. 2003; 23 5b:4235–4238

[18] Agrawal A, Hall NC, Ringel MD, Povoski SP, Martin EW, Jr. Combined use of perioperative TSH-stimulated (18)F-FDG PET/CT imaging and gamma probe

radioguided surgery to localize and verify resection of iodine scan-negative recurrent thyroid carcinoma. Laryngoscope. 2008; 118(12):2190–2194

[19] Saab G, Driedger AA, Pavlosky W, et al. Thyroid-stimulating hormone-stimulated fused positron emission tomography/computed tomography in the evaluation of recurrence in 131I-negative papillary thyroid carcinoma. Thyroid. 2006; 16(3):267–272

[20] Sriprapaporn J, Sethanandha C, Yingsa-nga T, Komoltri C, Thongpraparn T, Harnnanthawiwai C. Utility of adding SPECT/CT imaging to post-therapeutic radioiodine whole-body scan in patients with differentiated thyroid cancer. J Med Assoc Thai. 2015; 98(6):596–605

[21] Tharp K, Israel O, Hausmann J, et al. Impact of 131I-SPECT/CT images obtained with an integrated system in the follow-up of patients with thyroid carcinoma. Eur J Nucl Med Mol Imaging. 2004; 31(10):1435–1442

[22] Iwata M, Kasagi K, Misaki T, et al. Comparison of whole-body 18F-FDG PET, 99mTc-MIBI SPET, and post-therapeutic 131I-Na scintigraphy in the detection of metastatic thyroid cancer. Eur J Nucl Med Mol Imaging. 2004; 31 (4):491–498

[23] Atkins HL, Richards P. Assessment of thyroid function and anatomy with technetium-99 m as pertechnetate. J Nucl Med. 1968; 9(1):7–15

[24] de Geus-Oei LF, Oei HY, Hennemann G, Krenning EP. Sensitivity of 123I whole-body scan and thyroglobulin in the detection of metastases or recurrent differentiated thyroid cancer. Eur J Nucl Med Mol Imaging. 2002; 29 (6):768–774

[25] Haugen BR. Radioiodine remnant ablation: current indications and dosing regimens. Endocr Pract. 2012; 18(4):604–610

[26] Zeuren R, Biagini A, Grewal RK, et al. RAI thyroid bed uptake after total thyroidectomy: a novel SPECT-CT anatomic classification system. Laryngoscope. 2015; 125(10):2417–2424

[27] Stack BC, Jr, Lowe VJ, Hardeman S. Radioguided surgical advancements for head and neck oncology. South Med J. 2000; 93(4):360–363

[28] Nalley C, Wiebeck K, Bartel TB, Bodenner D, Stack BC, Jr. Intraoperative radiation exposure with the use of (18)F-FDG-guided thyroid cancer surgery. Otolaryngol Head Neck Surg. 2010; 142(2):281–283

[29] Desai DC, Arnold M, Saha S, et al. Correlative whole-body FDG-PET and intraoperative gamma detection of FDG distribution in colorectal cancer. Clin Positron Imaging. 2000; 3(5):189–196

[30] Higashi T, Saga T, Ishimori T, et al. What is the most appropriate scan timing for intraoperative detection of malignancy using 18F-FDG-sensitive gamma probe? Preliminary phantom and preoperative patient study. Ann Nucl Med. 2004; 18(2):105–114

[31] Andersen PA, Chakera AH, Klausen TL, et al. Radiation exposure to surgical staff during F-18-FDG-guided cancer surgery. Eur J Nucl Med Mol Imaging. 2008; 35(3):624–629

[32] Povoski SP, Sarikaya I, White WC, et al. Comprehensive evaluation of occupational radiation exposure to intraoperative and perioperative personnel from 18F-FDG radioguided surgical procedures. Eur J Nucl Med Mol Imaging. 2008; 35(11):2026–2034

[33] Kohn HI, Fry RJ. Radiation carcinogenesis. N Engl J Med. 1984; 310(8):504–511

[34] Prichard RDL. Reoperation for benign disease. In: Randolph GW, ed. Surgery of the Thyroid and Parathyroid Glands. Philadelphia, PA: Saunders; 2013:95–106

[35] Policeni BA, Smoker WR, Reede DL. Anatomy and embryology of the thyroid and parathyroid glands. Semin Ultrasound CT MR. 2012; 33(2):104–114

[36] Sasou S, Nakamura S, Kurihara H. Suspensory ligament of Berry: its relationship to recurrent laryngeal nerve and anatomic examination of 24 autopsies. Head Neck. 1998; 20(8):695–698

[37] Mete O, Rotstein L, Asa SL. Controversies in thyroid pathology: thyroid capsule invasion and extrathyroidal extension. Ann Surg Oncol. 2010; 17(2):386–391

[38] Portinari M, Carcoforo P. Radioguided sentinel lymph node biopsy in patients with papillary thyroid carcinoma. Gland Surg. 2016; 5(6):591–602

[39] Creach KM, Gillanders WE, Siegel BA, Haughey BH, Moley JF, Grigsby PW. Management of cervical nodal metastasis detected on I-131 scintigraphy after initial surgery of well-differentiated thyroid carcinoma. Surgery. 2010; 148 (6):1198–1204, discussion 1204–1206

[40] Quillo AR, Bumpous JM, Goldstein RE, Fleming MM, Flynn MB. Minimally invasive parathyroid surgery, the Norman 20% rule: is it valid? Am Surg. 2011; 77(4):484–487

24 Intraoperative Neural Monitoring in Neck Dissection

Bradley R. Lawson, Dipti Kamani, and Gregory W. Randolph

Abstract

Intraoperative nerve visualization is the accepted gold standard for prevention of neural injury during neck dissection. However, a structurally intact nerve does not always correlate with a postoperatively functioning nerve. Intraoperative neural monitoring has emerged as an adjunctive and additive tool for nerve identification and prognostication of postoperative function. While much of the existing data focus on surgery of the central neck compartment, we present emerging applications for monitoring of the nerves at risk in lateral compartment neck dissection.

Keywords: neural monitoring, thyroidectomy, central neck dissection, lateral neck dissection

24.1 Introduction

Neck dissection is a technically demanding operation that may present risk to numerous nerves during the course of a single procedure. Nerve visualization during surgery has long been considered the gold standard for the prevention of neural injury. However, an intraoperatively visualized and structurally intact nerve does not always correlate with a postoperatively functioning nerve. Neural monitoring has garnered increasing attention from thyroid and parathyroid surgeons worldwide, largely due to its prognostic information regarding postoperative nerve function. This technology has also been applied to lateral neck dissection. Emerging data are beginning to support the hypothesis that neural monitoring can reduce the incidence of neural injury. This chapter focuses on the history of intraoperative neural monitoring (IONM), its impact on surgical practice, standards of IONM, and application of IONM to lateral neck dissection.

24.2 Historical Overview

In 1848, Du Bois-Reymond became the first to demonstrate nerve action potentials and describe electrical activity of muscle with electromyography (EMG).[1] IONM allows for localization of neural structures, tests the function of these structures, and provides early detection of neural injury. The goal of IONM is to identify neural injury prior to the onset of irreparable damage, thereby allowing immediate corrective actions to be taken.[1] Historically, IONM has been most commonly used by spine surgeons, with neurosurgeons, vascular surgeons, orthopedic surgeons, urologists, and otolaryngologists all utilizing monitoring to some extent. The most common procedures in which IONM is applied include spine surgery, carotid endarterectomy, selected brain surgeries, and ENT procedures such as vestibular schwannoma resection, parotidectomy, thyroidectomy, parathyroidectomy, and neck dissection. Shedd and Durham in 1966 published the first report of electrical stimulation of the recurrent laryngeal nerve (RLN) and superior laryngeal nerve (SLN) in a canine model via endolaryngeal balloon spirography. A pressure recording from a balloon in the larynx consistently demonstrated recognizable changes upon stimulation of the RLN, thereby providing a means for its electrical identification. The authors were then able to confirm in two human patients that the endolaryngeal balloon pressure recording provided a clear signal of RLN and SLN stimulation.[2] In 1970, Riddell published a 23-consecutive-year experience of electrical identification of the RLN, with the addition of laryngeal palpation as a confirmatory safety measure.[3]

Different IONM techniques have been developed over the past four decades, including laryngeal palpation, glottic observation, intramuscular vocal cord electrodes, postcricoid surface electrodes, anterior laryngeal electrodes, and endotracheal tube (ETT)-based surface electrodes.[4,5] Due to the ease of setup and use as well as their noninvasive nature, ETT-based surface electrodes have become popular for IONM in central neck surgery.[4,5,6,7] While intramuscular electrodes deliver higher amplitudes, they are more complicated to insert, may be placed in the wrong location, may migrate during surgery, and may even break in some cases.

In light of these many different techniques for IONM, standardization became a priority in order to promote uniform application of this emerging technology. The International Neural Monitoring Study Group (INMSG) was founded in 2006 to guide the emerging field of neurophysiologic monitoring, particularly of the vagus and laryngeal nerves in thyroid and parathyroid surgery.[8]

Vagal and RLN monitoring have gained widespread acceptance within the global surgical community. A recent study from Pennsylvania State University indicates that IONM is used by 80% of otolaryngologists and 48% of general surgeons who perform thyroid and parathyroid surgery at academic centers in the United States.[9] Neural monitoring has become the standard of care in Germany; 93% of thyroidectomies were performed with RLN monitoring according to a national survey in 2010.[10] Exposure to IONM during training is associated with a 3.1 times greater likelihood of using it in practice.[11] Of note, use of IONM is actually more common among high-volume thyroid surgeons (> 100 cases per year). This suggests that IONM is not being used as a substitute for anatomical knowledge and surgical skill, but rather as a useful adjunctive tool to those who are most surgically experienced.[11,12]

Data continue to be discordant regarding the impact of neural monitoring on rates of neural injury in thyroid and parathyroid surgery. In a study of more than 850 patients undergoing revision surgery, Barczyński et al found transient and permanent RLN injuries in 2.6 and 1.4% of nerves with IONM versus 6.3 and 2.4% of nerves without IONM, respectively. The rate of transient paralysis was statistically significantly reduced when neural monitoring was used.[13] Thomusch et al compared visual RLN identification with neural monitoring in over 5,000 procedures; they found rates of transient and permanent paralysis of 1.4 and 0.4% of nerves at risk with IONM versus 2.1 and 0.8% of nerves at risk with visual identification alone. A multivariate logistic regression confirmed that use of neural monitoring decreased the rate of postoperative transient ($p < 0.008$) and permanent ($p < 0.004$) RLN palsy as an independent factor by 0.58 and 0.30, respectively.[14] However, Pisanu et al performed a meta-analysis of over 35,500 nerves at risk and found no statistically significant difference in the rates of transient and permanent RLN paralysis with and without neural monitoring.[15]

Dralle et al looked into this issue and found that an adequately powered study would require 9 million patients per arm for benign goiter and 40,000 patients per arm for thyroid malignancy surgery to detect statistical differences in the rate of RLN palsy with or without IONM.[16] The argument for selective versus routine use of IONM continues to evolve among the community of surgeons who use it. We perform IONM in all cases in order to distribute the benefit of this additional information to all patients. Dionigi et al have also articulated the point that difficult cases may not always be apparent preoperatively.[7] Routine use of IONM provides greater experience in interpreting the data, along with improved troubleshooting skills with the device itself should difficulties arise during a particularly challenging case. Current INMSG guidelines recommend the routine use of IONM for thyroid and parathyroid surgery, including central neck dissection.[4] Currently, no guidelines exist for the use of IONM in lateral neck dissection.

24.3 Benefits of Intraoperative Neural Monitoring Application

The discussion relating to rates of RLN paralysis represents a single and rather limited perspective for evaluation of the use of IONM and its benefits to patients. Overall benefits offered by IONM include (1) nerve identification/neural mapping, (2) aid in dissection following nerve identification, and (3) injury identification/postoperative neural prognostication. When one appreciates the electrical information provided by IONM as additive and confirmatory to visual information, these benefits become rather apparent. Neural monitoring does not replace but adds to anatomic knowledge and surgical skill, and it provides a new functional dynamic. The need for visual identification of the nerve is not replaced by IONM; this technology is not intended to be used as a "divining rod."

24.3.1 Neural Identification and Mapping

The RLN can be mapped out in the paratracheal region through linear stimulation with the neural probe. Visual identification then follows using directed dissection in the process referred to as neural mapping. Multiple studies report nerve identification rates of 98 to 100% using such neural mapping.[5] Chiang et al reported a 100% identification rate, including nerves (25% of the total) that were classified as difficult to identify visually because of their complex anatomy.[17] The previsualization neural mapping allows for rational and directed dissection, which may be a substantial advantage in scarred operative fields and cases with complex anatomy (such as ramified nerves, large goiters, revision surgeries, etc.).[18]

24.3.2 Aid in Neural Dissection

After the nerve has been visually identified, intermittent stimulation of the nerve versus adjacent nonnerve tissue can be helpful in tracing the nerve and its branches through the surgical field. This is analogous to intermittent facial nerve stimulation during parotidectomy. Accurate delineation of the medial border of the RLN can be very useful during ligament of Berry's dissection.

24.3.3 Injury Identification and Prognostication of Postoperative Function

While monitoring is helpful in neural identification and is an excellent adjunct during nerve dissection, the key utility of IONM is the intraoperative prediction of postoperative function. A structurally intact nerve is not necessarily equivalent to a functional nerve. Blunt and stretch injury to the nerve may not always be visually detectable. Several studies have suggested that the visualization of the nerve by the surgeon is a poor judgment of RLN injury intraoperatively. Only 10 to 14% of injured nerves are identified as being such during the course of the surgery.[19,20] Bergenfelz et al, when reviewing the Scandinavian endocrine quality register in over 3,660 cases, noted that they were able to intraoperatively identify nerve injury only in 11.3% of injured nerves. In addition, bilateral RLN injury was only identified during the operation in 16% of cases when it occurred.[21] Snyder et al have also recently concluded that the majority of injured nerves are judged to be visually intact during surgery.[22] Thus, visual examination is vastly insufficient to prognosticate postoperative RLN function.

In contrast, postoperative neural function prediction with IONM has been associated with uniformly high negative predictive values for injury ranging from 92 to 100%.[23] Criteria supported by the INMSG for neurapraxic injury include a 50% or greater decline in amplitude and a 10% or greater increase in latency. In the absence of these conditions, the nerve is judged to retain normal physiologic function. This predictive ability of IONM is of particular importance in bilateral thyroid surgery, because both nerves governing the laryngeal airway introitus are at risk with one surgery. If neurapraxic injury identified on the initial side of surgery does not quickly recover, operative strategy may be rationally changed. Goretzki et al found that when loss of signal was identified on the first side, surgery could be terminated and a staged contralateral procedure performed at a later date with complete avoidance of bilateral nerve paralysis. However, when the surgeon continued to contralateral side surgery after loss of signal on the first side, 19% of patients developed bilateral vocal cord paralysis.[24] The prognostic ability of IONM in the avoidance of the major morbidity of bilateral vocal cord paralysis is evident. This advantage is not amenable to statistical analysis but is likely one of the main reasons for IONM application.

24.3.4 Prognostic Testing Errors and Their Avoidance

As discussed previously, multiple recent studies report very high negative predictive value, making IONM vastly superior to visual identification of nerve injury. However, the following categories of errors may occur and should be considered by all monitoring surgeons. In these terms, we define positive (+) test as EMG loss of signal at the end of surgery (i.e., the test for the disease of postoperative vocal cord paralysis is positive), and we define negative (-) test as maintained EMG at the end of surgery (i.e., the test for vocal cord paralysis is negative).

1. False positives (i.e., loss of signal with intact neural function postoperatively). The causes of false positives include the following:
   a) Various equipment problems on both the stimulation (i.e., faulty probe, inaccurate probe connection to monitor) and recording (i.e., ETT malposition or displacement) sides.

b) Neuromuscular blockade.

c) Blood or fascia obscuring the stimulated nerve segment.

d) Early-response elimination due to the monitor's latency cutoff period for recording artifact suppression.

e) Vocal cord paralysis with early neural recovery.

Note that the majority of prognostic testing false positives relate to tube malpositioning.

2. False negatives (i.e., a good EMG with postoperative vocal cord paralysis).

a) Stimulation distal to the injured nerve segment (canine models suggest distal segments maintain electrical stimulability for up to 3 days). This is the primary rationale for vagal stimulation at the end of surgery.

b) Injuries subsequent to the final neural stimulation such as during wound irrigation, suctioning, and closure.

c) Delayed neurapraxia. One hypothesis is that progressive edema may affect the RLN at an intralaryngeal location such as the cricothyroid joint articulation.

d) Posterior RLN branch injury. Robust ETT electrode waveform confirms anterior branch RLN integrity. Posterior branches may be disrupted despite strong amplitude with stimulation, and such patients may have an abduction deficit postoperatively.[25,26]

e) Vocal cord immobility secondary to nonneural issues such as arytenoid cartilage dislocation or laryngeal edema.

24.4 Intraoperative Neural Monitoring Standards Guidelines

Despite the increasingly broad use of IONM, a review of the literature and clinical experience demonstrates there is significant variability in the application of neural monitoring across different centers. Variation exists in the use of pre- and postoperative laryngeal examination, a variety of stimulation probes and recording electrodes, and in monitor output with some providing only audio tone and others generating quantitative laryngeal EMG waveforms. Heterogeneity also exists regarding technique of ETT placement and the troubleshooting algorithm enacted when loss of signal occurs. The literature suggests that this nonstandard application of monitoring techniques leads to a significant rate of monitoring inaccuracies, most notably due to equipment-related problems such as ETT malposition in 3.8 to 23% of patients.[27,28,29,30,31]

24.4.1 Basic System Setup

Recording ground and nerve stimulator anode electrodes are placed on the patient's shoulder and are interfaced with the monitor through a connector box (▶ Fig. 24.1). The recording electrodes from the right and left vocal cords exit the ETT proximally and are also interfaced with the connector box. Finally, the nerve stimulator cathode electrode (i.e., the probe) is placed on the sterile surgical field and connected to the box underneath the sterile drapes.

24.4.2 Anesthesia

Close partnership with anesthesiology is absolutely essential in a successful neural monitoring program.[32,33] Anesthetic needs must be discussed prior to the case. Since IONM requires accurate and robust EMG response, neuromuscular blockade must be avoided without exception. Any neuromuscular blockade after induction could interfere with EMG activity; therefore, it is advisable to utilize short-acting neuromuscular blockade and to allow this to wear off following intubation.[34,35]

The ETT should be inserted without the use of lidocaine or any lubricant jelly. Pooled saliva may obscure the EMG signals, and using suction and possibly a drying agent may be helpful. The electrodes should abut very closely to the vocal cords; hence, the largest possible size tube for intubation

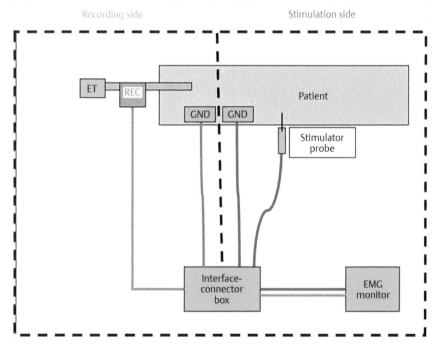

Fig. 24.1 Standard Monitoring Equipment Set-up (ref 2011 guidelines). ET, endotracheal tube; GND, ground electrodes; REC, recording electrodes.

should be used. Appropriate ETT electrode contact with the vocal cords must be confirmed after the patient is fully positioned. The INMSG has suggested two options for confirmation of optimal tube position prior to the start of surgical dissection. The first is to observe spontaneous respiratory variation, which is defined as the spontaneous bilateral EMG waveforms between 30 and 70 microvolts which is observed after the paralytic induction agent has worn off but before the inhalational plane of anesthesia becomes deep. Respiratory variation is typically present as the patient resumes spontaneous breathing and may be observed in conjunction with spontaneous movement or "bucking" (▶ Fig. 24.2). When respiratory variation is present unilaterally, this is an indication that the electrode has lost contact with the vocal cord due to rotation. Tube rotation may then be performed until bilateral waveforms are observed. The second option is to perform repeat laryngoscopy in order to visually ensure adequate ETT positioning. The video-laryngoscope may again be helpful for this post-positioning examination. Repeat laryngoscopy is recommended in all cases when respiratory variation cannot be identified. A recently published study by our unit found that identification of respiratory variation was possible in 91% of their patients, whereas the remaining 9% required a repeat laryngoscopy.[33,34,35]

After successful positioning of the ETT, the monitor setting should be assessed; low impedance values suggest good electrode–patient contact. The impedance of the electrodes should be less than 5 Ω and the imbalance between the two sides should be less than 1 Ω; monitor event threshold should be at 100 μV and the stimulator probe should be set to a pulsatile output of 4 per second with stimulating current set between 1 and 2 mA. At the onset of surgery, the stimulation of strap muscles resulting into a gross muscle twitch can be performed to confirm the absence of neuromuscular blockade as well as an intact stimulatory pathway. Vagal stimulation (V1) is performed prior to formal surgical dissection of the central neck compartment. It is only when the vagus nerve is stimulated and provides robust EMG activity that the surgeon may be assured that the system is fully functional and that the RLN can be safely sought after through the neural mapping technique. Only once the vagus nerve has been positively stimulated (true positive) can a subsequent negative response be regarded as a true negative. For each patient, IONM data must essentially include preoperative laryngeal exam (L1), an initial intraoperative suprathreshold vagal nerve stimulation (V1), an initial intraoperative RLN stimulation (R1), and also a similar set of events (R2 and V2) should be recorded at the end of the surgery followed by a postoperative laryngeal exam (L2).

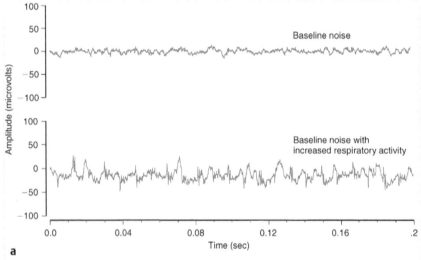

a

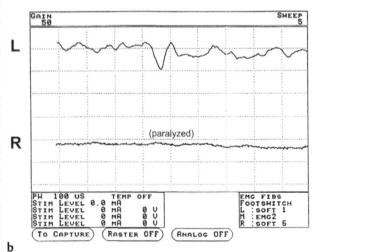

b

Fig. 24.2 Respiratory variation waveform: (a) Upper line—baseline noise (between 10 and 20 μV). *Lower line—baseline coarsening by* respiratory variation (30–70 μV) occurring when the patient is at the onset of bucking in the early anesthesia period). (b) Left and right baseline tracings in a patient with known right vocal cord palsy. The left vocal cord shows typical respiratory variation. The right vocal cord is electrically silent.

24.5 Monitoring Safety

Multiple studies have demonstrated the safety of repetitive stimulation of the facial nerve in neurotologic surgery, provided that the patient is appropriately isolated and grounded.[36,37,38] Multiple investigators have also demonstrated the safety of repetitive RLN stimulation during thyroidectomy/central neck dissection.[39,40,41,42,43,44,45,46] In the authors' experience, stimulation of individual nerves can be performed hundreds of times with constant current pulses of 1 to 2 mA without ill effects. Friedman et al have reported that in both dogs and humans, vagal and RLN stimulation in the 2- to 4-mA range at 10 to 25 Hz (with a pulse duration of 500 μs) was well tolerated without laryngeal or cardiorespiratory symptoms.[47] In both canine and porcine models, continuous, prolonged vagal stimulation has been shown not to be associated with any change in vagal or RLN stimulability or any significant cardiopulmonary effect.[48] On the basis of a literature review and the cumulative experience of its members, the INMSG has released a statement that repetitive stimulation of the RLN and vagus nerves is not associated with neural injury; the group specifically noted that vagal stimulation is not linked with bradyarrhythmias or bronchospasm.[24]

Several studies have supported the success and safety of neural monitoring performed with minimally invasive surgical approaches. A needle electrode placed through the cricothyroid membrane to monitor the bilateral vocal cords has been described and allows neural monitoring to be performed during local anesthesia (Snyder, personal communication, 2012).

24.6 Normative Human Monitoring Data

Normative data of RLN and vagus nerve stimulation during IONM is well reported in the literature.[48,49,50,51]

24.7 Threshold

Threshold is defined as the current that, applied to the nerve, initially starts to elicit recognizable EMG activity. The response amplitude produced at stimulation threshold is lower than the maximum amplitude that may be achieved as the stimulation current is increased. At a certain level of stimulation, all nerve fibers are depolarized, and maximum EMG amplitude is achieved. Beyond this point, increasing the stimulating current does not lead to further increases in recorded EMG amplitude. The human RLN maximally depolarizes at 0.8 mA. This serves as the rationale for stimulating at 1 mA during the bulk of the case since this represents safe suprathreshold stimulation. The use of 2 mA does not produce any higher EMG amplitude, but it depolarizes a larger sphere of tissue around the probe tip and can be quite useful during initial searching and mapping of the RLN.

24.8 Amplitude

The typically biphasic waveform represents the summated motor unit action potentials of the ipsilateral vocalis as recorded by vocal cord surface electrodes at the level of the glottis. Measures of amplitude may be correlated with the number of muscle fibers participating in the polarization during laryngeal EMG. Using existing standards in EMG monitoring physiology, we define amplitude as the vertical height from the apex of the positive waveform deflection to the nadir of the negative deflection (i.e., peak to peak). Mean RLN (both RLNs) amplitude is reported as 891.6 mV (± 731) and mean vagal amplitude as 739.7 mV (±433.9).[51]

24.9 Latency

Latency is generally believed to represent the speed of stimulation-induced depolarization and therefore depends on the distance of the stimulation point to the ipsilateral vocalis muscle. We define latency as the time from the stimulation spike to the first evoked waveform peak. Given the significant difference in length of the vagus nerve on both sides, latency is significantly longer on the left compared to the right side with vagal stimulation. This is evident in the study of normative EMG by Sritharan et al in which the difference between the mean left vagal latency (8.14 ms) and mean right vagal latency (5.47 ms) was statistically significant ($p < 0.0001$).[50] Analysis of normative data shows that RLN latencies are significantly shorter compared to vagal latencies.[44,52] In addition, the non-RLN has a shorter latency than the RLN. The non-RLN may be electrically identified when high vagal stimulation produces laryngeal response but more distal (i.e., caudal) stimulation does not.[44,52]

24.10 Monitor Problem Solving: Loss of Signal Algorithm

When loss of signal occurs, a surgeon must rule out equipment-related issues, and hence the surgeon's first response is to palpate the larynx while stimulating the vagus (▶ Fig. 24.3, ▶ Fig. 24.4). Laryngeal twitch is a simple method of intraoperative palpation of the posterior cricoarytenoid muscle.[40] Presence of laryngeal twitch confirms that the stimulation side of the monitoring system is adequately operational, and the majority of recording side issues are related to ETT malposition. The corrective maneuver consists of stimulation of the vagus as the anesthesiologist repositions the ETT until EMG signal is obtained.

If laryngeal twitch is not present during nerve stimulation, then the stimulation side connections should be inspected. The status of neuromuscular blockage should also be considered if stimulation current is absent. If the current in the range of 1 to 2 mA is being distributed to the patient, the strap or sternocleidomastoid (SCM) muscles are then stimulated. If the strap or SCM muscles respond, contralateral vagus stimulation should be attempted; if EMG response is present, consider ipsilateral neural injury.

An event must satisfy the following conditions to be labeled as true LOS:
1. Presence of a satisfactory EMG at the beginning (R1 = 500 μV) of the monitoring and prior to the event (> 100 μV).
2. No or low response (i.e., 100 μV or lower) with stimulation at 1 to 2 mA in a dry field.
3. Absence of laryngeal twitch on ipsilateral vagal stimulation.
4. Presence of contralateral nerve response on contralateral vagal stimulation.

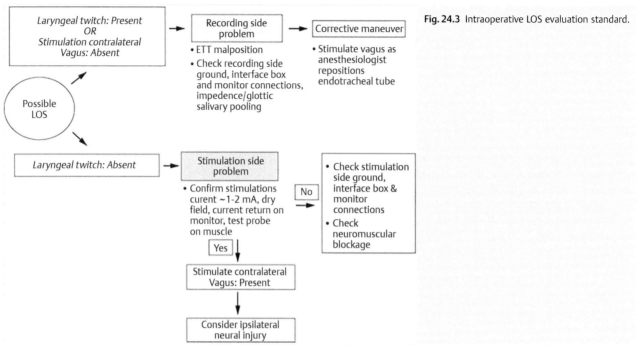

Fig. 24.3 Intraoperative LOS evaluation standard.

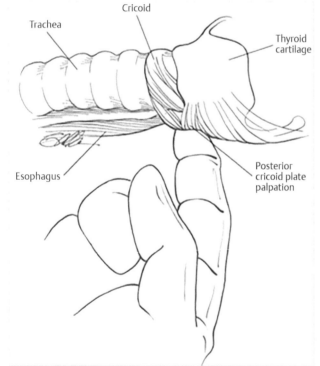

Fig. 24.4 Laryngeal palpation technique.

A true LOS should prompt the surgeon to identify the site of injury. It provides the opportunity to identify and treat the nerve injury if possible.

If signal is lost, the surgeon should stimulate the most distal point of the RLN (i.e., the laryngeal entry site) and serially stimulate proximally along the nerve to determine if a neurapraxic segment can be identified.[24] The identification of such a segment, termed "type I RLN injury—segmental injury," allows the surgeon to review the management of this portion of the nerve

as it relates to excessive traction, compression, clamping, or other injury. Should this method of retrograde mapping show the entire course of the RLN to be nonconductive, the injury is defined as type II RLN injury—global injury.[4] When true loss of signal occurs, the surgeon should then reconsider bilateral surgery in order to avoid the potential of bilateral nerve paralysis.

24.11 Continuous Neural Vagal Monitoring

The intermittent nature of intraoperative monitoring theoretically allows the nerve(s) to be at risk of damage between stimulations. Herein lies the principal methodological limitation of intermittent stimulation: it only allows the surgeon to identify neural injury once the damage has *already* been inflicted. Continuous vagal stimulation allows the establishment of baseline EMG amplitude and latency for each individual patient at the start of the case. A "combined event" involves concordant 50% or more decrease in baseline amplitude and 10% or more increase in initial baseline latency.[53,54] These combined electrophysiologic events typically precede postoperative vocal fold palsy, and they have been shown in a study of over 1,300 nerves at risk to be reversible in 82% of cases upon termination of the offending surgical maneuver.[55] Signal recovery to ≥ 50% of baseline amplitude during surgery signifies normal postoperative vocal fold function in all cases when a "combined event" does occur.[56] The current recommendation is to allow an injured nerve a minimum wait time of 20 minutes, prior to either moving on with contralateral surgery or terminating the operation.[56,52]

A major difference in continuous monitoring is that it requires opening of the carotid sheath for placement of a vagal electrode at the level of the cricoid cartilage. A variety of electrode configurations have been designed to allow the placement of a dedicated electrode on the vagus nerve for the purpose of continuous stimulation that provides ongoing amplitude and latency data.

These may be categorized according to the extent of dissection required around the vagus nerve for their placement. Repetitive pulsed stimulation (typically at 1 mA and ≤ 1 Hz) is performed via the vagal electrode, and there is no further need to interrupt surgery to stimulate the vagus nerve. Randolph et al demonstrated that a vagal electrode can be placed without complications in a matter of seconds.[52]

Implantable electrodes for the stimulation of the vagus nerve have been used for many years to treat a variety of chronic conditions such as epilepsy, depression, migraine, and Alzheimer's disease. No clinically relevant side effects have been observed with permanent vagus nerve stimulators.[57,58] Terris et al, in a small series conducted during the onset of use of CIONM in their group, reported a single episode of bradycardia; noticeably this study had a concomitant very high vagal electrode dislocation rate.[59] Numerous animal and human studies have supported the safety of continuous vagal monitoring for central neck surgery. Basic animal research has shown that a current of 1 mA recruits efferent type A motor fibers and myelinated type B autonomic fibers without activating thin, demyelinated vagal type C fibers. The vagal type C fibers are believed to mediate vasovagal symptoms causing cardiac (arrhythmias, bradycardia), pulmonary (bronchospasm), gastrointestinal (nausea, vomiting), or central (headache, numbness) side effects.[55,59,60]

24.12 Superior Laryngeal Nerve Monitoring

Damage to the external branch of the SLN can result in significant voice changes, particularly in singers, which are typically described as reduction in pitch, inability to reach higher registers, and decreased voice projection. Robinson et al, in a study of 35 patients with laryngeal EMG, found that SLN paresis/paralysis was associated with significant decreases in maximum phonation time and frequency range, along with increases in mean flow rate, jitter, shimmer, and noise-to-harmonic ratio.[61,62] Eisele reported estimated rates of SLN paralysis from 9 to 14%, and Cernea et al described rates up to 28%.[63,64]

Neural monitoring can be used to intraoperatively identify the external branch of the SLN. In 20% of cases, the external branch is hidden beneath the fascia of the inferior constrictor muscle and not seen directly.[64,65,66] Despite this, a nerve stimulator passed along the inferior constrictor can reliably elicit a discrete twitch. The laryngeal head of the sternothyroid muscle serves as an excellent landmark for the linear oblique path of the external branch as it traverses down along the inferior constrictor toward the cricothyroid muscle. The external branch of the SLN can be found within 1 to 2 mm of this obliquely oriented line (the laryngeal head of the sternothyroid, which inserts onto the thyroid cartilage lamina) with a high degree of certainty (▶ Fig. 24.5). Even when the nerve is deep to the fascia of the inferior constrictor, blind stimulation in this area will identify a linear path that results in discrete cricothyroid muscle contraction. Following this technique, neural stimulation should be able to identify the external branch of the SLN in 100% of cases.

EMG recording with ETT surface electrodes reveals a smaller amplitude and shorter latency with stimulation of the external branch of the SLN. On average, the average amplitude of the SLN is 34% of the ipsilateral RLN amplitude, consistent with canine

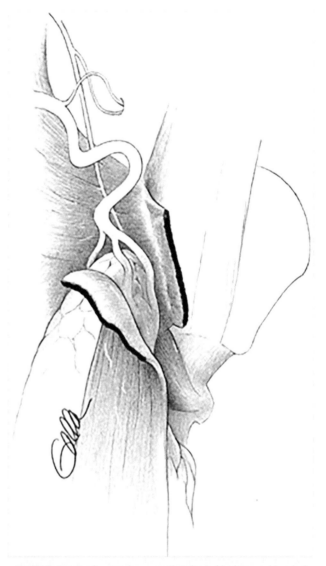

Fig. 24.5 Superior laryngeal nerve path indicated by laryngeal head of sternothyroid muscle.

data reported by Nasri et al.[67] It should be noted that the monitor's event threshold setting may need to be lowered and the stimulation rejection setting may need to be shortened in order to capture this early, low-amplitude waveform. Recent studies suggest that monitoring of the external branch of the SLN is associated with improved ability to identify the nerve and a lower rate of adverse voice parameters postoperatively.[68] To facilitate understanding and standardization of EBSLN monitoring, in 2013 INMSG has published guidelines for EBSLN monitoring.[69]

24.13 Nerve Monitoring in Lateral Compartment Dissection

As previously discussed, neck dissection may present risk to multiple nerves during the course of a single operation. Neural monitoring allows the surgeon to perform the function of neural mapping as previously discussed in relation to the RLN, in addition to assessing the functional status of motor nerves within the operative field in real time. There is currently no application for neural monitoring in relation to sensory nerves (i.e., lingual nerve) or special nerves (i.e., cervical sympathetic chain) that may be at risk of injury during neck dissection.

24.14 Marginal Mandibular Nerve

The marginal mandibular branch of the facial nerve faces injury during the approach to level I dissection. The rate of temporary paresis is reported at 10%, with permanent paralysis occurring in less than 1% of cases.[69] The result is asymmetric movement of the lower lip and possible oral incompetence. The marginal mandibular nerve travels in the superficial layer of the deep cervical fascia along the surface of the masseter muscle, passing over the facial vein and artery to innervate the lower lip. The inferior border of the submandibular gland serves as a landmark for the incision through the fascia in order to avoid marginal mandibular branch injury (▶ Fig. 24.6). A nerve stimulator passed along the fascia just inferior to the body of the mandible will elicit lower lip twitch with high reliability. The fascial incision is then placed inferior to the stimulated location of the nerve, and the fascia is elevated broadly along the caudal aspect of the mandibular body.

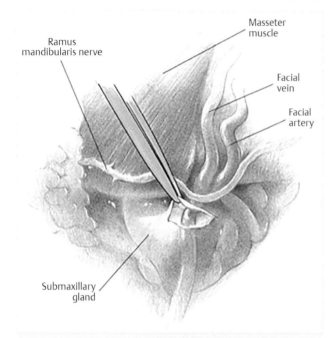

Fig. 24.6 Marginal mandibular nerve injury can be avoided by reflecting fascia along with the marginal mandibular nerve up and off the gland.

24.15 Hypoglossal Nerve

The hypoglossal nerve is at risk of injury during the course of level Ib dissection. It may also be at risk in level II dissection as the nodal specimen is dissected away from the anterior aspect of the carotid sheath. Injury to this nerve results in deviation of the tongue and atrophy of its intrinsic musculature. Oral phase dysphagia occurs due to difficulty with food bolus manipulation. The hypoglossal nerve passes deep to the posterior belly of the digastric muscle. It is typically identified on the surface of the hyoglossus muscle when the lateral border of the mylohyoid muscle is retracted anteriorly during level Ib dissection (▶ Fig. 24.7). In our experience, stimulation of the hypoglossal nerve is most beneficial to the surgeon as the nodal packet is dissected away from the carotid sheath in level II. Stimulation in a triangle defined by the internal jugular vein posteriorly, the superior thyroid artery inferiorly, and the posterior digastric belly superiorly reliably elicits contraction of the tongue and can help avoid inadvertent hypoglossal injury.

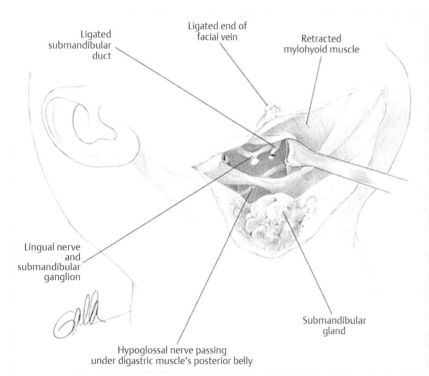

Fig. 24.7 Hypoglossal nerve exposed during lateral neck dissection.

24.16 Spinal Accessory Nerve

The spinal accessory nerve is at particular risk for traction injury during level II dissection (▶ Fig. 24.8). A recent study of neck dissection for thyroid cancer reports temporary spinal accessory nerve paresis in 27% of cases.[70,71] Injury leads to shoulder weakness when attempting to elevate the arm above the horizontal plane. Adhesive capsulitis of the glenohumeral joint and frozen shoulder may result if physical therapy is not initiated in a timely fashion. Transection of the spinal accessory nerve causes winged scapula. Stimulation of the spinal accessory nerve is particularly useful during lateral neck dissection, particularly when it is retracted for level IIb dissection. Periodic stimulation can be employed to monitor for possible neurapraxic traction injury, allowing for immediate reversal of an offending maneuver. Neural mapping may also be employed to allow for early identification of the spinal accessory nerve, as the anterior aspect of the SCM is freed from the superficial layer of the deep cervical fascia.

24.17 Phrenic Nerve

The phrenic nerve may be at risk of injury during dissection of levels III and IV. This nerve lies between the anterior scalene muscle and the overlying deep layer of the deep cervical fascia (▶ Fig. 24.8). The surgeon protects the phrenic nerve via preservation of the deep layer of the fascia. Phrenic nerve injury may result in hemidiaphragmatic paralysis and elevation, with up to a 25% reduction in lung capacity. Stimulation of the deep cervical fascia along the surface of the anterior scalene muscle will result in contraction of the diaphragm, which is palpable and often easily visible to the surgeon. Use of the neural mapping technique to trace the course of the phrenic nerve in the deep layer of fascia can be very useful for preservation of the fascia, notably when the surgeon is examining the compartment deep to the caudal aspect of the common carotid artery.

24.18 Vagus Nerve

Vagal nerve monitoring has been discussed in detail earlier in this chapter, but it merits mention that during dissection of levels II to IV, ligation and transection of the internal jugular vein presents particular risk to the vagus nerve. Continuous vagal nerve monitoring can provide significant benefit to the surgeon in the setting of retrocarotid nodal disease and invasion of the internal jugular vein.

24.19 Summary

Multimodality cranial nerve monitoring during neck procedures is rapidly becoming a new standard for safety and quality of care in head and neck surgery.

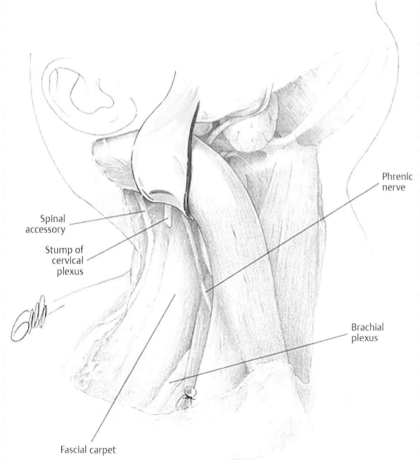

Fig. 24.8 Phrenic nerve and spinal accessory nerve preserved at the completion of lateral neck dissection.

Phrenic nerve

Spinal accessory

Stump of cervical plexus

Brachial plexus

Fascial carpet

References

[1] Sala F. Intraoperative neurophysiology is here to stay. Childs Nerv Syst. 2010; 26(4):413–417

[2] Shedd DP, Durham C. Electrical identification of the recurrent laryngeal nerve. I. Response of the canine larynx to electrical stimulation of the recurrent laryngeal nerve. Ann Surg. 1966; 163(1):47–50

[3] Riddell V. Thyroidectomy: prevention of bilateral recurrent nerve palsy. Results of identification of the nerve over 23 consecutive years (1946–69) with a description of an additional safety measure. Br J Surg. 1970; 57 (1):1–11

[4] Randolph GW, Dralle H, Abdullah H, et al. International Intraoperative Monitoring Study Group. Electrophysiologic recurrent laryngeal nerve monitoring during thyroid and parathyroid surgery: international standards guideline statement. Laryngoscope. 2011; 121 Suppl 1:S1–S16

[5] Randolph GW. Surgical anatomy of recurrent laryngeal nerve. In: Randolph GW, ed. Surgery of the Thyroid and Parathyroid Glands. Philadelphia, PA: Saunders; 2013

[6] Lamade W, Fogel W, Rieke K, Senninger N, Herfarth C. Intraoperative monitoring of the recurrent laryngeal nerve. A new method [in German]. Chirurg. 1996; 67(4):451–454

[7] Dionigi G, Lombardi D, Lombardi CP, et al. Working Group for Neural Monitoring in Thyroid and Parathyroid Surgery in Italy. Intraoperative neuromonitoring in thyroid surgery: a point prevalence survey on utilization, management, and documentation in Italy. Updates Surg. 2014; 66(4):269–276

[8] International Neural Monitoring Study Group (INMSG). Available at: http://www.inmsg.org. Accessed May 5, 2018

[9] Ho Y, Carr MM, Goldenberg D. Trends in intraoperative neural monitoring for thyroid and parathyroid surgery amongst otolaryngologists and general surgeons. Eur Arch Otorhinolaryngol. 2013; 270(9):2525–2530

[10] Dralle H, Sekulla C, Lorenz K, Nguyen Thanh P, Schneider R, Machens A. Loss of the nerve monitoring signal during bilateral thyroid surgery. Br J Surg. 2012; 99(8):1089–1095

[11] Horne SK, Gal TJ, Brennan JA. Prevalence and patterns of intraoperative nerve monitoring for thyroidectomy. Otolaryngol Head Neck Surg. 2007; 136 (6):952–956

[12] Sturgeon C, Sturgeon T, Angelos P. Neuromonitoring in thyroid surgery: attitudes, usage patterns, and predictors of use among endocrine surgeons. World J Surg. 2009; 33(3):417–425

[13] Barczyński M, Konturek A, Pragacz K, Papier A, Stopa M, Nowak W. Intraoperative nerve monitoring can reduce prevalence of recurrent laryngeal nerve injury in thyroid reoperations: results of a retrospective cohort study. World J Surg. 2014; 38(3):599–606

[14] Thomusch O, Machens A, Sekulla C, et al. Multivariate analysis of risk factors for postoperative complications in benign goiter surgery: prospective multicenter study in Germany. World J Surg. 2000; 24(11):1335–1341

[15] Pisanu A, Porceddu G, Podda M, Cois A, Uccheddu A. Systematic review with meta-analysis of studies comparing intraoperative neuromonitoring of recurrent laryngeal nerves versus visualization alone during thyroidectomy. J Surg Res. 2014; 188(1):152–161

[16] Dralle H, Timmerman W, Kruse E, et al. What Benefits Does Neural Monitoring Bring to Thyroid Surgery? Artz and Krankenhaus 2004:369–376

[17] Chiang FY, Lu IC, Chen HC, et al. Intraoperative neuromonitoring for early localization and identification of recurrent laryngeal nerve during thyroid surgery. Kaohsiung J Med Sci. 2010; 26(12):633–639

[18] Snyder SK, Hendricks JC. Intraoperative neurophysiology testing of the recurrent laryngeal nerve: plaudits and pitfalls. Surgery. 2005; 138(6):1183–1191, discussion 1191–1192

[19] Patow CA, Norton JA, Brennan MF. Vocal cord paralysis and reoperative parathyroidectomy. A prospective study. Ann Surg. 1986; 203(3):282–285

[20] Lo CY, Kwok KF, Yuen PW. A prospective evaluation of recurrent laryngeal nerve paralysis during thyroidectomy. Arch Surg. 2000; 135(2):204–207

[21] Bergenfelz A, Jansson S, Kristoffersson A, et al. Complications to thyroid surgery: results as reported in a database from a multicenter audit comprising 3,660 patients. Langenbecks Arch Surg. 2008; 393(5):667–673

[22] Snyder SK, Lairmore TC, Hendricks JC, Roberts JW. Elucidating mechanisms of recurrent laryngeal nerve injury during thyroidectomy and parathyroidectomy. J Am Coll Surg. 2008; 206(1):123–130

[23] Dralle H, Sekulla C, Lorenz K, Brauckhoff M, Machens A, German IONM Study Group. Intraoperative monitoring of the recurrent laryngeal nerve in thyroid surgery. World J Surg. 2008; 32(7):1358–1366

[24] Goretzki PE, Schwarz K, Brinkmann J, Wirowski D, Lammers BJ. The impact of intraoperative neuromonitoring (IONM) on surgical strategy in bilateral thyroid diseases: is it worth the effort? World J Surg. 2010; 34 (6):1274–1284

[25] Rea JL, Khan A. Clinical evoked electromyography for recurrent laryngeal nerve preservation: use of an endotracheal tube electrode and a postcricoid surface electrode. Laryngoscope. 1998; 108(9):1418–1420

[26] Marcus B, Edwards B, Yoo S, et al. Recurrent laryngeal nerve monitoring in thyroid and parathyroid surgery: the University of Michigan experience. Laryngoscope. 2003; 113(2):356–361

[27] Beldi G, Kinsbergen T, Schlumpf R. Evaluation of intraoperative recurrent nerve monitoring in thyroid surgery. World J Surg. 2004; 28(6):589–591

[28] Thomusch O, Sekulla C, Machens A, Neumann HJ, Timmermann W, Dralle H. Validity of intra-operative neuromonitoring signals in thyroid surgery. Langenbecks Arch Surg. 2004; 389(6):499–503

[29] Chan WF, Lo CY. Pitfalls of intraoperative neuromonitoring for predicting postoperative recurrent laryngeal nerve function during thyroidectomy. World J Surg. 2006; 30(5):806–812

[30] Dionigi G, Bacuzzi A, Boni L, Rovera F, Dionigi R. What is the learning curve for intraoperative neuromonitoring in thyroid surgery? Int J Surg. 2008; 6 Suppl 1:S7–S12

[31] Lu IC, Chu KS, Tsai CJ, et al. Optimal depth of NIM EMG endotracheal tube for intraoperative neuromonitoring of the recurrent laryngeal nerve during thyroidectomy. World J Surg. 2008; 32(9):1935–1939

[32] Deiner S. Highlights of anesthetic considerations for intraoperative neuromonitoring. Semin Cardiothorac Vasc Anesth. 2010; 14(1):51–53

[33] Macias AA, Eappen S, Malikin I, et al. Successful intraoperative electrophysiologic monitoring of the recurrent laryngeal nerve, a multidisciplinary approach: The Massachusetts Eye and Ear Infirmary monitoring collaborative protocol with experience in over 3000 cases. Head Neck. 2016; 38(10):1487–1494

[34] Marusch F, Hussock J, Haring G, Hachenberg T, Gastinger I. Influence of muscle relaxation on neuromonitoring of the recurrent laryngeal nerve during thyroid surgery. Br J Anaesth. 2005; 94(5):596–600

[35] Bragg P, Fisher DM, Shi J, et al. Comparison of twitch depression of the adductor pollicis and the respiratory muscles. Pharmacodynamic modeling without plasma concentrations. Anesthesiology. 1994; 80(2):310–319

[36] Cherng CH, Wong CS, Hsu CH, Ho ST. Airway length in adults: estimation of the optimal endotracheal tube length for orotracheal intubation. J Clin Anesth. 2002; 14(4):271–274

[37] Yap SJ, Morris RW, Pybus DA. Alterations in endotracheal tube position during general anaesthesia. Anaesth Intensive Care. 1994; 22(5):586–588

[38] Randolph GW, Kobler JB, Wilkins J. Recurrent laryngeal nerve identification and assessment during thyroid surgery: laryngeal palpation. World J Surg. 2004; 28(8):755–760

[39] Chiang FY, Lu IC, Kuo WR, Lee KW, Chang NC, Wu CW. The mechanism of recurrent laryngeal nerve injury during thyroid surgery–the application of intraoperative neuromonitoring. Surgery. 2008; 143(6):743–749

[40] Blitzer A, Crumley RL, Dailey SH, et al. Recommendations of the Neurolaryngology Study Group on laryngeal electromyography. Otolaryngol Head Neck Surg. 2009; 140(6):782–793

[41] Lorenz K, Sekulla C, Schelle J, Schmeiss B, Brauckhoff M, Dralle H, German Neuromonitoring Study Group. What are normal quantitative parameters of intraoperative neuromonitoring (IONM) in thyroid surgery? Langenbecks Arch Surg. 2010; 395(7):901–909

[42] Brauckhoff M, Walls G, Brauckhoff K, Thanh PN, Thomusch O, Dralle H. Identification of the non-recurrent inferior laryngeal nerve using intraoperative neurostimulation. Langenbecks Arch Surg. 2002; 386(7):482–487

[43] Prass RL. Iatrogenic facial nerve injury: the role of facial nerve monitoring. Otolaryngol Clin North Am. 1996; 29(2):265–275

[44] Rea JL, Khan A. Recurrent laryngeal nerve localisation in thyroid and parathyroid surgery: use of an indwelling laryngeal surface electrode with evoked electromyography. Oper Tech Otolaryngol Head and Neck Surg. 1994; 5:91

[45] Randolph G. Comparison of intraoperative recurrent laryngeal nerve monitoring techniques during recurrent laryngeal nerve surgery. Otolaryngol Head Neck Surg. 1994; 5(2):91–96

[46] Friedman M, Toriumi DM, Grybauskas VT, Applebaum EL. Implantation of a recurrent laryngeal nerve stimulator for the treatment of spastic dysphonia. Ann Otol Rhinol Laryngol. 1989; 98(2):130–134

[47] Phelan E, Kamani D, Shin J, Randolph GW. Neural monitored revision thyroid cancer surgery: surgical safety and thyroglobulin response. Otolaryngol Head Neck Surg. 2013; 149(1):47–52

[48] Caragacianu D, Kamani D, Randolph GW. Intraoperative monitoring: normative range associated with normal postoperative glottic function. Laryngoscope. 2013; 123(12):3026–3031

[49] Dionigi G, Chiang FY, Rausei S, et al. Surgical anatomy and neurophysiology of the vagus nerve (VN) for standardised intraoperative neuromonitoring (IONM) of the inferior laryngeal nerve (ILN) during thyroidectomy. Langenbecks Arch Surg. 2010; 395(7):893–899

[50] Sritharan N, Chase M, Kamani D, Randolph M, Randolph GW. The vagus nerve, recurrent laryngeal nerve, and external branch of the superior laryngeal nerve have unique latencies allowing for intraoperative documentation of intact neural function during thyroid surgery. Laryngoscope. 2015; 125(2): E84–E89

[51] Kamani D, Potenza AS, Cernea CR, Kamani YV, Randolph GW. The nonrecurrent laryngeal nerve: anatomic and electrophysiologic algorithm for reliable identification. Laryngoscope. 2015; 125(2):503–508

[52] Randolph GW, Kamani D. Intraoperative electrophysiologic monitoring of the recurrent laryngeal nerve during thyroid and parathyroid surgery: Experience with 1,381 nerves at risk. Laryngoscope. 2017; 127(1):280–286

[53] Schneider R, Randolph GW, Sekulla C, et al. Continuous intraoperative vagus nerve stimulation for identification of imminent recurrent laryngeal nerve injury. Head Neck. 2013; 35(11):1591–1598

[54] Van Slycke S, Gillardin JP, Brusselaers N, Vermeersch H. Initial experience with S-shaped electrode for continuous vagal nerve stimulation in thyroid surgery. Langenbecks Arch Surg. 2013; 398(5):717–722

[55] Schneider R, Sekulla C, Machens A, Lorenz K, Thanh PN, Dralle H. Dynamics of loss and recovery of the nerve monitoring signal during thyroidectomy predict early postoperative vocal fold function. Head Neck. 2016; 38 Suppl 1: E1144–E1151

[56] Schneider R, Lorenz K, Sekulla C, Machens A, Nguyen-Thanh P, Dralle H. Surgical strategy during intended total thyroidectomy after loss of EMG signal on the first side of resection [in German]. Chirurg. 2015; 86(2):154–163

[57] Groves DA, Brown VJ. Vagal nerve stimulation: a review of its applications and potential mechanisms that mediate its clinical effects. Neurosci Biobehav Rev. 2005; 29(3):493–500

[58] Ben-Menachem E, Revesz D, Simon BJ, Silberstein S. Surgically implanted and non-invasive vagus nerve stimulation: a review of efficacy, safety and tolerability. Eur J Neurol. 2015; 22(9):1260–1268

[59] Terris DJ, Chaung K, Duke WS. Continuous vagal nerve monitoring is dangerous and should not routinely be done during thyroid surgery. World J Surg. 2015; 39(10):2471–2476

[60] Schneider R, Przybyl J, Pliquett U, et al. A new vagal anchor electrode for real-time monitoring of the recurrent laryngeal nerve. Am J Surg. 2010; 199 (4):507–514

[61] Ben-Menachem E. Vagus-nerve stimulation for the treatment of epilepsy. Lancet Neurol. 2002; 1(8):477–482

[62] Robinson JL, Mandel S, Sataloff RT. Objective voice measures in nonsinging patients with unilateral superior laryngeal nerve paresis. J Voice. 2005; 19 (4):665–667

[63] Eisele D. Complications of thyroid surgery. In: Eisele D, ed. Complications in Head and Neck Surgery. St. Louis: Mosby; 1993

[64] Cernea CR, Ferraz AR, Nishio S, Dutra A, Jr, Hojaij FC, dos Santos LR. Surgical anatomy of the external branch of the superior laryngeal nerve. Head Neck. 1992; 14(5):380–383

[65] Cernea CR, Ferraz AR, Furlani J, et al. Identification of the external branch of the superior laryngeal nerve during thyroidectomy. Am J Surg. 1992; 164(6):634–639

[66] Lennquist S, Cahlin C, Smeds S. The superior laryngeal nerve in thyroid surgery. Surgery. 1987; 102(6):999–1008

[67] Nasri S, Beizai P, Ye M, Sercarz JA, Kim YM, Berke GS. Cross-innervation of the thyroarytenoid muscle by a branch from the external division of the superior laryngeal nerve. Ann Otol Rhinol Laryngol. 1997; 106(7, Pt 1):594–598

[68] Barczyński M, Randolph GW, Cernea CR, et al. International Neural Monitoring Study Group. External branch of the superior laryngeal nerve monitoring during thyroid and parathyroid surgery: International Neural Monitoring Study Group standards guideline statement. Laryngoscope. 2013; 123(Suppl 4):S1–S14

[69] Lifante JC, McGill J, Murry T, Aviv JE, Inabnet WB, III. A prospective, randomized trial of nerve monitoring of the external branch of the superior laryngeal nerve during thyroidectomy under local/regional anesthesia and IV sedation. Surgery. 2009; 146(6):1167–1173

[70] Lewis CM, Weber RS. Lateral neck dissection: technique. In: Randolph GW, ed. Surgery of the Thyroid and Parathyroid Glands. Philadelphia, PA: Saunders; 2013

[71] Kupferman ME, Patterson DM, Mandel SJ, LiVolsi V, Weber RS. Safety of modified radical neck dissection for differentiated thyroid carcinoma. Laryngoscope. 2004; 114(3):403–406

25 Management of the Neck with Radiation Therapy

Catherine E. Mercado and William M. Mendenhall

Abstract

Patients with a clinically negative neck undergo elective neck treatment if the risk of subclinical disease is 15% or higher. Elective neck dissection is employed if the primary site is treated with definitive radiotherapy (RT). Patients with clinically positive nodes who are treated with definitive RT undergo a post-RT neck dissection if the nodes do not completely respond. Patients who undergo definitive surgery receive postoperative RT for close or positive margins, 2 or more positive nodes, extracapsular extension, perineural invasion, ≥ 1 cm subglottic extension, and involvement of the apex of the pyriform sinus.

Keywords: radiotherapy, neck dissection, head and neck cancer, elective neck treatment

25.1 Introduction

The management of lymph node metastases is influenced by several factors, including the location, histologic differentiation, the size of the primary tumor, and the availability of capillary lymphatics.[1,2,3,4] The estimated risk of subclinical disease in the clinically negative neck as a function of primary site and tumor (T) stage is shown in ▶ Table 25.1.[1] Recurrent tumors have a higher risk of lymphatic involvement with a less predictable drainage pattern than untreated tumors.

Computed tomography (CT), magnetic resonance imaging (MRI), fluorodeoxyglucose–positron emission tomography (FDG-PET), and ultrasound may be used to evaluate cervical metastatic disease.[5] At the University of Florida, CT remains the primary method of examination of most carcinomas arising in the upper aerodigestive tract and the regional lymphatic system. MRI is the primary study only in patients with nasopharyngeal malignancies.

Table 25.1 Risk of subclinical disease in the neck

Group	Estimated risk of subclinical neck disease	Stage	Site
I: Low risk	< 20%	T1	Floor of mouth, retromolar trigone, gingiva, hard palate, buccal mucosa
II: Intermediate risk	20–30%	T1	Oral tongue, soft palate, pharyngeal wall, supraglottic larynx, tonsil
		T2	Floor mouth, oral tongue, retromolar trigone, gingiva, hard palate, buccal mucosa
III: High risk	> 30%	T1–T4	Nasopharynx, pyriform sinus, base of tongue
		T2–T4	Soft palate, pharyngeal wall, supraglottic larynx, tonsil
		T3–T4	Floor of mouth, oral tongue, retromolar trigone, gingiva, hard palate, buccal mucosa

Source: Adapted from Mendenhall and Million.[1]

Radiation therapy (RT) can be used in the treatment of cervical lymph node metastases as elective treatment when there is no clinically positive adenopathy, as the only treatment for clinically positive lymph nodes,[6] or as adjuvant preoperative or postoperative treatment in combination with neck dissection.[7] RT treatment planning of the neck is guided by several factors, including the location of the primary lesion, the estimated risk of subclinical disease in clinically negative lymph nodes, and the size, location, and number of clinically positive nodes.

Intensity-modulated RT (IMRT) is the most common RT technique used to treat head and neck squamous cell cancers of the mucosa; however, a low anterior neck field can be used to better limit the dose to the larynx when treating the lower neck nodes (▶ Fig. 25.1, ▶ Fig. 25.2). Advantages of IMRT over conventional RT include parotid sparing to reduce the risk of long-term xerostomia, avoiding a low-neck match in patients with a low-lying larynx, and improved coverage of the poststyloid parapharyngeal space in patients with nasopharyngeal cancer.[8] The most important disadvantage of using IMRT versus conventional RT is the increased risk of a marginal miss.[8] Additionally, the utilization of IMRT versus conventional RT results in increased treatment costs. A summary of typical IMRT treatment volumes when treating patients with head and neck squamous cell cancers is detailed in ▶ Table 25.2.

25.2 Elective Radiation Therapy of Cervical Lymph Nodes When the Primary Tumor Is Treated by Radiation Therapy

Several factors influence the decision to irradiate the neck electively. The most important factors are the site and size of the primary lesion. Other factors that influence this decision include histologic grade of the tumor, relative morbidity for adding lymph node coverage, likelihood of the patient's returning for follow-up examinations, and suitability of the patient for a neck dissection if the tumor recurs. If a patient has a primary lesion that is to be treated with RT and the risk of subclinical neck disease is 15% or greater, elective neck irradiation to a minimum dose equivalent to 45 to 50 Gy over 4.5 to 5 weeks is indicated (▶ Table 25.1).

Patients with lesions arising in the lip, nasal vestibule, nasal cavity, or paranasal sinuses have a low risk of subclinical neck disease, and the neck is not treated electively unless the lesion is recurrent, advanced, or poorly differentiated. Similarly, the risk of occult neck disease is essentially 0% for T1 and 1.7% for T2 glottic carcinomas, and elective neck RT is not indicated.[11,12]

Patients with lesions arising from the oral cavity, oropharynx, nasopharynx, subglottic larynx, and hypopharynx who have indications for RT at the primary site do receive elective neck irradiation due to the risk of clinically lymph node–negative subclinical

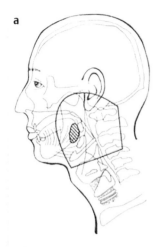
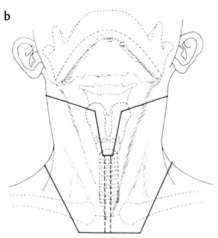

Fig. 25.1 Lateral and anterior fields are used to irradiate a patient with a carcinoma limited to the base of tongue. (a) Parallel-opposed fields include the primary lesion with a 2–3-cm inferior margin. The lower border of the field is placed at the thyroid notch and slants superiorly as the junction line proceeds posteriorly. This substantially reduces the amount of mucosa larynx and spinal cord included in the primary treatment portals. (b) En face low-neck portal with tapered midline larynx and tapered midline larynx block. It is not necessary to treat the supraclavicular fossa unless clinically positive nodes are found in that particular hemineck. A 5-mm midline tracheal block may be placed in the low-neck portal (dashed line). (Reproduced with permission of Mendenhall et al.[9])

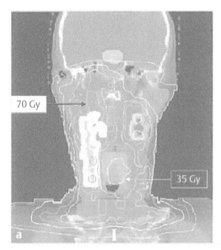
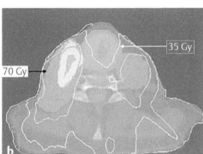

Fig. 25.2 Dose distribution using intensity-modulated radiation therapy as described in the text to treat the model patient with a stage T2N2b carcinoma of the tonsil with positive nodes on the right side at the level of the larynx. The plan was optimized to minimize the dose to the larynx while delivering 70 Gy to gross disease and 59.4 Gy to areas at risk for subclinical disease. (a) Coronal projection near the middle of the larynx. (b) Axial projection at the level of the true vocal cords. A comparison of (a) and (b) shows that sparing of the central portion of the larynx is shielded in an anterior low-neck field. (Reproduced with permission of Amdur et al.[10])

Table 25.2 Intensity-modulated radiation therapy target definitions at the University of Florida

Target	Definition
GTV primary	Gross tumor in primary site or post-op bed
GTV node	Gross tumor in lymph nodes
CTV HR	GTV primary + 1-cm isotropic expansion AND GTV node + 5-mm isotropic expansion
CTV IR	CTV HR + completion of positive and adjacent nodal stations
CTV SR	CTV IR + elective nodal regions
PTV HR, IR, SR	3-mm isotropic margin of each CTV

Abbreviations: CTV, clinical target volume; GTV, gross tumor volume; HR, high risk; IR, intermediate risk; PTV, planning target volume; SR, standard risk.

disease. Elective neck irradiation for oral cavity tumors includes the bilateral level Ib, II, III, and IV lymph nodes. For primary lesions located in the oropharynx, nasopharynx, and supraglottic larynx, level V nodes are also included. Patients with hypopharyngeal cancers and those with T3–T4 glottic carcinomas also receive RT to level VI nodes.

25.3 Treatment of Clinically Positive Cervical Lymph Nodes When the Primary Tumor Is Treated by Radiation Therapy

Clinically positive cervical lymph nodes require a higher dose of radiation to achieve local control when compared to subclinical disease. The required dose to these nodes is directly correlated with the size of the lymph node[6,13] and whether concomitant chemotherapy is administered.

Relatively recent data suggest that advanced disease has a better chance of cure after altered fractionation or concomitant chemotherapy.[14] Patients treated at the authors' institution routinely receive hyperfractionation or simultaneous integrated boost (SIB) combined with weekly cisplatin 30 mg/m². SIB consists of 70 Gy in 35 fractions over 30 treatment days in 6 weeks with 1 twice-daily fraction during the last 5 weeks with a minimum 6-hour interfraction interval. The high-risk planning treatment volume (PTV) receives 70 Gy at 2 Gy per fraction, intermediate PTV receives 63 Gy at 1.8 Gy per fraction, and the standard risk PTV receives 56 Gy at 1.6 Gy per fraction. Other dose regimens that are acceptable include IMRT with a sequential boost, or hyperfractionation with twice-daily fractionation. Positive nodes receive approximately 70 to 74 Gy, regardless of size or rate of regression. Acceptable dose regimens are detailed in ▶ Table 25.3.

The decision to add a neck dissection after RT for multiple unilateral positive nodes or bilateral lymph node disease is individualized and is based on the diameter of the largest node, node fixation, and number of clinically positive nodes in the neck. If clinically positive lymph nodes disappear completely during RT, the likelihood of control by RT alone is improved and a neck dissection may be withheld.[15,16,17,18] At the authors' institution, at PET-CT scan is obtained 12 weeks post-RT to evaluate for residual nodal disease. If a patient has PET-avid cervical adenopathy at this time, a neck dissection is recommended.

Johnson et al[19] reported on 81 patients with node-positive stages III and IV squamous cell carcinoma (SSC) of the head and neck treated with concomitant boost accelerated hyperfractionated RT at the Medical College of Virginia (Richmond). A total of 58 patients (72%) had a complete response in the neck and were followed; 3 patients (5%) subsequently developed an isolated recurrence in the neck, and 1 additional patient developed recurrent cancer in the neck and in the primary site. The 3-year neck disease control rates were 94% for nodes 3 cm or less compared with 86% for those more than 3 cm. Peters et al[20] reported on 100 node-positive patients with SSC of the oropharynx treated with concomitant boost RT between 1984 and 1993 at the MD Anderson Cancer Center (Houston, TX). Sixty-two patients had a complete response in the neck and received no further therapy. Three patients (5%) subsequently developed an isolated recurrence in the neck and four patients (6%) developed a recurrence in the neck in conjunction with other sites of relapse. The 2-year neck disease control rates did not vary significantly with pretreatment nodal size: 3 cm or less, 87%; and more than 3 cm, 85%. The incidence of subcutaneous fibrosis was similar following RT alone compared with another group of patients who underwent a neck dissection in addition to RT.

Multiple subsequent studies evaluating neck control rates after RT alone or combined with chemotherapy suggest that the likelihood of an isolated failure in the neck is low if there is a complete response after treatment.[7,21,22]

Liauw et al[23] evaluated a series of 550 patients treated with definitive RT at the University of Florida between 1990 and 2002; 341 patients (62%) underwent a post-RT planned neck dissection. CT images obtained at approximately 4 weeks post-RT were reviewed for 211 patients; radiographic complete response (rCR) was defined as no nodes greater than 1.5 cm and no focal abnormalities such as focal lucency, enhancement, or calcification.[23] The outcomes are depicted in ▶ Table 25.4. Thirty-two patients who had an rCR were followed, and did not undergo a neck dissection; the neck control rate was 97%. Recent data published by Yeung et al[24] suggest that for those who have a partial response to RT, neck dissection may be safely limited to only those levels that remain suspicious after RT.

Goenka et al[25] reported on 302 patients with node-positive oropharyngeal SCCs treated with IMRT and concomitant chemotherapy at the Memorial Sloan Kettering Cancer Center between 2002 and 2009. Patients underwent a PET-CT following treatment to assess response. A clinical and radiographic complete response was observed in 260 (86.1%) patients, and the patients were observed. The neck control rate was 97.7%. Three of four patients who recurred in the neck were successfully salvaged. Patients who underwent a neck dissection had the following rates of pathologically visible tumor: PET-CT positive, 52%; and PET-CT negative, 25%.

Mehanna et al[26] reported on a prospective trial where 564 node-positive patients were randomized to chemoradiation followed by PET-CT and either planned neck dissection (282 patients) or observation in the event of a CR (282 patients). Patients in the latter group underwent fewer neck dissections: the 2-year survival rates were comparable.

Table 25.3 Dose regimens for head and neck cancer

Standard fractionation: one fraction per day	PTV SR: 56 Gy at 1.6 Gy/fx
IMRT SIB	PTV IR: 63 Gy at 1.8 Gy/fx
Total treatment days: 35	PTV HR: 70 Gy at 2 Gy/fx
Accelerated fractionation: one fraction per day with two fractions 1 day per week starting on week 2	PTV SR: 56 Gy at 1.6 Gy/fx
IMRT SIB	PTV IR: 63 Gy at 1.8 Gy/fx
Total treatment days: 30	PTV HR: 70 Gy at 2 Gy/fx
Accelerated fractionation: two fractions per day	PTV SR: 50.4 Gy at 1.2 Gy/fx
IMRT sequential boost	PTV IR: 9.6 Gy at 1.2 Gy/fx boost (total dose 60 Gy)
Total treatment days: 31	PTV HR: 14.4 Gy at 1.2 Gy/fx boost (total dose 74.4 Gy)

Abbreviations: fx, fraction; HR, high risk; IMRT, intensity-modulated radiation therapy; IR, intermediate risk; PTV, planning target volume; SIB, simultaneous integrated boost; SR, standard risk.
Note: Accelerated fractionation is preferred

Table 25.4 Predictive value of postradiotherapy computed tomography findings at 4 weeks in the hemineck correlated with neck dissection pathology (N = 193 heminecks)

Findings	NPV		PPV	
	Number/ total number	Percent	Number/ total number	Percent
Any lymph node > 1.5 cm	85/118	72	24/75	32
Any lymph node with focal lucency	49/57	86	49/136	36
Any focally abnormal lymph nodes	75/98	77	34/95	36
Any lymph node with enhancement	111/147	76	21/46	46
Any lymph node with calcification	102/144	71	15/49	31
Two or more focally abnormal lymph nodes[a]	90/113	80	34/80	43
Any lymph node > 1.5 cm and any focally abnormal lymph node	32/34	94	55/159	35

Abbreviations: NPV, negative predictive value; PPV, positive predictive value.
[a]Focally abnormal lymph nodes equal grade 3 or 4 focal lucency, focal enhancement, or focal calcification.

At the University of Florida, all patients with clinically positive nodes are evaluated with a PET-CT at 3 months after the completion of RT. This time period between the completion of RT and the PET-CT minimizes the risk of a false-positive scan. Neck dissection is withheld in the subset of patients with a complete response, who are thought to have 5% or less risk of residual disease; the remainder of patients undergo a neck dissection.

If a neck dissection is planned to follow RT in patients with clinically positive lymph nodes, the preoperative dose can vary with the size and location of the lymph node, fixation, and response to RT. At the authors' institution, clinically positive lymph nodes regardless of morphology are treated within in the high-risk PTV to a dose of 70 to 75 Gy.

Large lymph nodes may not show much regression during the course of RT but often show significant regression from completion of treatment to the time the patient returns for neck dissection, usually after 4 to 6 weeks. The mass frequently has a thick capsule that facilitates its removal at the time of neck dissection. Performing a unilateral versus bilateral neck dissection requires individualized treatment planning jointly by the radiation oncologist and the surgeon. RT alone may be sufficient to control the disease on the side of the neck with minimal disease, and a neck dissection may be used on the side with more disease. If major bilateral disease is present, bilateral neck dissection should follow RT.

25.4 Treatment of the Neck After Incisional or Excisional Biopsy

Incisional or excisional biopsy of a clinically positive lymph node prior to definitive treatment can potentially spill malignant cells along tissue planes precluding the ability for the removal of all tumor cells with radical neck dissection. Therefore, an open biopsy before definitive treatment of the neck is strongly discouraged. McGuirt and McCabe[27] reported that incisional or excisional biopsy of positive neck nodes before definitive surgery increased the risk of neck failure and worsened the prognosis for patients with SCC of the head and neck. Parsons et al[28] reported their experience with incisional or excisional biopsy of positive neck nodes followed by RT as the initial step in the treatment of the patient; these data were updated by Mack et al.[29] After excisional biopsy of a single lymph node, RT alone to the primary lesion and to the neck resulted in a 95% rate of neck control.[29] If residual disease remained in the neck after biopsy, RT followed by neck dissection was more successful than RT alone for controlling neck disease (▶ Table 25.5).

If there is indication to treat the primary tumor surgically, the patient will undergo a complete neck dissection followed by RT. Alternatively, the patient is treated with preoperative RT followed by resection of the primary site and a neck dissection. If the primary lesion is to be treated with definitive RT, the patient's neck is treated with RT followed by a neck dissection if residual cervical adenopathy is present at the completion of RT. The dose of RT preceding a neck dissection depends on the amount of gross disease in the neck and the degree of fixation.

25.5 Ipsilateral Neck Irradiation

In patients without a history of previous neck surgery, the right and left lymphatic networks do not usually shunt from one side to the other. The utilization of ipsilateral radiation therefore can be considered in highly selected patients. Ipsilateral neck irradiation minimizes dose to the contralateral normal structures and potentially decreases acute and long-term morbidity from RT. However, a concern of ipsilateral therapy is the potential for contralateral neck nodal relapse. Therefore, this modality is primarily used in patients with well-lateralized T1–T2, N0–N2 stage tonsillar cancers without base of tongue or soft palate involvement.[31]

Kennedy et al[32] reported their experience with ipsilateral neck RT for early-stage SCC of the tonsillar area with no base of tongue or soft palate extension. Definitive RT to the primary site and ipsilateral neck resulted in a 5-year local-regional control rate of 92.6%. Of the 76 patients treated, only 1 patient failed in the contralateral, nonirradiated neck 3 years after primary RT (▶ Fig. 25.3).

Huang et al[31] from Princess Margaret Hospital reported on their experience of treatment of T1–T2, N0–N2b tonsillar cancer patients who received ipsilateral RT and bilateral RT between 1999 and 2014. At a median follow-up of 5 years, the overall survival, local control, and regional control rates were similar for the ipsilateral versus bilateral RT group. Contralateral neck failure occurred in 2 of the 86 patients (2.3%) who received ipsilateral RT.

At the authors' institution, unilateral RT is recommended for patients with tonsillar SSC when their risk of cancer in the contralateral lymph nodes is less than 10%. This subset includes patients with T1–T2, N0–N2b tonsillar fossa or anterior tonsillar pillar tumors with no soft palate or base of tongue invasion. Concurrent chemotherapy with weekly cisplatin (30 mg/m^2) is given to patients with two or more positive lymph nodes.

Table 25.5 Effect of neck node biopsy on 5-year rate of neck control (660 heminecks)

| Hemineck stage | No neck biopsy | | Neck biopsy | | |
	Number of heminecks	Probability of hemineck control (%)	Number of heminecks	Probability hemineck of control (%)	Significance of difference between curves
N1	253	87 ± 3	12	100	$p = 0.22$
N2A	53	73 ± 8	15	93 ± 6	$p = 0.18$
N2B	218	78 ± 3	23	72 ± 11	$p = 0.86$
N3A	69	54 ± 7	17	81 ± 10	$p = 0.30$

Source: Adapted from Ellis et al.[30]

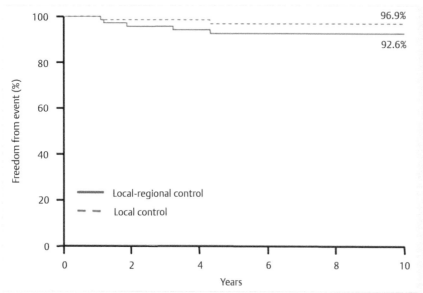

Fig. 25.3 Kaplan–Meier curve illustrating local control and local-regional control rates at 10 years of patients treated with definitive ipsilateral RT for early-stage squamous cell carcinoma of the tonsillar region. (Reproduced with permission of Kennedy et al.[32])

25.6 Treatment of the Neck After Surgery

Patients who are treated with primary surgery for their head and neck mucosal cancer generally undergo resection of their primary tumor and a unilateral or bilateral neck dissection. The surgical management of the neck is dependent on the location, extent of the primary tumor, and the extent of positive neck nodes. Indications for postoperative RT include positive or close (< 5 mm) margins, initially positive margins with negative, separately submitted margins, extracapsular extension, multiple positive nodes, perineural invasion, bone or cartilage invasion, extension into the soft tissues of the neck, invasion of the apex of the pyriform sinus, and subglottic extension of 1 cm or more.[33] The highest risk indications are positive margins and extracapsular extension and require the addition of concomitant cisplatin during the course of postoperative RT.

Potentially hypoxic tissues secondary to surgery can increase the risk of the radio resistance of tumor cells; hence, the minimum postoperative radiation dose recommended is 60 Gy at 2 Gy per once-daily fraction. Areas within the neck that are at the highest risk for microscopic disease should receive a higher dose in the range of 66 to 70 Gy. Treating the primary site alone if the neck nodes are pathologically negative may be considered, particularly for frail patients and those with significant postoperative complications. However, postoperative RT is not employed for the indication to electively treat the clinically negative neck in lieu of a neck dissection.

25.7 Complications of Neck Irradiation

The complications of neck irradiation include subcutaneous fibrosis and lymphedema of the larynx and submentum. The probability of complications is directly related to the radiation dose delivered and the location of the irradiated tumor relative

to normal structures, such as the mandible and hearing apparatus. There is little, if any, morbidity observed with the doses used for elective RT of the neck.

Complications of neck treatment in patients who receive RT in conjunction with resection of the primary lesion and a neck dissection are essentially the same as those occurring after neck dissection. However, they occur with an increased incidence depending on the RT dose and extent of surgery.

25.8 Results of Treatment

25.8.1 Clinically Negative Nodes

Elective neck dissection and elective neck irradiation are equivalent in locally controlling subclinical disease. In addition, elective neck irradiation is equally efficacious for SCC arising from various head and neck primary sites. The decision whether to use surgery or RT for the purpose of electively treating the neck nodes depends on the method used to treat the primary lesion. Patients with a relatively early primary lesion and clinically negative nodes should be treated with one modality. Patients who receive definitive RT to their primary lesion should be considered for elective neck irradiation, while those who are primarily treated surgically should undergo an elective neck dissection if indicated. Patients who develop a local recurrence or a metachronous second primary after RT for an SCC with a cN0 neck in whom the neck has been irradiated may be treated with surgery to the primary site alone and the neck observed because the likelihood of subclinical disease in the cervical lymphatics is less than 10%.[34,35]

The University of Florida has reported its results of elective neck irradiation for patients with SSC of the head and neck in whom the primary lesion was treated with definitive RT. The results are illustrated in ► Table 25.6.[1] Patients were divided into three risk categories based on the estimated risk of subclinical disease in the neck as follows: group I, low risk (< 20% likelihood of occult disease); group II, moderate risk (20–30% risk of occult disease); and group III, high risk (more than 30% likelihood of occult disease). There were 6 neck failures (21%) in 28 patients who did not receive elective neck irradiation and 8 neck failures (5%)

in 162 patients who received elective neck irradiation. Of the eight failures in patients receiving elective neck irradiation, two occurred within the irradiation fields, one at the field margin, and five in out-of-field areas. No correlation was found between the rate of tumor control in the first-echelon lymph nodes and the irradiation dose for doses ranging from 40 to 55 Gy or greater.[1] Only one failure occurred in the first-echelon lymph nodes, and this was after 48 Gy in 25 fractions using continuous-course irradiation.[1] The low neck, defined as that part of the neck located below the treatment portals used to treat the primary lesion, received either 50 Gy in 25 fractions or 40.5 Gy in 15 fractions, specified at D_{max} (0.5-cm depth). Both dose-fractionation protocols were equally effective in sterilizing subclinical disease in the low neck.[36]

Vandenbrouck et al[37] and Fakih et al[38] have conducted randomized trials comparing elective neck dissection with no elective neck treatment for patients with oral cavity carcinoma and oral tongue cancer, respectively. No survival advantage was noted for patients undergoing elective neck dissection in either study. However, because of the small number of patients in both trials, it is likely that even if a survival difference existed, it would have been missed. Subsequently, a randomized trial was conducted at the Tata Memorial Hospital (Mumbai) where 596 patients with T1–T1 N0 SCCs of the oral cavity were randomized to resection of the primary and observation of the neck or to resection of the primary and elective neck dissection. Those in the latter group had significantly improved overall survival at 3 years (80 vs. 68%; $p = 0.01$).[39]

Although elective neck irradiation significantly reduces the risk of recurrence in the neck, there is no definite evidence that it improves survival. A large randomized trial would be necessary to detect a survival difference, if one exists. Additionally, it is likely that if elective neck dissection improves survival, elective neck irradiation would as well.

Patients treated with primary RT who have a local recurrence in addition to a recurrence in the neck have a very poor chance of surgical salvage (< 10%). In patients in whom the primary lesion is controlled with RT and in whom disease recurs in the initially negative neck, the chances of salvage with neck dissection are approximately 50 to 60%.

25.8.2 Clinically Positive Nodes

The rate of controlling clinically positive cervical nodes with RT alone or with combined RT and neck dissection is directly correlated with a patient's volume of neck disease. The rate of control for neck nodes treated with RT alone as a function of node size, treatment scheme, and dose is shown in ▶ Table 25.7. RT alone is sufficient for patients with N1 (up to 2 cm) disease if the total dose is sufficient.[40] However, RT followed by neck dissection has provided better rates of disease control than RT alone for patients with more advanced neck disease. The incidence of treatment failure in the neck by N stage and treatment category has been reported by the MD Anderson Cancer Center (▶ Table 25.8) and the University of Florida (▶ Table 25.9).

In patients in whom the neck is treated with combined modalities, RT precedes surgery when the primary site is to be treated with irradiation or when the node is incompletely resectable. Surgery precedes RT when the primary site is to be treated operatively and the nodes are resectable.

Table 25.6 Control of disease in the clinically negative neck with elective neck irradiation (number controlled/number treated)

Risk group	No ENI (%)	Partial ENI (%)	Total ENI (%)
I (< 20%)	13/15 (87)	16/17 (94)	1/1 (100)
II (20–30%)	6/9 (67)	34/38 (89)	10/11 (91)
III (> 30%)	3/4 (75)	32/33 (97)	61/62 (98)

Abbreviation: ENI, elective neck irradiation.
Source: Adapted from Mendenhall and Million.[1]

Table 25.7 Lymph node disease control by radiation treatment technique (number controlled/number treated)

Node size (cm)	Continuous course (%)	Split course (%)	Excluded[a]	Total (%)
< 1.0	5/5	2/2	1/1	8/8
1.0	29/35 (83)	19/23 (85)	3/4	51/62 (82)
1.5–2.0	43/49 (88)	20/24 (83)	5/9	68/82 (83)
2.5–3.0	14/19 (74)	10/18 (56)	0/3	24/40 (60)
3.5–6.0	14/20 (70)	10/17 (59)	0/1	24/38 (63)
≥ 7.0	0/2	0/5	0/1	0/8

Source: Modified from Mendenhall et al.[40]
[a]Less than 50 Gy for nodes equal to 1.0 cm and < 55 Gy for nodes equal to 1.5 cm.

Table 25.8 Failure of initial ipsilateral neck treatment: 596 patients with carcinoma of the tonsillar fossa, base of tongue, supraglottic larynx, or hypopharynx

Treatment[a]	N0			N1 (%)	N2A (%)	N2B (%)	N3A (%)	N3B (%)
	No treatment	Partial treatment	Complete treatment					
Irradiation		15%	2%	15	27	27	38	34
Surgery	55% (16/29)	35%	7%	11	8	23	42	41
Combined		1/5	0/6	0	0	0	23	25

Source: Modified from Barkley et al.[41]
[a]MD Anderson Cancer Center data; patients treated in 1948–1967.

Table 25.9 Five-year rate of neck control by 1983 AJCC stage and treatment (459 patients; 593 heminecks)[a]

Stage	Irradiation alone		Irradiation + neck dissection		Significance
	Number heminecks	Control (%)	Number heminecks	Control (%)	
N1	215	86	38	93	$p = 0.28$
N2A	29	79	24	68	$p = 0.6$
N2B	138	70	80	91	$p < 0.01$
N3A	29	33	40	69	$p < 0.01$

Abbreviation: AJCC, American Joint Committee on Cancer.
Note: University of Florida data; patients treated from October 1964 to October 1985; analysis in December 1988 by Eric R. Ellis, MD.
[a]Excludes 67 heminecks on which incisional or excisional biopsy was done before treatment.

Table 25.10 Cervical metastasis appearing in the contralateral N0 neck: 596 patients with the carcinoma of tonsillar fossa, base of tongue, supraglottic larynx, or hypopharynx

Treatment[a]	Stage				
	N0 (%)	N1 (%)	N2A (%)	N2B (%)	N3A (%)
Irradiation	4	2	9	7	0
Surgery	25	17	23	43	33
Combined	0	0	0	11	0

Source: Adapted from Barkley et al.[41]
[a]MD Anderson Hospital data; patients treated in 1948–1967.

Table 25.11 Prognostic factors, in order of their importance, for predicting the time to occurrence of various events

Event	Rank order	Factor	Level of significance
Recurrence in neck ($N = 660$ heminecks)	1	Increasing N stage	$p = 0.0001$
	2	Treatment of neck with RT alone	$p = 0.0001$
	3	Fixed nodes	$p = 0.0001$
	4	T stage[a]	$p = 0.0350$
Death with disease present ($N = 508$ patients)	1	Recurrence above clavicles	$p = 0.0001$
	2	Increasing N stage	$p = 0.0003$
	3	Fixed nodes	$p = 0.0053$
	4	Treatment of neck RT alone	$p = 0.0121$
For occurrence of distant metastasis ($N = 508$ patients)	1	Recurrence above clavicles	$p = 0.0001$
	2	Increasing N stage	$p = 0.0003$
	3	Fixed nodes	$p = 0.0704$
	4	Nodes below thyroid notch	$p = 0.1032$

Abbreviations: RT, radiotherapy.
Source: Adapted from Ellis et al.[30]
[a]This factor is thought to be correlated with the censoring pattern.

When the initial treatment is surgery, a neck dissection is sufficient treatment for patients with a single positive lymph node less than 3 cm unless there is extracapsular spread of disease. RT may be added for control of subclinical disease in the contralateral side of the neck (▶ Table 25.10).[41] The presence of multiple positive nodes in the surgical specimen is an indication for postoperative RT of the neck, especially when positive nodes are found at more than one level.

The postoperative dose prescribed is usually 60 Gy in 30 fractions to 66 Gy in 33 fractions over 6 to 7 weeks for patients with negative margins; higher doses to 70 to 75 Gy may be prescribed when residual disease is present in the neck. If RT is to be added after surgery, it is usually initiated within 4 to 6 weeks after the operation. The likelihood of disease control in each side of the neck treated with irradiation and neck dissection is decreased when the node is fixed before treatment or when residual tumor is found in the pathologic specimen. The dose for clinically positive lymph nodes in the preoperative or definitive RT setting is 70 to 75 Gy.

25.8.3 Results After Incisional or Excisional Biopsy

Open biopsy is not recommended prior to the definitive treatment of metastatic cervical lymph nodes due to the increased risk of tumor cell spillage. Patients in this scenario do not have an increased risk of neck failure or decreased cure rate if RT is the next step in treatment.[28] However, the possibility of regional control in this situation likely diminishes if an operation without prior RT is performed because surgery is unable to remove all microscopic malignant cells into disrupt tissues not removed by neck dissection.

Ellis et al[30] reported on 508 patients with 660 positive heminecks treated at the University of Florida with RT alone or followed by a planned neck dissection. Pretreatment node biopsy did not influence outcome when RT was the next step in treatment (▶ Table 25.5).[30] The results of the forward stepwise log-rank tests of prognostic factors for predicting time to recurrence are shown in ▶ Table 25.11.[30]

Zenga et al[42] reported on 45 patients treated between 1998 and 2012 who underwent open biopsy for human papillomavirus–positive oropharyngeal cancer. All patients underwent definitive surgical treatment. Disease specific survival was 98 versus 99% in a control group who did not undergo an open biopsy. Approximately 7% of patients in the open biopsy group were found to have dermal metastases in the excised skin—thus illustrating the importance of excision of the skin in the biopsied area along with a neck dissection if surgery is the primary treatment for patients with previously violated cervical nodes. In these scenarios, adjuvant RT with 60 to 70 Gy is recommended to minimize the likelihood of regional recurrence.

References

[1] Mendenhall WM, Million RR. Elective neck irradiation for squamous cell carcinoma of the head and neck: analysis of time-dose factors and causes of failure. Int J Radiat Oncol Biol Phys. 1986; 12(5):741–746

[2] Lindberg R. Distribution of cervical lymph node metastases from squamous cell carcinoma of the upper respiratory and digestive tracts. Cancer. 1972; 29 (6):1446–1449

[3] Richard JM, Sancho-Garnier H, Micheau C, Saravane D, Cachin Y. Prognostic factors in cervical lymph node metastasis in upper respiratory and digestive tract carcinomas: study of 1,713 cases during a 15-year period. Laryngoscope. 1987; 97(1):97–101

[4] McLaughlin MP, Mendenhall WM, Mancuso AA, et al. Retropharyngeal adenopathy as a predictor of outcome in squamous cell carcinoma of the head and neck. Head Neck. 1995; 17(3):190–198

[5] Mancuso AA, Hanafee WN. Head and Neck Radiology. Philadelphia, PA: Williams & Wilkins; 2011

[6] Dubray BM, Bataini JP, Bernier J, et al. Is reseeding from the primary a plausible cause of node failure? Int J Radiat Oncol Biol Phys. 1993; 25(1):9–15

[7] Mendenhall WM, Villaret DB, Amdur RJ, Hinerman RW, Mancuso AA. Planned neck dissection after definitive radiotherapy for squamous cell carcinoma of the head and neck. Head Neck. 2002; 24(11):1012–1018

[8] Mendenhall WM, Mancuso AA. Radiotherapy for head and neck cancer–is the "next level" down? Int J Radiat Oncol Biol Phys. 2009; 73(3):645–646

[9] Mendenhall WM, Parsons JT, Million RR. Unnecessary irradiation of the normal larynx. Int J Radiat Oncol Biol Phys. 1990; 18(6):1531–1533

[10] Amdur RJ, Li JG, Liu C, Hinerman RW, Mendenhall WM. Unnecessary laryngeal irradiation in the IMRT era. Head Neck. 2004; 26(3):257–263, discussion 263–264

[11] Mendenhall WM, Parsons JT, Stringer SP, Cassisi NJ, Million RR. T1-T2 vocal cord carcinoma: a basis for comparing the results of radiotherapy and surgery. Head Neck Surg. 1988; 10(6):373–377

[12] Mendenhall WM, Parsons JT, Brant TA, Stringer SP, Cassisi NJ, Million RR. Is elective neck treatment indicated for T2N0 squamous cell carcinoma of the glottic larynx? Radiother Oncol. 1989; 14(3):199–202

[13] Taylor JM, Mendenhall WM, Lavey RS. Time-dose factors in positive neck nodes treated with irradiation only. Radiother Oncol. 1991; 22(3):167–173

[14] Mendenhall WM, Riggs CE, Vaysberg M, Amdur RJ, Werning JW. Altered fractionation and adjuvant chemotherapy for head and neck squamous cell carcinoma. Head Neck. 2010; 32(7):939–945

[15] Bartelink H, Breur K, Hart G. Radiotherapy of lymph node metastases in patients with squamous cell carcinoma of the head and neck region. Int J Radiat Oncol Biol Phys. 1982; 8(6):983–989

[16] Bartelink H. Prognostic value of the regression rate of neck node metastases during radiotherapy. Int J Radiat Oncol Biol Phys. 1983; 9(7):993–996

[17] Bataini JP, Bernier J, Jaulerry C, Brunin F, Pontvert D, Lave C. Impact of neck node radioresponsiveness on the regional control probability in patients with oropharynx and pharyngolarynx cancers managed by definitive radiotherapy. Int J Radiat Oncol Biol Phys. 1987; 13(6):817–824

[18] Maciejewski B. Regression rate of metastatic neck lymph nodes after radiation treatment as a prognostic factor for local control. Radiother Oncol. 1987; 8(4):301–308

[19] Johnson CR, Silverman LN, Clay LB, Schmidt-Ullrich R. Radiotherapeutic management of bulky cervical lymphadenopathy in squamous cell carcinoma of the head and neck: is postradiotherapy neck dissection necessary? Radiat Oncol Investig. 1998; 6(1):52–57

[20] Peters LJ, Weber RS, Morrison WH, Byers RM, Garden AS, Goepfert H. Neck surgery in patients with primary oropharyngeal cancer treated by radiotherapy. Head Neck. 1996; 18(6):552–559

[21] Ferlito A, Corry J, Silver CE, Shaha AR, Thomas Robbins K, Rinaldo A. Planned neck dissection for patients with complete response to chemoradiotherapy: a concept approaching obsolescence. Head Neck. 2010; 32(2):253–261

[22] Corry J, Peters L, Fisher R, et al. N2-N3 neck nodal control without planned neck dissection for clinical/radiologic complete responders-results of Trans Tasman Radiation Oncology Group Study 98.02. Head Neck. 2008; 30 (6):737–742

[23] Liauw SL, Mancuso AA, Amdur RJ, et al. Postradiotherapy neck dissection for lymph node-positive head and neck cancer: the use of computed tomography to manage the neck. J Clin Oncol. 2006; 24(9):1421–1427

[24] Yeung AR, Liauw SL, Amdur RJ, et al. Lymph node-positive head and neck cancer treated with definitive radiotherapy: can treatment response determine the extent of neck dissection? Cancer. 2008; 112(5):1076–1082

[25] Goenka A, Morris LG, Rao SS, et al. Long-term regional control in the observed neck following definitive chemoradiation for node-positive oropharyngeal squamous cell cancer. Int J Cancer. 2013; 133(5):1214–1221

[26] Mehanna H, Wong WL, McConkey CC, et al. PET-NECK Trial Management Group. PET-CT surveillance versus neck dissection in advanced head and neck cancer. N Engl J Med. 2016; 374(15):1444–1454

[27] McGuirt WF, McCabe BF. Significance of node biopsy before definitive treatment of cervical metastatic carcinoma. Laryngoscope. 1978; 88(4):594–597

[28] Parsons JT, Million RR, Cassisi NJ. The influence of excisional or incisional biopsy of metastatic neck nodes on the management of head and neck cancer. Int J Radiat Oncol Biol Phys. 1985; 11(8):1447–1454

[29] Mack Y, Parsons JT, Mendenhall WM, Stringer SP, Cassisi NJ, Million RR. Squamous cell carcinoma of the head and neck: management after excisional biopsy of a solitary metastatic neck node. Int J Radiat Oncol Biol Phys. 1993; 25 (4):619–622

[30] Ellis ER, Mendenhall WM, Rao PV, et al. Incisional or excisional neck-node biopsy before definitive radiotherapy, alone or followed by neck dissection. Head Neck. 1991; 13(3):177–183

[31] Huang SH, Waldron J, Bratman SV, et al. Re-evaluation of ipsilateral radiation for T1-T2N0-N2b tonsil carcinoma at the Princess Margaret Hospital in the human papillomavirus era, 25 years later. Int J Radiat Oncol Biol Phys. 2017; 98(1):159–169

[32] Kennedy WR, Herman MP, Deraniyagala RL, et al. Ipsilateral radiotherapy for squamous cell carcinoma of the tonsil. Eur Arch Otorhinolaryngol. 2016; 273 (8):2151–2156

[33] Amdur RJ, Parsons JT, Mendenhall WM, Million RR, Stringer SP, Cassisi NJ. Postoperative irradiation for squamous cell carcinoma of the head and neck: an analysis of treatment results and complications. Int J Radiat Oncol Biol Phys. 1989; 16(1):25–36

[34] Dagan R, Morris CG, Kirwan JM, et al. Elective neck dissection during salvage surgery for locally recurrent head and neck squamous cell carcinoma after radiotherapy with elective nodal irradiation. Laryngoscope. 2010; 120 (5):945–952

[35] Falchook AD, Dagan R, Morris CG, Mendenhall WM. Elective neck dissection for second primary after previous definitive radiotherapy. Am J Otolaryngol. 2012; 33(2):199–204

[36] Mendenhall WM, Parsons JT, Million RR. Elective lower neck irradiation: 5000 cGy/25 fractions versus 4050 cGy/15 fractions. Int J Radiat Oncol Biol Phys. 1988; 15(2):439–440

[37] Vandenbrouck C, Sancho-Garnier H, Chassagne D, Saravane D, Cachin Y, Micheau C. Elective versus therapeutic radical neck dissection in epidermoid carcinoma of the oral cavity: results of a randomized clinical trial. Cancer. 1980; 46(2):386–390

[38] Fakih AR, Rao RS, Borges AM, Patel AR. Elective versus therapeutic neck dissection in early carcinoma of the oral tongue. Am J Surg. 1989; 158(4):309–313

[39] D'Cruz AK, Vaish R, Kapre N, et al. Head and Neck Disease Management Group. Elective versus therapeutic neck dissection in node-negative oral cancer. N Engl J Med. 2015; 373(6):521–529

[40] Mendenhall WM, Million RR, Bova FJ. Analysis of time-dose factors in clinically positive neck nodes treated with irradiation alone in squamous cell carcinoma of the head and neck. Int J Radiat Oncol Biol Phys. 1984; 10 (5):639–643

[41] Barkley HT, Jr, Fletcher GH, Jesse RH, Lindberg RD. Management of cervical lymph node metastases in squamous cell carcinoma of the tonsillar fossa, base of tongue, supraglottic larynx, and hypopharynx. Am J Surg. 1972; 124 (4):462–467

[42] Zenga J, Graboyes EM, Haughey BH, et al. Definitive surgical therapy after open neck biopsy for HPV-related oropharyngeal cancer. Otolaryngol Head Neck Surg. 2016; 154(4):657–666

26 Systemic Therapies in the Management of Head and Neck Cancer

Andrew J. Johnsrud and Konstantinos Arnaoutakis

Abstract

Systemic therapy in head and neck cancer has been an evolving field over the last several years. Its utility in the locally advanced setting as an induction treatment, as an integral part of combined modality therapy, and in the adjuvant setting is well documented. Systemic therapy in the more advanced setting has also been studied and evolved to introduce more novel approaches such as monoclonal antibodies against the epidermal growth factor receptor and immunotherapy, particularly checkpoint inhibitors such as PD-1 inhibitors. In this chapter, we review the current treatment options utilizing systemic therapy, as well as future directions including the utilization of targeted agents and immune therapy.

Keywords: systemic therapies, chemotherapy, head and neck cancer

26.1 Introduction

The role of systemic treatment (i.e., chemotherapy) in the management of head and neck squamous cell carcinoma (HNSCC) has been an evolving topic over the past few decades. Though historically its use has been limited to palliative settings, chemotherapy is now established as an essential component of multimodal treatment in the setting of both early and locally advanced disease. Its utility in this setting is most recognized as a radiosensitizing component given concurrently with radiotherapy.

Several agents have demonstrated activity against HNSCC, including platinum compounds (cisplatin, carboplatin), taxanes (docetaxel, paclitaxel), and antimetabolites (5-fluorouracil [5-FU], methotrexate). Cisplatin, a potent radiosensitizer, is established as a standard agent in combination with radiation or coupled with other chemotherapeutic agents. It remains a preferred option over other platinum agents such as carboplatin, which has demonstrated improved tolerability at the expense of less activity in HNSCC. In 2009, a large meta-analysis was updated including 87 trials and more than 17,000 patients, evaluating the benefit of chemotherapy in HNSCC given as concurrent chemoradiotherapy (CRT), induction chemotherapy (ICT), or adjuvant treatment. The included trials compared locoregional treatment plus chemotherapy versus locoregional treatment alone. The total observed benefit from chemotherapy was an absolute 4.5% higher 5-year survival, confirming the benefits of chemotherapy in locally advanced HNSCC. A more pronounced absolute benefit of 6.5% was observed in trials of concurrent CRT, whereas there was no clear survival benefit seen for ICT or adjuvant chemotherapy.[1]

The current treatment options utilizing systemic therapy will be reviewed here, as well as future directions including the utilization of targeted agents and immune therapy.

26.2 Induction Chemotherapy

The rationale behind the use of ICT prior to definitive therapy includes several considerations. One aim is to improve locoregional control, though in theory the additive systemic therapy may obviate the progression of metastatic disease and prevent distant relapses. It is indeed estimated that at least 50% of patients treated for locally advanced HNSCC will develop locoregional or distant relapse within 2 years of treatment despite receiving adequate local control with surgery and/or radiotherapy.[2] It is also pertinent to consider that increased tumor volume and hypoxic tumor volume may have a deleterious effect on local therapies, particularly radiotherapy, considering its dependence on oxygen-derived free radicals. This is supported by several studies of laryngeal cancer, which have demonstrated an inverse relationship between tumor size and local control with radiotherapy.[3,4,5] As such, in cases with relatively large tumor burden, ICT can be expected to reduce tumor volume and afford more adequate responses to locoregional therapy by enhancing radiosensitivity or resectability. Others have adopted the use of ICT as a basis for organ preservation, by inducing better responses to locoregional control with nonsurgical methods. By the same token, inadequate responses may permit salvage surgery to occur in a nonirradiated tissue environment and prevent complications such as fistula formation or poor wound healing.

As mentioned previously, several agents have demonstrated activity against HNSCC. Platinum-based regimens have generally shown the most anticancer activity and continue to be the most commonly used agents in the first-line setting. Many of the initial investigations in the 1980s and 1990s evaluating ICT followed by locoregional therapy could show a decrease in the rate of distant metastases, but were unable to consistently demonstrate a survival benefit. Cisplatin plus 5-FU became a standard regimen for ICT based on the observed high response rates and its ability to eliminate the need for surgical resection in some trials, though only a limited number of these were able to show a benefit in overall survival (OS).[6,7,8] Though the previously described meta-analysis of chemotherapy in head and neck cancer (MACH-NC) revealed only a modest and statistically insignificant OS benefit from ICT (2.4%; *p* = 0.18), it should be considered that these trials included a heterogeneous collection of chemotherapy regimens, and when limited to those utilizing platinum and 5-FU, a statistically significant hazard ratio (HR) of 0.90 was obtained.[1] Importantly, the analysis also demonstrated a meaningful reduction in the rate of distant metastasis, with an absolute difference of 4.3% (HR, 0.73; 95% confidence interval [CI], 0.61–0.88) at 5 years. Improvement in this parameter provided critical support for the idea that ICT can improve distant control, and implied a clear benefit for its addition to locoregional treatment. Though controversial and not universally accepted, these findings have continued to justify the investigation of ICT in HNSCC.

In the 1990s, taxane therapy (docetaxel or paclitaxel) began to garner immense interest as a new drug in the treatment for HNSCC. This was spurred in large part by a phase II trial which enrolled patients with recurrent, metastatic, or locally advanced incurable HNSCC to receive paclitaxel, noting an impressive response rate of 40%.[9] The early success of taxane therapy inspired efforts to investigate its role in the setting of ICT. Ultimately, a benefit from the addition of a taxane to PF (cisplatin, 5-FU) regimens was demonstrated in three landmark phase III studies. The TAX323 study compared TPF (docetaxel, cisplatin, 5-FU) with PF as ICT in patients with locoregionally advanced, unresectable disease. In this study, 358 patients were randomized to receive TPF or PF followed by concurrent chemoradiation. At a median follow-up of 32.5 months, median progression-free survival PFS was 11.0 months in the TPF group compared to 8.2 months in the PF group (HR, 0.72; $p = 0.007$). Median survival was 18.8 months in TPF compared to 14.5 months with PF ($p = 0.02$).[10] In the TAX324 study, 501 patients with locoregionally advanced disease were randomized to receive either PF or TPF. The TPF group achieved better locoregional control than in the PF group ($p = 0.04$). Median OS in the TPF group was 71 months, compared to 30 months in the PF group ($p = 0.006$). No significant difference was seen in the rate of distant metastases.[11] Lastly, the GORTEC group for organ preservation randomized 213 patients with larynx and hypopharynx cancer requiring total laryngectomy, to receive three cycles of TPF or PF. Those who responded to chemotherapy received radiotherapy with or without additional chemotherapy, and those who did not respond to chemotherapy underwent total laryngectomy followed by radiotherapy with or without additional chemotherapy. The 3-year larynx preservation rate was 70.3% with TPF compared to 57.5% with PF ($p = 0.03$), showing a superior response rate and higher likelihood of larynx preservation with the TPF regimen.[12] Together, these trials created a new standard for ICT by demonstrating that the inclusion of a taxane (TPF) was superior to the previously established PF regimen. A subsequent meta-analysis including 1,772 patients comparing PF with TPF supported this notion, showing an absolute survival benefit at 5 years of 7.4% (HR, 0.79; 95% CI, 0.70–0.89; $p < 0.001$), as well as a significant reduction in progression, locoregional failure, and distant failure with the use of TPH compared to its PF counterpart as ICT.[13] These findings came with an important criticism that they were comparing two experimental arms, as ICT was not established as a standard treatment. Moreover, questions remained based on the aforementioned MACH-NC meta-analysis, which failed to demonstrate a meaningful survival benefit from the use of ICT. It is worth noting, however, that these trials did not include TPF regimens.

Despite these criticisms, the enthusiasm for ICT and the success of these trials ultimately provided the basis for its measurement against concurrent CRT alone as definitive therapy for HNSCC. In a phase III trial conducted by Hitt et al, patients with locally advanced HNSCC were assigned to ICT with either docetaxel, cisplatin, and 5-FU (TPF) or cisplatin and 5-FU (PF) followed by concurrent chemoradiation (cisplatin + RT) or chemoradiation alone. The results showed a median PFS of 14.6, 14.3, and 13.8 months in the TPF + CRT, PF + CRT, and CRT groups, respectively (95% CI, 11–17.5; $p = 0.56$).[14] They were unable to demonstrate statistically significant differences in time to treatment failure or in OS. In the PARADIGM trial, a phase III study, 145 patients with untreated, nonmetastatic head and neck cancer were randomized to receive ICT with TPF followed by concurrent CRT (weekly carboplatin + RT) or concurrent CRT alone (with standard two doses of cisplatin + RT). Three-year OS was 73% in the ICT + CRT group and 78% in the CRT alone group (HR, 1.09; 95% CI, 0.59–2.03; $p = 0.77$).[15] The DeCIDE trial was a phase II trial comparing ICT with TPF versus

CRT in patients with locally advanced HNSCC and high nodal stage disease (N2 or N3). At 3 years, no significant difference in OS was found, noting 72% in the induction arm and 69% in CRT arm ($p = 0.69$). There was a difference in rate of distant failure at 3 years with ICT (10 vs. 19%) but this difference was not statistically significant ($p = 0.11$).[16] A meta-analysis in 2014 evaluating ICT followed by CRT concluded that ICT with TPF before CRT does not improve OS (HR, 1.008; 95% CI, 0.816–1.246; $p = 0.94$) and suggested only a mild, insignificant benefit in PFS (HR, 0.881; 95% CI, 0.723–1.073; $p = 0.207$).[17] Of note, the slow rate of accrual in both studies led to premature termination after far less of the expected patients were enrolled (285 of expected 400 in PARADIGM, and 145 of expected 300 in DeCIDE). Therefore, though no difference in survival was noted between those treated with ICT followed by CRT and those receiving CRT alone, the deficiency of statistical power made it inherently difficult to detect any benefit to ICT.

In summary, the role of ICT prior to locoregional therapy in HNSCC remains controversial, and no consensus guidelines are available to guide its use. Despite the negative findings from these pertinent trials and meta-analyses, flaws in methodological design and heterogeneity in chemotherapy regimens employed limit any conclusive answer to the question of whether ICT has a definite role. Until stronger evidence is available, its use in locally advanced disease should be limited to unique scenarios and clinical trials, while concurrent CRT remains the standard of care. Some experts suggest considering ICT when delays in CRT therapy are expected, as a larynx-preserving approach, and in patients who are at high risk for distant relapse (such as those with N2c or low-neck disease). It is important to consider that in addition to the lack of efficacy achieved in the DeCIDE and PARADIGM trials, sequential treatment also caused more toxicity than CRT alone. In DeCIDE, severe adverse events were significantly higher in the ICT arm (47 vs. 28%, $p = 0.002$).[16] In PARADIGM, the incidence of grade III–IV febrile neutropenia was 23 versus. 1%, and grade III–IV mucositis was 47 versus 16% in the ICT arm.[15]

26.3 Concurrent Chemoradiotherapy

The primary benefits of chemotherapy in the setting of nonmetastatic HNSCC stem from its utility as a radiosensitizing agent. Therefore, the focus has been on agents with known activity in head and neck cancer, as well as established radiosensitizing properties including cisplatin, cetuximab, and 5-FU. The use of radiotherapy has been established with two main strategies, including concomitant chemotherapy (single or multiagent) with continuous radiotherapy or multiagent chemotherapy with split-course radiotherapy. Other acceptable approaches now include radiotherapy with altered fractionation. As mentioned, historically, chemotherapy was used exclusively for unresectable disease. The demonstration that chemotherapy could improve locoregional control compared to radiotherapy alone ultimately led to its study in other groups of patients including those with resectable disease and with organ preservation intent, and as adjuvant therapy after surgical resection in those with high-risk features. In 1992, Merlano et al randomized 157 patients with untreated, unresectable HNSCC to receive either cisplatin plus 5-FU plus radiotherapy or radiotherapy alone, and showed an increase in the frequency of complete response (43 vs. 22%, respectively; $p = 0.037$), increased PFS at 5 years (21 vs. 9%, respectively; $p = 0.008$), and increased 5-year survival benefit (24 vs. 10%, respectively; $p = 0.01$) in the combined treatment group.[18] This study represents a turning point in the interest in concurrent CRT for HNSCC. In 2003, a phase III study by Adelstein et al assigned 295 patients to radiotherapy alone, radiotherapy with concurrent cisplatin, or split-course radiotherapy given with 5-FU and cisplatin. Surgical resection was available to all three arms if appropriate after treatment was completed. Three-year OS for patients who received radiation alone was 23%, compared to 37% for those who received radiotherapy + cisplatin ($p = 0.014$), and 27% for those who received split-course radiotherapy given with 5-FU and cisplatin ($p =$ not significant).[19] This study established concurrent CRT with cisplatin as the standard of care for locally advanced, unresectable head and neck cancer. The meta-analysis by Pignon et al again highlighted the favorable results seen with this approach. Albeit with variable chemotherapy regimens, concurrent CRT showed an absolute survival benefit of 8% compared with radiation alone.[1]

Given that epidermal growth factor receptor (EGFR) is highly expressed in most HNSCC, and inversely associated with prognosis, EGFR inhibitors have garnered much interest in the treatment of HNSCC. In a study by Bonner et al, 424 patients were randomized to receive radiotherapy alone or radiotherapy with weekly cetuximab. The median duration of locoregional control was 24.4 months in those treated with cetuximab plus radiotherapy compared to 14.9 months in those treated with radiotherapy alone (HR, 0.68; $p = 0.005$). OS was 49 months compared to 29.3 months in those treated with combined therapy versus radiation alone, respectively (HR, 0.74; $p = 0.03$).[20] These findings led to the FDA approval for the use of cetuximab in combination with radiotherapy for patients with advanced head and neck cancer. It is important to note that the use of cetuximab with concurrent radiotherapy has not been compared directly with cisplatin, and indications for its use at this time remain limited to the treatment of patients whose age, performance status, or comorbidities preclude the use of cisplatin-based treatment.

Panitumumab, another monoclonal antibody against EGFR, was studied in the phase II CONCERT-2 study. A total of 152 patients with locally advanced HNSCC were randomized to receive CRT with two cycles of cisplatin 100 mg/m^2 during radiotherapy or to radiotherapy plus panitumumab (three cycles of 9 mg/kg every 3 weeks). Locoregional control at 2 years was 61 versus 51% in the CRT (cisplatin) group versus radiotherapy plus panitumumab group, respectively. The two groups showed no difference in OS.[21]

A few trials have investigated the utility of using concurrent CRT with the addition of EGFR inhibition to standard chemotherapy, without showing any significant advantage to date from the inclusion of EGFR inhibition. The RTOG-0522 trial compared cetuximab + cisplatin + radiotherapy to cisplatin/radiotherapy alone. At 3 years, there was no improvement noted in PFS (61.2 vs. 58.9%; $p = 0.76$), OS (72.9 vs. 75.8%; $p = 0.32$), or distant metastasis (13 vs. 9.7%; $p = 0.08$) in the cetuximab group compared to cisplatin/radiotherapy alone group, respectively.[22] In the CONCERT-1 trial, a phase II study, 150 patients with locally advanced HNSCC were randomized to receive CRT with

high-dose cisplatin, or CRT plus panitumumab. They failed to show any benefit in locoregional control at 2 years in the panitumumab + CRT group compared to CRT alone.[23] In a similar fashion, the addition of erlotinib (a tyrosine kinase inhibitor [TKI] acting on EGFR) to CRT did not show any improvement compared with CRT alone.[24]

26.4 Adjuvant Chemoradiation

The decision to provide adjuvant radiation or chemoradiation is based on pathologic features. The use of chemoradiation has been studied in two main trials, which together have provided some clarification of the indications for its use.

The EORTC trial randomized 167 patients with stage III or IV head and neck cancer to receive either radiotherapy alone or radiotherapy combined with cisplatin after undergoing surgery with curative intent. They demonstrated improvement in both PFS at 60 months (47 vs. 36%; HR, 0.75; $p = 0.04$) and 5-year OS (53 vs 40%; $p = 0.02$) in the combined therapy group compared to radiotherapy alone. The cumulative incidence of local or regional relapses was significantly lower in the combined therapy group ($p = 0.007$).[25] The RTOG trial employed the same two study arms, comparing combined CRT with cisplatin to radiotherapy alone after surgical resection in 231 patients with high-risk disease. At 45.9 months, the combined treatment group showed an improvement in locoregional control compared to radiotherapy alone (HR, 0.61; 95% CI, 0.41–0.91; $p = 0.01$), and longer disease free survival (DFS; HR, 0.78; 95% CI, 0.61–0.99; $p = 0.04$). Unlike the EORTC trial, no significant difference in OS was found in the RTOG trial.[26]

Though similar in their methodology, each of these trials employed slightly different definitions of high-risk pathologic features, which may explain some of the differences in their results. The RTOG defined high-risk disease to include the presence of multiple positive nodes, extracapsular extension of tumor, or a positive margin. The EORTC trial definition of high-risk disease included positive margins, extracapsular extension of nodal disease, vascular embolism, or perineural disease; for oral cavity or oropharyngeal tumors, high risk was defined as positive nodes at level IV or V. A pooled analysis of the two trials was carried out for clarification of these definitions, and concluded that the subsets of patients from both trials who benefited from combined therapy approach had either positive margins or extracapsular extension.[27] Hence, patients with either or both of these features are considered to have a clear indication for adjuvant CRT. On the other hand, radiotherapy alone is usually recommended for patients at intermediate risk of recurrence, such as those with T3–T4/N0 disease, multiple positive nodes (without extracapsular extension), perineural or lymphovascular invasion, or oropharyngeal cancers with cervical nodes at level IV or V.

As expected, the addition of chemotherapy to radiotherapy in this setting comes with an increased incidence of adverse events. In the aforementioned trials, serious adverse events were increased in the combined-treatment groups by as much as 43% in RTOG[26] and 20% in EORTC.[25] Moreover, an updated result of the RTOG trial at 10-year follow-up failed to show a statistically significant survival benefit, even when limited to subset analysis of patients with positive margins or extracapsular extension.[28]

26.5 Adjuvant Chemotherapy

A role for adjuvant chemotherapy has been undetermined, with relatively few trials executed largely due to the successes of concomitant radiotherapy dating back to the 1970s. These early studies have compared postsurgical management for HNSCC with or without chemotherapy, and failed to establish any efficacy.[29,30,31] Moreover, the recent MACH-NC meta-analysis failed to demonstrate a survival benefit in this subset of patients.[1] One trial analyzed 442 patients with completely resected tumors or the oral cavity, oropharynx, hypopharynx, or larynx, who were then randomized to receive either three cycles of cisplatin and 5-FU, followed by postoperative CRT, or postoperative CRT alone. Patients with both high-risk and low-risk treatment volumes were included. They were unable to show any significant difference in locoregional failure, DFS, or OS, but did show a decreased incidence of distant metastases in the chemotherapy arm (15 vs. 23%; $p = 0.03$).[31] Nevertheless, adjuvant chemotherapy alone has not been consistently shown to provide a clinical benefit and therefore is not indicated for postoperative HNSCC patients.

26.6 Metastatic or Incurable Recurrent Disease

Systemic therapy remains the mainstay of treatment in metastatic or incurable recurrent HNSCC. As described previously, several agents have shown activity in HNSCC and are available for use. Combination chemotherapy versus single-agent chemotherapy has been evaluated extensively, and although the multiagent approach tends to demonstrate higher response rates, these do not translate into significant survival benefits. Moreover, increased toxicities often a limit its use. A meta-analysis in 1994 analyzed trials comparing cisplatin plus 5-FU to single-agent therapy in this setting. It demonstrated a significant improvement in response with combination therapy, but only a 2-week difference in median survival (odds ratio, 0.43; 95% CI, 0.29–0.63) and increased toxicities for those who received combination therapy.[32] This approach should therefore be limited to patients with good performance status who may better tolerate increased treatment-related toxicity. Methotrexate has been used frequently as single-agent therapy due to its ease of administration, favorable toxicity profile, and low cost. Despite showing efficacy in early-stage disease, the use of taxanes has not proven to be beneficial in metastatic disease. Trials comparing paclitaxel versus methotrexate[33] and cisplatin plus paclitaxel versus cisplatin plus 5-FU[34] have failed to show any survival benefit from the addition of taxane therapy. In the phase III EXTREME trial, 440 patients with metastatic disease were assigned to receive cisplatin or carboplatin/5-FU/cetuximab or cisplatin or carboplatin/5-FU. They were able to show that the addition of cetuximab increased the response rate from 20 to 36% ($p < 0.001$), and prolonged PFS from 3.3 to 5.6 months (HR, 0.54; $p < 0.001$) as well as median OS from 7.4 to 10.1 months (HR, 0.80; $p = 0.04$).[23] This remains the standard approach in patients able to tolerate combination chemotherapy.

26.7 Novel Agents and Future Directions

The past few decades have yielded promising therapies in the treatment of early-stage and locally advanced HNSCC, most of which now involve multimodal therapy including systemic treatment with chemotherapy. Despite these advancements, many patients will develop local or distant failure after treatment. Ongoing efforts to improve outcomes will rely on further understanding of the biology of HNSCC and novel ideas for more targeted therapies. EGFR activity plays a central role in the development and progression of HNSCC, and its overexpression has been associated with poor outcomes. Several agents have been developed with anti-EGFR activity including monoclonal antibodies to EGFR (cetuximab, panitumumab) and TKIs (afatinib, dacomitinib, gefitinib, erlotinib, lapatinib, and vandetanib). As described previously, cetuximab concurrent with radiotherapy has been approved for use in the treatment of locally advanced HNSCC based on results of a phase III trial by Bonner et al,[20] and in recurrent/metastatic disease based on the EXTREME trial.[36] Panitumumab has been similarly investigated in the SPECTRUM trial, a phase III trial which randomized 657 patients with recurrent/metastatic HNSCC to receive cisplatin and 5-FU with or without panitumumab. No significant difference was demonstrated in OS, the primary endpoint, but a modest increase in PFS of 1.2 months was observed in the panitumumab group (5.8 vs. 4.6 months; $p = 0.004$).[35] At this time, there is no indication for the use of panitumumab in head and neck cancer.

Afatinib, a TKI which interrupts EGFR signaling, has been compared with methotrexate in recurrent/metastatic HNSCC in the phase III LUX-Head & Neck1 trial showing improved PFS in the afatinib group (2.6 vs. 1.7 months; HR, 0.80; $p = 0.030$) but no benefit in OS.[37] Less mature trials involving other TKI agents have shown largely negative results. Buparlisib, a phosphoinositide 3-kinase inhibitor, has been investigated as a potential option. The BERIL-1 study was a multicenter, phase II trial which randomized 158 patients with recurrent or metastatic HNSCC to receive buparlisib and paclitaxel versus placebo and paclitaxel for second-line treatment. The buparlisib/paclitaxel group showed improvement in PFS (4.5 vs. 3.5 months; HR, 0.65; $p = 0.01$), OS (10.4 vs. 6.5 months; HR, 0.72; $p = 0.04$), and overall response rate (ORR; 39.6 vs. 13.9%; $p < 0.001$).[38]

Immune therapy has garnered a great deal of interest in the treatment of both solid and hematologic malignancies based on the premise that tumors can be recognized as foreign and eradicated by effective immune responses. While an understanding of the interplay between tumor and immune cells remains rather rudimentary, this field is rapidly evolving and preclinical advancements have continued to reveal new insights which propel their integration into clinical practice. It is hypothesized that a normal host employs *immune surveillance*, where premalignant cells are continually sought and destroyed by a healthy immune system, precluding the establishment or progression of advanced disease. Accordingly, tumor progression depends on the acquisition of traits that allow cancer cells to evade immune surveillance and effective immune responses. A recent therapeutic approach involves modulation of T-cell activation, a process requiring a critical combination of T-cell receptor co-stimulation, as well as inhibitory stimulation to preserve appropriate, controlled activity levels in the normal host. Inhibition of these checkpoints has been confirmed to promote anticancer immune activity. One such checkpoint inhibitor, pembrolizumab, is a monoclonal antibody directed against programmed cell death-1 (PD-1), a cell surface receptor that plays an important role in downregulating the immune system. Data from the phase Ib KEYNOTE-012 trial demonstrated the efficacy of pembrolizumab in the treatment of recurrent or metastatic HNSCC, showing an ORR of 18%.[39] A pooled analysis of the trial was later presented after long-term follow-up of patients enrolled in KEYNOTE-012, showing an ORR of 17.7%. Median follow-up duration in responders was 12.5 months. Median duration or response had not yet been reached at the time of data cutoff, and among responders 76% had ongoing responses.[40] Based on these results, pembrolizumab was granted accelerated FDA approval for the treatment of recurrent/metastatic HNSCC in August 2016. Another anti-PD-1 monoclonal antibody, nivolumab, has been approved for use based on the CHECKMATE-141 trial, a phase III trial exploring the use of nivolumab in patients with recurrent/metastatic HNSCC. In this trial, 361 patients were randomized to receive nivolumab or standard, single-agent systemic therapy (methotrexate, docetaxel, or cetuximab). The results showed an improvement in OS (HR, 0.70; $p = 0.01$) in the nivolumab group compared to those who received standard therapy.[41]

While immune therapy has been established as a safe and effective approach in the treatment of recurrent/metastatic disease, it is conceivable that its greatest utility may exist in the management of early or locally advanced disease. For example, preclinical data have demonstrated a synergistic effect with the combination of checkpoint inhibitors and radiotherapy. In murine models, it has been observed that their concurrent administration can result in antitumor immune responses both in the radiation field and outside of it. This synergism is known as the abscopal effect.[42] PD-1 blockade has also been shown to induce rejection of persistent tumors in mouse models as adjuvant treatment after completion of radiotherapy. It is important to note that human papillomavirus (HPV) positivity, a favorable prognostic factor in HNSCC, engenders better responses to radiation, chemotherapy, or both. Interestingly it has been shown that HPV-positive tumors are more infiltrated by CD8 T-cells than HPV-negative tumors, and may have a particularly robust response to immune therapy. This is the result of checkpoint inhibitors induced by active exposure to tumor-specific antigens during radiation- or chemotherapy-induced cell death. The role for systemic treatment in HPV-positive HNSCC remains unclear and needs to be addressed in future trials.

In conclusion, the past several decades of research have unveiled a critical role for systemic therapy in the treatment of head and neck cancer. It can be expected that continued progress with novel, targeted agents and the rapidly growing field of immunotherapy will continue to provide new insight into this disease, and that these developments will augment complex, multimodality approaches with the hope of increasing cure rates by enhancing systemic treatment.

References

[1] Pignon JP, le Maître A, Maillard E, Bourhis J, MACH-NC Collaborative Group. Meta-Analysis of Chemotherapy in Head and Neck Cancer (MACH-NC): an update on 93 randomised trials and 17,346 patients. Radiother Oncol. 2009; 92(1):4–14

[2] Argiris A, Karamouzis MV, Raben D, Ferris RL. Head and neck cancer. Lancet. 2008; 371(9625):1695–1709

[3] Lee WR, Mancuso AA, Saleh EM, Mendenhall WM, Parsons JT, Million RR. Can pretreatment computed tomography findings predict local control in T3 squamous cell carcinoma of the glottic larynx treated with radiotherapy alone? Int J Radiat Oncol Biol Phys. 1993; 25(4):683–687

[4] Stadler P, Becker A, Feldmann HJ, et al. Influence of the hypoxic subvolume on the survival of patients with head and neck cancer. Int J Radiat Oncol Biol Phys. 1999; 44(4):749–754

[5] Dunst J, Stadler P, Becker A, et al. Tumor volume and tumor hypoxia in head and neck cancers. The amount of the hypoxic volume is important. Strahlenther Onkol. 2003; 179(8):521–526

[6] Wolf GT, Fisher SG, Hong WK, et al. Department of Veterans Affairs Laryngeal Cancer Study Group. Induction chemotherapy plus radiation compared with surgery plus radiation in patients with advanced laryngeal cancer. N Engl J Med. 1991; 324(24):1685–1690

[7] Domenge C, Hill C, Lefebvre JL, et al. French Groupe d'Etude des Tumeurs de la Tête et du Cou (GETTEC). Randomized trial of neoadjuvant chemotherapy in oropharyngeal carcinoma. French Groupe d'Etude des Tumeurs de la Tête et du Cou (GETTEC). Br J Cancer. 2000; 83(12):1594–1598

[8] Paccagnella A, Orlando A, Marchiori C, et al. Phase III trial of initial chemotherapy in stage III or IV head and neck cancers: a study by the Gruppo di Studio sui Tumori della Testa e del Collo. J Natl Cancer Inst. 1994; 86 (4):265–272

[9] Forastiere AA, Shank D, Neuberg D, Taylor SG, IV, DeConti RC, Adams G. Final report of a phase II evaluation of paclitaxel in patients with advanced squamous cell carcinoma of the head and neck: an Eastern Cooperative Oncology Group trial (PA390). Cancer. 1998; 82(11):2270–2274

[10] Vermorken JB, Remenar E, van Herpen C, et al. Long-term results of EORTC24971/TAX323: Comparing TPF to PF in patients with unresectable squamous cell carcinoma of the head and neck. Preliminary results of a modern integrated approach. J Clin Oncol. 2011; 29 suppl 15:5530

[11] Posner MR, Hershock DM, Blajman CR, et al. TAX 324 Study Group. Cisplatin and fluorouracil alone or with docetaxel in head and neck cancer. N Engl J Med. 2007; 357(17):1705–1715

[12] Pointreau Y, Garaud P, Chapet S, et al. Randomized trial of induction chemotherapy with cisplatin and 5-fluorouracil with or without docetaxel for larynx preservation. J Natl Cancer Inst. 2009; 101(7):498–506

[13] Blanchard P, Bourhis J, Lacas B, et al. Meta-Analysis of Chemotherapy in Head and Neck Cancer, Induction Project, Collaborative Group. Taxane-cisplatin-fluorouracil as induction chemotherapy in locally advanced head and neck cancers: an individual patient data meta-analysis of the meta-analysis of chemotherapy in head and neck cancer group. J Clin Oncol. 2013; 31(23):2854–2860

[14] Hitt R, Grau JJ, Lopez-Pousa A, et al. Final results of a randomized phase III trial comparing induction chemotherapy with cisplatin/5-FU or docetaxel/cisplatin/5-FU followed by chemoradiotherapy (CRT) vs. CRT alone as first line treatment of unresectable locally advanced head and neck cancer (LAHNC). J Clin Oncol. 2009; 27 suppl 15:6009

[15] Haddad RI, Rabinowits G, Tishler RB, et al. The PARADIGM trial: a phase III study comparing sequential therapy to concurrent chemoradiotherapy in locally advanced head and neck cancer. J Clin Oncol. 2012; 30 suppl 15:5501

[16] Cohen EE, Karrison T, Kocherginsky M, et al. DeCIDE: A phase II randomized trial of docetaxel, cisplatin, 5FU induction chemotherapy in patients with N2 N3 locally advanced squamous cell cancer of the head and neck. J Clin Oncol. 2012; 30 suppl 15:5500

[17] Budach W, Boelke E, Kammers K, Gripp S, Matuschek C. Induction chemotherapy followed by chemoradiotherapy versus chemoradiotherapy as treatment of unresected locally advanced head and neck squamous cell cancer (HNSCC): A meta-analysis of randomized trials. J Clin Oncol. 2014; 32(suppl 15):6012

[18] Merlano M, Benasso M, Corvò R, et al. Five-year update of a randomized trial of alternating radiotherapy and chemotherapy compared with radiotherapy alone in treatment of unresectable squamous cell carcinoma of the head and neck. J Natl Cancer Inst. 1996; 88(9):58:3–589

[19] Adelstein DJ, Li Y, Adams GL, et al. An intergroup phase III comparison of standard radiation therapy and two schedules of concurrent chemoradiotherapy in patients with unresectable squamous cell head and neck cancer. J Clin Oncol. 2003; 21(1):92–98

[20] Bonner JA, Harari PM, Giralt J, et al. Radiotherapy plus cetuximab for squamous-cell carcinoma of the head and neck. N Engl J Med. 2006; 354(6):567–578

[21] Giralt J, Trigo J, Nuyts S, et al. Panitumumab plus radiotherapy versus chemoradiotherapy in patients with unresected, locally advanced squamous-cell

carcinoma of the head and neck (CONCERT-2): a randomised, controlled, open-label phase 2 trial. Lancet Oncol. 2015; 16(2):221–232

[22] Ang KK, Zhang Q, Rosenthal DI, et al. Randomized phase III trial of concurrent accelerated radiation plus cisplatin with or without cetuximab for stage III to IV head and neck carcinoma: RTOG 0522. J Clin Oncol. 2014; 32 (27):2940–2950

[23] Mesía R, Henke M, Fortin A, et al. Chemoradiotherapy with or without panitumumab in patients with unresected, locally advanced squamous-cell carcinoma of the head and neck (CONCERT-1): a randomised, controlled, open-label phase 2 trial. Lancet Oncol. 2015; 16(2):208–220

[24] Martins RG, Parvathaneni U, Bauman JE, et al. Cisplatin and radiotherapy with or without erlotinib in locally advanced squamous cell carcinoma of the head and neck: a randomized phase II trial. J Clin Oncol. 2013; 31(11):1415–1421

[25] Bernier J, Domenge C, Ozsahin M, et al. European Organization for Research and Treatment of Cancer Trial 22931. Postoperative irradiation with or without concomitant chemotherapy for locally advanced head and neck cancer. N Engl J Med. 2004; 350(19):1945–1952

[26] Cooper JS, Pajak TF, Forastiere AA, et al. Radiation Therapy Oncology Group 9501/Intergroup. Postoperative concurrent radiotherapy and chemotherapy for high-risk squamous-cell carcinoma of the head and neck. N Engl J Med. 2004; 350(19):1937–1944

[27] Bernier J, Cooper JS, Pajak TF, et al. Defining risk levels in locally advanced head and neck cancers: a comparative analysis of concurrent postoperative radiation plus chemotherapy trials of the EORTC (# 22931) and RTOG (# 9501). Head Neck. 2005; 27(10):843–850

[28] Cooper JS, Zhang Q, Pajak TF, et al. Long-term follow-up of the RTOG 9501/intergroup phase III trial: postoperative concurrent radiation therapy and chemotherapy in high-risk squamous cell carcinoma of the head and neck. Int J Radiat Oncol Biol Phys. 2012; 84(5):1198–1205

[29] Taylor SGIV, IV, Applebaum E, Showel JL, et al. A randomized trial of adjuvant chemotherapy in head and neck cancer. J Clin Oncol. 1985; 3(5):672–679

[30] Rentschler RE, Wilbur DW, Petti GH, et al. Adjuvant methotrexate escalated to toxicity for resectable stage III and IV squamous head and neck carcinomas–a prospective, randomized study. J Clin Oncol. 1987; 5(2):278–285

[31] Laramore GE, Scott CB, al-Sarraf M, et al. Adjuvant chemotherapy for resectable squamous cell carcinomas of the head and neck: report on Intergroup Study 0034. Int J Radiat Oncol Biol Phys. 1992; 23(4):705–713

[32] Browman GP, Cronin L. Standard chemotherapy in squamous cell head and neck cancer: what we have learned from randomized trials. Semin Oncol. 1994; 21(3):311–319

[33] Vermorken J, Catimel G, Mulder PD, et al. Randomized phase II trial of weekly methotrexate (MTX) versus two schedules of triweekly paclitaxel (Taxol [trade]) in patients with metastatic or recurrent squamous cell carcinoma of the head and neck (SCCHN). [abstract]. Proc Am Soc Clin Oncol. 1999; 18:395

[34] Gibson MK, Li Y, Murphy B, et al. Eastern Cooperative Oncology Group. Randomized phase III evaluation of cisplatin plus fluorouracil versus cisplatin plus paclitaxel in advanced head and neck cancer (E1395): an intergroup trial of the Eastern Cooperative Oncology Group. J Clin Oncol. 2005; 23 (15):3562–3567

[35] Vermorken JB, Stöhlmacher-Williams J, Davidenko I, et al. SPECTRUM investigators. Cisplatin and fluorouracil with or without panitumumab in patients with recurrent or metastatic squamous-cell carcinoma of the head and neck (SPECTRUM): an open-label phase 3 randomised trial. Lancet Oncol. 2013; 14 (8):697–710

[36] Vermorken JB, Mesia R, Rivera F, et al. Platinum-based chemotherapy plus cetuximab in head and neck cancer. N Engl J Med. 2008; 359(11):1116–1127

[37] Machiels JP, Haddad RI, Fayette J, et al. LUX-H&N 1 investigators. Afatinib versus methotrexate as second-line treatment in patients with recurrent or metastatic squamous-cell carcinoma of the head and neck progressing on or after platinum-based therapy (LUX-Head & Neck 1): an open-label, randomised phase 3 trial. Lancet Oncol. 2015; 16(5):583–594

[38] Soulières D, Faivre S, Mesía R, et al. Buparlisib and paclitaxel in patients with platinum-pretreated recurrent or metastatic squamous cell carcinoma of the head and neck (BERIL-1): a randomised, double-blind, placebo-controlled phase 2 trial. Lancet Oncol. 2017; 18(3):323–335

[39] Uppaluri R, Zolkind P, Lin T, Nussenbaum B, Paniello R, Rich J. Immunotherapy with pembrolizumab in surgically resectable head and neck squamous cell carcinoma. Paper presented at: the American Society of Clinical Oncology Annual Meeting; June 3–7, 2016; Chicago, IL

[40] Mehra R, Seiwert TY, Mahipal A, et al. Efficacy and safety of pembrolizumab in recurrent/metastatic head and neck squamous cell carcinoma (R/M HNSCC): pooled analyses after long-term follow up in KEYNOTE-012. Paper presented at: the American Society of Clinical Oncology Annual Meeting; June 3–7, 2016; Chicago, IL

[41] Ferris RL, Blumenschein G, Jr, Fayette J, et al. Nivolumab for recurrent squamous-cell carcinoma of the head and neck. N Engl J Med. 2016; 375 (19):1856–1867

[42] Demaria S, Kawashima N, Yang AM, et al. Immune-mediated inhibition of metastases after treatment with local radiation and CTLA-4 blockade in a mouse model of breast cancer. Clin Cancer Res. 2005; 11(2, Pt 1):728–734

27 Histopathologic Evaluation of Neck Dissections

Chien Chen

Abstract

The purpose of histopathologic evaluation of neck dissections is to identify metastatic disease to locoregional lymph nodes. The standard protocol for processing neck dissections is effective for the evaluation of macrometastases and works well for clinically positive necks, but clinically negative necks (cN0) present a clinicopathologic dilemma. While many clinically negative necks harbor occult macroscopic and microscopic disease, intensive histopathologic evaluation of neck dissections to identify microscopic disease is neither economically nor technically feasible. Sentinel node biopsy is a sensitive strategy for identifying cN0 patients who require neck dissection and also provides a potential target for more intensive histologic evaluation. Despite relatively low sensitivities, intraoperative evaluation of sentinel lymph nodes is beneficial because it has high specificity and can facilitate neck dissection in roughly half of patients who require one. Although micrometastases and even isolated tumor cells are clinically important, there is no consensus standard protocol for intensive evaluation of sentinel lymph nodes in the head and neck literature. We propose a protocol for the evaluation of sentinel lymph nodes of the head and neck based on the current evidence. Thyroid cancer is discussed separately as it does not require comparable aggressive surgical management of microscopic nodal disease. The pathologic evaluation and workup of nodal metastases of unknown primary is also discussed.

Keywords: neck dissection, pathology, lymph node, sentinel, macrometastasis, micrometastasis, isolated tumor cells, occult primary

27.1 Introduction

The purpose of the neck dissection is to assess for lymph node metastases and excise regional disease. This chapter will discuss the pathologic processing and evaluation of neck dissections, its limitations, and possible solutions for these limitations. Pathologic nodal staging (pN) is based on the American Joint Committee on Cancer (AJCC) staging guidelines.[1] For head and neck tumors, the principal criteria that determine nodal staging and therefore prognosis are (1) the presence or absence of metastases, (2) the size of the largest metastasis, (3) the presence or absence of extranodal extension, and (4) the laterality of involvement. Interestingly, the number of involved lymph nodes has relatively little impact on the pathologic nodal stage, although it is a reflection of the burden of disease. Of these criteria, the single most significant driver of prognosis for all head and neck sites is the presence or absence of lymph node metastases.[2,3,4] The purpose of histopathologic evaluation is to answer each of these questions regarding nodal involvement.

27.2 Processing and Reporting of Neck Dissections

To understand the histopathologic evaluation of neck dissections, it is important to understand how they are processed.

The processing of neck dissections requires cooperation between the surgeon and the pathologist. Radical neck dissections have anatomic landmarks, which allow the pathologist to orient and separate the neck dissection into individual nodal levels at the grossing bench. However, these landmarks are absent in both modified neck dissections and selective neck dissections; thus, it is important for the surgeon to aid in the orientation of these specimens. This may be readily achieved in two ways. The entire neck dissection can be pinned out on a cork board and oriented by the surgeon using a surgical marker, either in the operating room or subsequently in the surgical pathology gross room. Alternatively, the specimen can be divided into individual levels in the operating room and the individual levels can be sent separately. Orientation by the surgeon ensures that the specimen will be properly separated into the correct nodal levels for pathologic evaluation.

Once separated into individual levels, the pathologic processing and evaluation of neck dissections follows a generic protocol applicable to lymph node dissections in general.[5] Specimens should be received and processed fresh rather than in formalin fixative. Fresh tissue is softer than fixed tissue and the difference in the consistency of the lymph nodes and the surrounding soft tissue is more readily appreciable, making them easier to identify. Once identified, each lymph node should be blunt dissected from the surrounding tissue. Fresh processing is particularly relevant for neck dissections as they often contain significant amounts of fibromuscular tissue which can become quite firm after fixation, making blunt dissection difficult. A thorough search for lymph nodes should be made with the intent to identify all lymph nodes in the dissection. Despite the fact that a minimum lymph node count is not part of pathologic nodal staging, it is important to have an accurate lymph node count because it is a surrogate measure of the quality of the neck dissection and is an independent predictor of the risk of recurrence.[6,7,8] If lymph nodes are not identified by palpation, the tissue should be submitted in toto. While this may compromise the integrity of the lymph node count, lymph nodes that are grossly undetectable are unlikely to harbor tumor and in toto submission increases the sensitivity for detecting lymph nodes, which is paramount. All identified lymph nodes should be submitted for evaluation. For lymph nodes grossly involved by tumor, measurement of largest metastasis and evaluation for extranodal extension for each lymph node with one or more gross sections are generally sufficient.

Grossly uninvolved lymph nodes should be serially sectioned at 2-mm intervals and submitted in toto (▶ Fig. 27.1). Smaller lymph nodes (< 2 cm) should be sectioned perpendicular to the shortest axis (longitudinal), whereas larger lymph nodes should be sectioned perpendicular to the longest axis (transverse). Care should be taken to place the sections in the cassette sequentially such that different surfaces are presented for cutting to ensure that the lymph node is consistently being evaluated at 2-mm intervals. While the Association of Directors of Anatomic and Surgical Pathology (ADASP) recommendations accept a thicker section (3–4 mm),[5] this risks missing small macrometastases (> 2 mm) and current guidance from the College of

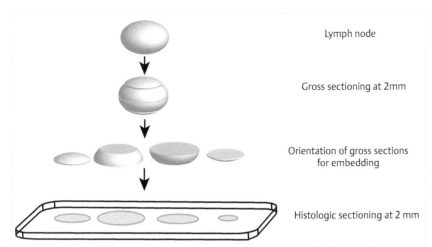

Fig. 27.1 Protocol for histologic processing of nonsentinel lymph nodes.

Lymph node

Gross sectioning at 2mm

Orientation of gross sections for embedding

Histologic sectioning at 2 mm

American Pathologists favors the 2-mm gross section thickness.[9] If multiple lymph nodes are submitted in a cassette, the surface of the lymph node should be differentially inked prior to sectioning to identify which sections belong to which lymph node so that positive lymph nodes are only counted once.

Only lymph nodes from the same nodal level/sublevel should be submitted together in a cassette. Lymph nodes too small to be grossly sectioned should be submitted whole with similarly sized lymph nodes from the same nodal level. Cassette summaries should indicate how many lymph nodes are present in each cassette, if and how they have been inked and sectioned, and from which nodal level they originate. One hematoxylin and eosin (H&E) slide containing multiple histologic sections cut at 2- μm thickness is generally considered sufficient for histologic evaluation. If a submandibular gland is identified, it should be serially sectioned and grossly evaluated for abnormalities, and a representative section should be taken to document the presence of the salivary gland and any identified abnormality.

Pathologic reports should include the following information: the total number of lymph nodes identified in each nodal level and the number involved by tumor, the presence of extranodal extension, the size of the largest metastasis (not the size of the involved lymph node), the presence of any soft-tissue deposits without evidence of lymph node architecture, and the presence of submandibular glands and associated pathology.[5]

27.3 Limitations of Histopathologic Evaluation

The greatest limitation of histologic evaluation of neck dissection specimens is that it only evaluates a minute fraction of the tissue received. When tissue is received from the operating room, based on gross evaluation, only representative gross sections are usually taken to evaluate critical information such as margin status, histologic type and grade, lymphovascular invasion, and mitotic activity. Because of this, the taking of representative gross sections requires both judgment and experience to maximize yield. It is a testament to the importance of nodal status that grossly uninvolved lymph nodes are generally submitted in toto. Even then, only a tiny fraction of the submitted tissue is ever histologically

evaluated. Given 2-mm gross sections, the fact that a histologic section is 2 μm means that only 0.1% of the tissue is evaluated in each histologic section. The standard protocol essentially takes a representative "snapshot" of the tissue at 2-mm intervals, and can therefore identify all lesions larger than 2 mm in *smallest* dimension *if* the gross section thickness is 2 mm and the sections are properly oriented and embedded. Smaller lesions may never enter the plane of sectioning and can therefore be missed altogether.

So why do we accept this limitation? Essentially, complete histologic evaluation is impractical. True complete histologic evaluation of even a single 1 cm × 0.6 cm × 0.6 cm lymph node would require 3,000 histologic sections, more than the entire daily workload of the average academic surgical pathology laboratory and would thus be both prohibitively expensive and technically infeasible. Even with representative histologic evaluation, each incremental improvement in sensitivity increases the histopathologic workload geometrically. This is a big deal because the typical neck dissection contains approximately 20 lymph nodes which currently require 20 to 40 H&E slides to evaluate so workloads can quickly spiral out of control. The current processing protocol is a tradeoff between yield and resource utilization and can identify all macrometastases (> 2 mm) but have a significant risk of missing micrometastasis (2 to 0.2 mm) and largely miss isolated tumor cells (ITCs; < 0.2 mm).

Another limitation of standard processing is the difficulty of identifying small tumor deposits on routine H&E stain. Small groups and single tumor cells may resemble histiocytes or endothelial cells, which are normal components of the lymph node. Similarly, basaloid and small round blue cell tumors can blend into the background lymphoid tissue at scanning power. This limitation can usually be overcome by careful examination and judicious use of immunohistochemical (IHC) stains. However, routine use of IHC stains to evaluate lymph nodes is cost prohibitive and can generate false-positive results.

Despite these limitations, standard processing and reporting works well for neck dissections in which gross disease is evident. Once gross tumor is identified in a lymph node, the main additional pieces of information needed are the size of the largest metastasis and whether there is contralateral involvement. Since the standard grossing protocol can find all macrometastases, high N stage disease can be readily assessed in this manner.

27.4 The Dilemma of the cN0 Neck

Clinical N0 necks (cN0) present a problem. It is well documented that a significant portion of cN0 necks contain tumor on pathologic evaluation.[3,10] The risk of involvement is dependent on tumor site, tumor (T) stage, and tumor thickness. In high T stage cancers (T3 and T4), a substantial fraction of cN0 necks contain tumor and elective neck dissection is generally considered to be prudent regardless of the clinical nodal status.[4,10] The real challenge lies with low T stage (T1 and T2) lesions, which are estimated to have an approximately 20 to 50% risk of nodal metastases despite being cN0, depending on primary site.[4] That these clinically unapparent nodal metastases affect survival has been amply demonstrated both by comparison of watchful waiting versus elective prophylactic neck dissection[11,12] and by comparison of pN0 and pN1 patients given elective neck dissection despite cN0 status.[13] In these low T stage patients, routine elective neck dissection risks overtreatment with its associated morbidity and expense but watchful waiting risks undertreatment and worse disease-free and overall survival. This has led to significant research into strategies to predict the risk factors for nodal metastases in low T stage tumors, clinically, radiologically, and pathologically.

27.5 Sentinel Node Biopsy

The premise of sentinel lymph node biopsy is that the lymphatic drainage of a tumor can be identified using tracers (radioactive, colorimetric, fluorescent, etc.), which, if injected into the tumor site, will enter the lymphatics around the tumor and accumulate in the first lymph node(s)—the sentinel lymph node(s)—that drain the tumor site. Tumor cells travelling through the lymphatics either take residence in the first lymph node(s) they encounter or "skip" metastasizes, i.e. bypass the first encountered lymph nodes. Skip metastases are rare. If the "sentinel lymph nodes" are negative, the likelihood of nodal involvement in the entire nodal basin is low. This strategy has been used successfully in other cancers and has in fact become the standard of care in breast cancer and melanoma. While not widely used for squamous cell carcinoma of the head and neck in the United States, many studies, mostly in the European and Asian literature, suggest that this strategy has the potential to solve the dilemma of the cN0 neck in low T stage head and neck tumors.[14,15,16,17]

There are a number of theoretical limitations to sentinel lymph node biopsy in head and neck tumors that may explain its slow adoption in the United States.[10,17] It has been asserted that the proximity of the lymph node basins to the tumor site, and therefore to the site of tracer injection, can obscure the detection of the sentinel lymph node, particularly in floor-of-mouth tumors. Also, mass effect by a tumor might obstruct draining lymphatics and redirect tracers to nonsentinel lymph nodes. Additionally, some studies suggest that there is a high false-negative rate if only a single sentinel lymph node is evaluated and more extended tracer injections identify multiple lymph nodes, typically two to three, the removal of which may not be superior to an ultraselective nodal dissection in terms of morbidity and expense. Furthermore, the small surgical window used to extract the sentinel lymph nodes might risk injury to adjacent structures, which would not occur with a larger operative field. Despite these limitations, several multicenter randomized clinical trials have shown that sentinel lymph node biopsy is safe and highly reproducible, and has high sensitivities and negative predictive values.[14,15,16,17,18,19]

27.5.1 Intraoperative Evaluation of Sentinel Lymph Nodes

Ideally, once a sentinel lymph node is identified, intraoperative evaluation could allow for immediate triage to neck dissection if tumor is identified. The two primary mechanisms for intraoperative evaluation are frozen section and touch imprint cytology. For frozen section, the sentinel lymph node is bisected perpendicular to the shortest axis and the tissue is embedded in optimum cutting temperature compound and frozen in a cryostat. Two to three frozen sections are cut at 5- to 10- μm thickness and are H&E stained for evaluation. For touch imprint cytology, the sentinel lymph node is bisected or serially sectioned longitudinally, the cut surfaces are touched to a glass slide, and the slide is H&E stained.

Much of the literature regarding the performance of frozen section versus touch imprint cytology is derived from the breast cancer literature,[9] but the findings are likely applicable to the head and neck. Frozen section benefits from greater general familiarity in the general surgical pathology community but it is both more expensive and time consuming (15–20 minutes per frozen section block processed). This significantly limits the number of sections that can be evaluated within the real-time constraints of a surgery. Additionally, frozen section artifact can both compromise permanent H&E evaluation and interfere with ancillary IHC studies.

Touch imprint cytology is significantly faster (a few minutes) to process, allows rapid evaluation of multiple cut surfaces, and could potentially evaluate a much larger volume of the sentinel lymph node if it is serially sectioned. Unfortunately, it suffers from less familiarity in the surgical pathology community, resulting in a slightly decreased overall sensitivity for touch imprint cytology as compared to frozen section.

Both frozen section and touch imprint cytology techniques have broad range of reported sensitivities, ranging from 50 to 90%, likely as a result of variable sectioning protocols, patient populations, tumor sites, types and sizes, and overall experience of the evaluating pathologists.[9] It is therefore important to recognize the limitations of intraoperative evaluation and to communicate to the patient that the decision to perform a neck dissection may need to be deferred to permanent processing of the sentinel lymph node(s). Despite these limitations, the fact that intraoperative sentinel lymph node evaluation can triage roughly half of patients requiring nodal dissection to immediate dissection represents a substantial cost saving and justifies its use. Other modalities for intraoperative evaluation have been studied including one-step RT-PCR (reverse transcription polymerase chain reaction) and ultrafast immunohistochemistry, but these methods are both time consuming and expensive and are therefore not currently ready for routine clinical use.[9]

27.5.2 Permanent Evaluation of Sentinel Lymph Nodes

The use of sentinel lymph node biopsy is attractive from a histopathologic standpoint because it provides a smaller target to concentrate more extensive histologic evaluation. As previously discussed, intensive histologic evaluation of a full neck dissection is both technically and financially infeasible. However, if evaluation can be focused on one or a few sentinel lymph nodes, a more aggressive approach may be taken. How extensive this evaluation should be is dependent on the clinical significance of macrometastases, micrometastases, and ITCs. The prognostic significance of macrometastases and the therapeutic value of neck dissection in this setting are well documented and serve as the basis for both the current AJCC pathologic nodal staging system and the standard histopathologic grossing protocol.

A growing body of evidence suggests that micrometastases and even ITCs also have clinical prognostic significance.[20,21,22] Two main strategies have been employed to identify micrometastases and ITCs, step sectioning and IHC. Step sectioning is the process of taking histologic sections at discrete intervals through the paraffin-embedded gross section. Suggested intervals range from 50 to 500 μm. Obviously, smaller intervals increase sensitivity but this must be balanced with practical considerations. To avoid missing any micrometastases, the section interval would have to be 200 μm or less; to find all ITCs is technically infeasible. However, even a small lymph node with a shortest axis of 6 mm would require 30 histologic sections to evaluate at this interval. Given that an average of 3 sentinel lymph nodes are identified, this translates to 90 histologic sections, roughly the current histologic workload equivalent of a full neck dissection, per sentinel lymph node procedure. This would place a significant workload and financial burden on pathology departments given the current reimbursement environment, so its feasibility remains to be seen. IHC can detect smaller lesions than routine H&E but is more time consuming and expensive and thus becomes infeasible at even relatively large sectioning intervals.

27.5.3 Proposed Protocol for Evaluation of Sentinel Lymph Nodes of the Head and Neck

Work from the breast literature provides promise for a feasible histologic protocol for sentinel lymph nodes. In breast cancer, micrometastases and ITCs within lymph nodes tend to be multiple. In a classic study, sentinel lymph nodes initially called negative on routine H&E were completely serially sectioned at 150 μm to identify occult micrometastases and ITCs. In 95% of these sentinel lymph nodes, at least one micrometastasis or ITC was identified within the first three levels by immunohistochemistry. Importantly, much of this effect was due to additional sampling rather than the increased sensitivity of IHC because 80% of these micrometastases and ITCs would have been identifiable by H&E.[23] If the same holds true for head and neck tumors, it will provide a feasible strategy for histologic evaluation of sentinel lymph nodes.

The feasibility of representative sampling in head and neck tumors is further supported by a recent evaluation of the distribution of micrometastases in the sentinel lymph nodes of patients with head and neck squamous cell carcinoma.[24] This study shows metastatic foci are asymmetrically distributed and tend to aggregate near the afferent pole along the central axes

of the lymph node. As a result, representative sampling in this region of the lymph node identifies most occult metastases. In this study, at least 90% of micrometastases and 80% of ITCs were identified by evaluation of the first four slices of a sentinel lymph node sectioned at 150 μm along the shortest axis.

Based on these two studies, the following protocol (▸ Fig. 27.2) is recommended to evaluate sentinel lymph nodes in head and neck tumors. The sentinel lymph node should be grossly bisected or sectioned at 2-mm intervals (if larger than 5 mm in shortest diameter) perpendicular to the shortest axis with the plane of bisection as the central sectioning plane, and embedded to insure that the central slices are cut starting at the center at the plane of bisection and stepping outward but all other slices present a different surface for cutting. Note that this is different from the embedding protocol for nonsentinel lymph nodes. Two unstained slides at 2 to 4 μm should be cut at each of four levels at 150- μm intervals. One slide from each level should be routinely stained with H&E and evaluated. If all of these H&E slides are negative, one or more of the unstained slides should be subjected to IHC for evaluation. This strategy maximizes sensitivity within the confines of feasible representative sectioning and minimizes the use of more expensive and time-consuming IHC studies without loss of sensitivity. Studies by Broglie et al show 96% long-term neck control in patients with cN0 necks who have negative sentinel lymph nodes as assessed by a similar protocol.[20,21]

Once micrometastases and ITCs are identified histopathologically, the question is what to do about them. In the breast literature, there is convincing evidence that while small micrometastases and ITCs in sentinel lymph nodes predict a low but real risk of nonsentinel lymph node axillary involvement (13–26%),[25] they do not appear to affect overall survival.[26] The presence of micrometastases and ITCs in the sentinel lymph nodes of head and neck tumors also predicts a similar likelihood of involvement (13–20%)[27] of nonsentinel lymph nodes. While we know that microscopic disease in cervical lymph nodes affects survival in head and neck tumors, it is unclear if elective neck dissection in these cases would necessarily improve survival. However, the behavior of head and neck micrometastases and ITCs cannot be assumed to be analogous to those of the breast. Numerous systemic adjuvant chemotherapy options are used routinely for breast cancer, while surgical intervention or radiotherapy remains the mainstay of disease control in the head and neck. Therefore, until a reliable nomogram, analogous to those used in breast cancer, can be formulated to estimate the risk of additional nonsentinel lymph node metastases, elective neck dissection or adjuvant radiation to the neck is prudent for all cases with identified metastases to sentinel lymph nodes regardless of size.

27.6 Special Considerations for Thyroid Cervical Metastases

Unlike other head and neck sites, thyroid carcinoma (except anaplastic carcinoma) benefits from effective systemic therapy in the form of radioactive iodine (RAI), which can ablate microscopic metastatic disease. As such, the purpose of neck dissection is to de-bulk gross disease to maximize the effectiveness of RAI. Therefore, clinically positive necks are treated much as they would be

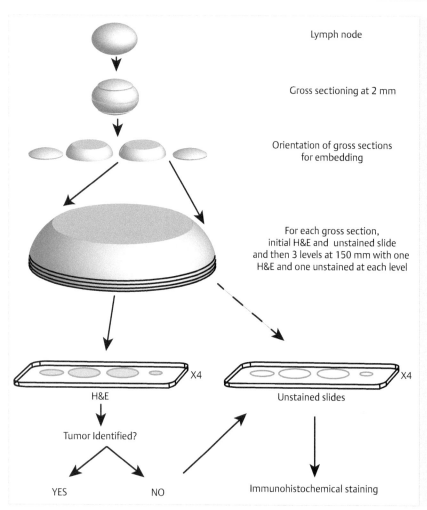

Lymph node

Gross sectioning at 2 mm

Orientation of gross sections
for embedding

For each gross section,
initial H&E and unstained slide
and then 3 levels at 150 mm with one
H&E and one unstained at each level

X4

X4

H&E

Unstained slides

Tumor Identified?

YES

NO

Immunohistochemical staining

Fig. 27.2 Proposed protocol for histologic processing of sentinel lymph nodes.

for any other head and neck site but cN0 necks are not aggressively pursued. The 2015 American Thyroid Association (ATA) guidelines[28] recommend ultrasound evaluation of the central and lateral neck compartments prior to surgery for well-differentiated thyroid carcinoma and biopsy of sonographically suspicious lymph nodes, but does not recommend sentinel lymph node biopsy in clinically and radiographically unremarkable necks. Postsurgical use of a scanning dose of RAI may help identify occult disease and a therapeutic dose of RAI may be used in patients with high-risk features, but prophylactic neck dissection for the cN0 neck is generally not warranted. The primary means of pathologic evaluation for clinically or radiologically suspicious lymph nodes is ultrasound-guided fine needle aspiration (▶ Fig. 27.4a, b) with or without thyroglobulin assay.

27.7 Cervical Metastases of Unknown Primary

In general, metastases to the cervical lymph nodes are largely from sites in the head and neck, particularly the mucosal surfaces, the thyroid, the skin, and the salivary glands. Less common considerations are metastases from the lung and breast; other sites are quite rare except in advanced disease. Additionally, lymphoma should be considered in patients with diffuse bulky lymphadenopathy.

True occult primaries, in which the initial clinical presentation is a positive cervical lymph node, are most commonly associated with squamous cell carcinomas arising in Waldeyer's ring (~ 90%) and to a much lesser extent papillary carcinomas of the thyroid and melanomas of the scalp. While they can be occult, cervical metastases from tumors of the salivary gland, breast, and lung tend to be a late finding in advanced disease. Nevertheless, it is sometimes necessary to differentiate among a number of possible known and suspected primary sites to appropriately stage and treat a patient. The standard means of initial evaluation for a neck mass of unknown primary is fine needle aspiration, although excisional biopsy may be warranted for more extensive workups.

27.7.1 Cytomorphology

The cytomorphology of the metastatic tumor is often helpful in narrowing the likely primary site (▶ Table 27.1).This cytomorphology can be broken down into five general categories: keratinizing squamous cell carcinoma, well/moderately differentiated adenocarcinoma, basaloid carcinoma, poorly differentiated carcinoma, and mononuclear malignancy. While spindle cell malignancies can metastasize to the cervical nodes, they are rare and almost always spindle cell variants of squamous cell carcinoma or melanoma. Metastases from true mesenchymal malignancies to the cervical neck are quite rare and almost never occult.

Table 27.1 Cytomorphology and immunophenotype of metastatic tumors to the cervical lymph nodes

Cytomorphology	Immunophenotype									Other findings	Primary site
	PanCK	CK7	TTF-1	Pax-8	Gata-3	p40/p63	S-100	CD56	CD20		
Keratinizing SCC	+	−	−	−	−	+	−	−	−	Mature squamous cells	Skin, mucosal surfaces of head and neck; lung
Well-to-moderately differentiated adenocarcinoma	+	+	+	+	−	−	−	+	−	Flat sheets, nuclear features	Thyroid papillary thyroid carcinoma
	+	+	+	+	−	−	−	+	−	Polygonal, dense cytoplasm	Thyroid Hurthle cell carcinoma
	+	+	−	−	−	−	−	−	−	Oncocytic, pseudopapillary	Salivary gland acinic cell
	+	+	−	−	−	+	−	−	−	Mucus cells, mucicarmine (+)	Salivary gland mucoepidermoid
	+	+	−	−	−	f	f	−	−	Cribriform, metachromatic matrix	Salivary gland adenoid cystic
	+	+	−	−	+	−	+	-	-	Oncocytic, GCDFP(+)	Salivary gland mammary analogue carcinoma
	+	+	−	−	+	−	−	−	−	GCDFP-15 (+), rarely occult	Breast ductal adenocarcinoma
	+	+	+	−	−	−	−	−	−	Napsin-A (+), rarely occult	Lung (pulmonary) adenocarcinoma
Basaloid carcinoma	+	−	−	−	−	+	−	−	−	Block p16 (+), HPV (+)	Basaloid SCC of Waldeyer's ring
	+	−	−	−	−	+	−	−	−	Wildtype p16, HPV (−)	Basaloid SCC (ENT or lung)
	+	−	−	−	−	+	−	−	−	Rarely occult	Basal cell carcinoma of skin
	+	+	−	−	−	f	f	−	−	Strong diffuse CD117 (+)	Solid variant of adenoid cystic
	+	+	−	−	−	+	+	−	−	Rare tumor	Basal cell adenocarcinoma
	+	v	+	−	−	−	−	+	−	Nuclear molding, crush artifact	Small cell carcinoma
Poorly differentiated carcinoma	+	−	−	−	−	+	−	−	-	EBER (+)	Nasopharyngeal carcinoma
	+	−	−	−	−	+	−	−	−	EBER (−)	Poorly differentiated SCC (ENT or lung)
	+	+	−	−	+	−	−	−	−	Rarely occult	Salivary duct carcinoma
	+	+	−	−	+	−	−	−	−	Rarely occult	Breast ductal carcinoma
	+	+	v	−	−	−	−	−	−	Rarely occult	Pulmonary adenocarcinoma
	+	v	−	+	−	−	−	−	−	Rarely occult	Thyroid anaplastic carcinoma
Mononuclear malignancy	−	−	−	−	−	−	+	−	−	HMB45 (+), Mart-1 (+), Sox-1 (+)	Melanoma
	−	−	−	−	−	−	−	−	+	Very high N/C ratio	B-cell lymphoma
	+	+	+	−	−	−	−	+	−	Plasmacytoid, uniform	Thyroid medullary carcinoma
	+	+	−	−	+	−	−	−	−	Uniform, mucicarmine (+)	Breast lobular carcinoma

Abbreviations: f, focal SCC, squamous cell carcinoma; v, variable.

Keratinizing squamous cell carcinoma morphology generally suggests a mucosal, skin, or pulmonary primary site (▶ Fig. 27.3). It is usually impossible to determine the site of origin of keratinizing squamous cell carcinomas pathologically because of extensive morphologic and immunophenotypic overlap, so careful clinical and radiologic evaluation is crucial.

A well-to-moderately differentiated adenocarcinoma suggests primaries of the thyroid, salivary gland, lung, or breast (▶ Fig. 27.4). Papillary thyroid carcinoma tends to be a well-differentiated adenocarcinoma with sheetlike cytological architecture and distinctive nuclear features including elongation, clearing, grooves, and pseudoinclusions (▶ Fig. 27.4a), whereas Hurthle cell carcinoma is composed of sheets of oncocytic cells with dense granular cytoplasm, sharp cytoplasmic borders, and prominent nucleoli (▶ Fig. 27.4b). Follicular carcinoma (non–Hurthle cell type) rarely metastasizes to the cervical lymph nodes, and poorly differentiated and undifferentiated thyroid carcinoma metastases in lymph nodes are rare. Salivary gland primaries often have distinctive cytologic appearances (▶ Fig. 27.4c–e) but more poorly differentiated ones may overlap with breast and lung primaries, which are generally moderately to poorly differentiated adenocarcinomas with three-dimensional architecture (▶ Fig. 27.4f, g). These can often be differentiated on the basis of immunophenotype.

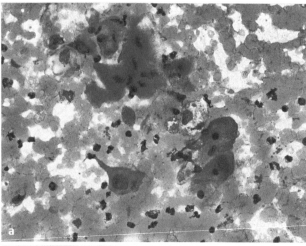

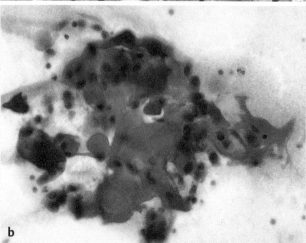

Fig. 27.3 Keratinizing squamous cell carcinoma. **(a)** Diff-Quik stain, 400×. **(b)** Papanicolaou stain, 400×.

Basaloid malignancies include basaloid squamous cell carcinoma of the head and neck, basal cell carcinoma of the skin, the solid variant of adenoid cystic carcinoma, and basal cell adenocarcinoma of the salivary gland, and sometimes small cell carcinoma of the lung (▶ Fig. 27.5). The presence of a magenta metachromatic matrix may suggest basal cell adenocarcinoma (▶ Fig. 27.5d) or a solid variant of adenoid cystic but the first four entities are otherwise quite difficult to differentiate cytologically. In contrast, small cell carcinoma is more dyscohesive and shows nuclear molding, single-cell necrosis, and crush artifact (▶ Fig. 27.5c). IHC studies can be quite helpful in differentiating these entities.

Poorly differentiated carcinomas include poorly differentiated squamous cell carcinoma of the head and neck or lung, and poorly differentiated adenocarcinomas of the salivary gland, lung, and breast (▶ Fig. 27.6). Statistically, a poorly differentiated squamous cell carcinoma of the head and neck is the most likely source but this must be proven. Immunoprofiling may be helpful, but poorly differentiated malignancies often lose tissue-specific markers and, as a result, immunophenotypes are often equivocal.

Mononuclear dyscohesive tumors include melanoma, medullary carcinoma of the thyroid, lobular carcinoma of the breast, small cell carcinoma of the lung, and lymphoma (▶ Fig. 27.7). Melanoma and medullary carcinoma are often described as "great mimickers" due to their variable appearance but, classically, melanoma cells tend to be pleomorphic, with moderate cytoplasm and prominent nucleoli, whereas medullary carcinoma tends to be relatively bland with a plasmacytoid appearance, neuroendocrine chromatin, and indistinct nucleoli. Lobular carcinoma of the breast tends to be bland and can have cytoplasmic vacuoles. Small cell carcinoma has a very high nuclear-to-cytoplasmic (N/C) ratio, shows nuclear molding, and significant crush artifact. Lymphoma is the most dyscohesive of the mononuclear malignancies, but otherwise is similar to small cell carcinoma in its N/C ratio, propensity to crush, and overall uniformity. As cytologic evaluation is relatively insensitive for detecting low-grade lymphomas (▶ Fig. 27.7e, f), patients older than 45 years with enlarged cervical lymph nodes but without overt evidence of other malignancy on fine needle aspiration should be evaluated by flow cytometry to exclude lymphoma.

27.7.2 Immunophenotyping

IHC stains can often further narrow down the primary site in each cytomorphologic category (▶ Table 27.1). For squamous cell carcinomas, positivity for HPV or p16 coupled with basaloid morphology is strongly suggestive of a primary arising from Waldeyer's ring[29] (▶ Fig. 27.5a), whereas EBER positivity and a poorly differentiated morphology would suggest a nasopharyngeal primary (▶ Fig. 27.6a). For adenocarcinomas, TTF-1 positivity suggests either a thyroid or lung primary and PAX-8 positivity suggests a thyroid primary. Strong diffuse CK7 positivity is seen in thyroid, salivary, lung, and breast primaries but not in squamous cell carcinomas of the head and neck. GATA-3 is seen primarily in breast primaries and some salivary gland primaries (mostly salivary duct carcinomas and mammary analogue carcinomas). CD56 is useful for identifying tumors of the thyroid and small cell carcinoma of the lung. For basaloid malignancies, CK7 reactivity can distinguish salivary gland primaries and small cell

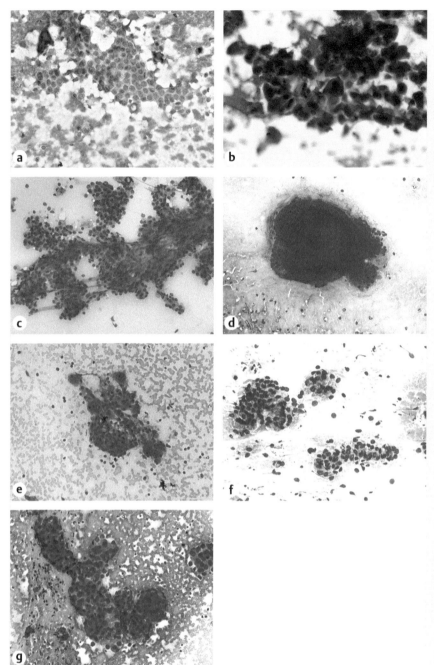

Fig. 27.4 Cervical lymph node metastases with well/moderately differentiated adenocarcinoma cytomorphology. **(a)** Papillary thyroid carcinoma (Papanicolaou stain, 400 ×). **(b)** Hurthle cell carcinoma (Papanicolaou stain, 400 ×). **(c)** Acinic cell carcinoma (Diff-Quik stain, 200 ×). **(d)** Adenoid cystic carcinoma (Diff-Quik stain, 200 ×). **(e)** Mucoepidermoid carcinoma, well differentiated (Diff-Quik stain, 200 ×). **(f)** Pulmonary non–small cell adenocarcinoma well differentiated (Diff-Quik stain, 200 ×). **(g)** Breast ductal carcinoma, well differentiated (Diff-Quik stain, 200 ×).

carcinoma from squamous cell carcinoma and basal cell carcinoma. Strong diffuse CD117 positivity can be quite helpful for identifying the solid variant of adenoid cystic carcinoma and CD56 positivity can identify small cell carcinoma. For poorly differentiated carcinomas, p63 and p40 are very sensitive for squamous differentiation but also stain many salivary gland tumors; this can often be solved using CK7, which usually strongly stains salivary gland tumors but is either negative or focally positive in squamous cell carcinomas of the head and neck. In contrast, breast and lung primaries would be p63 negative and CK7 positive. Among mononuclear malignancies, S-100 is a sensitive marker for melanoma but HMB-45 and Melan-A are more specific. Calcitonin can identify the vast majority of medullary carcinomas and CD20 will identify most B-cell lymphomas. As such,

judicious use of immunohistochemistry can be very helpful in narrowing the search for the primary site within each cytomorphologic grouping. However, since neither the cytomorphology nor the immunoprofile are entirely specific, they cannot substitute for a careful clinical and radiologic examination.

27.8 Conclusion

In short, histopathologic evaluation of neck dissections serves the purpose of assessing for regional nodal involvement by metastatic lesions of the head and neck. This evaluation is limited by the necessity of representative histologic sampling even though all lymph nodes are entirely grossly submitted. This problem is particularly significant for cN0 necks but sentinel

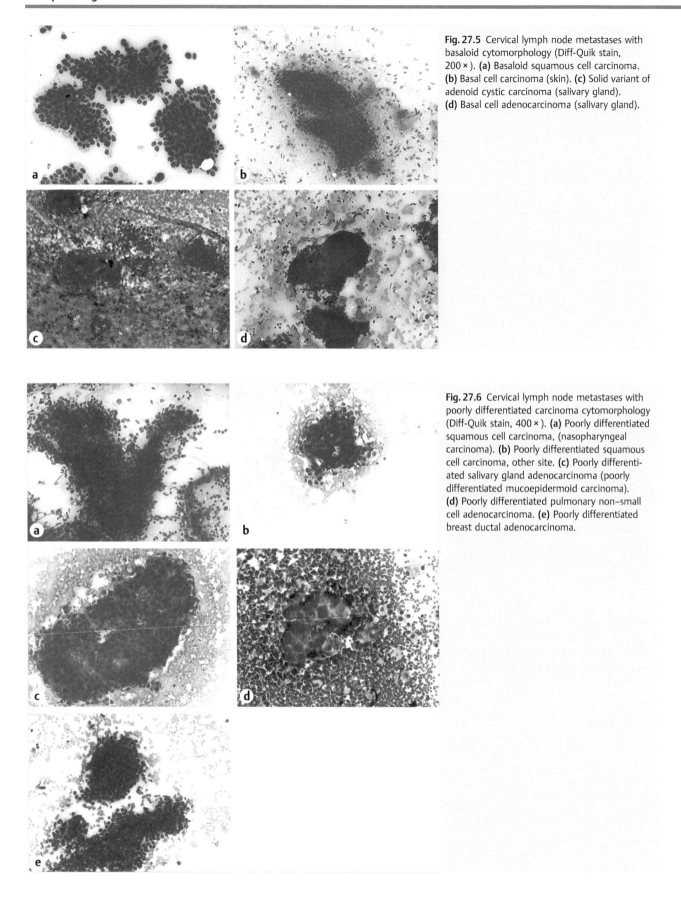

Fig. 27.5 Cervical lymph node metastases with basaloid cytomorphology (Diff-Quik stain, 200 ×). (a) Basaloid squamous cell carcinoma. (b) Basal cell carcinoma (skin). (c) Solid variant of adenoid cystic carcinoma (salivary gland). (d) Basal cell adenocarcinoma (salivary gland).

Fig. 27.6 Cervical lymph node metastases with poorly differentiated carcinoma cytomorphology (Diff-Quik stain, 400 ×). (a) Poorly differentiated squamous cell carcinoma, (nasopharyngeal carcinoma). (b) Poorly differentiated squamous cell carcinoma, other site. (c) Poorly differentiated salivary gland adenocarcinoma (poorly differentiated mucoepidermoid carcinoma). (d) Poorly differentiated pulmonary non–small cell adenocarcinoma. (e) Poorly differentiated breast ductal adenocarcinoma.

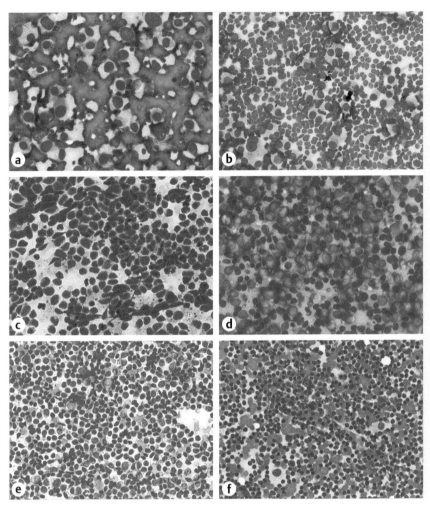

Fig. 27.7 Cytomorphology of metastatic mononuclear malignancies (Diff-Quik stain, 200 ×). **(a)** Melanoma. **(b)** Thyroid medullary carcinoma. **(c)** Lung small cell carcinoma. **(d)** High-grade lymphoma (diffuse large B-cell lymphoma). **(e)** Low-grade lymphoma (chronic lymphocytic lymphoma). **(f)** Reactive lymph node.

lymph node biopsy may provide a viable target for more intensive sampling. Based on the current evidence, we propose a protocol for evaluation of sentinel lymph nodes. Thyroid primaries represent an exception to the need to intensive evaluation of the neck because RAI is an effective adjunct to treat microscopic disease with minimal and acceptable morbidity. Finally, cytomorphologic evaluation and immunohistochemistry can help narrow down possible primary sites for occult metastases to the cervical lymph nodes but cannot substitute for a careful and thorough clinical and radiologic evaluation.

References

[1] Amin MB, Edge S, Greene F, et al. AJCC Cancer Staging Manual. 8th ed. New York, NY: Springer; 2016

[2] Coskun HH, Medina JE, Robbins KT, et al. Current philosophy in the surgical management of neck metastases for head and neck squamous cell carcinoma. Head Neck. 2015; 37(6):915–926

[3] Sharma D, Koshy G, Grover S, Sharma B. Sentinel lymph node biopsy: a new approach in the management of head and neck cancers. Sultan Qaboos Univ Med J. 2017; 17(1):e3–e10

[4] Kapoor C, Vaidya S, Wadhwan V, Malik S. Lymph node metastasis: a bearing on prognosis in squamous cell carcinoma. Indian J Cancer. 2015; 52 (3):417–424

[5] ADASP Committee. The Association of Directors of Anatomic and Surgical Pathology. ADASP recommendations for processing and reporting of lymph node specimens submitted for evaluation of metastatic disease. Mod Pathol. 2001; 14(6):629–632

[6] Divi V, Chen MM, Nussenbaum B, et al. Lymph node count from neck dissection predicts mortality in head and neck cancer. J Clin Oncol. 2016; 34 (32):3892–3897

[7] Pou JD, Barton BM, Lawlor CM, Frederick CH, Moore BA, Hasney CP. Minimum lymph node yield in elective level I-III neck dissection. Laryngoscope. 2017; 127(9):2070–2073

[8] Kuo P, Mehra S, Sosa JA, et al. Proposing prognostic thresholds for lymph node yield in clinically lymph node-negative and lymph node-positive cancers of the oral cavity. Cancer. 2016; 122(23):3624–3631

[9] Maguire A, Brogi E. Sentinel lymph nodes for breast carcinoma: a paradigm shift. Arch Pathol Lab Med. 2016; 140(8):791–798

[10] Teymoortash A, Werner JA. Current advances in diagnosis and surgical treatment of lymph node metastasis in head and neck cancer. GMS Curr Top Otorhinolaryngol Head Neck Surg. 2012; 11:Doc04

[11] D'Cruz AK, Vaish R, Kapre N, et al. Head and Neck Disease Management Group. Elective versus therapeutic neck dissection in node-negative oral cancer. N Engl J Med. 2015; 373(6):521–529

[12] Tsushima N, Sakashita T, Homma A, et al. The role of prophylactic neck dissection and tumor thickness evaluation for patients with cN0 tongue squamous cell carcinoma. Eur Arch Otorhinolaryngol. 2016; 273(11):3987–3992

[13] Barroso Ribeiro R, Ribeiro Breda E, Fernandes Monteiro E. Prognostic significance of nodal metastasis in advanced tumors of the larynx and hypopharynx. Acta Otorrinolaringol Esp. 2012; 63(4):292–298

[14] Liu M, Wang SJ, Yang X, Peng H. Diagnostic efficacy of sentinel lymph node biopsy in early oral squamous cell carcinoma: a meta-analysis of 66 studies. PLoS One. 2017; 12(1):e0170322

[15] Green B, Blythe J, Brennan PA. Sentinel lymph node biopsy for head and neck mucosal cancers - an update on the current evidence. Oral Dis. 2016; 22 (6):498–502

[16] Monroe MM, Lai SY. Sentinel lymph node biopsy for oral cancer: supporting evidence and recent novel developments. Curr Oncol Rep. 2014; 16(5):385

[17] Seim NB, Wright CL, Agrawal A. Contemporary use of sentinel lymph node biopsy in the head and neck. World J Otorhinolaryngol Head Neck Surg. 2016; 2(2):117–125

[18] Schilling C, Stoeckli SJ, Haerle SK, et al. Sentinel European Node Trial (SENT): 3-year results of sentinel node biopsy in oral cancer. Eur J Cancer. 2015; 51 (18):2777–2784

[19] Farmer RW, McCall L, Civantos FJ, et al. Lymphatic drainage patterns in oral squamous cell carcinoma: findings of the ACOSOG Z0360 (Alliance) study. Otolaryngol Head Neck Surg. 2015; 152(4):673–677

[20] Broglie MA, Haerle SK, Huber GF, Haile SR, Stoeckli SJ. Occult metastases detected by sentinel node biopsy in patients with early oral and oropharyngeal squamous cell carcinomas: impact on survival. Head Neck. 2013; 35 (5):660–666

[21] Broglie MA, Haile SR, Stoeckli SJ. Long-term experience in sentinel node biopsy for early oral and oropharyngeal squamous cell carcinoma. Ann Surg Oncol. 2011; 18(10):2732–2738

[22] Cho JH, Lee YS, Sun DI, et al. Prognostic impact of lymph node micrometastasis in oral and oropharyngeal squamous cell carcinomas. Head Neck. 2016; 38 Suppl 1:E1777–E1782

[23] Fréneaux P, Nos C, Vincent-Salomon A, et al. Histological detection of minimal metastatic involvement in axillary sentinel nodes: a rational basis for a sensitive methodology usable in daily practice. Mod Pathol. 2002; 15(6):641–646

[24] Denoth S, Broglie MA, Haerle SK, et al. Histopathological mapping of metastatic tumor cells in sentinel lymph nodes of oral and oropharyngeal squamous cell carcinomas. Head Neck. 2015; 37(10):1477–1482

[25] Bargehr J, Edlinger M, Hubalek M, Marth C, Reitsamer R. Axillary lymph node status in early-stage breast cancer patients with sentinel node micrometastases (0.2–2 mm). Breast Care (Basel). 2013; 8(3):187–191

[26] Giuliano AE, Hawes D, Ballman KV, et al. Association of occult metastases in sentinel lymph nodes and bone marrow with survival among women with early-stage invasive breast cancer. JAMA. 2011; 306(4):385–393

[27] Den Toom IJ, Bloemena E, van Weert S, Karagozoglu KH, Hoekstra OS, de Bree R. Additional non-sentinel lymph node metastases in early oral cancer patients with positive sentinel lymph nodes. Eur Arch Otorhinolaryngol. 2017; 274(2):961–968

[28] Haugen BR, Alexander EK, Bible KC, et al. 2015 American Thyroid Association Management Guidelines for Adult Patients with Thyroid Nodules and Differentiated Thyroid Cancer: The American Thyroid Association Guidelines Task Force on Thyroid Nodules and Differentiated Thyroid Cancer. Thyroid. 2016; 26(1):1–133

[29] El-Mofty SK, Zhang MQ, Davila RM. Histologic identification of human papillomavirus (HPV)-related squamous cell carcinoma in cervical lymph nodes: a reliable predictor of the site of an occult head and neck primary carcinoma. Head Neck Pathol. 2008; 2(3):163–168

28 Quality Outcome Measures in Neck Dissection

Vasu Divi and Misha Amoils

Abstract

Although neck dissection is one of the most common procedures in head and neck surgery, there are no well-accepted quality outcome measures for this operation. There are many opportunities to develop measures that demonstrate the quality and value of care provided and allow for benchmarking and improvement initiatives. This chapter explores the evidence behind potential metrics and the strengths and weaknesses of using them on a national scale. Finally, it discusses the steps needed to develop them for use across diverse practices.

Keywords: quality, outcomes, metrics, lymph node yield, quality of life, complication rates, regional recurrence

28.1 Introduction

As health care costs continue to escalate and health care reform has been unable to change the nature of the incentive system, addressing value in health care has become even more urgent. In January 2015, the Department of Health and Human Services outlined specific goals in transitioning health care from rewarding volume to value. One of the key objectives is that 90% of Medicare payments be tied to quality or value by 2018.[1] The provisions of the Medicare Access and CHIP Reauthorization Act of 2015 (MACRA) have defined the framework for how this will occur for Medicare physicians.

One difficulty with a value-based health care system is effectively defining what we mean by "high-quality" care. One of the most well-known frameworks for quality was first proposed in 1966 by Avedis Donabedian, MD, MPH, a professor at the University of Michigan School of Public Health. His framework defined three domains of quality: structure, process, and outcomes.

Structural measures assess the overall context where care is delivered and includes the facilities, resources, and organization of care. Process measures are the individual actions that occur in the course of patient care, such as whether a patient received a recommended treatment. Outcomes measures are the end result of care and can be evaluated by a clinical outcome or change in health status.

In the context of neck dissection in head and neck cancer (HNC), structural quality measures could include the number of neck dissections performed (volume) at a given institution or by a given surgeon. Subspecialty training of the surgeon is also a structural measure. Process measures could include adherence to clinical guidelines for when a neck dissection is indicated, performing the correct levels of neck dissection or correct laterality. Process measures may also comprise more generic measures of quality such as administration of preoperative antibiotics.

Quality outcomes measures in neck dissections can be broadly categorized into intermediate outcomes and end outcomes. End outcomes are the most important ones to patients and affect them directly. Important end outcomes include perioperative complications, function and quality of life (QOL), and regional recurrence rates.

Intermediate outcomes are results that are on the pathway to the desired end outcome. One example is measuring hemoglobin A1c on a patient whose end outcome may be the number of diabetic complications. These are particularly important since they may provide a more tangible way to affect the end outcomes, and can be more frequently monitored or modified. Intermediate outcomes in neck dissections include lymph node yield (LNY) from neck dissections.

28.2 Lymph Node Yield in Neck Dissection

Using the number of lymph nodes counted and analyzed in a regional nodal basin dissection was first popularized in colorectal cancer, where studies demonstrated that in patients with stage II or III colorectal cancer, the removal of 12 or more lymph nodes is associated with increased overall survival.[2,3,4] Since then, additional disease sites have investigated this concept and established quality metrics around LNYs. These metrics have been adopted by the American College of Surgeons Commission on Cancer Measures for Quality of Cancer Care, with recommended minimum nodal yields now established for bladder, gastric, kidney, and lung cancer.[5]

In neck dissections, the concept of a minimum nodal yield was introduced into the American Joint Cancer Commission (AJCC) staging manual. The manual states that "*a selective neck dissection will ordinarily include 10 or more lymph nodes, and a radical or modified radical neck dissection will ordinarily include 15 or more lymph nodes.*" This was increased from the 6 and 10 nodes, respectively, recommended in the seventh edition.[6,7] The purpose of achieving these nodal counts was to adequately stage the neck for prognostic and treatment purposes.

The above numbers, however, were not based on statistical evidence of an appropriate cutoff for minimum number of nodes. The first study in head and neck surgery to look at the idea of a cutoff was by Ebrahimi et al in 2011. They analyzed 225 patients from a single institution who had elective neck dissections performed for N0 disease. They found that an LNY less than 18 was associated with reduced overall survival (hazard ratio [HR], 2.0; 95% confidence interval [CI], 1.1–3.6; $p = 0.020$) and lower disease-specific survival.[8] This was followed by a multi-institutional study with 1,567 patients, which again demonstrated reduced overall survival (HR, 1.69; 95% CI, 1.22–2.34; $p = 0.002$) in patients with less than 18 nodes.[9]

Divi et al performed the first study in node-positive disease. Using data from the RTOG 9501 and RTOG 0234 trials, the authors analyzed 572 patients with 98% N + disease who underwent therapeutic neck dissection. An overall survival benefit (HR, 1.38; 95% CI, 1.09–1.74; $p = 0.007$) was shown for patients with 18 nodes or more, and this was largely driven by higher rates of local-regional failure. Interestingly, this study independently calculated the optimal cut-point for survival difference and also found 18 nodes as the best threshold.[10] In a subsequent analysis of the National Cancer Database, instead of calculating a new optimal cutoff, Divi et al tested the 18 LNY cutoff across 63,978 patients. In both N0 and N + patient populations, achieving LNY of 18 nodes or more was associated with a significant improvement in overall survival[11] (► Fig. 28.1).

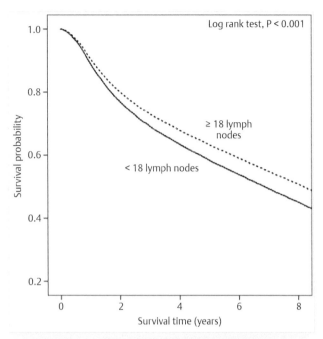

Fig. 28.1 Adjusted overall survival probability for adult patients with head and neck cancer stratified by < 18 and ≥ 18 lymph nodes examined. Survival curves adjusted for sex, age group, race, comorbidities, pathologic stage, head and neck subsite, margins, extracapsular extension, positive nodes, adjuvant therapy, insurance, socioeconomic status, hospital volume, and hospital type.[13,14,15,16]

Several other studies have supported this LNY metric. For example, Graboyes et al performed a retrospective analysis of their patients with clinically N0 oral cavity cancer, and found that LNY was one of four quality metrics associated with improved outcomes.[12] A few other studies with limited analyses did not find the same correlation; however, these authors were evaluating lymph node ratios and did not design studies to identify an optimal LNY for improved outcomes.[13,14,15,16]

While the evidence is fairly consistent across single institutional, multi-institutional, and large database studies, there remains some controversy when discussing implementation of LNY as a quality metric. The most notable is that LNY is a function of both the surgeon and the pathologist analyzing the specimen. Therefore, one must be careful to not attribute the entire performance on this metric to the surgeon. The LNY is only associated with improved overall survival and no causative mechanism can be assumed, since there are many components of care which may also be associated with higher LNY. In particular, patients who are treated by surgeons with higher LNY may also receive better perioperative care or better adjuvant treatment, both of which may have a survival impact. However, even in single institution studies which have more consistent process of care, the LNY was seen to associate with survival.[8,12]

Patient biology may also theoretically contribute. Patients with higher lymph node counts may have a more robust immune response to the tumor, leading to both higher lymph node counts and potentially better outcomes. Finally, patients with matted nodes with gross extranodal extension may have a lower nodal count if multiple nodes make a single conglomerate mass. These patients are known to have a worse outcome, although this is a minority of patients in these studies.

It is important to emphasize that all of the prior studies have been done in untreated necks, and therefore use of the metric would be limited to this patient population since prior radiation therapy is known to decrease LNY.

Ultimately, how a quality metric is implemented has a significant impact on its utility. Expecting that all patients would achieve a minimum of 18 nodes is not reasonable since—as discussed above—patient factors and tumor factors may impact the ultimate nodal yield. LNY should likely be evaluated at a hospital level, with a benchmark or minimum performance threshold for the percentage of cases that meet the metric. The Quality Integration Committee of the ACS Commission on Cancer establishes expected estimated performance rates (EPRs) for metrics monitored by their quality program. In colorectal cancer, the EPR is 85% for LNY, meaning that this percentage of eligible patients at the hospital has 12 or more lymph nodes removed and analyzed. For gastric cancer, the EPR is 80%.[17] While there is no standard set for neck dissections, there is some evidence that an 80% threshold at the hospital level is an appropriate cutoff. Patients treated at hospitals meeting this threshold had better survival outcomes than those treated at hospitals that fell below this threshold.[18]

28.3 Intraoperative and Postoperative Complications

During and after a neck dissection, there are a number of potential complications that can occur. Intraoperatively, unexpected injury of a major vessel or nerve can potentially leave a patient with significant sequela. Postoperatively, patients may develop a hematoma, surgical site infection, or chyle leak. While these are known risks of the surgery, and can potentially be avoided, the risks of each complication are highly dependent on the patient and the disease, in addition to the skill of the surgeon.

For the rates of postoperative complications to be used as a quality measure, a formal process of "operationalizing" the measure needs to be undertaken. One example of how to do this is outlined by the Measures Management System (MMS) Blueprint maintained by the Center for Medicare and Medicaid Services.[19] Prior to developing a measure, a known performance gap must first be identified, and the strength of evidence and business case (cost of implementation vs. anticipated benefit) must be evaluated. Measures should be considered for feasibility, reliability, and validity. In order to develop the measure, specifications must be determined, which include the measure description, population the metric applies to (denominator), expected outcome or process (numerator), sampling method, risk adjustment, and calculation algorithm. Testing and implementation of the measure then follow.

This process highlights some of the important challenges in developing new quality measures. In particular, deciding which patients meet inclusion criteria and performing appropriate risk adjustment is important, and would need to take into account additional factors such as disease type. A neck dissection for thyroid cancer would have very different risks and outcomes than a postradiation salvage neck dissection. Converting rates of postoperative complications into true quality measures is possible, but would require a more in-depth analysis of the data, and once implemented, each patient would need to be risk adjusted before reporting the metric. Comparing raw, unadjusted rates would likely have little face validity to clinicians, who may feel their patients are different than the "average" case.

28.4 Functional Outcomes and Quality of Life

Most QOL tools in HNC research rely on questionnaires to assess disease or treatment-related symptoms. Examples of general surveys used in cancer populations include the Medical Outcomes Study-Short Form 36 (MOS SF-36) and the Sickness Impact Profile (SIP).[20,21] Instruments specific to HNC include the head and neck subscale of the Functional Assessment of Cancer Therapy (FACT-HN), the University of Washington QOL Questionnaire (UWQOL), and the 35-item head and neck questionnaire from the European Organization for Research and Treatment of Cancer Quality of Life Questionnaire (EORTC QLQ-H&N35).[21,22,23,24] These types of surveys focus on domains specific to HNC such as speech, swallowing, and eating. However, while these are useful tools to assess QOL in patients with HNC in general, none were specifically developed to focus on QOL assessment in patients after neck dissection.

Important variables to consider in QOL measurement after neck dissection include nerve injury (great auricular, marginal mandibular branch, hypoglossal, and spinal accessory nerves), lymphedema, scar appearance or cosmetic disfigurement, sensory function, and shoulder function. Shoulder function represents one of the most commonly studied QOL outcomes given its potential to result in significant morbidity and interference with many activities of daily living. A number of studies have suggested improved QOL in patients who undergo more limited neck dissections, related to better shoulder function.[21,25,26,27]

Tools that have been used to evaluate postoperative shoulder function include the Neck Dissection Impairment Index (NDII) and Constant's Shoulder Assessment. The NDII is a validated questionnaire that consists of 10 items with a 5-point Likert scale; lower scores correspond with worse QOL impairment. Questions focus on neck or shoulder pain, stiffness, difficulty with self-care, ability to lift objects or reach overhead, overall activity level, participation in social activities, ability to participate in leisure or recreational activities, and ability to work.[28] The Constant Shoulder Assessment is a test that combines patient symptom scores with objective measures of active shoulder function, such as range of movement, rotation, and strength. Patient symptoms represent 35% of the sum and include pain, sleep, recreation, and vocational activities; active shoulder function represents 65%.[22,25,28]

Similar to the NDII and Constant's Assessment, the self-administered neck dissection questionnaire (NDQ) and arm abduction test (ABT) are tools that Japanese authors have used to focus on postoperative QOL after neck dissection. QOL variables taken into account for NDQ questions included neck stiffness, constriction, pain, numbness, shoulder drop, reach, and neck appearance. The ABT requires patients to rate their arm abduction on a scale of 0 to 5. Similar to other authors, these tools suggest that preservation of the spinal accessory nerve and sternocleidomastoid muscle results in significantly improved QOL.[29,30]

Consistent evaluation of shoulder dysfunction after neck dissection using tools such as the NDII and Constant's Assessment,

or NDQ and ABT, may provide a QOL score that is amenable to comparison across providers. Outcomes would also need to take into account factors such as the level of disease burden, and the extent of neck dissection for appropriate risk adjustment. Implementation of this metric would require widespread adoption of these tools by providers, and additional resources to collect and record survey data, which may significantly limit their use.

28.5 Regional Recurrence Rates

The most important oncologic outcome of a neck dissection is long-term regional control of disease. Similar to creating quality metrics around perioperative complications, developing an outcome measure around regional recurrence rates poses a few challenges. First, rates of regional recurrence would need to take into account different histologies, nodal stage, local recurrence, and cancer biology (e.g., extracapsular extension). In addition, adjuvant treatment with radiation—with or without chemotherapy—would also affect regional recurrence rates. Therefore, a more careful study and risk adjustment of patients would be required. While it is a worthwhile goal to create nationally recognized benchmarks for regional recurrence rates, ultimate implementation would be challenging. Each patient would need to be risk adjusted prior to comparing their outcomes, requiring significant data collection and reporting by providers. Regional recurrence rates for the nodal basin at risk would need to be reported, along with any concurrent local recurrence. Another possible approach would be to use the regional recurrence rates of a single disease (e.g., T1/T2N0 oral cavity disease) as a marker for all sites and stages. This would allow for easier risk adjustment, but it would be harder for any individual provider to generate sufficient case numbers to provide feedback in this setting.

28.6 Conclusion

There are many potential outcome quality measures for neck dissection. Many of these measures would require significant development to allow for comparison across different providers and different institutions. Nevertheless, in an era of value-based medicine, it is important for head and neck surgeons to define what constitutes high-quality care in their field.

References

[1] Burwell SM. Setting value-based payment goals–HHS efforts to improve U.S. health care. N Engl J Med. 2015; 372(10):897–899

[2] Prandi M, Lionetto R, Bini A, et al. Prognostic evaluation of stage B colon cancer patients is improved by an adequate lymphadenectomy: results of a secondary analysis of a large scale adjuvant trial. Ann Surg. 2002; 235 (4):458–463

[3] Le Voyer TE, Sigurdson ER, Hanlon AL, et al. Colon cancer survival is associated with increasing number of lymph nodes analyzed: a secondary survey of intergroup trial INT-0089. J Clin Oncol. 2003; 21(15):2912–2919

[4] Swanson RS, Compton CC, Stewart AK, Bland KI. The prognosis of T3N0 colon cancer is dependent on the number of lymph nodes examined. Ann Surg Oncol. 2003; 10(1):65–71

[5] National Cancer Database. CoC Quality of Care Measures. Available at: https://www.facs.org/quality-programs/cancer/ncdb/qualitymeasures

[6] Edge SB, Byrd DR, Compton CC, et al. AJCC Cancer Staging Manual. 7th ed. New York, NY: Springer; 2010

[7] Amin MB, Edge S, Greene F, et al. AJCC Cancer Staging Manual. 8th ed. New York, NY: Springer; 2017

[8] Ebrahimi A, Zhang WJ, Gao K, Clark JR. Nodal yield and survival in oral squamous cancer: defining the standard of care. Cancer. 2011; 117(13):2917–2925

[9] Ebrahimi A, Clark JR, Amit M, et al. Minimum nodal yield in oral squamous cell carcinoma: defining the standard of care in a multicenter international pooled validation study. Ann Surg Oncol. 2014; 21(9):3049–3055

[10] Divi V, Harris J, Harari PM, et al. Establishing quality indicators for neck dissection: correlating the number of lymph nodes with oncologic outcomes (NRG Oncology RTOG 9501 and RTOG 0234). Cancer. 2016; 122(12):3464–3471

[11] Divi V, Chen MM, Nussenbaum B, et al. Lymph node count from neck dissection predicts mortality in head and neck cancer. J Clin Oncol. 2016; 34 (32):3892–3897

[12] Graboyes EM, Gross J, Kallogjeri D, et al. Association of compliance with process-related quality metrics and improved survival in oral cavity squamous cell carcinoma. JAMA Otolaryngol Head Neck Surg. 2016; 142(5):430–437

[13] Gil Z, Carlson DL, Boyle JO, et al. Lymph node density is a significant predictor of outcome in patients with oral cancer. Cancer. 2009; 115(24):5700–5710

[14] Ryu IS, Roh JL, Cho KJ, Choi SH, Nam SY, Kim SY. Lymph node density as an independent predictor of cancer-specific mortality in patients with lymph node-positive laryngeal squamous cell carcinoma after laryngectomy. Head Neck. 2015; 37(9):1319–1325

[15] Shrime MG, Bachar G, Lea J, et al. Nodal ratio as an independent predictor of survival in squamous cell carcinoma of the oral cavity. Head Neck. 2009; 31 (11):1482–1488

[16] Patel SG, Amit M, Yen TC, et al. International Consortium for Outcome Research (ICOR) in Head and Neck Cancer. Lymph node density in oral cavity cancer: results of the International Consortium for Outcomes Research. Br J Cancer. 2013; 109(8):2087–2095

[17] Commission on Cancer. A Quality Program of the American College of Surgeons. CoC Standards 4.4 and 4.5 Implementation for Surveys in 2017. October 2016. https://www.facs.org/~/media/files/quality%20programs/cancer/ncdb/standard%204%204_4%205_2017%20implementation.ashx

[18] Schoppy DW, Yifei M, Rhoads KF, et al. Association of surgical quality metrics and hospital-level overall survival for patients with head and neck squamous cell carcinoma. J Clin Oncol. 2017; 35(8):206

[19] CMS. Blueprint for the CMS Measures Management System. Version 13.0. Available at: https://www.cms.gov/Medicare/Quality-Initiatives-Patient-Assessment-Instruments/MMS/Downloads/Blueprint-130.pdf. Accessed July 24, 2017

[20] Terrell JE, Ronis DL, Fowler KE, et al. Clinical predictors of quality of life in patients with head and neck cancer. Arch Otolaryngol Head Neck Surg. 2004; 130(4):401–408

[21] Murphy BA, Ridner S, Wells N, Dietrich M. Quality of life research in head and neck cancer: a review of the current state of the science. Crit Rev Oncol Hematol. 2007; 62(3):251–267

[22] Schiefke F, Akdemir M, Weber A, Akdemir D, Singer S, Frerich B. Function, postoperative morbidity, and quality of life after cervical sentinel node biopsy and after selective neck dissection. Head Neck. 2009; 31(4):503–512

[23] Chaukar DA, Walvekar RR, Das AK, et al. Quality of life in head and neck cancer survivors: a cross-sectional survey. Am J Otolaryngol. 2009; 30(3):176–180

[24] Sayed SI, Elmiyeh B, Rhys-Evans P, et al. Quality of life and outcomes research in head and neck cancer: a review of the state of the discipline and likely future directions. Cancer Treat Rev. 2009; 35(5):397–402

[25] Murer K, Huber GF, Haile SR, Stoeckli SJ. Comparison of morbidity between sentinel node biopsy and elective neck dissection for treatment of the n0 neck in patients with oral squamous cell carcinoma. Head Neck. 2011; 33 (9):1260–1264

[26] Terrell JE, Welsh DE, Bradford CR, et al. Pain, quality of life, and spinal accessory nerve status after neck dissection. Laryngoscope. 2000; 110(4):620–626

[27] Shah S, Har-El G, Rosenfeld RM. Short-term and long-term quality of life after neck dissection. Head Neck. 2001; 23(11):954–961

[28] Taylor RJ, Chepeha JC, Teknos TN, et al. Development and validation of the neck dissection impairment index: a quality of life measure. Arch Otolaryngol Head Neck Surg. 2002; 128(1):44–49

[29] Nibu K, Ebihara Y, Ebihara M, et al. Quality of life after neck dissection: a multicenter longitudinal study by the Japanese Clinical Study Group on Standardization of Treatment for Lymph Node Metastasis of Head and Neck Cancer. Int J Clin Oncol. 2010; 15(1):33–38

[30] Inoue H, Nibu K, Saito M, et al. Quality of life after neck dissection. Arch Otolaryngol Head Neck Surg. 2006; 132(6):662–666

Index

295